M000195142

Health Informatics

(formerly Computers in Health Care)

Kathryn J. Hannah   Marion J. Ball
Series Editors

Springer
New York
Berlin
Heidelberg
Barcelona
Hong Kong
London
Milan
Paris
Singapore
Tokyo

Health Informatics Series

(formerly Computers in Health Care)

Series Editors
Kathryn J. Hannah   Marion J. Ball

Dental Informatics
Integrating Technology into the Dental Environment
L.M. Abbey and J. Zimmerman

Aspects of the Computer-based Patient Record
M.J. Ball and M.F. Collen

Performance Improvement Through Information Management
Health Care's Bridge to Success
M.J. Ball and J.V. Douglas

Strategies and Technologies for Healthcare Information
Theory into Practice
M.J. Ball, J.V. Douglas, and D.E. Garets

Nursing Informatics
Where Caring and Technology Meet, Third Edition
M.J. Ball, K.J. Hannah, S.K. Newbold, and J.V. Douglas

Healthcare Information Management Systems
A Practical Guide, Second Edition
M.J. Ball, D.W. Simborg, J.W. Albright, and J.V. Douglas

Clinical Decision Support Systems
Theory and Practice
E.S. Berner

Strategy and Architecture of Health Care Information Systems
M.K. Bourke

Information Networks for Community Health
P.F. Brennan, S.J. Schneider, and E. Tornquist

Introduction to Clinical Informatics
P. Degoulet and M. Fieschi

Patient Care Information Systems
Successful Design and Implementation
E.L. Drazen, J.B. Metzger, J.L. Ritter, and M.K. Schneider

Introduction to Nursing Informatics, Second Edition
K.J. Hannah, M.J. Ball, and M.J.A. Edwards

Information Technology for the Practicing Physician
J.M. Kiel

Computerizing Large Integrated Health Networks
The VA Success
R.M. Kolodner

(continued after Index)

Edward H. Shortliffe Leslie E. Perreault
Editors

Gio Wiederhold Lawrence M. Fagan
Associate Editors

Medical Informatics

Computer Applications in Health Care and Biomedicine

Second Edition

With 199 Illustrations

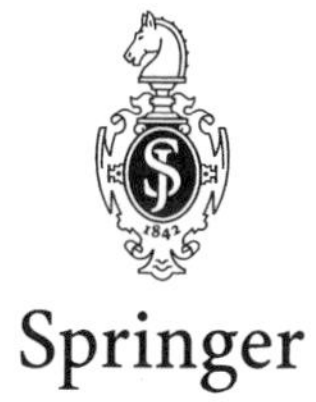

Springer

Edward H. Shortliffe, MD, PhD, FACP, FACMI
Professor and Chair
Department of Medical Informatics in Medicine
Professor of Medicine and Computer Science Vanderbilt Clinic
Columbia University College of Physicians and Surgeons
Columbia-Presbyterian Medical Center
New York, NY 10032-3720, USA

Leslie E. Perreault, MS
Director
First Consulting Group
New York, NY 10019-4105, USA

Gio Wiederhold, PhD, FIEEE, FACM, FACMI
Professor of Computer Science, Electrical Engineering, and Medicine
Stanford University
Stanford, CA 94305-9040, USA

Lawrence M. Fagan, MD, PhD, FACMI
Senior Research Scientist and Associate Director, Stanford Medical Informatics
Co-Director, Medical Information Sciences Training Program
Director, Medical Informatics Short Course
Stanford University School of Medicine
Stanford, CA 94305-5479, USA

Series Editors:
Kathryn J. Hannah, RN, PhD
Professor, Department of Community Health Science
Faculty of Medicine
The University of Calgary
Calgary, Alberta T2N 4N1, Canada

Marion J. Ball, EdD
Professor, The Johns Hopkins University School of Nursing
Baltimore, MD, USA
and
Vice President
First Consulting Group
Baltimore, MD 21210, USA

Cover illustration: Robert Schuster

Library of Congress Cataloging-in-Publication Data
Medical informatics : computer applications in health care and biomedicine / editors, Edward H. Shortliffe, Leslie E. Perreault ; associated editors, Gio Wiederhold, Lawrence M. Fagan—2nd ed.
p. cm. — (Health informatics series)
Includes bibliographical references and index.
ISBN 0-387-98472-0 (hardcover : alk. paper)
1. Medical informatics. I. Shortliffe, Edward Hance. II. Health informatics.
R858.M397 2000
610′.285—dc21 99-089476

Printed on acid-free paper.

The first edition of this book was published by Addison-Wesley Publishing Company, Inc. © 1990 by Addison-Wesley Publishing Company, Inc.

Production coordinated by Chernow Editorial Services, Inc., and managed by Timothy Taylor, manufacturing supervised by Erica Bresler.
Typeset by Matrix Publishing Services, Inc., York, PA.
Printed and bound by Maple-Vail Book Manufacturing Group, York, PA.
Printed in the United States of America.

9 8 7 6 5 4 3 2 1

ISBN 0-387-98472-0 SPIN 10664767

Springer-Verlag New York Berlin Heidelberg
A member of BertelsmannSpringer Science+Business Media GmbH

Where is the knowledge we have lost in information?
Where is the wisdom we have lost in knowledge?
—T.S. Elliot, "The Rock"

To the memory of Scott Blois, innovator, philosopher, and scholar, who showed us how to look beyond technology to the concepts and perspectives that help to define the scientific underpinnings for the field of medical informatics.

Series Preface

This series is directed to healthcare professionals who are leading the transformation of health care by using information and knowledge. Launched in 1988 as Computers in Health Care, the series offers a broad range of titles: some addressed to specific professions such as nursing, medicine, and health administration; others to special areas of practice such as trauma and radiology. Still other books in the series focus on interdisciplinary issues, such as the computer-based patient record, electronic health records, and networked healthcare systems.

Renamed Health Informatics in 1998 to reflect the rapid evolution in the discipline now known as health informatics, the series continues to add titles that contribute to the evolution of the field. In the series, eminent experts, serving as editors or authors, offer their accounts of innovations in health informatics. Increasingly, these accounts go beyond hardware and software to address the role of information in influencing the transformation of healthcare delivery systems around the world. The series also increasingly focuses on "peopleware" and the organizational, behavioral, and societal changes that accompany the diffusion of information technology in health services environments.

These changes will shape health services in the new millennium. By making full and creative use of the technology to tame data and to transform information, health informatics will foster the development of the knowledge age in health care. As co-editors, we pledge to support our professional colleagues and the series readers as they share advances in the emerging and exciting field of health informatics.

Kathryn J. Hannah
Marion J. Ball

Preface

Just as banks cannot practice modern banking without financial software, and airlines cannot manage modern travel planning without shared databanks of flight schedules and reservations, it has become impossible to practice modern medicine without information technologies. Health professionals recognize that a large percentage of their activities relates to *information management*—for example, obtaining and recording information about patients, consulting colleagues, reading the scientific literature, planning diagnostic procedures, devising strategies for patient care, interpreting results of laboratory and radiologic studies, or conducting case-based and population-based research. It is complexity and uncertainty, plus society's overriding concern for patient well-being and the resulting need for optimal decision-making, that set medicine apart from many other information-intensive fields. Our desire to provide the best possible health and health care for our society gives a special significance to the effective organization and management of the huge bodies of data with which health professionals must deal. It also suggests the need for specialized approaches and for skilled scientists who are knowledgeable about both medicine and information technologies.

Information Management in Biomedicine

Although the application of computers to biomedicine is recent, the clinical and research influence of medical-computing systems is already remarkably broad. Clinical information systems, which provide communication and information-management functions, are now installed in essentially all healthcare institutions. Physicians can search entire drug indexes in a few seconds, using the information provided by a computer program to anticipate harmful side effects or drug interactions. Electrocardiograms often are analyzed initially by computer programs, and similar techniques are being applied for interpretation of pulmonary-function tests and a variety of laboratory and radiologic abnormalities. Microprocessor systems routinely monitor patients and provide warnings in critical-care settings, such as the intensive-care unit or the operating room. Both biomedical researchers and clinicians regularly use computer programs to search the medical literature, and modern clinical research would be severely hampered without computer-based data-storage techniques and statistical-analysis systems. Advanced decision-support tools also are emerging from research laboratories, are being integrated with patient-care systems, and are likely to have a profound effect on the way medicine is practiced in the future.

Despite this growing use of computers in healthcare settings and the resulting expansion of interest in learning more about medical computing, many health students and professionals have found it difficult to obtain a comprehensive and rigorous, but nontechnical, overview of the field. Both practitioners and basic scientists are recognizing that thorough preparation for their professional futures requires that they gain an understanding of the state of the art in biomedical computing, of the current and future capabilities *and* limitations of the technology, and of the way in which such developments fit within the scientific, social, and financial context of biomedicine. In turn, the future of the medical-computing field will be largely determined by how well health professionals and other people are prepared to guide the discipline's development. This book is intended to meet this growing need for well-equipped professionals.

The first edition appeared in 1990 and has been used throughout the world in courses on medical informatics. Like the first edition, this new version provides a conceptual framework for learning about computer applications in medical care, for critiquing existing systems, and for anticipating future directions that the field may take. In many respects, however, this new edition is very different from its predecessor. Most importantly, it reflects the remarkable changes in computing and communications that have occurred in the past decade. For example, the Internet was barely mentioned in the first edition, but it and the World Wide Web are now discussed in almost every chapter in light of their pervasive societal influence in recent years. In addition, new chapters are included, and others have been deleted or revamped. We include new chapters on bioinformatics, standards development, systems evaluation, technology assessment, legal topics, and ethical considerations. The former chapter on "hospital information systems" has now given way to a discussion of enterprise computing for integrated delivery networks. Those who are familiar with the first edition will find that the organization and philosophy are unchanged, but the content is almost entirely new.[1]

This book differs from other introductions to the field in its broad coverage and in its emphasis on the field's conceptual underpinnings. Our book does not presume that readers have a health-science or computer-science background, but

[1]As in the first edition, the book tends to draw both its examples and its contributors from North America. There is excellent work in other parts of the world as well, although variations in healthcare systems, and especially in financing, do tend to change the way in which systems evolve from one country to the next. The basic concepts are identical, however, so the book is intended to be useful in educational programs in other parts of the world as well.

it does assume that they are interested in a comprehensive summary of the field that stresses the underlying concepts, and it introduces technical details only to the extent that they are necessary to meet the principal goal. It thus differs from an impressive early text in the field (Ledley, 1965) that emphasized technical details but did not dwell on the broader social and clinical context in which medical computing systems are developed and implemented.

Overview and Guide to Use of This Book

This book is written as a text so that it can be used in formal courses, but we have adopted a broad view of the population for whom it is intended. Thus, it may be used not only by students of medicine and of the other health professions but also by future medical-computing professionals as an introductory text as well as a text for self-study and for reference by practitioners. The book is probably too detailed for use in a 2- or 3-day continuing-education course, although it could be introduced as a reference for further independent study.

Our principal goal in writing this text is to teach *concepts* in medical informatics—the study of biomedical information and its use in decision-making—and to illustrate them in the context of descriptions of representative systems that are in use today or that taught us lessons in the past. As you will see, medical informatics is more than the study of computers in medicine, and we have organized the book to emphasize this point. Chapter 1 first sets the stage for the rest of the book by providing a glimpse of the future, defining important terms and concepts, describing the content of the field, explaining the connections between medical informatics and related disciplines, and discussing the forces that have influenced research in medical informatics and its integration into medical practice.

Broad issues regarding the nature of data, information, and knowledge pervade all areas of application, as do concepts related to optimal decision-making. Chapters 2 and 3 focus on these topics but mention computers only in passing. They serve as the foundation for all that follows.

Chapters 4 and 5 introduce the central ideas of computer hardware and software that are important for understanding the applications described later. Also included is a discussion of computer-system design, with explanations of important issues for you to consider when you read about specific applications and systems throughout the remainder of the book.

Chapter 6 summarizes the issues of standards development, focusing in particular on data exchange and issues related to sharing of clinical data. This important and rapidly evolving topic was not covered in our first edition but warrants inclusion here given the increasingly central role of standards in enabling clinical systems to have their desired influence on healthcare practices.

Chapter 7 addresses the key legal and ethical issues that have arisen when health information systems are considered. Then, in Chapter 8, the challenges associated with technology assessment and the evaluation of clinical information systems are introduced.

Chapters 9 through 18 survey many of the key biomedical areas in which computers are being used. Each chapter explains the conceptual and organizational issues in building that type of system, reviews the pertinent history, and examines the barriers to successful implementations.

Chapter 19 provides a historical perspective on changes in the way society pays for health care. It discusses alternative methods for evaluating the costs and the benefits of health care and suggests ways in which financial considerations affect medical computing. The book concludes in Chapter 20 with a look to the future—a vision of how informatics concepts, computers, and advanced communication devices one day may pervade every aspect of medical practice.

The Study of Computer Applications in Medicine

The actual and potential uses of computers in medical care form a remarkably broad and complex topic. Just as you do not need to understand how a telephone works to make good use of it and to tell when it is functioning poorly, however, we believe that technical medical-computing skills are not needed by health workers who simply wish to become effective computer users. On the other hand, such technical skills are of course necessary for individuals with career commitment to developing computer systems for medical environments. Thus, this book will neither teach you to be a programmer nor show you how to fix a broken computer (although it might motivate you to learn how to do both). It also will not tell you about every important medical-computing system or application; we shall direct you to a wealth of literature where review articles and individual project reports can be found. We describe specific systems only as examples that can provide you with an understanding of the conceptual and organizational issues to be addressed in building systems for such uses. Examples also help to reveal the remaining barriers to successful implementations. Some of the application systems described in the book are well established, even in the commercial marketplace. Others are just beginning to be used broadly in biomedical settings. Several are still largely confined to the research laboratory.

Because we wish to emphasize the concepts underlying this field, we generally limit the discussion of technical implementation details. The computer-science issues can be learned from other courses and other textbooks. One exception, however, is our emphasis on the details of decision science as they relate to medical problem-solving (Chapters 3 and 16). These topics generally are not presented in computer-science courses, yet they play a central role in the intelligent use of medical data and knowledge. Sections on medical decision-making and computer-assisted decision support accordingly include more technical detail than you will find in other chapters.

All chapters include annotated Suggested Readings to which you can turn if you have a particular interest in a topic, and there is a comprehensive Bibliography at the end of the book. We use **boldface** print to indicate the key terms of each chapter; the definitions of these terms are included in the Glossary at the end of the book. Because many of the issues in medical informatics are conceptual, we have included Questions for Discussion at the end of each chapter. You will quickly discover that most of these questions do not have "right" answers. They are intended to illuminate key issues in the field and to motivate you to examine additional readings and new areas of research.

It is inherently limiting to learn about computer applications solely by reading about them. We accordingly encourage you to complement your studies by seeing real systems in use—ideally by using them yourself. Your understanding of system limitations and of what *you* would do to improve a medical-computing system will be greatly enhanced if you have personal experience with representative applications. Be aggressive in seeking opportunities to observe and use working systems.

In a field that is changing as rapidly as computer science is, it is difficult ever to feel that you have knowledge that is completely current. The conceptual basis for study, however, changes much more slowly than do the detailed technological issues. Thus, the lessons you learn from this volume will provide you with a foundation on which you can continue to build in the years ahead.

The Need for a Course in Medical Computing Applications

Suggesting that new courses are needed in the curricula for students of the health professions does not increase your popularity. If anything, educators and students have been clamoring for *reduced* lecture time, for more emphasis on small group sessions, and for more free time for problem-solving and reflection. A 1984 national survey by the Association of American Medical Colleges found that both medical students and their educators severely criticized the current emphasis on lectures and memorization. Yet the analysis of a panel on the General Professional Education of the Physician [Association of American Medical Colleges, 1984] specifically identified medical informatics, including computer applications, as an area in which new educational opportunities needed to be developed so that physicians would be better prepared for the practice of medicine. The report recommended the formation of new academic units in medical informatics in our medical schools, and subsequent studies and reports have continued to stress the importance of the field and the need for its inclusion in the educational environments of health professionals.

The reason for this strong recommendation is clear: *The practice of medicine is inextricably entwined with the management of information.* In the past, practitioners handled medical information through resources such as the nearest hospital or medical-school library; personal collections of books, journals, and reprints; files of patient records; consultation with colleagues; manual office bookkeeping; and (all-too-often flawed) memorization. Although all these techniques continue to be valuable, the computer now offers new methods for finding, filing, and sorting information: online bibliographic-retrieval systems, including full-text publications; personal computers, with database software to maintain personal information and reprint files; office-practice and clinical information systems to capture, communicate, and preserve key elements of the medical record; consultation systems to provide assistance when colleagues are inaccessible or unavailable; practice-management systems to integrate billing and receivable functions with other aspects of office or clinic organization; and other online information resources that help to reduce the pressure to memorize in a field that defies total mastery of all but its narrowest aspects. With such a pervasive and inevitable role for computers in clinical practice, and with a growing failure of traditional techniques to deal with the rapidly increasing information-management needs of practitioners, it has become obvious to many people that a new and essential topic has emerged for study in schools that train medical and other health professionals.

What are less clear are how the subject should be taught and to what extent it should be left for postgraduate education. We believe that topics in medical computing are best taught and learned in the context of health-science training, which allows concepts from both medicine and computer science to be integrated. Medical-computing novices are likely to have only limited opportunities for intensive study of the material once their health-professional training has been completed.

The format of medical-informatics education is certain to evolve as faculty members are hired to develop it at more health-science schools and as the emphasis on lectures as the primary teaching method diminishes. Computers will be used increasingly as teaching tools and as devices for communication, problem-solving, and data sharing among students and faculty. In the meantime, medical informatics will be taught largely in the classroom setting. This book is designed to be used in that kind of traditional course, although the Questions for Discussion also could be used to focus conversation in small seminars and working groups. As resources improve in schools, integration of medical-computing topics into clinical experiences also will become more common. The eventual goal should be to provide instruction in medical informatics whenever this field is most relevant to the topic the student is studying. This aim requires educational opportunities throughout the years of formal training, supplemented by continuing-education programs after graduation.

The goal of integrating medicine and computer science is to provide a mechanism for increasing the sophistication of health professionals so that they know and understand the available resources. They also should be familiar with medical computing's successes and failures, its research frontiers, and its limitations so that they can avoid repeating the mistakes of the past. Study of medical computing also should improve their skills in information management and problem-solving. With a suitable integration of hands-on computer experience, computer-based learning, courses in clinical problem-solving, and study of the material in this volume, health-science students will be well prepared to make effective use of computer-based tools and information management in health-care delivery.

The Need for Specialists in Medical Informatics

As mentioned, this book also is intended to be used as an introductory text in programs of study for people who intend to make their professional careers in medical informatics. If we have persuaded you that a course in medical informatics is needed, then the requirement for trained faculty to teach the courses will be obvious. Some people, however, might argue that a course on this subject could be taught by a computer scientist who has an interest in medical computing or by a physician who has taken a few computing courses. Indeed, in the past, most teaching—and research—has been undertaken by faculty trained primarily in one of the fields and later drawn to the other. Today, however, schools are beginning to realize the need for professionals trained specifically at the interfaces among medicine, computer science, and related disciplines such as statistics, cognitive science, health economics, and medical ethics. This book outlines a first course for students training for careers in the medical-informatics field. We specifically address the need for an educational experience in which computing and information-science concepts are synthesized with biomedical issues regarding research, training, and clinical practice. It is the *integration* of the related disciplines that traditionally has been lacking in the educational opportunities available to students with career interests in medical informatics. If schools are to establish such courses and training programs (and there are already a few examples of each), they clearly need educators who have a broad familiarity with the field and who can develop curricula for students of the health professions as well as of engineering and computer science.

The increasing introduction of computing techniques into medical environments will require that well-trained individuals be available not only to teach students but also to design, develop, select, and manage the medical-computing systems of tomorrow. There is a wide range of context-dependent computing issues that people can appreciate only by working on problems defined by the healthcare setting and its constraints. The field's development has been hampered because there are relatively few trained personnel to design research programs, to carry out the experimental and developmental activities, and to provide academic leadership in medical computing. A frequently cited problem is the difficulty a health professional and a technically trained computer scientist experience when they try to communicate with one another. The vocabularies of the two fields are complex and have little overlap, and there is a process of acculturation to medicine that is difficult for computer scientists to appreciate through distant observation. Thus, interdisciplinary research and development projects are more likely to be successful when they are led by people who can effectively bridge the medical and computing fields. Such professionals often can facilitate sensitive communication among program personnel whose backgrounds and training differ substantially.

It is exciting to be working in a field that is maturing and that is having a beneficial effect on society. There is ample opportunity remaining for innovation as new technologies evolve and fundamental computing problems succumb to the creativity and hard work of our colleagues. In light of the increasing sophistication and specialization required in computer science in general, it is hardly surprising that a new discipline should arise at that field's interface with medicine. This book is dedicated to clarifying the definition and to nurturing the effectiveness of that new discipline: medical informatics.

Edward H. Shortliffe
Leslie E. Perreault

Acknowledgments

When Larry Fagan, Gio Wiederhold, and I decided to compile the first comprehensive textbook on medical informatics, none of us predicted the enormity of the task we were about to undertake. Our challenge was to create a multi-authored textbook that captured the collective expertise of leaders in the field yet was cohesive in content and style. The concept for the book was first developed in 1982. We had begun to teach a course on computer applications in health care at Stanford University School of Medicine and had quickly determined that there was no comprehensive introductory text on the subject. Despite several collections of research descriptions and subject reviews, none had been developed with the needs of a rigorous introductory course in mind.

The thought of writing a textbook was daunting due to the diversity of topics. None of us felt he was sufficiently expert in the full range of important subjects for us to write the book ourselves. Yet we wanted to avoid putting together a collection of disconnected chapters containing assorted subject reviews. Thus, we decided to solicit contributions from leaders in the respective fields to be represented but to provide organizational guidelines in advance for each chapter. We also urged contributors to avoid writing subject reviews but, instead, to focus on the key conceptual topics in their field and to pick a handful of examples to illustrate their didactic points.

As the draft chapters began to come in, we realized that major editing would be required if we were to achieve our goals of cohesiveness and a uniform orientation across all the chapters. We were thus delighted when, in 1987, Leslie Perreault, a graduate of our training program, assumed responsibility for reworking the individual chapters to make an integral whole and for bringing the project to completion. The final product, published in 1990, was the result of many compromises, heavy editing, detailed rewriting, and numerous iterations. We were gratified by the positive response to the book when it finally appeared and especially by the students of medical informatics who have often come to us at scientific meetings and told us about their appreciation of the book.

As the 1990s progressed, however, we began to realize that, despite our emphasis on basic concepts in the field (rather than a survey of existing systems), the volume was beginning to show its age. A great deal had changed since the initial chapters were written, and it became clear that a new edition would be required. The original editors discussed the project and decided to redesign the book, solicit updated chapters, and publish a new edition. Leslie Perreault by this time was a busy Director at First Consulting Group in New York City and would not have as much time to devote to the project as she had when we did the first edition. With trepidation, in light of our knowledge of the work that would be involved, we embarked on the new project.

As before, the chapter authors have done a marvelous job, trying their best to meet our deadlines, putting up with editing changes that were designed to bring a uniform style to the book, and contributing excellent chapters that nicely reflect the changes in the field in the last decade. We are all extremely appreciative of their commitment and for the excellence of their work on behalf of the book and the field.

The completed volume reflects the work and support of many people in addition to the editors and chapter authors. Particular gratitude is once again owed to Lyn Dupré, our developmental editor, whose rigorous attention to detail is reflected on every page. We also appreciate the kindness and professionalism of Peter Gordon from Addison-Wesley, who worked with us to effect a smooth transition in the transfer of the book to a new publisher for the second edition. At Springer-Verlag we have been delighted to work with the responsible editors, first with Bill Day and, more recently, with Nhora Cortes-Comerer. Marion Ball and Kathy Hannah have also been extremely supportive in working with us to move this volume into their Springer-Verlag informatics series.

Members of the administrative staff in our group at Stanford have also been remarkably supportive during what has at times been an exhausting and time-consuming process. Rosalind Ravasio competently managed the administrative details so that we could attend to our writing and editing. We are also grateful for the support of the Computing Resources Group at Stanford Medical Informatics. Under the direction of Farhad Shafabaksh, the Computing Resources Group maintains a smoothly functioning computing environment that has been crucial to the production of this book in its electronic format and to the distribution of chapters and revisions among the authors and editors via the World Wide Web.

The unsung hero of the effort is our assistant, Barbara Morgan, who has shouldered the lion's share of the burden for online editing of the chapters, maintaining a system for keeping track of new versions, managing permissions and figures, and somehow keeping a good natured disposition throughout it all. We are all sincerely grateful to Barbara for accepting this new set of responsibilities—clearly *not* in her job description—and doing a marvelous job in ushering this volume to a successful completion. Thank you, Barbara!

Edward H. Shortliffe
Leslie E. Perreault

Contents

UNIT II MEDICAL COMPUTING APPLICATIONS

UNIT III MEDICAL INFORMATICS IN THE YEARS AHEAD

Contributors

Russ B. Altman, MD, PhD, FACP, FACMI
Associate Professor of Medicine and of Computer Science, Stanford University School of Medicine, Stanford, CA 94305-5479, USA (russ.altman@stanford.edu)

Suzanne Bakken, RN, DNSc, FAAN, FACMI
Professor of Nursing and of Medical Informatics, Columbia University College of Physicians and Surgeons, New York, NY 10032-3720, USA (sue.bakken@dmi.columbia.edu)

G. Octo Barnett, MD, FACP, FACMI
Professor of Medicine, Harvard Medical School, Director, Laboratory of Computer Science, Massachusetts General Hospital, Boston, MA 02114, USA (barnett.octo@mgh.harvard.edu)

Marsden S. Blois, MD, PhD[†]
Formerly Professor of Medical Informatics and of Dermatology, University of California, San Francisco, USA

Patricia Flatley Brennan, RN, PhD, FAAN, FACMI
Lillian S. Moehlman Bascom Professor, School of Nursing and College of Engineering, University of Wisconsin-Madison, Madison, WI 53706, USA (pbrennan@engr.wisc.edu)

James F. Brinkley, MD, PhD, FACMI
Research Associate Professor of Biological Structure, Computer Science and Engineering, and Medical Education, University of Washington, Seattle, Washington 98195, USA (brinkley@u.washington.edu)

James J. Cimino, MD, FACP, FACMI
Associate Professor of Medical Informatics in Medicine, Columbia University College of Physicians and Surgeons, Columbia-Presbyterian Medical Center, New York, NY 10032, USA (james.cimino@columbia.edu)

[†]Deceased

William M. Detmer, MD, MS, FACP
Clinical Assistant Professor, Department of Health Evaluation Sciences, University of Virginia, Health Sciences Center, Charlottesville, VA 22908, USA (bdetmer@virginia.edu)

Parvati Dev, PhD, FACMI
Director, SUMMIT Laboratory, and Senior Research Scientist, Stanford Medical Informatics, Stanford University School of Medicine, Stanford, CA 94305-5466, USA (parvati.dev@stanford.edu)

Alain C. Enthoven, PhD
Professor of Public and Private Management, Graduate School of Business, Stanford University, Stanford CA 94305-5015, USA (enthoven_alain@gsb.stanford.edu)

Lawrence M. Fagan, MD, PhD, FACMI
Senior Research Scientist and Associate Director, Stanford Medical Informatics, Co-Director, Medical Information Sciences Training Program, Director, Medical Informatics Short Course, Stanford University School of Medicine, Stanford, CA 94305-5479, USA (fagan@smi.stanford.edu)

Andrew Friede, MD, MPH
Physician Executive, Cerner Corporation, Atlanta GA 30328, USA (AFriede@cerner.com)

Charles P. Friedman, PhD, FACMI
Professor of Medicine and Director, Center for Biomedical Informatics, University of Pittsburgh, Pittsburgh, PA 15213-2582, USA (cpf@cbmi.upmc.edu)

Mark E. Frisse, MD, MS, MBA, FACMI
Vice President, Clinical Information Services, Express Scripts, Maryland Heights, Missouri 63043, USA (mfrisse@express-scripts.com)

Alan M. Garber, MD, PhD, FACP
Professor of Medicine, Economics, and Health Research and Policy, Director, Center for Primary Care and Outcomes Research, Director, Center for Health Policy, Stanford University, Stanford, CA 94305-6019, USA (garber@stanford.edu)

Reed M. Gardner, PhD, FACMI
Professor and Chair, Department of Medical Informatics, University of Utah, Co-Director of Medical Informatics, LDS Hospital, School of Medicine, Salt Lake City, UT 84132, USA (reed.gardner@hsc.utah.edu)

Kenneth W. Goodman, PhD
Director, Forum for Bioethics and Philosophy, University of Miami
Miami, FL 33101, USA (kwg@cs.miami.edu)

Robert A. Greenes, MD, PhD, FACR, FACMI
Professor of Radiology, Harvard Medical School, Professor of Health Sciences and Technology, Harvard-MIT Division of Health Sciences and Technology, Professor of Health Policy and Management, Harvard School of Public Health, Radiologist, Brigham and Women's Hospital,
Director, Decision Systems Group, Brigham and Women's Hospital, Boston, MA 02115, USA (greenes@harvard.edu)

W. Edward Hammond, PhD, FACMI
Professor of Community and Family Medicine and Chief, Division of Medical Informatics, Duke University School of Medicine, Duke University, Durham, NC 27710, USA (hammo001@mc.duke.edu)

William R. Hersh, MD, FACP, FACMI
Associate Professor and Chief, Division of Medical Informatics and Outcomes Research, Oregon Health Sciences University, Portland, OR 97201, USA (hersh@ohsu.edu)

Edward P. Hoffer MD, FACP, FRCP(C), FACMI
Associate Clinical Professor of Medicine, Harvard Medical School
Senior Physician, Lahey Clinic, Senior Scientist and Assistant Director, Laboratory of Computer Science, Massachusetts General Hospital, Framingham, MA 01702, USA (ehoffer@partners.org)

Clement J. McDonald, MD, FACP, FACMI
Director, Regenstrief Institute and Distinguished Professor of Medicine, Indiana University School of Medicine, Indianapolis, IN 46202, USA (clem@regen.rg.iupui.edu)

Randolph A. Miller, MD, FACMI
Professor and Chairman, Division of Biomedical Informatics, Vanderbilt University Medical Center, Nashville, TN 37232-8340, USA (randy.miller@mcmail.vanderbilt.edu)

Mark A. Musen, MD, PhD, FACP, FACMI
Associate Professor of Medicine and of Computer Science, Head, Stanford Medical Informatics, Stanford University School of Medicine, Stanford, CA 94305- 5479, USA (musen@stanford.edu)

Douglas K. Owens, MD, MS
Health Services Research and Development Senior Research Associate, VA Palo Alto Health Care System, Associate Professor of Medicine and Health Research and Policy, Stanford University School of Medicine, Center for Primary Care and Outcomes Research, Stanford, CA 94305-6019, USA (owens@stanford.edu)

Judy G. Ozbolt, PhD, RN, FAAN, FACMI
Independence Foundation Professor of Nursing and Professor of Biomedical Informatics, Vanderbilt University, Nashville, TN 37240-0008, USA (judy.ozbolt@mcmail.vanderbilt.edu)

Leslie E. Perreault, MS
Director, First Consulting Group, New York, NY 10019-4105, USA (perreault@smi.stanford.edu)

Thomas C. Rindfleisch, MS, FACMI
Director, Lane Medical Library, Senior Research Scientist, Stanford Medical Informatics, Stanford University School of Medicine, Stanford, CA 94305-5123, USA (rindfleisch@stanford.edu)

Charles Safran, MD, MS, FACP, FACMI
Associate Clinical Professor of Medicine, Harvard Medical School, Chief Executive Officer, Clinician Support Technology, Framingham, MA 01701, USA (csafran@harvard.edu)

M. Michael Shabot, MD, FACMI
Associate Director of Surgery and Director, Surgical Critical Care, Cedars-Sinai Medical Center, Los Angeles, CA 90048, USA (shabot@csmc.edu)

Yuval Shahar, MD, PhD
Assistant Professor of Medicine/Medical Informatics and of Computer Science, Stanford Medical Informatics, Stanford University School of Medicine, Stanford, CA 94305-5479, USA (shahar@smi.stanford.edu)

Edward H. Shortliffe, MD, PhD, FACP, FACMI
Professor and Chair, Department of Medical Informatics, Professor of Medicine and of Computer Science, Columbia University College of Physicians and Surgeons, Columbia-Presbyterian Medical Center, New York, NY 10032-3720, USA (shortliffe@dmi.columbia.edu)

Sara J. Singer, MBA
Executive Director, Center for Health Policy, Institute for International Studies, Stanford University, Stanford, CA 94305, USA (singer@healthpolicy.stanford.edu)

Harold C. Sox, Jr., MD, MACP
Joseph M. Huber Professor and Chair, Department of Medicine, Dartmouth-Hitchcock Medical Center, Lebanon, NH 03756, USA (harold.c.sox.jr@hitchcock.org)

Paul C. Tang, MD, FACP, FACMI
Vice President, Epic Research Institute, Medical Director, Clinical Informatics, Palo Alto Medical Foundation, Mountain View, CA 94041, USA (tang@smi.stanford.edu)

Gio Wiederhold, PhD, FIEEE, FACM, FACMI
Professor of Computer Science, Electrical Engineering, and Medicine, Stanford University, Stanford, CA 94305-9040, USA (gio@cs.stanford.edu)

Jeremy C. Wyatt, DM(Oxon), FRCP(UK), FACMI(US), MB BS(Lon)
Director, Health Knowledge Management Centre, School of Public Policy, University College London, London, WC1H 9EZ, UK (uctqjwy@ucl.ac.uk)

Unit I
Recurrent Themes in Medical Informatics

1
The Computer Meets Medicine and Biology: Emergence of a Discipline

EDWARD H. SHORTLIFFE AND MARSDEN S. BLOIS†

After reading this chapter, you should know the answers to these questions:

- Why is information management a central issue in biomedical research and clinical practice?
- What are integrated information-management environments, and how might we expect them to affect the practice of medicine and biomedical research in coming years?
- What do we mean by the terms *medical computer science, medical computing, medical informatics, clinical informatics, nursing informatics, bioinformatics,* and *health informatics*?
- Why should health professionals and students of the health professions learn about medical-informatics concepts and informatics applications?
- How has the development of minicomputers, microprocessors, and the Internet changed the nature of biomedical computing?
- How is medical informatics related to clinical practice, biomedical engineering, molecular biology, decision science, information science, and computer science?
- How does information in clinical medicine and health differ from information in the basic sciences?
- How can changes in computer technology and the way medical care is financed influence the integration of medical computing into clinical practice?

1.1 Integrated Information Management: Technology's Promise[1]

After scientists had developed the first digital computers in the 1940s, society was told that these new machines would soon be serving routinely as memory devices, assisting with calculations and with information retrieval. Within the

---

[1]Portions of this section are adapted from a paper presented at Medinfo98 in Seoul, Korea (Shortliffe, 1998c).
†Deceased.

next decade, physicians and other health workers had begun to hear about the dramatic effects that such technology would have on medical practice. More than four decades of remarkable progress in computing have followed those early predictions, and many of the original prophesies have come to pass. Stories regarding the "information revolution" fill our newspapers and popular magazines, and today's children show an uncanny ability to make use of computers as routine tools for study and entertainment. Similarly, clinical workstations are now available on hospital wards and in outpatient offices. Yet many observers cite the healthcare system as being slow to understand information technology, to exploit it for its unique practical and strategic functionalities, and to incorporate it effectively into the work environment. Nonetheless, the enormous technological advances of the last two decades—personal computers and graphical workstations, new methods for human-computer interactions, innovations in mass storage of data, personal digital assistants, the Internet and the World Wide Web, wireless communications—have all combined to make routine use of computers by all health workers and biomedical scientists inevitable. A new world is already with us, but its greatest influence is yet to come. This book will teach you both about our present resources and accomplishments *and* about what we can expect in the years ahead.

It is remarkable to realize that the first microprocessors, enabling personal computers, did not appear until the late 1970s, and the World Wide Web dates only to the early 1990s. This dizzying rate of change, combined with equally pervasive and revolutionary changes in almost all international healthcare systems during the past decade, makes it difficult for healthcare planners and institutional managers to try to deal with both issues at once. Yet many observers now believe that the two topics are inextricably related and that planning for the new healthcare environments of the twenty-first century requires a deep understanding of the role that information technology is likely to play in those environments.

What might that future hold for the typical practicing clinician? As we shall discuss in detail in Chapter 9, no clinical computing topic is gaining more attention currently than is the issue of electronic medical records (EMRs). Healthcare organizations are finding that they do not have systems in place that allow them to answer questions that are crucially important for strategic planning and for their better understanding of how they compare with other provider groups in their local or regional competitive environment. In the past, administrative and financial data were the major elements required for such planning, but comprehensive clinical data are now also important for institutional self-analysis and strategic planning. Furthermore, the inefficiencies and frustrations associated with the use of paper-based medical records have become increasingly clear (Dick & Steen, 1991 [revised 1997]), especially when inadequate access to clinical information is one of the principal barriers that clinicians encounter when trying to increase their efficiency in order to meet productivity goals for their practices.

1.1.1 Electronic Health Records: Anticipating the Future

Many healthcare institutions are seeking to develop integrated clinical workstations. These are single-entry points into a medical world in which computational tools assist not only with clinical matters (reporting results of tests, allowing direct entry of orders by clinicians, facilitating access to transcribed reports, and in some cases supporting telemedicine applications or decision-support functions) but also with administrative and financial topics (tracking of patients within the hospital, managing materials and inventory, supporting personnel functions, managing the payroll, and the like), research (e.g., analyzing the outcomes associated with treatments and procedures, performing quality assurance, supporting clinical trials, and implementing various treatment protocols), scholarly information (e.g., accessing digital libraries, supporting bibliographic search, and providing access to drug information databases), and even office automation (providing access to spreadsheets, word processors, and the like). The key idea, however, is that at the heart of the evolving clinical workstation lies the medical record in a new incarnation: electronic, accessible, confidential, secure, acceptable to clinicians and patients, and integrated with other types of nonpatient-specific information.

Inadequacy of the Traditional Paper Record

The paper-based medical record is woefully inadequate for meeting the needs of modern medicine. It arose in the nineteenth century as a highly personalized "lab notebook" that clinicians could use to record their observations and plans so that they could be reminded of pertinent details when they next saw that same patient. There were no bureaucratic requirements, no assumptions that the record would be used to support communication among varied providers of care, and few data or test results to fill up the record's pages. The record that met the needs of clinicians a century ago has struggled mightily to adjust over the decades and to accommodate to new requirements as health care and medicine have changed.

Difficulty in obtaining information, either about a specific patient or about a general issue related to patient management, is a frustrating but common occurrence for practitioners. With increasing pressures to enhance clinical productivity, practitioners have begun to clamor for more reliable systems that provide facile, intuitive access to the information they need at the time they are seeing their patients. The EMR offers the hope for such improved access to patient-specific information and should provide a major benefit both for the quality of care and for the quality of life for clinicians in practice.

Despite the obvious need for a new record-keeping paradigm, most organizations have found it challenging to try to move to a paperless, computer-based clinical record (see Chapters 9 and 10). This observation forces us to ask the questions "What *is* a health record in the modern world? Are the available products and systems well matched with the modern notions of a comprehensive health record?" Companies offer medical-record products, yet the packages are limited in their capabilities and seldom seem to meet the full range of needs defined within our complex healthcare organizations.

The complexity associated with automating medical records is best appreciated if one analyzes the *processes* associated with the creation and use of such records rather than thinking of the record as an object that can be moved around as needed within the institution. For example, on the input side (Fig. 1.1), the medical record requires the integration of processes for data capture and for merging information from diverse sources. The contents of the paper record have traditionally been organized chronologically—often a severe limitation when a clinician seeks to find a specific piece of information that could occur almost anywhere within the chart. To be useful, the record system must make it easy to access and display needed data, to analyze them, and to share them among colleagues and with secondary users of the record who are not involved in direct patient care (Fig. 1.2). Thus, the computer-based medical record is best viewed not as an object, or a product, but rather as a set of processes that an organization must put into place, supported by technology (Fig. 1.3). Implementing electronic records is inherently a systems-integration task; it is not possible to buy a

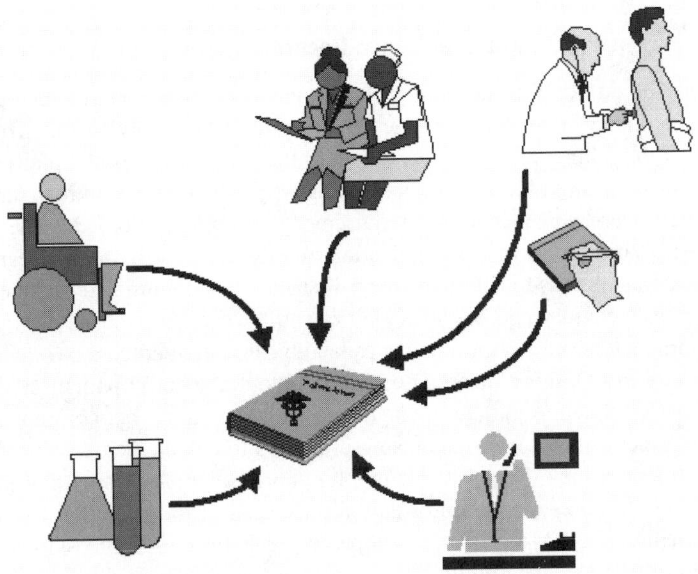

FIGURE 1.1. Inputs to the medical record. The traditional paper medical record is created by a variety of organizational processes that capture varying types of information (notes regarding direct encounters between health professionals and patients, laboratory or radiologic results, reports of telephone calls or prescriptions, and data obtained directly from patients). The record thus becomes a merged collection of such data, generally organized in chronological order.

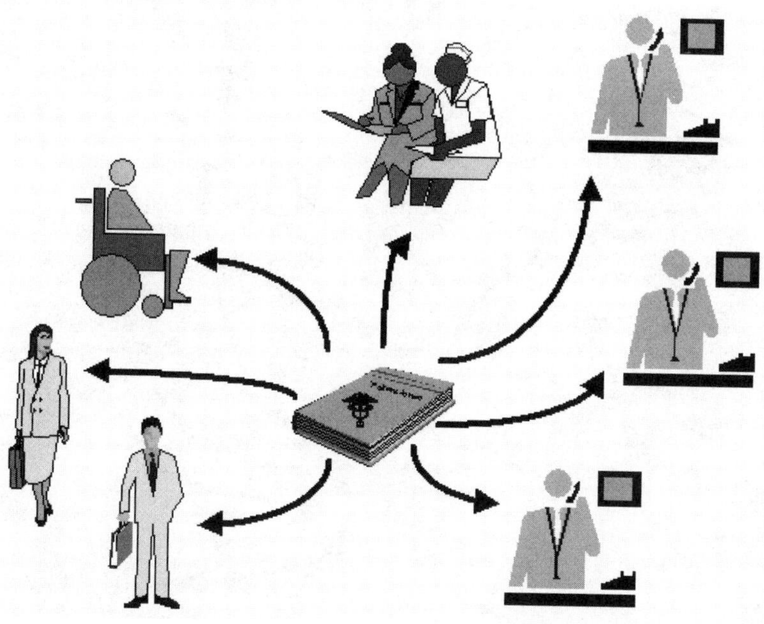

FIGURE 1.2. Outputs from the medical record. Once information is collected in the traditional paper medical record, it may be provided to a wide variety of potential users of the chart. These users include health professionals and the patients themselves but also a wide variety of "secondary users" (represented here by the individuals in business suits) who have valid reasons for accessing the record but who are not involved with direct patient care. Numerous providers are typically involved in a patient's care, so the chart also serves as a means for communicating among them. The mechanisms for displaying, analyzing, and sharing information from such records results from a set of processes that often vary substantially across several patient-care settings and institutions.

medical-record system for a complex organization as an off-the-shelf product. Joint development is crucial.

The Medical Record and Clinical Trials

The arguments for automating medical records are nicely summarized in Chapters 2 and 9 and in the Institute of Medicine's report on computer-based patient records (Dick & Steen, 1991 [revised 1997]). One argument that warrants emphasis is the importance of the electronic record in supporting **clinical trials**—experiments in which data from specific patient interactions are pooled and analyzed in order to learn about the safety and efficacy of new treatments or tests and to gain insight into disease processes that are not otherwise well understood. Medical researchers are constrained today by clumsy methods for acquiring the data needed for clinical trials, generally relying on manual capture of information onto datasheets that are later transcribed into computer databases for statis-

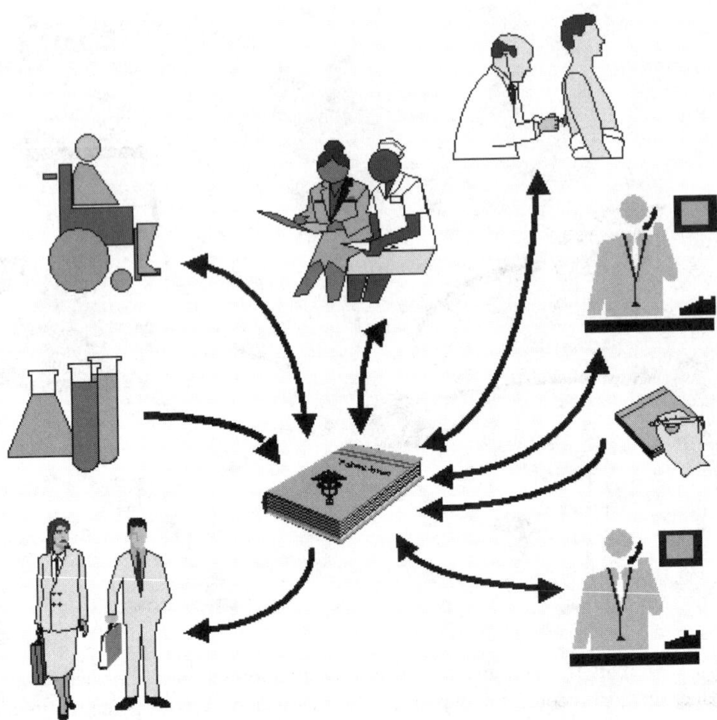

FIGURE 1.3. Complex processes demanded of the record. As shown in Figures 1.1 and 1.2, the medical record is the incarnation of a complex set of organizational processes that both gather information to be shared and then distribute that information to those who have valid reasons for accessing it. Paper-based documents are severely limited in meeting the diverse requirements for data collection and information access that are implied by this diagram.

tical analysis (Fig. 1.4). The approach is labor intensive, fraught with opportunities for error, and adds to the high costs associated with randomized prospective research protocols.

The use of EMRs offers many advantages to those carrying out clinical research. Most obviously, it helps to eliminate the manual task of extracting data from charts or filling out specialized datasheets. The data needed for a study can be derived directly from the EMR, thus making research data collection a by-product of routine clinical record keeping (Fig. 1.5). Other advantages accrue as well. For example, the record environment can help to ensure compliance with a research protocol, pointing out to a clinician when a patient is eligible for a study or when the protocol for a study calls for a specific management plan given the currently available data about that patient. We are also seeing the development of novel authoring environments for clinical-trial protocols that can help to

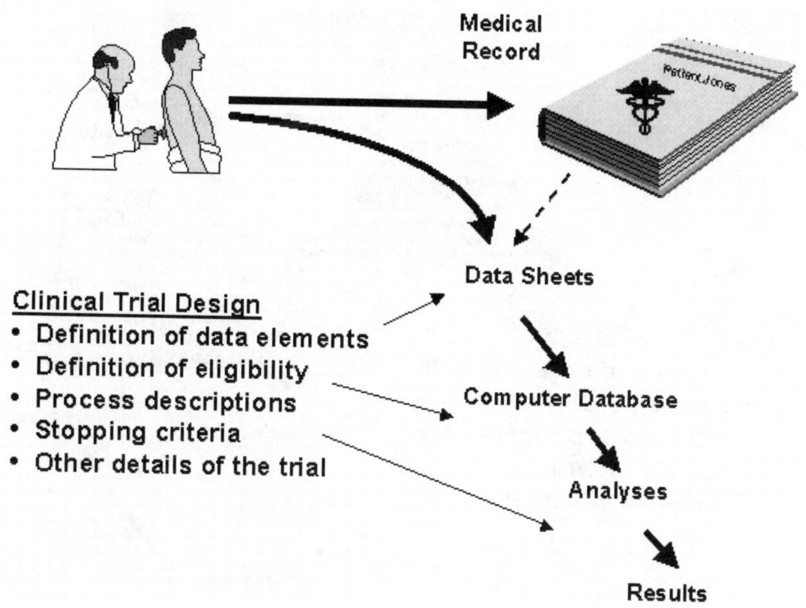

FIGURE 1.4. Conventional data collection for clinical trials. Although modern clinical trials routinely use computer systems for data storage and analysis, the gathering of research data is often a manual task. Physicians who care for patients enrolled in trials are often asked to fill out special datasheets for later transcription into computer databases. Alternatively, data managers are hired to abstract the relevant data from the traditional paper chart. The trials are generally designed to define data elements that are required and the methods for analysis, but it is common for the process of collecting those data in a structured format to be left to manual processes at the point of patient care.

ensure that the data elements needed for the trial are compatible with the local EMR's conventions for representing patient descriptors.

1.1.2 *Recurring Issues That Must Be Addressed*

There are at least four major issues that have consistently constrained our efforts to build effective patient-record systems: (1) the need for standards in the area of clinical terminology; (2) concerns regarding data privacy, confidentiality, and security; (3) challenges of data entry by physicians; and (4) difficulties associated with the integration of record systems with other information resources in the healthcare setting. The first of these issues is discussed in detail in Chapter 6, and privacy is one of the central topics in Chapter 7. Issues of direct data entry by clinicians are discussed in Chapter 2 and again in Chapter 9 and throughout many other chapters in this book as well. In the next section we examine recent trends in networking and ask how communications are changing the way in

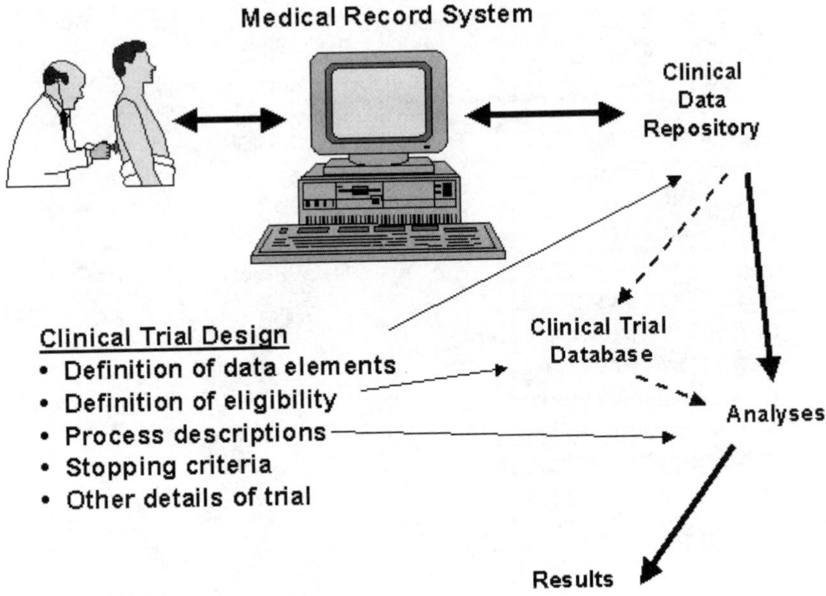

FIGURE 1.5. Role of EMRs in supporting clinical trials. With the introduction of computer-based patient record systems, the collection of research data for clinical trials can become a by-product of the routine care of the patients. Research data may be analyzed directly from the clinical data repository, or a secondary research database may be created by downloading information from the on-line patient records. The manual processes in Figure 1.4 are thereby eliminated. In addition, the interaction of the physician with the medical record permits two-way communication, which can greatly improve the quality and efficiency of the clinical trial. Physicians can be reminded when their patients are eligible for an experimental protocol, and the computer system can also remind the clinicians of the rules that are defined by the research protocol, thereby increasing compliance with the experimental plan.

which the patient-care record can be better integrated with other relevant information resources and clinical processes that are currently fragmented and poorly coordinated.

1.1.3 Integrating the Patient Record with Other Information Resources

Experience has shown that physicians are "horizontal" users of information technology (Greenes & Shortliffe, 1990). Rather than becoming "power users" of a narrowly defined software package, they tend to seek broad functionality across a wide variety of systems and resources. Thus, routine use of computers, and of EMRs, will be most easily achieved if the computing environment offers a critical mass of functionality that makes the system both smoothly integrated and useful for essentially every patient encounter.

With the introduction of networked systems within our healthcare organizations, there are new opportunities to integrate a wide variety of resources through single clinical workstations (see Chapter 10). The nature of the integration tasks is illustrated in Figure 1.6 in which various workstations are shown at the upper left (machines for use by patients, clinicians, or clerical staff) connected to an enterprise-wide network or **intranet**. In such an environment, diverse clinical, financial, and administrative databases all need to be accessed and integrated, typically by using both networks to tie them together and a variety of standards for sharing data among them. Thus the clinical data *repository* has developed as an increasingly common idea. This term refers to a central computer that gathers and integrates clinical data from diverse sources such as the chemistry and microbiology laboratories, the pharmacy, and the radiology department. As is suggested in the diagram, this clinical database can provide the nidus for what will evolve into an EMR as more and more clinical data become available in electronic form and the need for the paper documents shrinks and eventually vanishes.

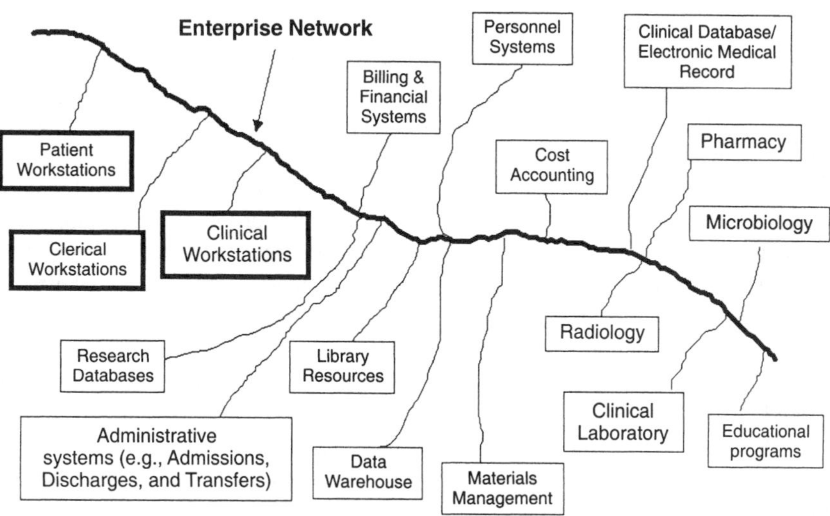

FIGURE 1.6. Networking the organization. The *enterprise intranet* is a locally controlled network that extends throughout a healthcare system. It allows specialized workstations to access a wide variety of information sources: educational, clinical, financial, and administrative. An EMR emerges from such an architecture if a system is implemented that gathers patient-specific data from multiple sources and merges them for ease of access by users such as those illustrated in Figure 1.2. Such systems are often called *clinical data repositories,* particularly if they do not yet contain the full range of information that would normally occur in a medical record.

Another theme in the changing world of health care is the increasing investment in the creation of clinical guidelines and pathways (see Chapter 16), generally in an effort to reduce practice variability and to develop consensus approaches to recurring management problems. Several government and professional organizations, as well as individual provider groups, have invested heavily in guideline development, often putting an emphasis on using clear evidence from the literature, rather than expert opinion alone, as the basis for the advice. Despite the success in creating such **evidence-based guidelines**, there is a growing recognition that we need better methods for delivering the decision logic to the point of care. Guidelines that appear in monographs or journal articles tend to sit on shelves, unavailable when the knowledge they contain would be most valuable to practitioners. Computer-based tools for implementing such guidelines, and integrating them with the EMR, present a potential means for making high-quality advice available in the routine clinical setting. Many organizations are accordingly attempting to integrate decision-support tools with their nascent electronic record systems.

Rethinking Common Assumptions

One of the first instincts of software developers is to create an electronic version of an object or process from the physical world. Some familiar notion provides the inspiration for a new software product. Once the software version has been developed, however, human ingenuity and creativity often lead to an evolution that extends the software version far beyond what was initially contemplated. The computer can thus facilitate paradigm shifts in how we think about such familiar concepts.

Consider, for example, the remarkable difference between today's word processors and the typewriter that was the original inspiration for their development. Although the early word processors were designed largely to allow users to avoid retyping papers each time a minor change was made to a document, the word processors of today bear little resemblance to a typewriter. Consider all the powerful desktop-publishing facilities, integration of figures, spelling correction, grammar aids, and the like. Similarly, today's spreadsheet programs bear little resemblance to the tables of numbers that we once created on graph paper. Also consider automatic teller machines and their facilitation of today's worldwide banking in ways that were never contemplated when the industry depended on human bank tellers.

It is accordingly logical to ask what the health record will become after it has been effectively implemented on computer systems and new opportunities for its enhancement become increasingly clear to us. It is unlikely that the computer-based health record a decade from now will bear much resemblance to the antiquated paper folder that still dominates many of our healthcare environments. One way to anticipate the changes that are likely to occur is to consider the potential role of wide-area networking and the Internet in the record's evolution.

Extending the Record Beyond the Single Institution

In considering ongoing trends in information technology that are likely to make changes inevitable, it would be difficult to start with any topic other than the Internet. The Internet began in 1968 as a United States research activity funded by the Advanced Research Projects Agency (ARPA) of the Department of Defense. Initially known as the ARPAnet, the network began as a novel mechanism for allowing a handful of defense-related mainframe computers, located mostly at academic institutions or in the defense industry, to share data files with each other and to provide remote access to computing power at other locations. The notion of electronic mail arose soon thereafter, and machine-to-machine electronic mail exchanges quickly became a major component of the network's traffic. As the technology matured, its value for nonmilitary research activities was recognized, and by 1973 the first medically related research computer had been added to the network (Shortliffe, 1998b).

During the 1980s the technology began to be developed in other parts of the world, and the National Science Foundation took over the task of running the principal high-speed **backbone network** in the United States. The first hospitals, mostly academic centers, began to be connected to what had by then become known as the Internet, and in a major policy move it was decided to allow commercial organizations to join the network as well. By April 1995 the Internet in the United States had become a fully commercialized operation, no longer depending on the U.S. government to support even the major backbone connections. Many people point to the Internet as a superb example of the facilitating role of federal investment in promoting innovative technologies. The Internet is a major societal force that arguably would never have been created if the research and development, plus the coordinating activities, had been left to the private sector.

The explosive growth of the Internet did not occur until the late 1990s, when the World Wide Web (which had been conceived initially by the physics community as a way of using the Internet to share preprints with photographs and diagrams among researchers) was introduced and popularized. The Web is highly intuitive, requires no special training, and provides a mechanism for access to multimedia information that accounts for its remarkable growth as a worldwide phenomenon.

The Internet Society[2] reports data on the growth of the international networking infrastructure, and they indicate that by 1998 there were close to 50 million host computers connected to the Internet worldwide (not counting all the end-user machines used to *access* the network). These machines were spread across more than 2 million host **domains**—unique corporate or institutional addresses that often account for multiple hosts. Given the current exponential growth, we should anticipate close to 200 million Internet host machines in the near future.

---

[2]See http://www.isoc.org/.

Such growth is not being ignored by the telecommunications industry. Data from MCI-Worldcom, Inc., one of the companies that is actively involved in the growth of high-speed networking, indicate that they experienced a 5,600 percent growth in Internet-related traffic between October 1994 and January 1996.[3] Between 1996 and 1999, growth was compounding at approximately 15 percent per month, which naturally led to questions about when market saturation would occur. Particularly impressive was the projection that MCI's Internet traffic would exceed their voice telephony, in terms of relative use of MCI's network capacity, by the year 2001. The business implications of such data for the telecommunications industry are clear.

The societal impact of this communications phenomenon cannot be overstated, especially given the international connectivity that has grown phenomenally in the past 5 years. Countries that once were isolated from information that was important to citizens, ranging from consumers to scientists to those interested in political issues, are now finding new options for bringing timely information to the desktop machines of individuals with an Internet connection.

There is accordingly a major upheaval underway in the telecommunications industry, with companies that used to be in different businesses now finding that their activities and technologies are beginning to merge. In the United States, legislation was passed in 1996 to allow new competition to develop and new industries to emerge. The full implications remain to be seen, especially as the business arguments for investments by the industry are refined and we see just how quickly changes will occur. There is, however, already ample evidence of the merging of technologies such as cable television, telephone, networking, and satellite communications. High-speed lines into homes and offices are increasingly available, and inexpensive mechanisms for connecting to the Internet without using a computer have also emerged. The impact on all individuals is likely to be great and hence on our patients and on their access to information and to their healthcare providers. Medicine cannot afford to ignore these rapidly occurring changes.

Envisioning the Enterprise Internet

Although we should always expect a medical record to be populated with data about a specific patient, in the electronic implementation of records we also expect to find data regarding populations of patients, *integrated* access to the biomedical literature, and interactive environments for offering clinical guidelines or frank consultative advice. We envision a world in which the enterprise intranet of Figure 1.6 is seamlessly connected to the full Internet beyond, with integrated access to a wide variety of information sources that are geographically distributed well beyond our local institutions (Fig. 1.7). To the extent that an individual's medical records are maintained in compatible electronic formats at all

---

[3]Data are taken from a presentation delivered by an MCI-Worldcom corporate vice president and Internet visionary, Vint Cerf, at the National Library of Medicine in March 1997.

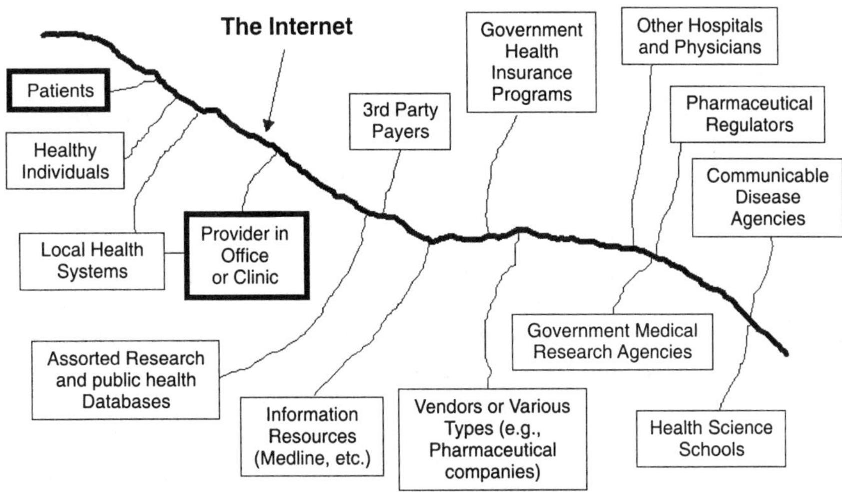

FIGURE 1.7. Moving beyond the organization. The *enterprise Internet* is the integration of an organization's intranet (Fig. 1.6, encapsulated in the box here labeled "Local Health System") with the full potential of the worldwide Internet. Both providers and patients increasingly access the Internet for a wide variety of information sources and functions suggested by this diagram (see text).

the institutions where they have been seen, the Internet provides the potential of creating "virtual medical records," the electronic compilation of a patient's health data from all the settings in which they have been seen. Although such a concept raises important issues regarding patient data privacy and confidentiality, there are technical and policy measures that can be taken to help to ensure that such virtual records are kept secure from prying eyes but can be made available at times of medical need (see Chapter 7) (National Research Council, 1997).

Implications for Patients

As the number of Internet users grows (estimates suggest that there were more than 50 million users in the United States alone by 1999), it is not surprising that increasing numbers of patients, as well as healthy individuals, are turning to the Internet for health information (see Fig. 1.7). It is a rare North American physician who has not encountered a patient who comes to an appointment armed with a question, or a stack of laser-printed pages, that arose due to medically related searches on the World Wide Web. The companies that provide search engines for the Internet report that medically related sites are among the most popular ones being explored by consumers. As a result, physicians and other care providers must be prepared to deal with information that patients discover on the Web and bring with them when they seek care from clinicians. Some of the information is timely and excellent; in this sense physicians can often learn about innovations from their patients and will need to be increasingly open to the kinds of questions that this enhanced access to information will generate from patients in their practices. On the other hand, much of the health information on the Web lacks peer review or is purely anecdotal. People who lack medical training can be misled by such information, just as they have been in the past by printed information in books and magazines dealing with fad treatments from anecdotal sources. In addition, some sites provide personalized advice, often for a fee, with all the attendant concerns about the quality of the suggestions and the ability to give valid advice based on an electronic mail or Web-based interaction.

In a more positive light, the new communications technologies offer clinicians creative ways to interact with their patients and to provide higher quality care. Years ago medicine adopted the telephone as a standard vehicle for facilitating patient care, and we now take this kind of interaction with patients for granted. If we extend the audio channel to include our visual sense as well, the notion of **telemedicine** emerges. Although there are major challenges to be overcome before telemedicine is likely to be widely adopted for direct patient care (Grigsby & Sanders, 1998), there are specialized settings in which it is already proving to be successful and cost effective (e.g., international medicine, teleradiology, and video-based care of patients in state and federal prisons). The challenges are largely regulatory and fiscal before telemedicine will be widely adopted.

A potentially more practical concept in the short term is to use computers and the Internet as the basis for communication between patients and providers. For example, there has been rapid growth in the use of electronic mail as a mechanism for avoiding "telephone tag" and allowing simple questions to be answered asynchronously (the telephone requires synchronous communication; electronic mail does not). More exploratory, but extremely promising, are communications methods based on the technology of the World Wide Web. For example, there are young companies that work with managed care organizations and healthcare systems to provide Web-based facilities for disease management. Patients log in to a private Web site, provide information about the status of their chronic disease (e.g., blood glucose readings in diabetes), and later obtain feedback from their physician or from disease managers who seek to keep the patients healthy at home, thereby decreasing the need for emergency-room or clinic visits.

Requirements for Achieving the Vision

Many of the concepts proposed above depend on the emergence of an Internet with much higher **bandwidth** and **reliability** decreased **latency** and financial models that make the applications cost effective and practical. Major research efforts are underway to address some of these concerns, including the federal **Next Generation Internet** activity in the United States.[4] In addition, academic institutions have banded together in a consortium designed to create new test beds for high-bandwidth communications in support of research and education.

[4]See http://www.ccic.gov/ngi/.

Incorporated as the University Consortium for Advanced Internet Development (UCAID[5]), their initial effort has built on existing federally funded or experimental networks and is known as **Internet 2**. Exploratory efforts that continue to push the state of the art in Internet technology all have significant implications for the future of healthcare delivery in general and of the computer-based health record in particular (Shortliffe, 1998a).

Education and Training There is a difference between computer literacy (familiarity with computers and their routine uses in our society) and knowledge of the role that computing and communications technology can and should play in our healthcare system. We are generally doing a poor job of training future clinicians in the latter area and are thereby leaving them poorly equipped for the challenges and opportunities they will face in the rapidly changing practice environments that surround them (Shortliffe, 1995a).

Furthermore, much of the future vision we have proposed here can be achieved only if educational institutions produce a cadre of talented individuals who not only understand computing and communications technologies but also have a deep understanding of the medical milieu and of the needs of practitioners and other health workers. Computer-science training alone is not adequate. Fortunately, we have begun to see the creation of formal training programs in medical informatics that provide custom-tailored educational opportunities. Many of the trainees are physicians, nurses, pharmacists, and other health professionals who see the career opportunities and challenges at the intersections of biomedicine, information science, computer science, and communications technologies. The demand for such individuals far outstrips the supply, however, both for academic and industrial career pathways (Greenes & Shortliffe, 1990). We need more training programs, expansion of those that already exist, plus support for junior faculty in health-science schools who may wish to seek additional training in this area.[6]

Organizational and Management Change Finally, as implied above, there needs to be a greater understanding among healthcare leaders regarding the role of process reengineering in successful software implementation. Health care provides some of the most complex organizational structures in society, and it is simplistic to assume that off-the-shelf products will be smoothly introduced into a new institution without major analysis, redesign, and cooperative joint-development efforts. Underinvestment and a failure to understand the requirements for process reengineering as part of software implementation, as well as problems with technical leadership and planning, account for many of the frustrating experiences that healthcare organizations report regarding their efforts to use computers more effectively in support of patient care and provider productivity.

---

[5]See http://www.ucaid.org/.

[6]A directory of some existing training programs is available on the Web at http://www.smi.stanford.edu/academics/informaticsprgms.html.

The vision of the future described here is meant to provide a glimpse of what lies ahead and to suggest the topics that need to be addressed in a book such as this one. You will find that essentially all of the chapters that follow touch on some aspect of the vision of integrated systems that extend beyond single institutions. Before embarking on these topics, however, let us emphasize two points. First, the vision presented in this section will become reality only if individual hospitals, academic medical centers, and national coordinating bodies provide the standards, infrastructure, and resources that are necessary. No individual system developer, vendor, or administrator can mandate the standards for connectivity and data sharing implied by an integrated environment such as the one illustrated in Figure 1.7. A national initiative of cooperative planning and implementation for computing and communications resources within single institutions and clinics is required before practitioners will have routine access to information. A uniform environment is required if transitions between resources are to be facile and uncomplicated.

Second, although our vision focused on the clinician's view of integrated information access, other workers in the field have similar needs that can be addressed in similar ways. The academic research community has already made use of much of the technology that needs to be coalesced if the clinical user is to have similar access to data and information.

With this discussion as background, let us now consider the discipline that has led to the development of many of the facilities that need to be brought together in the integrated medical-computing environment of the future. The remainder of this chapter deals with medical computing as a field and with medical information as a subject of study. It provides additional background needed to understand many of the subsequent chapters in this book.

1.2 The Use of Computers in Biomedicine

Biomedical applications of computers is a phrase that evokes different images depending on the nature of one's involvement in the field. To a hospital administrator, it might suggest the maintenance of medical records using computers; to a decision scientist, it might mean the assistance of computers in disease diagnosis; to a basic scientist, it might mean the use of computers for maintaining and retrieving gene-sequencing information. Many physicians immediately think of office-practice tools for tasks such as patient billing or appointment scheduling. The field includes study of all these activities and of a great many others too. More important, it includes the consideration of various external factors that affect the medical setting. Unless you keep in mind these surrounding factors, it may be difficult to understand how medical computing can help us to tie together the diverse aspects of health care and its delivery.

To achieve a unified perspective, we might consider three related topics: (1) the applications of computers in medicine, (2) the concept of medical information (why it is important in medical practice and why we might want to use computers to process it), and (3) the structural features of medicine, including all those subtopics to which computers might be applied. The first of these is the subject of this book. We mention the second and third topics briefly in this and the next chapter, and we provide references in the Suggested Readings section for those students who wish to learn more.

The modern computer is still a relatively young device. Because the computer as a machine is exciting, people may pay a disproportionate amount of attention to it as such—at the expense of considering what the computer can do given the numbers, concepts, ideas, and cognitive underpinnings of a field such as medicine. In recent years, computer scientists, philosophers, psychologists, and other scholars have *collectively* begun to consider such matters as the nature of information and knowledge and how humans process such concepts. These investigations have been given a sense of timeliness (if not urgency) by the simple existence of the computer. The cognitive activities of clinicians in practice probably have received more attention over the past two decades than in all previous history. Again, the existence of the computer and the possibilities of its extending a clinician's cognitive powers have motivated most of these studies: To develop computer-based tools to assist with decisions, we must understand more clearly such human processes as diagnosis, therapy planning, decision-making, and problem-solving in medicine.

1.2.1 Terminology

Since the 1960s, by which time almost anyone doing serious biomedical computation had access to some kind of computer system, people have been uncertain what name they should use for the medical application of computer-science concepts. The name *computer science* was itself new in 1960 and was only vaguely defined. Even today, *computer science* is used more as a matter of convention than as an explanation of the field's scientific content.

We use the phrase **medical computer science** to refer to the subdivision of computer science that applies the methods of the larger field to medical topics. As you will see, however, medicine has provided a rich area for computer-science research, and several basic computing insights and methodologies have been derived from applied medical-computing research.

The term **information science**, which is occasionally used in conjunction with *computer science*, originated in the field of library science and is used to refer, somewhat generally, to the broad range of issues related to the management of both paper-based and electronically-stored information. Much of what information science originally set out to be is now drawing renewed interest under the name **cognitive science**.

Information theory, in contrast, was first developed by scientists concerned about the physics of communication; it has evolved into what may be viewed as a new branch of mathematics. The results scientists have obtained with information theory have illuminated many processes in communications technology, but they have had little effect on our understanding of *human* information processing.

The term **biomedical computing** has been used for a number of years. It is nondescriptive and neutral, implying only that computers are employed for some purpose in biology or medicine. It often is associated with engineering applications of computers, however, in which computers are viewed more as tools for an engineering application than as the primary focus of research.

A term originally introduced in Europe is **medical informatics**, which is broader than **medical computing** (it includes such topics as medical statistics, record keeping, and the study of the nature of medical information itself) and deemphasizes the computer while focusing instead on the nature of the field to which computations are applied. Because the term *informatics* became widely accepted in the United States only during the 1990s, **medical information science** has often been used instead in this country; this term, however, may be confused with library science, and it does not capture the broader implications of the European term. As a result, the name *medical informatics* appears to have become the preferred term, even in the United States, although some people dislike the use of what they consider to be an awkward neologism. Others express concern that the adjective "medical" is too focused on physicians and fails to appreciate the relevance of this discipline to other health professionals, although most people in the field do not intend that the word "medical" be viewed as being specifically physician oriented or even illness oriented. Thus, the term *health informatics,* or *healthcare informatics,* has gained some popularity. We view it as an alternate term for *medical informatics,* but one which has the disadvantage of tending to exclude applications to biology (Chapter 18).

Despite these concerns, we believe that the broad range of issues in biomedical information management *does* require an appropriate name and we have used *medical informatics* for this purpose throughout this book. It is the most widely accepted term, has been adopted by the major professional societies in the field, and should be viewed as encompassing broadly all areas of application in health, clinical practice, and biomedical research. When we are speaking specifically about computers and their use within medical-informatics activities, we use the terms *medical computer science* (for the methodologic issues) or *medical computing* (to describe the activity itself). Note, however, that medical informatics has many other component sciences in addition to computer science. These include the decision sciences, cognitive science, information science, and even management sciences. We return to this point shortly when we discuss the basic versus applied nature of the field when it is viewed as a basic research discipline.

Although labels such as these are arbitrary, they are by no means insignificant. In the case of new fields of endeavor or branches of science, they are important both in designating the field and in defining or restricting its contents. The most distinctive feature of the modern computer is the generality of its application. The nearly unlimited range of computer uses complicates the business of naming the field. As a result, the nature of computer science is perhaps better illustrated by examples than by attempts at formal definition. Much of this book presents examples that do just this.

In summary, *we define medical informatics as the scientific field that deals with biomedical information, data, and knowledge—their storage, retrieval, and optimal use for problem-solving and decision-making*. It accordingly touches on all basic and applied fields in biomedical science and is closely tied to modern information technologies, notably in the areas of computing and communication (medical computer science). The emergence of medical informatics as a new discipline is due in large part to rapid advances in computing and communications technology, to an increasing awareness that the knowledge base of medicine is essentially unmanageable by traditional paper-based methods, and to a growing conviction that the *process* of informed decision-making is as important to modern biomedicine as is the collection of facts on which clinical decisions or research plans are made.

1.2.2 Historical Perspective

The modern digital computer grew out of developments in the United States and abroad during World War II, and general-purpose computers began to appear in the marketplace by the mid-1950s (Fig. 1.8). Speculation about what might be done with such machines (if they should ever become reliable) had, however,

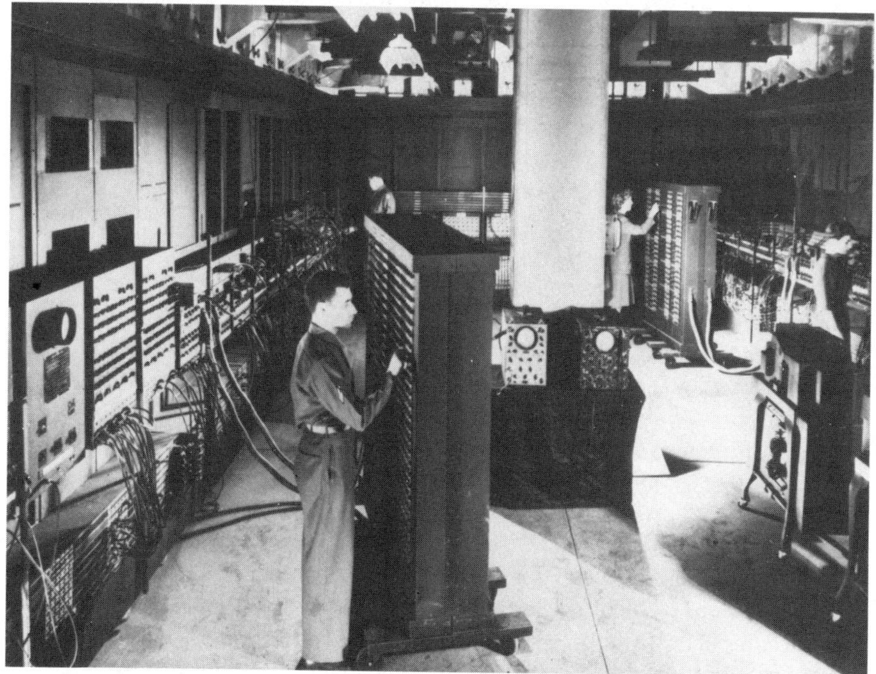

FIGURE 1.8. The ENIAC. Early computers, such as the ENIAC, were the precursors of today's personal computers and handheld calculators. (Photograph courtesy of Unisys Corporation.)

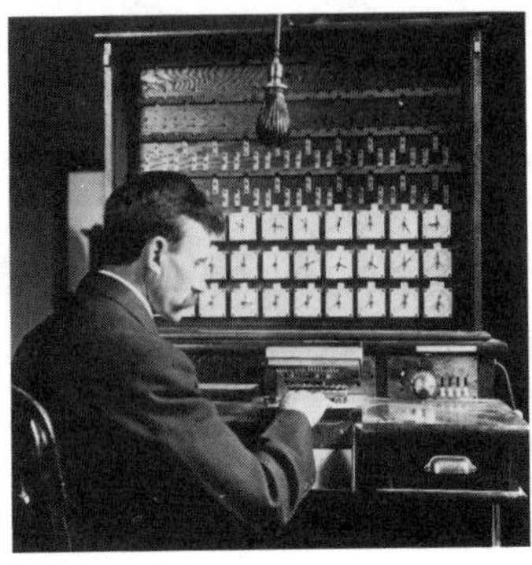

FIGURE 1.9. Tabulating machines. The Hollerith Tabulating Machine was an early data-processing system that performed automatic computation using punched cards. (Photograph courtesy of the Library of Congress.)

begun much earlier. Scholars at least as far back as the Middle Ages often had raised the question of whether human reasoning might be explained in terms of formal or algorithmic processes.[7] Gottfried Wilhelm von Leibnitz, a seventeenth-century German philosopher and mathematician, tried to develop a calculus that could be used to simulate human reasoning. The notion of a "logic engine" was subsequently worked out by Charles Babbage in the middle of the nineteenth century.

The first practical application of automatic computing relevant to medicine was Herman Hollerith's development of a punched-card data-processing system for the 1890 U.S. census (Fig. 1.9). His methods were soon adapted to **epidemiologic** and public health surveys, initiating the era of electromechanical punched-card data-processing technology, which matured and was widely adopted during the 1920s and 1930s. These techniques were the precursors of the stored-program and wholly electronic digital computers that began to appear in the late 1940s (Collen, 1995).

One early activity in medical computing was the attempt to construct systems that would assist a physician in decision-making (see Chapter 16). Not all medical-computing programs pursued this course, however. Many of the early ones instead investigated the notion of a total hospital information system (HIS; see Chapter 10). These projects were perhaps less ambitious in that they were more concerned with practical applications in the short term; the difficulties they encountered, however, were still formidable. The earliest work on HISs in the United States was probably that associated with the MEDINET project at General Electric, followed by work at Bolt, Beranek, Newman in Cambridge, Massachusetts, and then at the Massachusetts General Hospital (MGH) in Boston. A number of hospital application programs were developed at MGH by Barnett and his associates over three decades beginning in the early 1960s. Work on similar systems was undertaken by Warner at Latter Day Saints (LDS) Hospital in Salt Lake City, by Collen at Kaiser Permanente in Oakland, California, by Wieder-

[7]An algorithm is a well-defined procedure or sequence of steps for solving a problem.

hold at Stanford University in Stanford, California, and by scientists at Lockheed in Sunnyvale, California.[8]

The course of HIS applications bifurcated in the 1970s. One approach was based on the concept of an integrated or monolithic design in which a single, large, *time-shared computer* would be used to support an entire collection of applications. An alternative was a distributed design that favored the separate implementation of specific applications on smaller individual computers—minicomputers—thereby permitting the independent evolution of systems in the respective application areas. A common assumption was the existence of a single shared database of patient information. The multimachine model was not practical, however, until network technologies permitted rapid and reliable communication among distributed and (sometimes) heterogeneous types of machines. Such distributed HISs began to appear in the 1980s (Simborg et al., 1983).

Medical-computing activity broadened in scope and accelerated with the appearance of the *minicompute*r in the early 1970s. These machines made it possible for individual departments or small organizational units to acquire their own dedicated computers and to develop their own application systems (Fig. 1.10). In tandem with the introduction of general-purpose software tools that provided standardized facilities to individuals with limited computer training (such as the UNIX operating system and programming environment), the minicomputer put more computing power in the hands of more medical investigators than did any other single development until the introduction of the *microprocessor,* a central processing unit (CPU) contained on one or a few chips (Fig. 1.11).

Everything changed radically beginning in the late 1970s and early 1980s, when the microprocessor and the *personal computer* (PC) or *microcomputer* became available. Not only could hospital departments afford minicomputers, but now individuals could afford microcomputers. This change enormously broadened the base of computing in our society and gave rise to a new software industry. The first articles on computers in medicine had appeared in clinical journals in the late 1950s, but it was not until the late 1970s that the first advertisements dealing with computers and aimed at physicians began to appear (Fig. 1.12). Within a few years, a wide range of computer-based information-management tools was available as commercial products; their descriptions began to appear in journals alongside the traditional advertisements for drugs and other medical products. At present, individual physicians find it practical to employ personal computers in a variety of settings, including for *limited* applications in patient care or clinical investigation. There remains, however, a serious shortage of application software for most of the professional activities in which physicians are engaged.

The stage is now set with a wide range of hardware of various sizes, types, prices, and capabilities, all of which will continue to evolve in the new century.

---

[8]The latter system was subsequently taken over and further developed by the Technicon Corporation (subsequently TDS Healthcare Systems Corporation). The system is now part of the suite of products available from Eclipsys, Inc.

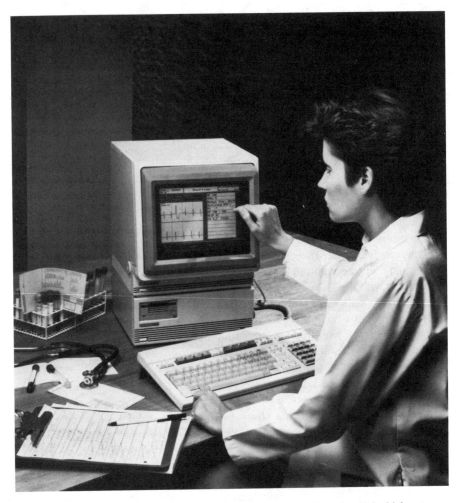

FIGURE 1.10. Departmental system. Hospital departments, such as the clinical laboratory, were able to implement their own custom-tailored systems when affordable minicomputers became available. Today, these departments often use microcomputers to support administrative and clinical functions. (Photograph courtesy Hewlett-Packard Company.)

The recent trend—reductions in size and cost of computers with simultaneous increases in power (Fig. 1.13)—shows no sign of slowing, although scientists are beginning to foresee the ultimate physical limitations to the miniaturization of computer circuits.

Progress in medical-computing research will continue to be tied to the availability of funding from either government or commercial sources. Because most medical-computing research is exploratory and is far from ready for commercial application, the federal government has played a key role in funding the work of the last three decades, mainly through the National Institutes of Health (NIH)

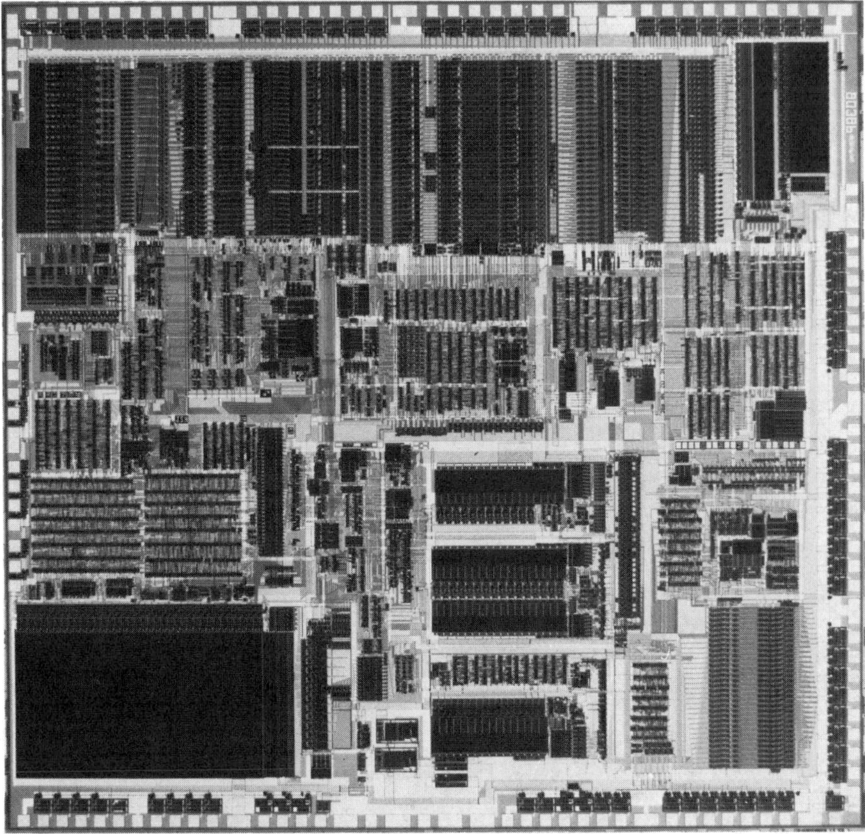

FIGURE 1.11. Miniature computer. The microprocessor, or "computer on a chip," revolutionized the computer industry in the 1970s. By installing chips in small boxes and connecting them to a computer terminal, engineers produced the personal computer (PC)—an innovation that made it possible for individual users to purchase their own systems.

and the Agency for Healthcare Research and Quality (AHRQ). The National Library of Medicine (NLM) has assumed a primary role for medical informatics, especially with support for basic research in the field (Fig. 1.14). As increasing numbers of applications prove to be cost effective (see Chapters 5 and 19), it is likely that more development work will shift to industrial settings and that university programs will focus increasingly on fundamental research problems viewed as too speculative for short-term commercialization.

1.2.3 Relationship to Biomedical Science and Medical Practice

The exciting accomplishments of medical informatics, and the implied potential for future benefits to medicine, must be viewed in the context of our society and

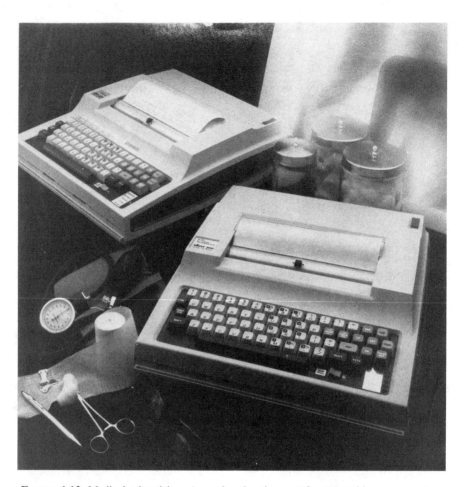

FIGURE 1.12. Medical advertising. An early advertisement for a portable computer terminal, which appeared in general medical journals in the late 1970s. The development of compact, inexpensive peripheral devices and personal computers inspired future experiments in marketing directly to clinicians. (Reprinted by permission of copyright holder Texas Instruments Incorporated © 1985.)

of the existing healthcare system. As early as 1970, one eminent clinician suggested that computers might in time have a revolutionary influence on medical care, on medical education, and even on the selection criteria for health-science trainees (Schwartz, 1970). The subsequent enormous growth in computing activity has been met with some trepidation by health professionals. They ask where it will all end. Will health workers gradually be replaced by computers? Will nurses and physicians need to be highly trained in computer science before they can practice their professions effectively? Will both patients and health workers eventually revolt rather than accept a trend toward automation that they believe may threaten the traditional humanistic values in healthcare delivery (see Chap-

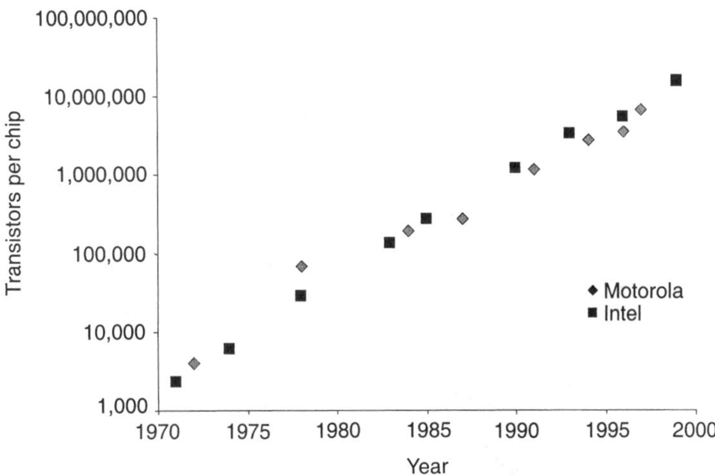

FIGURE 1.13. Moore's Law. Former Intel chairman Gordon Moore is credited with popularizing the "law" that the size and cost of microprocessor chips will half every 18 months while they double in computing power. This graph shows the exponential growth in the number of transistors that can be integrated on a single microprocessor by two of the major chip manufacturers. (*Source:* San Jose Mercury News, December 1997.)

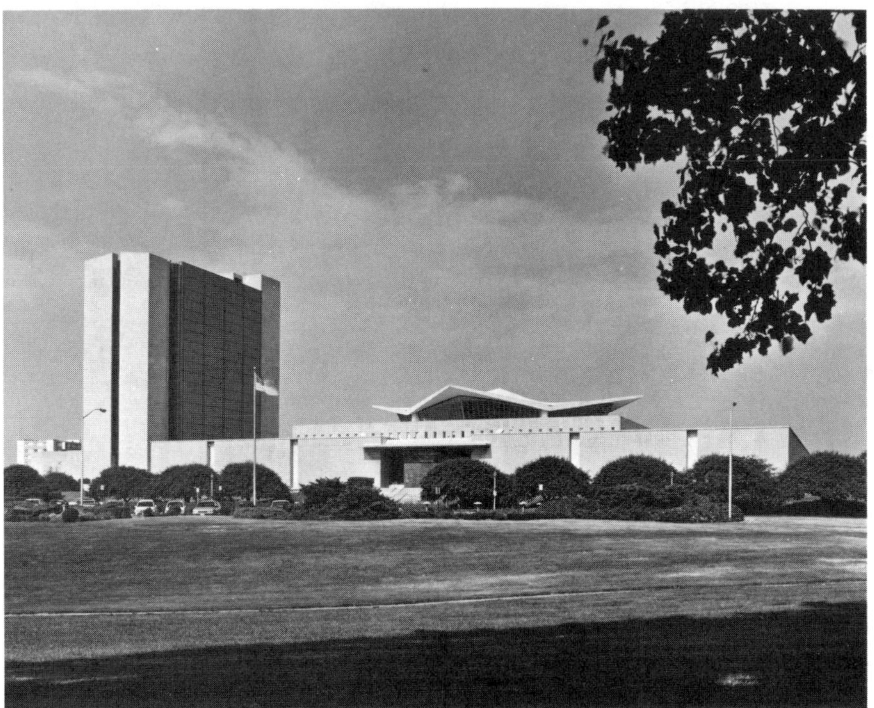

FIGURE 1.14. The National Library of Medicine (NLM). The NLM, on the campus of the National Institutes of Health in Bethesda, Maryland, is the principal biomedical library for the nation (see Chapter 15). It is also a major source of support for research in medical informatics. (Photograph courtesy of the National Library of Medicine.)

ter 7) (Shortliffe, 1993)? Will clinicians be viewed as outmoded and backward if they do not turn to computational tools for assistance with information management and decision-making (Fig. 1.15)?

Medical informatics is intrinsically entwined with the substance of biomedical science. It determines and analyzes the structure of medical information and

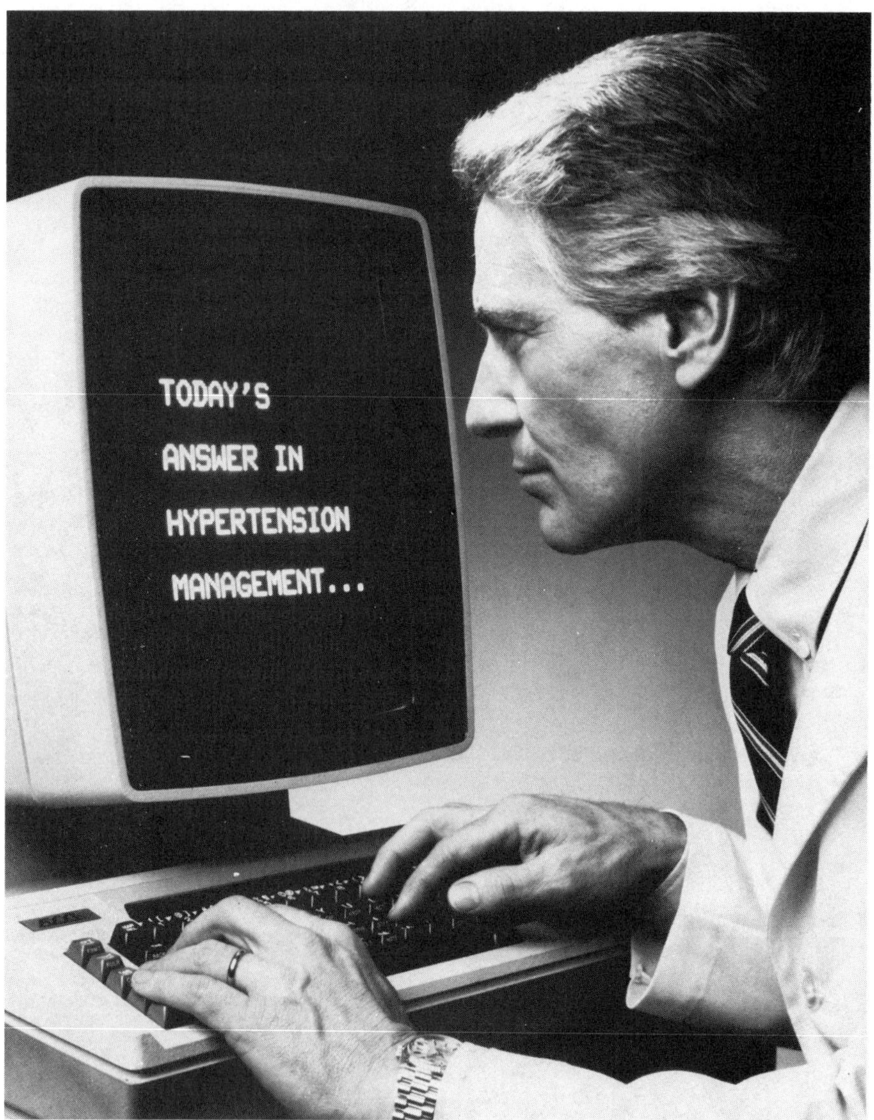

FIGURE 1.15. Doctor of the future. By the early 1980s, advertisements in medical journals began to use computer equipment as props. The suggestion in this photograph seems to be that an up-to-date physician feels comfortable using computer-based tools in his practice. (Photograph courtesy of ICI Pharma, Division of ICI Americas, Inc.)

knowledge, whereas medical science is constrained by that structure. Medical informatics melds the study of medical computer science with analyses of medical information and knowledge, thereby addressing specifically the interface between computer science and biomedical science. To illustrate what we mean by the "structural" features of medical information and knowledge, we can contrast the properties of the information and knowledge typical of such fields as physics or engineering with the properties of those typical of medicine (see Section 1.3).

Medical informatics is perhaps best viewed as a basic medical science, with a wide variety of potential areas of application (Fig. 1.16). The analogy with other **basic sciences** is that medical informatics uses the results of past experience to understand, structure, and encode objective and subjective medical findings and thus to make them suitable for processing. This approach supports the integration of the findings and their analyses. In turn, the selective distribution of newly created knowledge can aid patient care, health planning, and basic biomedical research.

Medical computing is, by its nature, an experimental science. An **experimental science** is characterized by posing questions, designing experiments, performing analyses, and using the information gained to design new experiments. One goal is simply to search for new knowledge, called **basic research**. A second goal is to use this knowledge for practical ends, called **applications research**. There is a continuity between these two endeavors (see Fig. 1.16). In medical informatics, there is an especially tight coupling between the application areas, some of which are indicated at the bottom of Figure 1.16, and the identification

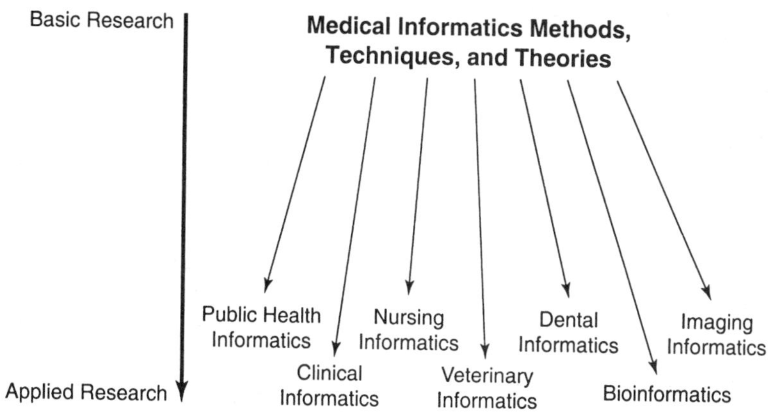

FIGURE 1.16. Medical informatics as basic science. We view the term *medical informatics* as referring to the basic-science discipline in which the development and evaluation of new methods and theories are a primary focus of activity. These core concepts and methods in turn have broad applicability in the health and biomedical sciences. The informatics subfields indicated by the names across the bottom of this figure are accordingly best viewed as *application* domains for a common set of concepts and techniques from the field of medical informatics (see text).

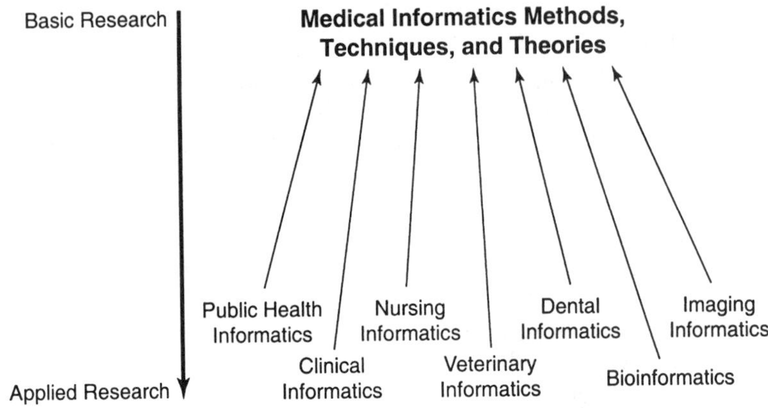

FIGURE 1.17. Applications-driven science. Work in medical informatics is motivated totally by the application domains that the field is intended to serve. Thus the basic-research activities in the field generally result from the identification of a problem in the real world of health or biomedicine for which an informatics solution is sought (see text).

of basic research tasks that characterize the scientific underpinnings of the field. In general, medical informatics researchers derive their inspiration from one of the application areas, identifying fundamental methodologic issues that need to be addressed and testing them in system prototypes or, for more mature methods, in actual systems that are used in clinical or biomedical research settings (Fig. 1.17). One important implication of this viewpoint is that the core discipline is identical, regardless of the area of application that a given individual is motivated to address. This argues for unified medical informatics educational programs, ones that bring together students with a wide variety of applications interests. Elective courses and internships in areas of specific interest are of course important complements to the basic core exposures that students should receive, but, given the need for teamwork and understanding in the field, it would be counterproductive and wasteful to separate trainees based on the application areas that may interest them.[9]

The scientific contributions of medical informatics also can be appreciated through its potential for benefiting the education of health professionals. For example, in the education of medical students, the various cognitive activities of physicians traditionally have tended to be considered separately and in isolation—they have been largely treated as though they are independent and dis-

---

[9]The medical informatics training program at Stanford University School of Medicine, for example, was designed with this perspective in mind. Students with interests in clinical, imaging, nursing, epidemiologic, and biologic applications are trained together and are required to learn something about each of the other application areas. Details of the curriculum can be found at http://www.smi.stanford.edu/academics (see also Shortliffe, 1995b).

tinct modules of performance. One activity attracting increasing interest is that of formal medical decision-making (see Chapter 3). The specific content of this area remains to be defined completely, but the discipline's dependence on formal methods and its use of knowledge and information reveal that it is one aspect of medical informatics.

A particular topic in the study of medical decision-making is **diagnosis**, which is often conceived and taught as though it were a free-standing and independent activity. Medical students may thus be led to view diagnosis as a process that physicians carry out in isolation before choosing therapy for a patient or proceeding to other modular tasks. A number of studies have shown that this model is oversimplified and that such a decomposition of cognitive tasks may be quite misleading (Elstein et al., 1978; Patel & Groen, 1986). Physicians seem to deal with several tasks at the same time. Although a diagnosis may be one of the first things physicians think about when they see a new patient, patient assessment (diagnosis, management, analysis of treatment results, monitoring of disease progression, and so on) is a process that never really terminates. A physician must be flexible and open minded. It is generally appropriate to alter the original diagnosis if it turns out that treatment based on it is unsuccessful or if new information weakens the evidence supporting the diagnosis or suggests a second and concurrent disorder.

When we speak of making a diagnosis, choosing a treatment, managing therapy, making decisions, monitoring a patient, or preventing disease, we are using labels for different aspects of *medical care*, an entity that has overall unity. The fabric of medical care is a continuum in which these elements are tightly interwoven. Regardless of whether we view computer and information science as a profession, as a technology, or as a science, there is no doubt about its importance to medicine. We can assume computers will be used increasingly in medical practice, in medical research, and in medical education.

1.2.4 Relationship to Computer Science

During its evolution as an academic entity in universities, computer science followed an unsettled course as involved faculty attempted to identify key topics in the field and to find the discipline's organizational place. Many computer-science programs were located in departments of electrical engineering, because major concerns of their researchers were computer architecture and design and the development of practical hardware components. At the same time, computer scientists were interested in programming languages and software, undertakings not particularly characteristic of engineering. Furthermore, their work with algorithm design, computability theory,[10] and other theoretical topics seemed more related to mathematics.

---

[10]Many interesting problems cannot be computed in a finite time and require heuristics. Computability theory is the foundation for assessing the feasibility and cost of computation to provide the complete and correct results to a formally stated problem.

Medical informatics draws from all of these activities—development of hardware, software, and computer-science theory. Medical computing generally has not had a large enough market to influence the course of major hardware developments; that is, computers have not been developed specifically for medical applications. Not since the early 1960s (when health-computing experts occasionally talked about and, in a few instances, developed special *medical* terminals) have people assumed that medical-computing applications would use hardware other than that designed for general use.

The question of whether medical applications would require specialized programming languages might have been answered affirmatively in the 1970s by anyone examining the MUMPS language (Massachusetts General Hospital Utility Multi-Programming System) (Greenes et al., 1970), which was specially developed for use in medical applications. For several years, MUMPS was the most widely used language for medical-record processing. Under its new name, M, it is still in widespread use. New implementations have been developed for each generation of minicomputers and microcomputers. M, however, like any programming language, is not equally useful for all computing tasks. In addition, the software requirements of medicine are better understood and no longer appear to be unique; rather, they are specific to the *kind* of task. A program for scientific computation looks pretty much the same whether it is designed for chemical engineering or for pharmacokinetic calculations.[11]

How, then, does medical informatics differ from medical computer science? Is the new discipline simply the study of computer science with a "medical flavor?" If you return to the definition of medical informatics that we provided in Section 1.2.1, and then refer to Figures 1.16 and 1.17, we believe you will begin to see why medical informatics is more than simply the biomedical application of computer science. The issues that it addresses not only have broad relevance to health, medicine, and biology, but the underlying sciences on which medical informatics professionals draw are inherently interdisciplinary as well. Thus, for example, successful medical informatics research will often draw on and contribute to computer science, but it may also be closely related to the decision sciences (probability theory, decision analysis, or the psychology of human problem-solving), to cognitive science, to information sciences, or to the management sciences (Fig. 1.18). Furthermore, a medical informatics researcher will be tightly linked to some underlying problem from the real world of health or biomedicine. As Figure 1.18 illustrates, for example, a medical informatics researcher working in the domain of clinical medicine will generally be seeking to contribute a solution to a recognized problem or need in the clinical world, thereby drawing inspiration from this applications perspective and feeding it back into the definition of the fundamental basic research problems that need to be addressed. A doctoral student in medical informatics will accordingly be moti-

---

[11]Pharmacokinetics is the study of the routes and mechanisms of drug disposition over time, from initial introduction into the body through distribution in body tissues, biotransformation, and ultimate elimination.

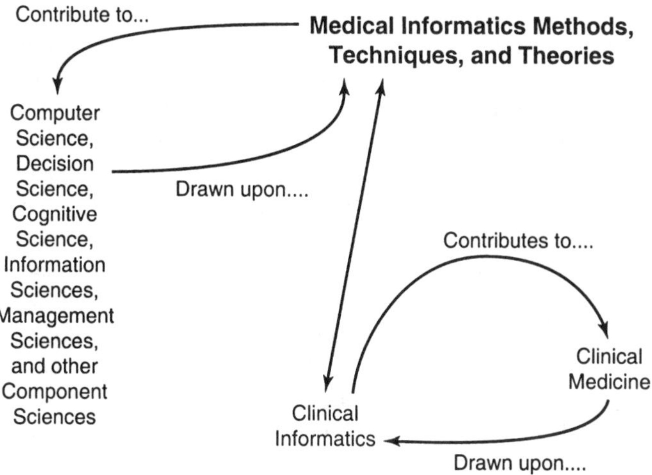

FIGURE 1.18. Component sciences in medical informatics. To use clinical informatics as an example, this application area is motivated by the needs of clinical medicine, to which it attempts to contribute solutions to problems. Thus clinical informatics draws upon clinical medicine for its inspiration, and in turn often leads to the delineation of basic research challenges in medical informatics that must be tackled if clinical medicine is ultimately to benefit. At the methodologic level, medical informatics draws on, and contributes to, a wide variety of component disciplines, of which computer science is only one. As Figures 1.16, 1.17, and 1.18 show explicitly, medical informatics is inherently multidisciplinary, both in its areas of application and in the component sciences on which it draws.

vated by one of the application areas, such as those shown at the bottom of Figures 1.16 and 1.17, but the dissertation worthy of a PhD in the field will usually be identified by a generalizable scientific result that also contributes to one of the component disciplines (Fig. 1.18) and on which other scientists can build in the future.

1.2.5 Relationship to Biomedical Engineering

If medical informatics is an emerging discipline, then by contrast biomedical engineering is a well-established one. Many engineering and medical schools have formal academic programs in the latter subject, often with departmental status and full-time faculty. How does medical informatics relate to biomedical engineering, especially in an era when engineering and computer science are increasingly intertwined?

Biomedical engineering departments emerged 30 to 40 years ago, when technology began to play an increasingly prominent role in medical practice. The emphasis in such departments has tended to be research on and development of instrumentation (e.g., as is discussed in Chapters 13 and 14, advanced monitoring systems, specialized transducers for clinical or laboratory use, and image-enhancement techniques for use in radiology), with an orientation toward the development of medical devices, prostheses,[12] and specialized research tools (Fig. 1.19). In recent years, computing techniques have been used both in the design and building of medical devices and in the medical devices themselves. For example, the "smart" devices increasingly found in most specialties are all dependent on microprocessor technology. Intensive-care monitors that generate blood-pressure records while calculating mean values and hourly summaries are examples of such "intelligent" devices.

The overlap between biomedical engineering and medical informatics suggests that it would be unwise for us to draw compulsively strict boundaries between the two fields. There are ample opportunities for interaction, and there are chapters in this book that clearly overlap with biomedical-engineering topics—for example, Chapter 13 on patient-monitoring systems and Chapter 14 on imaging systems. Even where they meet, however, the fields have differences in emphasis that can help you to understand their different evolutionary histories. In biomedical engineering, the emphasis is on medical *devices*; in medical informatics, the emphasis is on medical *information* and *knowledge* and their management using computers. In both fields, the computer is secondary, although both use

[12]Devices that replace body parts—for example, artificial hips or hearts.

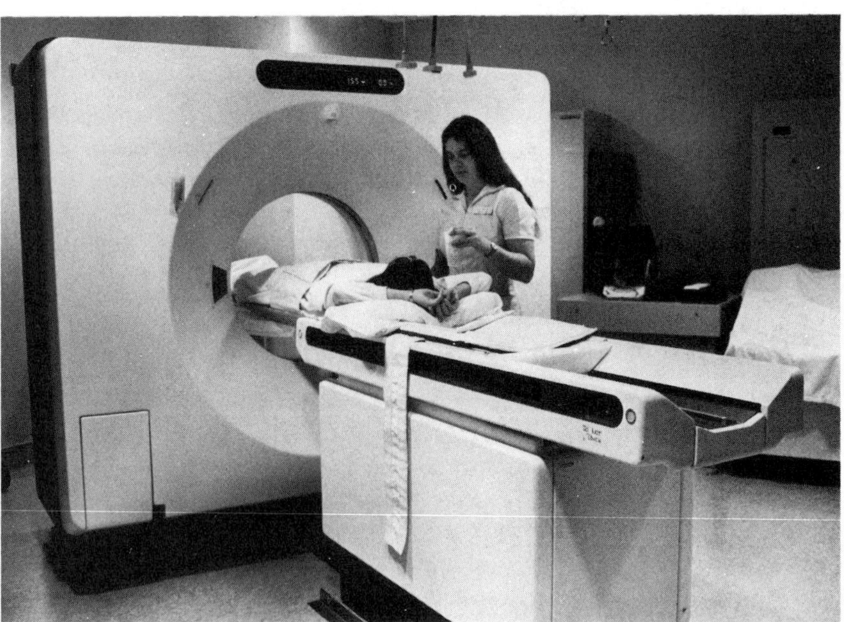

FIGURE 1.19. Advanced imaging device. Computed-tomography scanners and other imaging devices used in radiology are of interest to both medical computer scientists and biomedical engineers. (Photograph by Janice Anne Rohn.)

computing technology. The emphasis in this book is on the informatics end of the spectrum of medical computer science, so we shall not spend much time examining biomedical engineering topics.

1.3 The Nature of Medical Information

From the previous discussion, you might conclude that medical applications do not raise any unique problems or concerns. On the contrary, the medical environment raises several issues that, in interesting ways, are quite distinct from those encountered in most other domains of computer application. Clinical information seems to be systematically different from the information used in physics, engineering, or even clinical chemistry (which more closely resembles chemical applications generally than it does medical ones). Aspects of medical information include an essence of uncertainty—we can never know all about a physiological process, and this results in inevitable variability among individuals. These differences raise special problems. It is partly for this reason that some investigators suggest that medical computer science differs from conventional computer science in fundamental ways. We shall explore these differences only briefly here; for details, you can consult Blois' book on this subject (see Suggested Readings).

Let us examine an instance of what we will call a *low-level* (or readily formalized) science. Physics is a natural starting point; in any discussion of the hierarchical relationships among the sciences (from the fourth- century B.C. Greek philosopher Aristotle to the twentieth-century U.S. librarian Melvil Dewey), physics will be placed near the bottom of the hierarchy. Physics characteristically has a certain kind of simplicity, or generality. The concepts and descriptions of the objects and processes of physics, however, are necessarily used in all applied fields, including medicine. The laws of physics and the descriptions of certain kinds of physical processes are essential in representing or explaining functions that we regard as medical in nature. We need to know something about molecular physics, for example, to understand why water is such a good solvent; to explain how nutrient molecules are metabolized, we talk about the role of electron-transfer reactions.

Applying a computer (or any formal computation) to a physical problem in a medical context is no different from doing so in a physics laboratory or for an engineering application. The use of computers in various **low-level processes** (such as those of physics or chemistry) is similar and is independent of the application. If we are talking about the solvent properties of water, it makes no difference whether we happen to be working in geology, engineering, or medicine. Such low-level processes of physics are particularly receptive to mathematical treatment, so using computers for these applications requires only conventional numerical programming.

In medicine, however, there are other **higher level processes** carried out in more complex objects such as organisms (one type of which is patients). Many of the important informational processes are of this kind. When we discuss, describe, or record the properties or behavior of humans, we are using the descriptions of very high-level objects, the behavior of whom has no counterpart in physics or in engineering. The person using computers to analyze the descriptions of these high-level objects and processes encounters serious difficulties (Blois, 1984).

You might object to this line of argument by remarking that, after all, computers are used routinely in commercial applications in which human beings and situations concerning them are involved and that relevant computations are carried out successfully. The explanation is that, in these commercial applications, the descriptions of human beings and their activities have been so highly abstracted that the events or processes have been reduced to low-level objects. In medicine, abstractions carried to this degree would be clinically worthless.

For example, one instance of a human being in the banking business is the customer, who may deposit, borrow, withdraw, or invest money. To describe commercial activities such as these, we need only a few properties; the customer can remain an abstract entity. In clinical medicine, however, we could not begin to deal with a patient represented with such skimpy abstractions. We must be prepared to analyze most of the complex behaviors that humans display and to describe patients as completely as possible. We must deal with the rich descriptions occurring at high levels in the hierarchy, and we may be hard pressed to encode and process this information using the tools of mathematics and computer science, which work so well at low levels. In light of these remarks, the general enterprise known as **artificial intelligence** (AI) can be aptly described as the application of computer science to high-level, real-world problems.

Medical informatics thus includes computer applications that range from processing of very low-level descriptions, which are little different from their counterparts in physics, chemistry, or engineering, to processing of extremely high-level ones, which are completely and systematically different. When we study human beings in their entirety (including such aspects as human cognition, self-consciousness, intentionality, and behavior), we must use these high-level descriptions. We will find that they raise complex issues to which conventional logic and mathematics are less readily applicable. In general, the attributes of low-level objects appear sharp, crisp, and unambiguous (e.g., "length," "mass"), whereas those of high-level ones tend to be soft, or fuzzy, and inexact (e.g., example, "unpleasant scent," "good").

Just as we need to develop different methods to describe high-level objects, the inference methods we use with such objects may differ from those we use with low-level ones. In formal logic, we begin with the assumption that a given proposition must be either true or false. This feature is essential because logic is concerned with the preservation of truth value under various formal transformations. It is difficult or impossible, however, to assume that all propositions have truth values when we deal with the many high-level descriptions in medicine or, indeed, in everyday situations. Such questions as "Was Woodrow Wilson a good president?" cannot be answered "yes" or "no" (unless we limit the question to specific criteria for determining the goodness of presidents). Many common questions in medicine have the same property.

1.4 Integrating Medical Computing and Medical Practice

It should be clear from the previous discussion that medical informatics is a remarkably broad and complex topic. We have argued that information management is intrinsic to medical practice and that interest in using computers to aid in information management has grown over the last three decades. In this chapter and throughout the book, we emphasize the myriad ways in which computers are used in medicine to ease the burdens of information processing and the means by which new technology promises to change the delivery of health care. The rate at and degree to which such changes are realized will be determined in part by external forces that influence the costs of developing and implementing medical applications and the ability of the healthcare system to accrue the potential benefits.

We can summarize several global forces that are affecting medical computing and that will determine the extent to which computers are assimilated into medical practice: (1) new developments in computer hardware and software, (2) a gradual increase in the number of professionals who have been trained in both clinical medicine and medical informatics, and (3) ongoing changes in healthcare financing designed to control the rate of growth of medical expenditures. We touched on the first of these factors in Section 1.2.2, when we described the historical development of medical computing and the trend from mainframe computers to microcomputers and personal computers. The future view outlined in Section 1.1 similarly builds on the influence that the Internet has provided throughout society during the past decade. The new hardware technologies have made powerful computers inexpensive and thus available to hospitals, to departments within hospitals, and even to individual physicians. The broad selection of computers of all sizes, prices, and capabilities makes computer applications both attractive and accessible. Technological advances in information-storage devices—for example, optical disks—are facilitating the inexpensive storage of large amounts of data, thus improving the feasibility of data-intensive applications, such as the all-digital radiology department discussed in Chapter 14. Standardization of hardware and advances in network technology are making it easier to share data and to integrate related information-management functions within a hospital or other healthcare organization.

Computers are increasingly prevalent in all aspects of our lives, whether as an automatic bank-teller machine, as the microprocessor in a microwave oven, or as a word processor. Physicians trained in recent years may have used computer programs to learn diagnostic techniques or to manage the therapy of simulated patients. They may have learned to use a computer to search the medical literature, either directly or with the assistance of a specially trained librarian. Simple exposure to computers does not, however, guarantee an eagerness to embrace the machine. Medical personnel will be unwilling to use computer-based systems that are poorly designed, confusing, unduly time consuming, or lacking in clear benefit.

The second factor is the increase in the number of professionals who are being trained to understand the medical issues as well as the technical and engineering ones. Computer scientists who understand medicine are better able to design systems responsive to actual needs. Medical personnel who receive formal training in medical informatics are likely to build systems using well-established techniques while avoiding the past mistakes of other developers. As more professionals are trained in the special aspects of both fields, and as the programs they develop are introduced, healthcare professionals are more likely to have available useful and usable systems when they turn to the computer for help with information-management tasks.

The third factor affecting the integration of computing technologies into healthcare settings is managed care and the increasing pressure to control medical spending (Chapter 19). The escalating tendency to apply technology to all patient-care tasks is a frequently cited phenomenon in modern medical practice. Mere physical findings no longer are considered adequate for making diagnoses and planning treatments. In fact, medical students who are taught by more experienced physicians to find subtle diagnostic signs by examining various parts of the body nonetheless often choose to bypass or deemphasize physical examinations in favor of ordering one test after another. Sometimes, they do so without paying sufficient attention to the ensuing cost. Some new technologies replace less expensive, but technologically inferior, tests. In such cases, the use of the more expensive approach is generally justified. Occasionally, computer-related technologies have allowed us to perform tasks that previously were not possible. For example, the scans produced with computed tomography (see Chapter 14) have allowed physicians to visualize cross-sectional slices of the body for the first time, and medical instruments in intensive-care units perform continuous monitoring of patients' body functions that previously could be checked only episodically (see Chapter 13).

Yet the development of expensive new technologies, and the belief that more technology is better, helped to fuel the rapidly escalating healthcare costs of the 1970s and 1980s, leading to the introduction of managed care and capitation in recent years. Chapter 19 discusses the mechanisms that opened the door to rapid growth in health expenses and the changes in financing and delivery that were designed to curb spending in the new era of cost consciousness. Integrated computer systems potentially provide the means to capture data for detailed cost accounting, to analyze the relationship of costs of care to the benefits of that care, to evaluate the quality of care provided, and to identify areas of inefficiency. Systems that improve the quality of care while reducing the cost of providing that care clearly will be favored. The effect of cost-containment pressures on technologies that increase the cost of care while improving the quality are less clear. Medical technologies, including computers, will need to improve the delivery of medical care while either reducing costs or providing benefits that clearly exceed their costs.

Improvements in hardware and software make computers more suitable for medical applications. Designers of medical systems must, however, address satisfactorily many logistical and engineering questions before computers can be fully integrated into medical practice. For example, are computer terminals conveniently located? Could handheld devices effectively replace the tethered terminals and workstations of the past? Can users complete their tasks without excessive delays? Is the system reliable enough to avoid loss of data? Can users interact easily and intuitively with the computer? Are patient data secure and appropriately protected from prying eyes? In addition, cost-control pressures produce a growing reluctance to embrace expensive technologies that add to the high cost of health care. The net effect of these opposing trends will in large part determine the degree to which computers are integrated into the healthcare environment.

In summary, rapid advances in computer hardware and software, coupled with an increasing computer literacy of healthcare professionals, favor the implementation of effective computer applications in medical practice. Furthermore, in the increasingly competitive healthcare industry, providers have a greater need for the information-management capabilities supplied by computer systems. The challenge is to demonstrate the financial and clinical advantages of these systems.

Suggested Readings

Altman R.B. (1997). Informatics in the care of patients: Ten notable challenges. *Western Journal of Medicine,* 166(6):118–122.

This thoughtful article was written to introduce the concepts of medical informatics to clinicians while explaining a major set of challenges that help to define the goals and research programs for the field.

Blois M.S. (1984). *Information and Medicine: The Nature of Medical Descriptions.* Berkeley: University of California Press.

The author analyzes the structure of medical knowledge in terms of a hierarchical model of information. He explores the ideas of high- and low-level sciences and suggests that the nature of medical descriptions accounts for difficulties in applying computing technology to medicine.

Collen M.F. (1995). *A History of Medical Informatics in the United States: 1950 to 1990.* Bethesda, MD: American Medical Informatics Association, Hartman Publishing.

This comprehensive book traces the history of the field of medical informatics and identifies the origins of the discipline's name (which first appeared in the English-language literature in 1974).

Degoulet P., Phister B., Fieschi, M. (1997). *Introduction to Clinical Informatics.* New York: Springer-Verlag.

This introductory volume provides a broad view of medical informatics and carries the concepts forward with an emphasis on clinical applications.

Elstein A.S., Shulman L.S., Sprafka S.A. (1978). *Medical Problem Solving: An Analysis of Clinical Reasoning.* Cambridge, MA: Harvard University Press.

This classic collection of papers describes detailed studies that have illuminated several aspects of the ways in which expert and novice physicians solve medical problems.

Shortliffe E. (1993). Doctors, patients, and computers: Will information technology dehumanize health care delivery? *Proceedings of the American Philosophical Society*, 137(3):390–398.

In this paper, the author examines the frequently expressed concern that the introduction of computing technology into healthcare settings will disrupt the development of rapport between clinicians and patients and thereby dehumanize the therapeutic process. He argues, rather, that computers may have precisely the opposite effect on the relationship between clinicians and their patients.

van Bemmel J.H., Musen, M.A. (1997). *Handbook of Medical Informatics*. Heidelberg: Springer-Verlag.

This volume provides a comprehensive overview of the field of medical informatics and is an excellent starting reference point for many of the topics in the field.

Questions for Discussion

1. How do you interpret the phrase "logical behavior"? Do computers behave logically? Do people behave logically? Explain your answers.
2. What do you think it means to say that a computer program is "effective"? Make a list of a dozen computer applications with which you are familiar. List the applications in decreasing order of effectiveness, as you have explained this concept. Then, for each application, indicate your estimate of how well human beings perform the same tasks (this will require that you determine what it means for a *human being* to be effective). Do you discern any pattern? If so, how do you interpret it?
3. Discuss three society-wide factors that will determine the extent to which computers are assimilated into medical practice.
4. Reread the future vision presented in Section 1.1. Describe the characteristics of an integrated environment for managing medical information. Discuss two ways in which such a system could change medical practice.
5. Do you believe that improving the technical quality of health care entails the risk of dehumanization? If so, is it worth the risk? Explain your reasoning.

2
Medical Data: Their Acquisition, Storage, and Use

EDWARD H. SHORTLIFFE AND G. OCTO BARNETT

After reading this chapter, you should know the answers to these questions:

- What are medical data?
- How are medical data used?
- What are the drawbacks of the traditional paper medical record?
- What is the potential role of the computer in data storage, retrieval, and interpretation?
- What distinguishes a database from a knowledge base?
- How are data collection and hypothesis generation intimately linked in medical diagnosis?
- What are the meanings of the terms *prevalence*, *predictive value*, *sensitivity*, and *specificity*? How are the terms related?
- What are the alternatives for entry of data into a medical database?

2.1 What Are Medical Data?

From earliest times, the ideas of ill health and its treatment have been wedded to those of the observation and interpretation of data. Whether we consider the disease descriptions and guidelines for management in early Greek literature or the modern physician's use of complex laboratory and X-ray studies, it is clear that gathering data and interpreting their meaning are central to the healthcare process. A textbook on computers in medicine will accordingly refer time and again to issues in data collection, storage, and use. This chapter lays the foundation for this recurring set of issues that is pertinent to all aspects of the use of computers in medicine.

If data are central to all medical care, it is because they are crucial to the process of *decision-making* (as described in detail in Chapter 3). In fact, simple reflection will reveal that *all* medical-care activities involve gathering, analyzing, or using data. Data provide the basis for categorizing the problems a patient may be having or for identifying subgroups within a population of patients. They also help a physician to decide what additional information is needed and what actions should be taken to gain a greater understanding of a patient's problem or to treat most effectively the problem that has been diagnosed.

It is overly simplistic to view data as the columns of numbers or the monitored waveforms that are a product of our increasingly technological health-care environment. Although laboratory-test results and other numeric data are often invaluable, a variety of more subtle types of data may be just as important to the delivery of optimal care: the sidewards awkward glance by a patient who seems to be avoiding a question during the medical interview, information about a patient's family or economic setting, the subjective sense of disease severity that an experienced physician will often have within a few seconds of entering a patient's room. No physician disputes the importance of such observations in decision-making during patient assessment and management, yet the precise role of these data and the corresponding decision criteria are so poorly understood that it is difficult to record them in ways that convey their full meaning, even from one physician to another. Even with these limitations, we need to share computer-based information when we cannot interact directly with one another.

We consider a **medical datum** to be any single observation of a patient—for example, a temperature reading, a red-blood-cell count, a past history of rubella, or a blood-pressure reading. As the last example shows, it is a matter of perspective whether a single observation is in fact more than one datum. A blood pressure of 120/80 might well be recorded as a single datum point in a setting where knowledge that a patient's blood pressure is normal is all that matters. If the difference between diastolic (while the heart cavities are beginning to fill) and systolic (while they are contracting) blood pressures is important for decision-making or for analysis, however, the blood-pressure reading is best viewed as *two* pieces of information (systolic pressure = 120 mm Hg, diastolic pressure = 80 mm Hg). Human beings can glance at a written blood-pressure value and easily make the transition between its unitary view as a single datum point and the decomposed information about systolic and diastolic pressures. Such dual views can be much more difficult for computers, however, unless they are specifically allowed for in the design of the method for data storage and analysis. The idea of a *data model* for computer-stored medical data accordingly becomes an important issue in the design of medical data systems.

If a medical datum is a single observation about a patient, then medical data are multiple observations. Such data may involve several different observations made concurrently, the observation of the same patient parameter made at several points in time, or both. Thus, a single datum generally can be viewed as defined by four elements:

1. The *patient* in question
2. The *parameter* being observed (e.g., liver size, urine-sugar value, history of rheumatic fever, heart size on chest X-ray film)

3. The *value* of the parameter in question (e.g., weight is *70 kg*, temperature is *98.6°F*, profession is *steel worker*)
4. The *time* of the observation (e.g., 2:30 A.M. on 14FEB1997[1])

Time can particularly complicate the assessment and computer-based management of data. In some settings, the date of the observation is adequate—for example, in outpatient clinics or private offices where a patient generally is seen infrequently and the data collected need to be identified in time with no greater accuracy than a calendar date. In others, minute-to-minute variations may be important—for example, the frequent blood-sugar readings obtained for a patient in diabetic ketoacidosis[2] or the continuous measurements of mean arterial blood pressure for a patient in cardiogenic shock.[3]

It often also is important to keep a record of the circumstances under which a datum was obtained. For example, was the blood pressure taken in the arm or leg? Was the patient lying or standing? Was the pressure obtained just after exercise? During sleep? What kind of recording device was used? Was the observer reliable? Such additional information, sometimes called *modifiers*, can be of crucial importance in the proper interpretation of data.

A related issue is the *uncertainty* in the values of data. It is rare that an observation—even one by a skilled clinician—can be accepted with absolute certainty. Consider the following examples:

- An adult patient reports a childhood illness with fevers and a red rash in addition to joint swelling. Could he have had scarlet fever? The patient does not know what his pediatrician called the disease.
- A physician listens to the heart of an asthmatic child and thinks that she hears a heart murmur—but she is not certain because of the patient's loud wheezing.
- A radiologist looking at a shadow on a chest X-ray film is not sure whether it represents overlapping blood vessels or a lung tumor.
- A confused patient is able to respond to simple questions about his illness, but his physician is uncertain how much of his reported history is reliable.

As described in Chapter 3, there is a variety of possible responses to deal with the uncertainty in data and in their interpretation. One technique is to collect additional data that will either confirm or eliminate the concern raised by the initial observation. This solution is not always appropriate, however, because the *costs* of data collection must be considered. The additional observation might be expensive, risky for the patient, or wasteful of time during which treatment could

[1]Note that it was the tendency to record such dates in computers as "14FEB97" that led to the end-of-century complexities that we call the *Year 2000 problem*. It was short-sighted to think that it was adequate to encode the year of an event with only two digits.
[2]Ketoacidosis results from acid production due to poorly controlled blood sugar levels.
[3]Cardiogenic shock is dangerously low blood pressure due to failure of the heart.

have been instituted. The idea of *tradeoffs* in data collection thus becomes extremely important in guiding healthcare decision-making.

2.1.1 What Are the Types of Medical Data?

The examples in the previous section suggest that there is a broad range of data types in the practice of medicine and the allied health sciences. They range from narrative, textual data to numerical measurements, recorded signals, drawings, and even photographs.

Narrative data account for a large component of the information that is gathered in the care of patients. For example, the patient's description of his present illness, including responses to focused questions from the physician, generally is gathered verbally and is recorded as text in the medical record. The same is true of the patient's social and family history, the general review of systems that is part of most evaluations of new patients, and the clinician's report of physical examination findings. Such narrative data were traditionally handwritten by clinicians and then placed in the patient's medical record (Fig. 2.1). Increasingly, however, the narrative summaries are dictated and then transcribed by typists who work with word processors to produce printed summaries for inclusion in medical records. The electronic versions of such reports can also easily be integrated into electronic medical records and clinical data repositories so that clinicians can access important clinical information even when the paper record is not available. On-line transcriptions of dictated information often include not only patient histories and physical examinations but also other narrative descriptions such as reports of specialty consultations, surgical procedures, pathologic examinations of tissues, and hospitalization summaries when a patient is discharged.

Some narrative data are loosely coded with shorthand conventions known to health personnel, particularly data collected during the physical examination, in which recorded observations reflect the stereotypic examination process taught to all practitioners. It is common, for example, to find the notation "PERRLA" under the eye examination in a patient's medical record. This encoded form indicates that the patient's "Pupils are Equal (in size), Round, and Reactive to Light and Accommodation."[4]

Complete phrases have become loose standards of communication among medical personnel. Examples include "mild dyspnea [shortness of breath] on exertion," "pain relieved by antacids or milk," and "failure to thrive." Such standardized expressions are attempts to use conventional text notation as a form of summarization for otherwise heterogeneous conditions that together characterize a simple concept about a patient.

Many data used in medicine take on discrete numeric values. These include such parameters as laboratory tests, vital signs (such as temperature and pulse rate), and certain measurements taken during the physical examination. When such numerical data are interpreted, however, the issue of *precision* becomes important. Can a physician distinguish reliably between a 9-cm and a 10-cm liver

---

[4]Accommodation is the process of focusing on near objects.

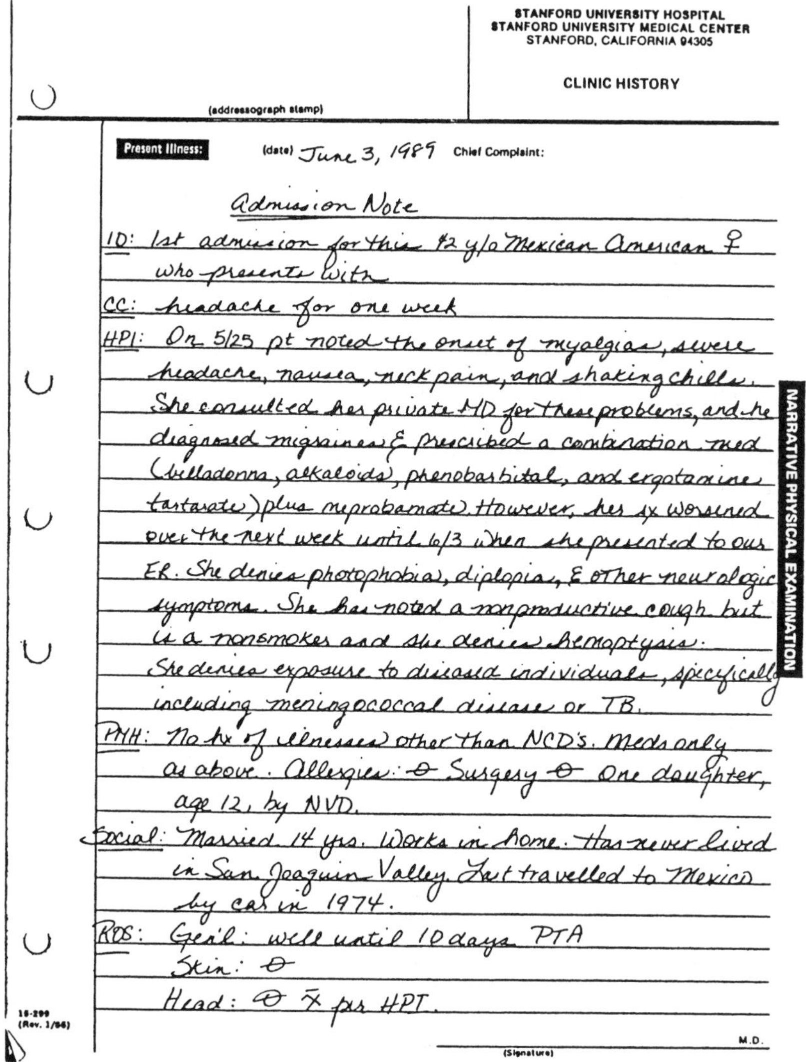

STANFORD UNIVERSITY HOSPITAL
STANFORD UNIVERSITY MEDICAL CENTER
STANFORD, CALIFORNIA 94305

CLINIC HISTORY

(addressograph stamp)

Present Illness: (date) June 3, 1989 Chief Complaint:

Admission Note

ID: 1st admission for this 42 y/o Mexican American ♀ who presents with

CC: headache for one week

HPI: On 5/25 pt noted the onset of myalgias, severe headache, nausea, neck pain, and shaking chills. She consulted her private MD for these problems, and he diagnosed migraines & prescribed a combination med (belladonna, alkaloids, phenobarbital, and ergotamine tartarate) plus meprobamate. However, her sx worsened over the next week until 6/3 when she presented to our ER. She denies photophobia, diplopia, & other neurologic symptoms. She has noted a nonproductive cough but is a nonsmoker and she denies hemoptysis. She denies exposure to diseased individuals, specifically including meningococcal disease or TB.

PMH: No hx of illnesses other than NCD's. Meds only as above. Allergies: ⊖ Surgery ⊖ One daughter, age 12, by NVD.

Social: Married 14 yrs. Works in home. Has never lived in San Joaquin Valley. Last travelled to Mexico by car in 1974.

ROS: Gen'l: well until 10 days PTA

Skin: ⊖

Head: ⊖ $\bar{x}$ per HPI.

NARRATIVE PHYSICAL EXAMINATION

M.D.
(Signature)

15-299
(Rev. 1/86)

FIGURE 2.1. Much of the information gathered during a physician-patient encounter is written in the medical record.

span when she examines the patient's abdomen? Does it make sense to report a serum-sodium level to two-decimal-place accuracy? Is a 1-kg fluctuation in weight from one week to the next significant? Was the patient weighed on the same scale both times (i.e., could the different values reflect variation between measurement instruments rather than changes in the patient)?

In some fields of medicine, analog data in the form of continuous signals are particularly important (see Chapter 13). Perhaps the best known example is an electrocardiogram (ECG), a tracing of the electrical activity from a patient's heart;

there are many similar examples. When such data are stored in medical records, a graphical tracing frequently is included, with a written interpretation of its meaning. There are clear challenges in determining how such data are best managed in computer storage systems.

Visual images—either acquired from machines or sketched by the physician—are another important category of data. Radiologic images are obvious examples. It also is common for a physician to draw simple pictures to represent abnormalities that she has observed; such drawings may serve as a basis for comparison when she or another physician next sees the patient. For example, a sketch is a concise way of conveying the location and size of a nodule in the prostate gland (Fig. 2.2).

As should be clear from these examples, the idea of data is inextricably bound to the idea of **data recording**. Physicians and other healthcare personnel are taught from the outset that it is crucial that they not trust their memory when caring for patients. They must record their observations, as well as the actions that they have taken and the rationales for those actions, for later communication to themselves and other people. A glance at a medical record will quickly reveal the wide variety of data-recording techniques that have evolved. The range goes from hand-written text to commonly understood shorthand notation to cryptic symbols that only specialists can understand; few physicians know how to interpret the data-recording conventions of an ophthalmologist, for example (Fig. 2.3). The notations may be highly structured records of brief text or numerical

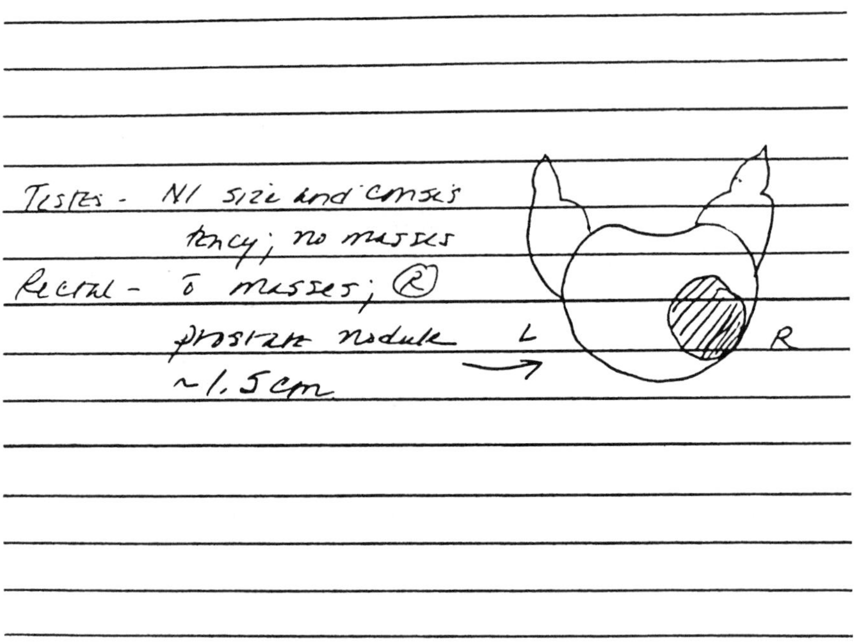

FIGURE 2.2. A physician's hand-drawn sketch of a prostate nodule. A drawing may convey precise information more easily and compactly than a textual description.

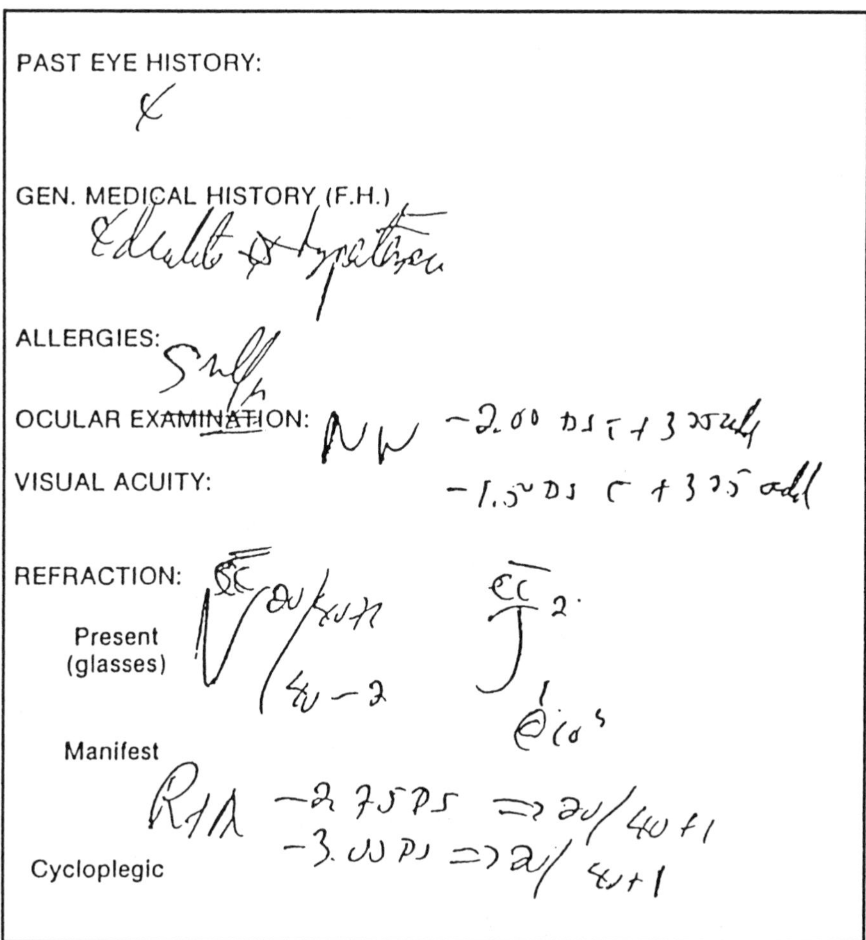

PAST EYE HISTORY:

GEN. MEDICAL HISTORY (F.H.)

ALLERGIES:

OCULAR EXAMINATION:

VISUAL ACUITY:

REFRACTION:

Present (glasses)

Manifest

Cycloplegic

FIGURE 2.3. An ophthalmologist's report of an eye examination. Most physicians trained in other specialties would have difficulty deciphering the symbols that the ophthalmologist has used.

information, hand-drawn sketches, machine-generated tracings of analog signals, or photographic images (of the patient or of his radiologic or other studies). This range of data-recording conventions presents significant challenges to the person implementing computer-based medical-record systems.

2.1.2 Who Collects the Data?

Health data on patients and populations are gathered by a variety of health professionals. Although conventional ideas of the **healthcare team** evoke images of co-workers treating ill patients, the team has much broader responsibilities than treatment per se; data collection and recording are a central part of its task.

Physicians are key players in the process of data collection and interpretation. They converse with a patient to gather narrative descriptive data on the chief complaint, past illnesses, family and social information, and the system review. They examine the patient, collecting pertinent data and recording them during or at the end of the visit. In addition, they generally decide what additional data to collect by ordering laboratory or radiologic studies and by observing the patient's response to therapeutic interventions (yet another form of data that contributes to patient assessment).

In both outpatient and hospital settings, nurses play a central role in making observations and recording them for future reference. The data that they gather contribute to nursing care plans as well as to the assessment of patients by physicians and by other healthcare staff. Thus, nurses' training includes instruction in careful and accurate observation, history taking, and examination of the patient. Because nurses typically spend more time with patients than physicians do, especially in the hospital setting, nurses often build relationships with patients that uncover information and insights that contribute to proper diagnosis, to understanding of pertinent psychosocial issues, or to proper planning of therapy or discharge management (Fig. 2.4). The role of information

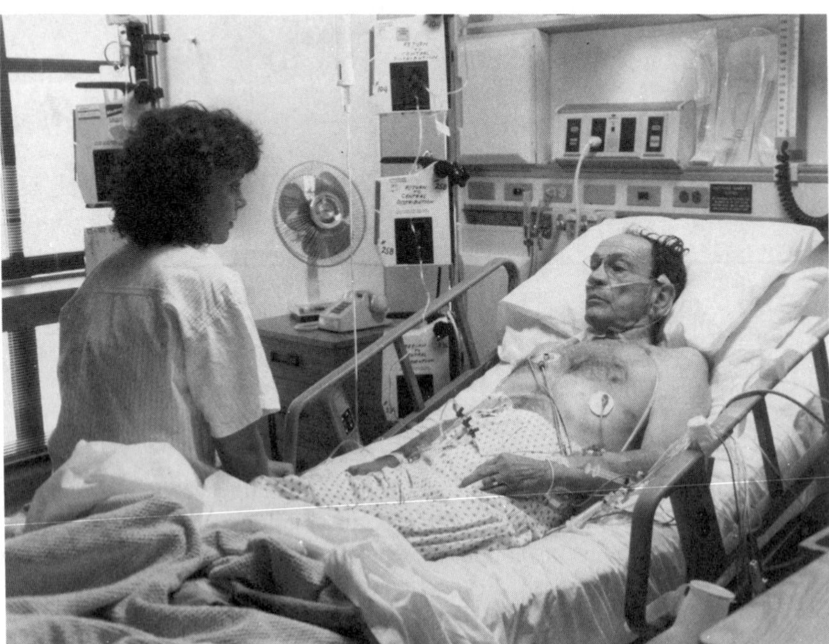

FIGURE 2.4. Nurses often develop close relationships with patients. These relationships may allow the nurse to make observations that are missed by other staff. This ability is just one of the ways in which nurses play a key role in data collection and recording. (*Source:* Photograph by Janice Anne Rohn.)

systems in contributing to patient-care tasks such as care planning by nurses is the subject of Chapter 12.

Various other healthcare workers contribute to the data-collection process. Office staff and admissions personnel gather demographic and financial information. Physical or respiratory therapists record the results of their treatments and often make suggestions for further management. Laboratory personnel perform tests on biological samples, such as blood or urine, and record the results for later use by physicians and nurses. Radiology technicians perform X-ray examinations; radiologists interpret the resulting data and report their findings to the patients' physicians. Pharmacists may interview patients about their medications or about drug allergies and then monitor the patients' use of prescription drugs. As these examples suggest, most people employed in healthcare settings gather, record, and make use of patient data in their work.

Finally, there are the technological devices that generate data—laboratory instruments, imaging machines, monitoring equipment in intensive-care units, and measurement devices that take a single reading (such as thermometers, ECG machines, sphygmomanometers for taking blood pressures, and spirometers for testing lung function). Sometimes such a device produces a paper report suitable for inclusion in a traditional medical record. Sometimes the device indicates a result on a gauge or traces a result that must be read by an operator and then recorded in the patient's chart. Sometimes a trained specialist must interpret the output. Increasingly, however, the devices feed their results directly into computer equipment so that the data can be analyzed or formatted for electronic storage as well as reported on paper. With the advent of comprehensive electronic medical records (see Chapter 9), the printing of such data summaries may no longer be required, and all access to information will be through computer workstations.

2.2 Uses of Medical Data

Medical data are recorded for a variety of purposes. They may be needed to support the proper care of the patient from whom they were obtained, but they also may contribute to the good of society through the aggregation and analysis of data regarding populations of individuals. One problem with traditional data-recording techniques has been that the paper record has worked reasonably well to support the proper care of individual patients but has made clinical research across populations of patients extremely cumbersome. Computer-based record keeping offers major advantages in this regard, as we discuss in more detail later in this chapter and in Chapters 9 and 11.

2.2.1 Create the Basis for the Historical Record

Any student of science has learned the importance of collecting and recording data meticulously when carrying out an experiment. Just as a laboratory notebook provides a record of precisely what a scientist has done, the experimental data observed, and the rationale for intermediate decision points, medical records are intended to provide a detailed compilation of information about individual patients:

- What is the patient's history (development of a current illness; other diseases that coexist or have resolved; pertinent family, social, and demographic information)?
- What symptoms has the patient reported?
- What physical signs have been noted on examination?
- How have signs and symptoms changed over time?
- What laboratory results have been or are now available?
- What radiologic and other special studies have been performed?
- What interventions have been undertaken?
- What is the reasoning behind those management decisions?

Each new patient complaint and its management can be viewed as a therapeutic experiment, inherently confounded by uncertainty, with the goal of answering three questions:

1. What was the nature of the disease or symptom?
2. What was the treatment decision?
3. What was the outcome of that treatment?

As is true for all experiments, one purpose is to learn from experience through careful observation and recording of data. The lessons learned in a given encounter may be highly individualized (e.g., the physician may learn how a specific patient tends to respond to pain or how family interactions tend to affect the patient's response to disease), or they may be best derived by pooling of data from many patients who have similar problems and analysis of the results of various treatment options to determine efficacy.

Although laboratory research has contributed dramatically to our knowledge of human disease and treatment, especially over the past half century, it is careful observation and recording by skilled healthcare personnel that has always provided the foundation for the generation of new knowledge about patient care. We learn from the aggregation of information from large numbers of patients; thus, the historical record for individual patients is of inestimable importance to clinical research.

2.2.2 *Support Communication Among Providers*

A central function of structured data collection and recording in healthcare settings is to assist personnel in providing coordinated care to a patient over time. Most patients who have significant medical conditions are seen over months or years on several occasions for one or more problems that require ongoing evaluation and treatment.

It was once common for patients to receive essentially all their care from a single provider: the family doctor who tended both children and adults, often seeing the patient over many or all the years of that person's life. We tend to picture such physicians as having especially close relationships with their patients—knowing the family and sharing in many of the patient's life events, especially in smaller communities. Such doctors nonetheless kept records of all encounters so that they could refer to data about past illnesses and treatments as a guide to evaluating future care issues.

In the world of modern medicine, the emergence of subspecialization and the increasing provision of care by *teams* of health professionals have placed new emphasis on the central role of the medical record (Fig. 2.5). Now the record not only contains observations by a physician for reference on the next visit but also serves as a communication mechanism among physicians and other medical personnel, such as physical or respiratory therapists, nursing staff, radiology technicians, social workers, or discharge planners. In many outpatient settings, patients receive care over time from a variety of physicians—colleagues covering for the primary physician, or specialists to whom the patient has been referred, or a managed care organization's case manager. It is not uncommon to hear com-

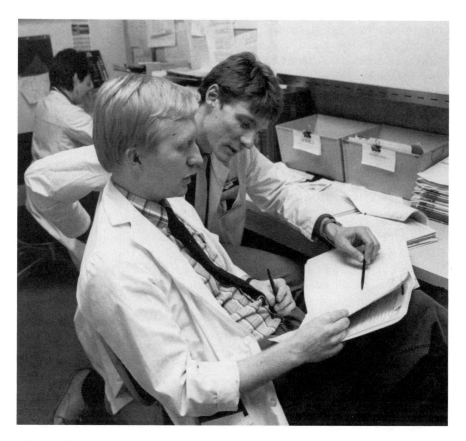

FIGURE 2.5. One role of the medical record: a communication mechanism among health professionals who work together to plan patient care. (*Source:* Photograph by Janice Anne Rohn.)

plaints from patients who remember the days when it was possible to receive essentially all their care from a single physician whom they had come to trust and who knew them well. Physicians are sensitive to this issue and therefore recognize the importance of the medical record in ensuring quality and **continuity of care** through adequate recording of the details and logic of past interventions and ongoing treatment plans. This idea is of particular importance in a healthcare system, such as ours in the United States, in which chronic diseases rather than care for trauma or acute infections increasingly dominate the basis for interactions between patients and their doctors.

2.2.3 Anticipate Future Health Problems

Providing high-quality medical care involves more than responding to patients' acute or chronic health problems. It also requires educating patients about the ways in which their environment and lifestyles can contribute to or reduce the risk of future development of disease. Similarly, data gathered routinely in the ongoing care of a patient may suggest that he is at high risk of developing a specific problem even though he may feel well and be without symptoms at present. Medical data therefore are important in screening for risk factors, following patients' risk profiles over time, and providing a basis for specific patient education or preventive interventions, such as diet, medication, or exercise. Perhaps the most common examples of such ongoing risk assessment in our society are routine monitoring for excess weight, high blood pressure, and elevated serum-cholesterol levels. In these cases, abnormal data may be predictive of later symptomatic disease; optimal care requires early intervention before the complications have an opportunity to develop fully.

2.2.4 Record Standard Preventive Measures

The medical record also serves as a source of data on interventions that have been performed to prevent common or serious disorders. The best examples of such interventions are immunizations: the vaccinations that begin in early childhood and may continue throughout life, including special treatments administered when a person will be at particularly high risk (e.g., injections of gamma globulin to protect people from hepatitis, administered before travel to areas where hepatitis is endemic). When a patient comes to his local hospital emergency room with a laceration, the physicians routinely check for an indication of when he most recently had a tetanus immunization. When easily accessible in the record (or from the patient), such data can prevent unnecessary treatments (in this case, an injection) that may be associated with risk or significant cost.

2.2.5 Identify Deviations from Expected Trends

Data often are useful in medical care only when viewed as part of a continuum over time. An example is the routine monitoring of children for normal growth and development by pediatricians (Fig. 2.6). Single data points regarding height and weight generally are not useful by themselves; it is the trend in such data points observed over months or years that may provide the first clue to a medical problem. It is accordingly common for such parameters to be recorded on special charts or forms that make the trends easy to discern at a glance. Women who want to get pregnant often keep similar records of body temperature. By measuring temperature daily and recording the values on special charts, women can identify the slight increase in temperature that accompanies ovulation and thus may discern the days of maximum fertility. Many physicians will ask a patient to keep such graphical records so that they can later discuss the data with the patient and include the record in the medical charts for ongoing reference.

2.2.6 Provide a Legal Record

Another use of medical data, once they are charted and analyzed, is as the foundation for a legal record to which the courts can refer if necessary. The medical record is a legal document; most of the clinical information that is recorded must be signed by the responsible individual. In addition, the chart generally should describe and justify both the presumed diagnosis for a patient and the choice of management.

We emphasized earlier the importance of recording data; in fact, data do not exist unless they are recorded. The legal system stresses this point as well. A provider's unsubstantiated memory of what she observed or why she took some action is of little value in the courtroom. The medical record is the foundation for determining whether proper care was delivered. Thus, a well-maintained record is a source of protection for both patients and their physicians.

2.2.7 Support Clinical Research

Although experience caring for individual patients provides physicians with special skills and enhanced judgment over time, it is only by formally analyzing data collected from large numbers of patients that researchers can develop and validate new clinical knowledge of general applicability. Thus, another use of medical data is to support clinical research through the aggregation and statistical analysis of observations gathered from populations of patients (see Section 1.1 and Figures 1.4 and 1.5).

Randomized clinical trials (RCTs) are a common method by which specific clinical questions are addressed experimentally. They typically involve the random assignment of matched groups of patients to alternate treatments when there is uncertainty about how best to manage the patients' problem. The variables that might affect a patient's course (e.g., age, gender, weight, coexisting medical problems) are measured and recorded. As the study progresses, data are gathered meticulously to provide a record of how each patient fared under treatment and precisely how the treatment was administered. By pooling such data, sometimes after years of experimentation (depending on the time course of the disease un-

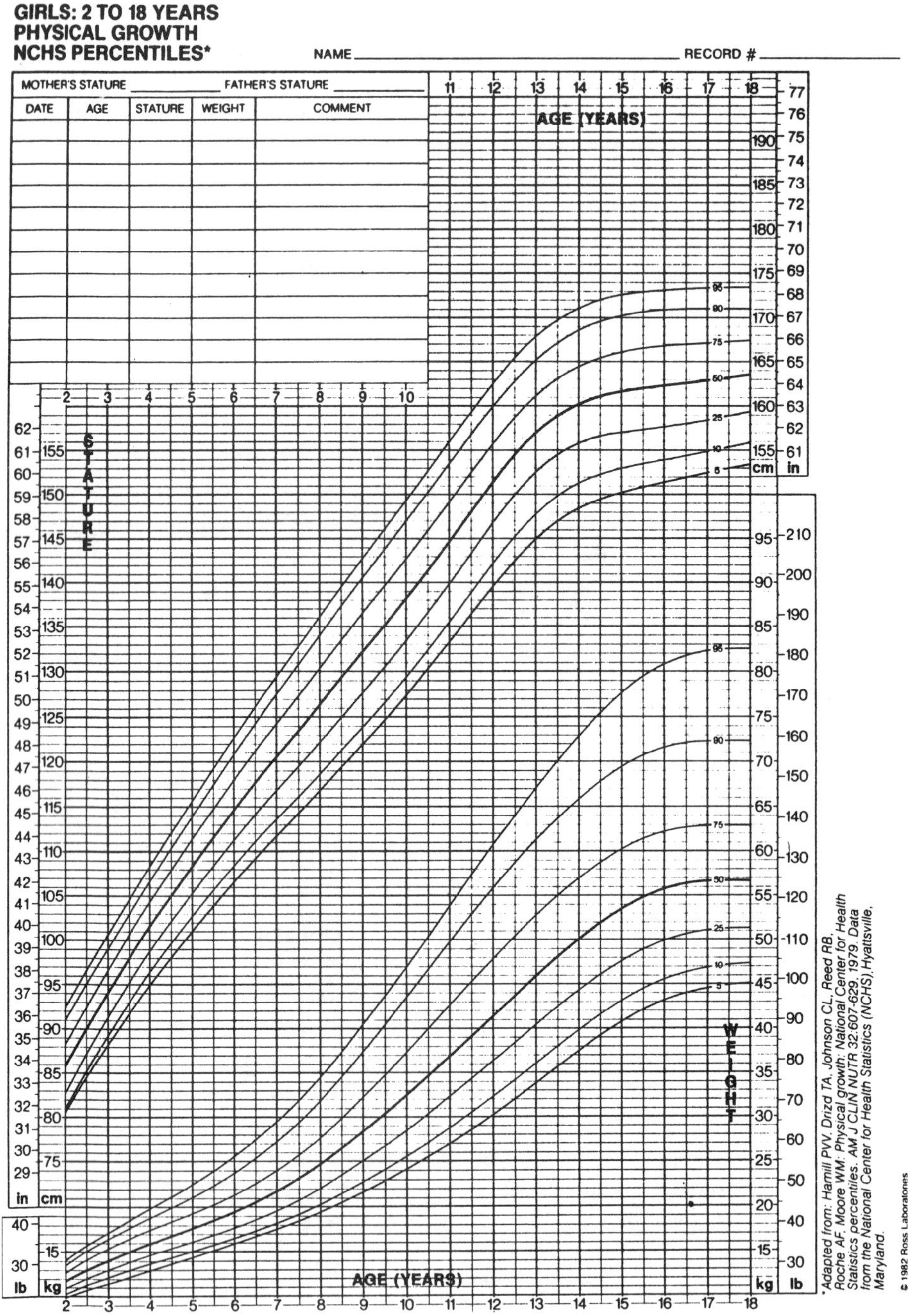
GIRLS: 2 TO 18 YEARS
PHYSICAL GROWTH
NCHS PERCENTILES*
NAME
RECORD #
MOTHER'S STATURE
FATHER'S STATURE
DATE
AGE
STATURE
WEIGHT
COMMENT
AGE (YEARS)
STATURE
WEIGHT
in
cm
kg
lb
AGE (YEARS)
*Adapted from: Hamill PVV, Drizd TA, Johnson CL, Reed RB, Roche AF, Moore WM: Physical growth: National Center for Health Statistics percentiles. AM J CLIN NUTR 32:607-629, 1979. Data from the National Center for Health Statistics (NCHS), Hyattsville, Maryland.
© 1982 Ross Laboratories

FIGURE 2.6. A pediatric growth chart. Single datum points would not be useful; it is the changes in values over time that indicate whether development is progressing normally. (*Source:* Used with permission of Ross Laboratories, Columbus, OH 43216.)

der consideration), researchers may be able to demonstrate a statistical difference among the study groups depending on precise characteristics present when patients entered the study or on the details of how patients were managed. Such results then help investigators to define the standard of care for future patients with the same or similar problems.

Medical knowledge also can be derived from the analysis of large patient data sets even when the patients were not specifically enrolled in an RCT. Much of the research in the field of epidemiology involves analysis of population-based data of this type. Our knowledge of the risks associated with cigarette smoking, for example, is based on irrefutable statistics derived from large populations of individuals with and without lung cancer, other pulmonary problems, and heart disease.

2.3 Weaknesses of the Traditional Medical-Record System

The preceding description of medical data and their uses emphasizes the positive aspects of information storage and retrieval in the paper record. All medical personnel, however, quickly learn that use of the medical record is complicated by a bevy of logistical and practical realities that greatly limit the record's effectiveness for its intended uses.

2.3.1 Pragmatic and Logistical Issues

Recall, first, that data cannot effectively serve the delivery of health care unless they are recorded. Their optimal use depends on positive responses to the following questions:

- Can I find the data I need when I need them?
  - Can I find the medical record in which they are recorded?
  - Can I find the data within the record?
  - Can I find what I need quickly?
- Can I read and interpret the data once I find them?
- Can I update the data reliably with new observations in a form consistent with the requirements for future access by myself or other people?

All too frequently, the traditional paper-record system creates situations in which people answer such questions negatively. For example

- The patient's chart may be unavailable when the healthcare professional needs it. It may be in use by someone else at another location; it may have been misplaced despite the hospital's, clinic's, or office's record-tracking system (Fig. 2.7); or it may have been taken by someone unintentionally and is now buried on a desk.
- Once the chart is in hand, it might still be difficult to find the information required. The data may have been known previously but never recorded due to

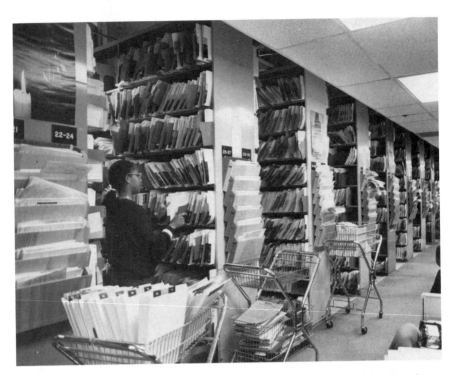

FIGURE 2.7. A typical storage room for medical records. It is not surprising that charts sometimes are mislaid. (*Source:* Photograph by Janice Anne Rohn.)

an oversight by a physician or other health professional. Poor organization in the chart may lead to the user spending an inordinate time searching for the data, especially in the massive paper charts of patients who have long and complicated histories.

- Once the healthcare professional has located the data, he may find them difficult to read. It is not uncommon to hear one physician asking another as they peer together into a chart: "What is that word?" "Is that a two or a five?" "Whose signature is that?" Illegible and sloppy entries can be a major obstruction to effective use of the chart (Fig. 2.8).
- When a chart is unavailable, the healthcare professional still must provide medical care. Thus, providers make do without past data, basing their decisions instead on what the patient can tell them and on what their examination reveals. They then write a note for inclusion in the chart—when the chart is located. In a large institution with thousands of medical records, it is not surprising that such loose notes often fail to make it to the patient's chart or are filed out of sequence so that the actual chronology of management is disrupted in the record.
- When patients who have chronic or frequent diseases are seen over months or years, their records grow so large that the charts must be broken up into mul-

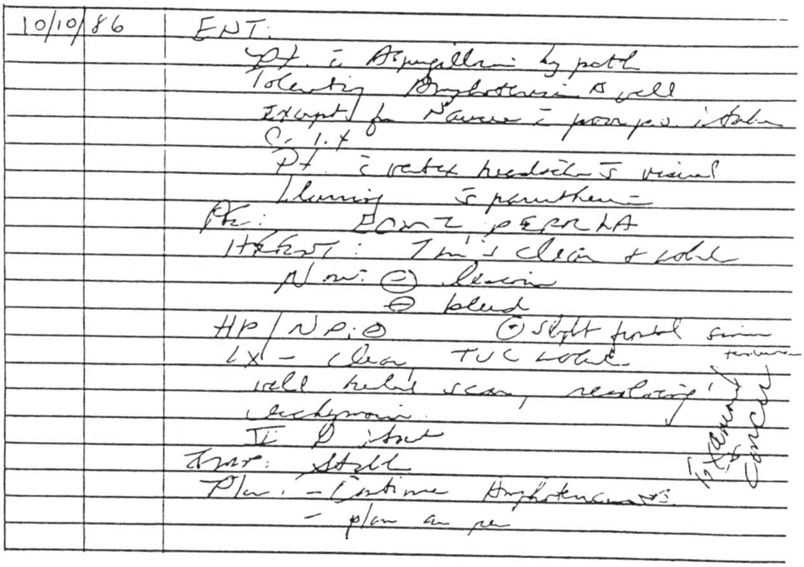

FIGURE 2.8. Written entries are standard in paper records, yet handwritten notes may be illegible. Notes that cannot be interpreted by other people may cause delays in treatment or inappropriate care.

tiple volumes. When a hospital clinic or emergency room orders the patient's chart, only the most recent volume typically is provided. Old but pertinent data may be in early volumes that are stored offsite or are otherwise unavailable.

As described in Chapter 9, computer-based medical-record systems offer potential solutions to all these practical problems in the use of the paper record.

2.3.2 *Redundancy and Inefficiency*

To be able to find data quickly in the chart, health professionals have developed a variety of techniques that provide redundant recording to match alternate modes of access. For example, the result of a radiologic study typically is entered on a standard radiology reporting form, which is filed in the portion of the chart labeled "X-ray." For complicated procedures, the same data often are summarized in a brief note by the radiologist in the narrative part of the chart, which she enters at the time of the study because she knows that the formal report will not make it back to the chart for 1 or 2 days. In addition, the study results often are mentioned in notes written by the patient's admitting and consulting physicians and by the nursing staff. Although there may be good reasons for recording such information multiple times in different ways and in different locations within the chart, the combined bulk of these notes accelerates the physical growth of the document and, accordingly, complicates the task of the chart's logistical management. Furthermore, it becomes increasingly difficult to locate specific patient

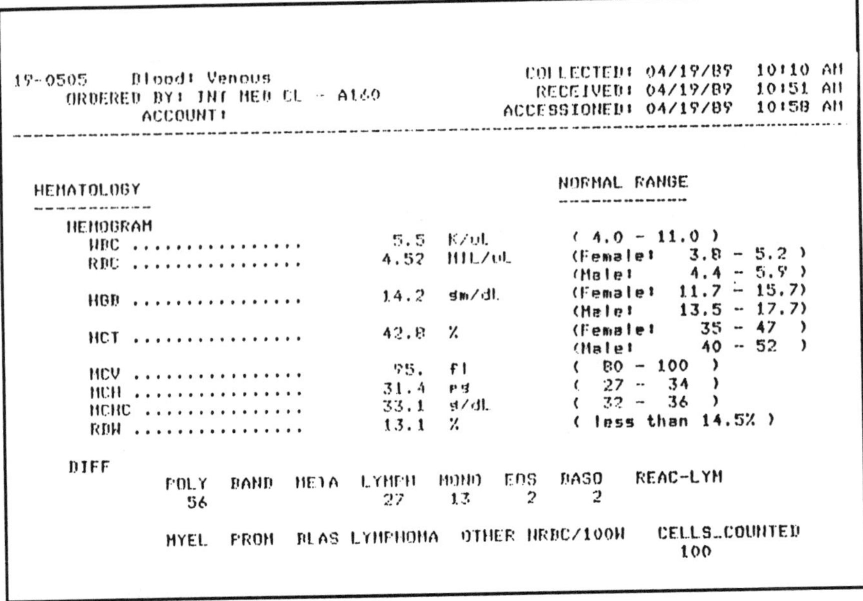

19-0505 Blood: Venous
ORDERED BY: INT MED CL - A160
ACCOUNT:

COLLECTED: 04/19/89 10:10 AM
RECEIVED: 04/19/89 10:51 AM
ACCESSIONED: 04/19/89 10:58 AM

HEMATOLOGY

HEMOGRAM

Test	Result	Units	NORMAL RANGE
WBC	5.5	K/uL	(4.0 - 11.0)
RBC	4.52	MIL/uL	(Female: 3.8 - 5.2) (Male: 4.4 - 5.9)
HGB	14.2	gm/dL	(Female: 11.7 - 15.7) (Male: 13.5 - 17.7)
HCT	42.8	%	(Female: 35 - 47) (Male: 40 - 52)
MCV	95.	fl	(80 - 100)
MCH	31.4	pg	(27 - 34)
MCHC	33.1	g/dL	(32 - 36)
RDW	13.1	%	(less than 14.5%)

DIFF

POLY	BAND	META	LYMPH	MONO	EOS	BASO	REAC-LYM
56			27	13	2	2	

MYEL	PROM	BLAS	LYMPHOMA	OTHER	NRBC/100W	CELLS_COUNTED
						100

FIGURE 2.9. Laboratory reporting forms record medical data in a consistent, familiar format.

data as the chart succumbs to obesity. The predictable result is that someone writes yet another redundant entry, summarizing information that it took her hours to track down.

A similar inefficiency occurs because of a tension between opposing goals in the design of reporting forms used by many laboratories. Most health personnel prefer a consistent, familiar paper form, often with color coding, because it helps them to find information more quickly (Fig. 2.9). For example, a physician may know that a urinalysis report form is printed on yellow paper and records the bacteria count halfway down the middle column of the form. This knowledge allows the physician to work backward quickly in the laboratory section of the chart to find the most recent urinalysis sheet and to check at a glance the bacterial count. The problem is that such forms typically store only sparse information. It is clearly suboptimal if a rapidly growing physical chart is filled with sheets of paper that report only a single datum.

2.3.3 *Influence on Clinical Research*

Anyone who has participated in a clinical research project based on chart review can attest to the tediousness of flipping through myriad medical records. For all the reasons described in Section 1.1 (see Fig. 1.4), it is arduous to sit with stacks of patients' charts, extracting data and formatting them for structured statistical analysis, and the process is vulnerable to transcription errors. Observers often wonder how much medical knowledge is sitting untapped in medical records because there is no easy way to analyze experience across large populations of patients without first extracting pertinent data from the paper records.

Suppose, for example, that a physician notices that patients receiving a certain common oral medication for diabetes (call it drug X) seem to be more likely to have significant postoperative hypotension (low blood pressure) than do surgical patients receiving other medications for diabetes. The doctor has based his hypothesis—that drug X influences postoperative blood pressure—on only a few recent observations, however, so he decides to look in existing hospital records to see whether this correlation has occurred with sufficient frequency to warrant a formal investigation. The best way to follow up on his theory from existing medical data would be to examine the hospital charts of all patients who have diabetes and also have been admitted for surgery. The task would then be to examine those charts and to note for all patients (1) whether they were taking drug X when admitted and (2) whether they had postoperative hypotension. If the statistics showed that patients receiving drug X were more likely to have low blood pressure after surgery than were similar diabetic patients receiving alternate treatments, then a controlled trial (prospective observation and data gathering) might well be appropriate.

Note the distinction between **retrospective chart review** to investigate a question that was not a subject of study at the time the data were collected and **prospective studies** in which the clinical hypothesis is known in advance and the **research protocol** is designed specifically to collect future data that are relevant to the question under consideration. Subjects are assigned **randomly** to different study groups to help prevent researchers—who are bound to be biased, having developed the hypothesis—from unintentionally skewing the results by assigning a specific class of patients all to one group. For the same reason, to the extent possible, the studies are **double blind**; that is, neither the researchers nor the subjects know which treatment is being administered. Such blinding is of course impractical when it is obvious to patients or physicians what therapy is being given (such as surgical procedures versus drug therapy). Prospective, randomized, double-blind studies are considered the best method for determining optimal management of disease.

Returning to our example, consider the problems in chart review that the researcher would encounter in addressing the postoperative-hypotension question retrospectively. First, he would have to identify the charts of interest: the subset of medical records dealing with surgical patients who are also diabetic. In a hospital record room filled with thousands of charts, the task of chart selection can be overwhelming. Medical records departments generally do keep indexes of diagnostic and procedure codes cross-referenced to specific patients (see Section 2.4.1). Thus, it might be possible to use such an index to find all charts in which the discharge diagnoses included diabetes and the procedure codes included major surgical procedures. The researcher might compile a list of patient identification numbers and have the individual charts pulled from the file room for review.

The researcher's next task is to examine each chart serially to find out what treatment the patient was receiving for diabetes at the time of the surgery *and* to determine whether the patient had postoperative hypotension. Finding such information may be extremely time consuming. Where should the researcher look for it? The admission drug orders might show what the patient received for diabetes control, but it would also be wise to check the medication sheets to see whether the therapy was also administered (as well as ordered) and the admission history to see whether a routine treatment for diabetes, taken right up until the patient entered the hospital, was not administered during the inpatient stay. Information about hypotensive episodes might be similarly difficult to locate. The researcher might start with nursing notes from the recovery room or with the anesthesiologist's data sheets from the operating room, but the patient might not have been hypotensive until after leaving the recovery room and returning to the ward. So the nursing notes from the ward need to be checked too, as well as vital-signs sheets, physicians' progress notes, and the discharge summary.

It should be clear from this example that retrospective chart review is a laborious and tedious process and that people performing it are prone to make transcription errors and to overlook key data. One of the great appeals of computer-based medical records is their potential ability to facilitate the chart-review process. They obviate the need to retrieve hard copy charts; instead, researchers can use computer-based data retrieval and analysis techniques to do most of the work (finding relevant patients, locating pertinent data, and formatting the information for statistical analyses). Researchers can use similar techniques to harness computer assistance with data management in prospective clinical trials.

2.3.4 *The Passive Nature of Paper Records*

The traditional manual system has another limitation that would have been meaningless until the emergence of the computer age. A manual archival system is inherently passive; the charts sit waiting for something to be done with them. They are insensitive to the characteristics of the data recorded within their pages, such as legibility, accuracy, or implications for patient management. They cannot take an active role in responding appropriately to those implications.

Increasingly, computer-based record systems have changed our perspective on what health professionals can expect from the medical chart. Automated record systems introduce new opportunities for dynamic responses to the data that are recorded in them. As described in many of the chapters to follow, computational techniques for data storage, retrieval, and analysis make it feasible to develop record systems that (1) monitor their contents and generate warnings or advice for providers based on single observations or on logical combinations of data; (2) provide automated quality control, including the flagging of potentially erroneous data; or (3) provide feedback on patient-specific or population-based deviations from desirable standards.

2.4 The Structure of Medical Data

Scientific disciplines generally develop a precise terminology or notation that is standardized and accepted by all workers in the field. Consider, for example, the universal language of chemistry embodied in chemical formulae, the precise definitions and mathematical equations used by physicists, the predicate calculus used by logicians, or the conventions for describing circuits used by electrical engineers. Medicine is remarkable for its failure to develop a standardized vocabulary and **nomenclature**, and many observers believe that a true scientific basis for the field will be impossible until this problem is addressed. Other people argue that common references to the "art of medicine" reflect an important distinction between medicine and the "hard" sciences; these people question whether it is possible to introduce too much standardization into a field that prides itself in humanism.

The debate has been accentuated by the introduction of computers for data management, because such machines tend to demand conformity to data standards and definitions. Otherwise, issues of data retrieval and analysis are confounded by discrepancies between the meanings intended by the observers or recorders and those intended by the individuals retrieving information or doing data analysis. What is an "upper respiratory infection"? Does it include infections of the trachea or of the mainstem bronchi? How large does the heart have to be before we can refer to "cardiomegaly"? How should we deal with the plethora of disease names based on eponyms (e.g., Alzheimer's disease, Hodgkin's disease) that are not descriptive of the illness and may not be familiar to all practitioners? What do we mean by an "acute abdomen?" Are the boundaries of the abdomen well agreed on? What are the time constraints that correspond to "acuteness" of abdominal pain? Is an "ache" a pain? What about "occasional" cramping?

Imprecision and the lack of a standardized vocabulary are particularly problematic when we wish to aggregate data recorded by multiple health professionals or to analyze trends over time. Without a controlled, predefined vocabulary, data interpretation is inherently complicated, and the automatic summarization of data may be impossible. For example, one physician might note that a patient has "shortness of breath." Later, another physician might note that she has "dyspnea." Unless these terms are designated as synonyms, an automated flowcharting program will fail to indicate that the patient had the same problem on both occasions.

Regardless of arguments regarding the "artistic" elements in medicine, the need for health personnel to communicate effectively is clear both in acute-care settings and when patients are seen over long periods. Both high-quality care and scientific progress depend on *some* standardization in terminology. Otherwise, differences in intended meaning or in defining criteria will lead to miscommunication, improper interpretation, and potentially negative consequences for the patients involved.

Given the lack of formal definitions for many medical terms, it is remarkable that medical workers communicate as well as they do. Only occasionally is the care for a patient clearly compromised by miscommunication. If computer-based records are to become dynamic and responsive manipulators of patient data, however, their encoded logic must be able to presume a specific meaning for the terms and data elements entered by the observers. This point is discussed in greater detail in Chapter 6, which deals with the multiple efforts to develop healthcare computing standards, including a shared, controlled terminiology for biomedicine.

2.4.1 *Coding Systems*

We are used to seeing figures regarding the growing incidences of certain types of tumors, deaths from influenza during the winter months, and similar health statistics that we tend to take for granted. How are such data accumulated? Their role in health planning and healthcare financing is clear, but if their accumulation required chart review through the process described earlier in this chapter, we would know much less about the health status of the populations in various communities (see Chapter 11).

Because of the needs to know about health trends for populations and to recognize epidemics in their early stages, there are various health-reporting requirements for hospitals (as well as other public organizations) and practitioners. For example, cases of gonorrhea, syphilis, and tuberculosis generally must be reported to local public-health organizations, which code the data to allow trend analyses over time. The Centers for Disease Control and Prevention in Atlanta then pool regional data and report national as well as local trends in disease incidence, bacterial-resistance patterns, and the like.

Another kind of reporting involves the coding of all discharge diagnoses for hospitalized patients, plus coding of certain procedures (e.g., type of surgery) that were performed during the hospital stay. Such codes are reported to state and federal health-planning and analysis agencies and also are used internally at the institution for case-mix analysis (determining the relative frequencies of various disorders in the hospitalized population and the average length of stay for each disease category) and for research. For such data to be useful, the codes must be well defined as well as uniformly applied and accepted.

The government publishes a national diagnostic coding scheme called the International Classification of Disease (ICD). Its current version is used by all nonmilitary hospitals in the United States for discharge coding, and must be reported on the bills submitted to most insurance companies (Fig. 2.10). Pathologists have developed another widely used diagnostic coding scheme; originally known as SNOP (Systematized Nomenclature of Pathology), it has been expanded to form SNOMED (Systematized Nomenclature of Medicine) (American College of Pathologists, 1982; Côté & Robboy, 1980). Another coding scheme developed by the American Medical Association is the Current Procedural Terminology (CPT) (Finkel, 1977) and is similarly widely used in producing bills for services

CHRONIC OBSTRUCTIVE PULMONARY DISEASE AND ALLIED CONDITIONS (490-496)

490 Bronchitis, not specified as acute or chronic

491 Chronic bronchitis

491.0 Simple chronic bronchitis
491.1 Mucopurulent chronic bronchitis
491.2 Obstructive chronic bronchitis
491.8 Other chronic bronchitis
491.9 Unspecified chronic bronchitis

492 Emphysema

492.0 Emphysematous bleb
492.8 Other emphysema

493 Asthma

493.0 Extrinsic asthma
493.1 Intrinsic asthma
493.9 Asthma, unspecified

494 Bronchiectasis

495 Extrinsic allergic alveolitis

495.0 Farmer's lung
495.1 Bagassosis
495.2 Bird-fanciers' lung
495.3 Suberosis
495.4 Malt workers' lung
495.5 Mushroom workers' lung
495.6 Maple bark-strippers' lung
495.7 "Ventilation" pneumonitis
495.8 Other specified allergic alveolitis and pneumonitis
Cheese-washers' lung, Coffee workers' lung, Fish-meal workers' lung, Furriers' lung, Grain-handlers' disease or lung, Pituitary snuff-takers' disease, Sequoiosis or red-cedar asthma, Wood asthma
495.9 Unspecified allergic alveolitis and pneumonitis

FIGURE 2.10. A small subset of the disease categories identified by the Ninth International Classification of Disease, Clinical Modification (ICD-9-CM). (*Source:* Health Care Financing Administration [1980]. *The International Classification of Diseases, 9th Revision, Clinical Modification, ICD-9-CM.* U.S. Department of Health and Human Services, Washington, D.C. DHHS Publication No. [PHS] 80-1260.)

rendered to patients. More details on such schemes are provided in Chapter 6. What warrants emphasis here, however, is the motivation for the codes' development: Healthcare personnel need standardized terms that can support pooling of data for analysis and can provide criteria for determining charges for individual patients.

The historical roots of a coding system reveal themselves as limitations or idiosyncrasies when the system is applied in more general clinical settings. For example, the ICD-9 code was derived from a classification scheme developed for epidemiologic reporting. Consequently, it has more than 50 separate codes for describing tuberculosis infections. SNOMED permits coding of pathologic findings in exquisite detail but only recently has begun to introduce codes for expressing the dimensions of a patient's functional status. In a particular clinical setting, no one of the common coding schemes is likely to be completely satisfactory. In some cases, the granularity of the code will be too coarse; a hematologist (person who studies blood diseases) may want to distinguish among a variety of hemoglobinopathies (disorders of the structure and function of hemoglobin) lumped under a single code in ICD. On the other hand, another practitioner may prefer to aggregate many individual codes—for example, those for active tuberculosis—into a single category to simplify the coding and retrieval of data.

Such schemes cannot be effective unless they are accepted by healthcare providers. There is an inherent tension between the need for a coding system that is general enough to cover many different patients and the need for precise and unique terms that accurately apply to a specific patient and do not unduly constrain physicians' attempts to describe what they observe. Yet if physicians view the computer-based medical record as a blank sheet of paper on which any unstructured information can be written, the data they record will be unsuitable for dynamic processing, clinical research, and health planning. The challenge is to learn how to meet all these needs. Researchers at many institutions have worked for over a decade to develop a unified medical language system (UMLS), a common structure that ties together the various vocabularies that have been created. At the same time, the developers of specific terminologies are continually working to refine and expand their independent coding schemes (Humphreys & Lindberg, 1993) (see Chapter 6).

2.4.2 The Data-to-Knowledge Spectrum

A central focus in medical informatics is the information base that constitutes the "substance of medicine." Workers in the field have tried to clarify the distinctions among three terms frequently used to describe the content of computer-based systems: *data*, *information*, and *knowledge* (Blum, 1986b). These terms are often used interchangeably. In this volume, we shall refer to a **datum** as a single observational point that characterizes a relationship.[5] It generally can be regarded as the value of a specific parameter for a particular object (e.g., a patient) at a given point in time. **Knowledge**, then, is derived through the formal or informal analysis (or interpretation) of data. Thus, it includes the results of

[5]Note that *data* is a plural term, although it is often erroneously used in speech and writing as though it were singular.

formal studies and also common sense facts, assumptions, heuristics (strategic rules of thumb), and models—any of which may reflect the experience or biases of people who interpret the primary data. The term **information** is more generic in that it encompasses both organized data and knowledge, although data are not information until they have been organized in some way for analysis or display.

The observation that patient Brown has a blood pressure of 180/110 is a *datum*, as is the report that the patient has had a myocardial infarction (heart attack). When researchers pool and analyze such data, they may determine that patients with high blood pressure are more likely to have heart attacks than are patients with normal or low blood pressure. This data analysis has produced a piece of *knowledge* about the world. A physician's belief that prescribing dietary restriction of salt is unlikely to be effective in controlling high blood pressure in patients of low economic standing (because the latter are less likely to be able to afford special low-salt foods) is an additional personal piece of *knowledge*—a **heuristic** that guides that physician in her decision-making. Note that the appropriate interpretation of these definitions depends on the context. Knowledge at one level of abstraction may be considered data at higher levels. A blood pressure of 180/110 mm Hg is a raw piece of data; the statement that the patient has hypertension is an interpretation of that data and thus represents a higher level of knowledge. As input to a diagnostic decision aid, however, the presence or absence of hypertension may be requested, in which case the presence of hypertension is treated as a data item.

A **database** is a collection of individual observations without any summarizing analysis. A computer-based medical record system is thus primarily viewed as a database—the place where patient data are stored. A **knowledge base**, on the other hand, is a collection of facts, heuristics, and models that can be used for problem-solving and analysis of data. If the knowledge base provides sufficent structure, including semantic links among knowledge items, the computer itself may be able to apply that knowledge as an aid to case-based problem-solving. Many decision-support systems have been called *knowledge-based systems*, reflecting this distinction between knowledge bases and databases (see Chapter 16).

2.5 Strategies of Medical Data Selection and Use

It is illusory to conceive of a "complete medical data set." All medical databases, and medical records, are necessarily incomplete because they reflect the selective collection and recording of data by the healthcare personnel responsible for the patient. There can be marked interpersonal differences in both style and problem-solving that account for variations in the way practitioners collect and record data for the same patient under the same circumstances. Such variations do not necessarily reflect good practices, however, and much of medical education is directed at helping physicians and other health professionals to learn what observations to make, how to make them (generally an issue of technique), how to interpret them, and how to decide whether they warrant formal recording.

An example of this phenomenon is the difference between the first medical history, physical examination, and written report developed by a medical student and the similar process undertaken by a seasoned clinician examining the same patient. Medical students tend to work from comprehensive mental outlines of questions to ask, physical tests to perform, and additional data to collect. Because they have not developed skills of selectivity, the process of taking a medical history and performing a physical examination may take more than 1 hour, after which the student writes an extensive report of what she observed and how she has interpreted her observations. It clearly would be impractical, inefficient, and inappropriate for physicians in practice to spend this amount of time assessing every new patient. Thus, part of the challenge for the neophyte is to learn how to ask only the questions that are necessary, to perform only the examination components that are required, and to record only those data that will be pertinent in justifying the ongoing diagnostic approach and in guiding the future management of the patient.

What do we mean by **selectivity** in data collection and recording? It is precisely this process that often is viewed as a central part of the "art of medicine," an element that accounts for individual styles and the sometimes marked distinctions among clinicians. As is discussed with numerous clinical examples in Chapter 3, the idea of selectivity implies an ongoing decision-making process that guides data collection and interpretation. Attempts to understand how expert clinicians internalize this process, and to formalize the ideas so that they can better be taught and explained, are central in medical-informatics research. Improved guidelines for such decision-making, derived from research activities in medical informatics, not only are enhancing the teaching and practice of medicine but also are providing insights that suggest methods for developing computer-based decision-support tools.

2.5.1 The Hypothetico-Deductive Approach

Studies of medical decision-makers have shown that strategies for data collection and interpretation may be imbedded in an iterative process known as the **hypothetico-deductive approach** (Elstein et al., 1978; Kassirer & Gorry, 1978). As medical students learn this process, their data collection becomes more focused and efficient, and their medical records become more compact. The central idea is one of sequential, staged data collection, followed by data interpretation and the generation of hypotheses, leading to hypothesis-directed selection of the next most appropriate data to be collected. As data are collected at each stage, they are added to the growing database of observations and are used to reformulate or refine the active hypotheses. This process is iterated until one hypothesis reaches a threshold level of certainty (e.g., it is proved to be true, or at least the uncertainty is reduced to a satisfactory level). At that point, a management, disposition, or therapeutic decision can be made.

This process is clarified by the diagram in Figure 2.11. As is shown, data collection begins when the patient presents to the physician with some complaint (a

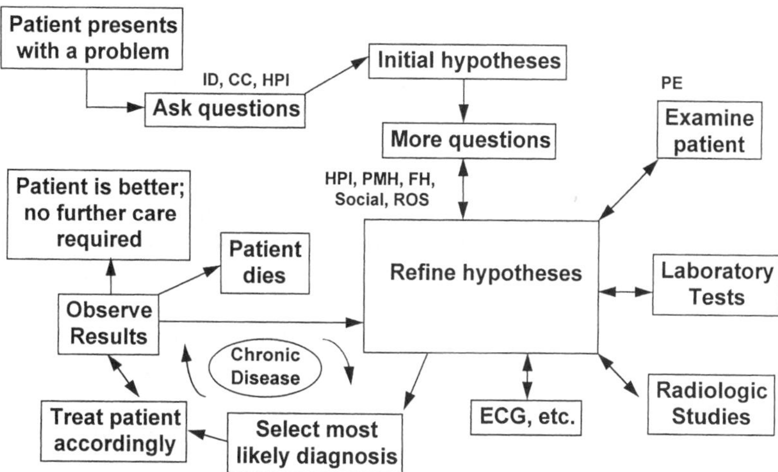

FIGURE 2.11. A schematic view of the hypothetico-deductive approach. The process of medical data collection and treatment is intimately tied to an ongoing process of hypothesis generation and refinement. See text for full discussion. ID = patient identification; CC = chief complaint; HPI = history of present illness; PMH = past medical history; FH = family history; Social = social history; ROS = review of systems; PE = physical examination.

symptom or disease). The physician generally responds with a few questions that allow her to focus rapidly on the nature of the problem. In the written report, the data collected with these initial questions typically are recorded as the patient identification, chief complaint, and initial portion of the history of the present illness. Studies have shown that an experienced physician will have an initial set of hypotheses (theories) in mind after hearing the patient's response to the first six or seven questions (Elstein et al., 1978). These hypotheses then serve as the basis for selecting additional questions. As shown in Figure 2.11, answers to these additional questions allow the physician to refine her hypotheses about what is the source of the patient's problem. Physicians refer to the set of active hypotheses as the differential diagnosis for a patient; the **differential diagnosis** comprises the set of possible diagnoses among which the physician must distinguish to determine how best to administer treatment.

Note that the question-selection process is inherently *heuristic;* for example, it is personalized and efficient, but it is not guaranteed to collect every piece of information that might be pertinent. Human beings use heuristics all the time in their decision-making because it often is impractical or impossible to use an exhaustive problem-solving approach. A common example of heuristic problem-solving is the playing of a complex game such as chess. Because it would require an enormous amount of time to define all the possible moves and countermoves that could ensue from a given board position, expert chess players develop personal heuristics for assessing the game at any point and then selecting a strategy for how best to proceed. Differences among such heuristics account in part for variations in observed expertise.

Physicians have developed safety measures, however, to help them avoid missing important issues that they might not discover when collecting data in a hypothesis-directed fashion during the history taking for the present illness (Pauker et al., 1976). These measures tend to be focused in four general categories of questions that follow the collection of information about the chief complaint: past medical history, family history, social history, and a brief **review of systems** in which the physician asks some general questions about the state of health of each of the major organ systems in the body. Occasionally, the physician discovers entirely new problems or finds important information that modifies the hypothesis list or modulates the treatment options available (e.g., if the patient reports a serious past drug reaction or allergy).

When the physician has finished asking questions, the refined hypothesis list (which may already be narrowed to a single diagnosis) then serves as the basis for a focused physical examination. By this time, the physician may well have expectations of what she will find on examination or may have specific tests in mind that will help her to distinguish among still active hypotheses about diseases based on the questions that she has asked. Once again, as in the question-asking process, focused hypothesis-directed examination is augmented with general tests that occasionally turn up new abnormalities and generate hypotheses that the physician did not expect on the basis of the medical history alone. In addition, unexplained findings on examination may raise issues that require additional history taking. Thus, the asking of questions generally is partially integrated with the examination process.

When the physician has completed the physical examination, her refined hypothesis list may be narrowed sufficiently that she can undertake specific treatment. It often is necessary to gather additional data, however. Such testing is once again guided by the current hypotheses. The options available include laboratory tests (of blood, urine, other body fluids, or biopsy specimens), radiologic studies (X-ray examinations, nuclear-imaging scans, computed-tomography studies, magnetic-resonance scans, sonograms, or any of a number of other imaging modalities), and other specialized tests (electrocardiograms, electroencephalograms, nerve-conduction studies, and many others). As the results of such studies become available, the physician constantly revises and refines her hypothesis list.

Ultimately, the physician is sufficiently certain about the source of a patient's problem to be able to develop a specific management plan. Treatments are administered, and the patient is observed. Note that the response to treatment is itself a datum point that may affect the hypotheses about a patient's illness. If the patient does not respond to treatment, it may mean that the disease is resistant to that therapy and that the physician should try an alternate approach, or it may mean that the initial diagnosis was incorrect and that she should consider alternate explanations for the patient's complaint.

The patient may remain in a cycle of treatment and observation for a long time, as shown in Figure 2.11. This long cycle reflects the nature of chronic-disease management—an aspect of medical care that is accounting for an increasing proportion of the healthcare community's work (and an increasing proportion of the healthcare dollar). Alternatively, the patient may recover and no longer need therapy, or he may die. Although the process outlined in Figure 2.11 is oversimplified in many regards, it is generally applicable to the process of data collection, diagnosis, and treatment in most areas of medicine.

Note that the hypothesis-directed process of data collection, diagnosis, and treatment is inherently *knowledge based.* It is dependent not only on a significant fact base that permits proper interpretation of data and selection of appropriate follow-up questions and tests but also on the effective use of heuristic techniques that characterize individual expertise.

Another important issue, addressed in Chapter 3, is the need for physicians to balance financial costs and health risks of data collection against the perceived benefits to be gained when those data become available. It costs nothing but time to examine the patient at the bedside or to ask an additional question, but if the data being considered require, for example, X-ray exposure, coronary angiography, or a computed tomogram of the head (all of which have associated risks and costs), then it may be preferable to proceed with treatment in the absence of full information. Differences in the assessment of cost-benefit trade-offs in data collection often account for differences of opinion among collaborating physicians.

2.5.2 The Relationship Between Data and Hypotheses

We wrote rather glibly in the preceding section about the "generation of hypotheses from data"; now we need to ask: What precisely is the nature of that process? Researchers with a psychological orientation have spent much time trying to understand how expert problem-solvers evoke hypotheses (Elstein et al., 1978; Pauker et al., 1976; Pople, 1982) and the traditional probabilistic decision sciences have much to say about that process as well. We provide only a brief introduction to these ideas here; they are discussed in greater detail in Chapter 3.

When an observation evokes a hypothesis (e.g., when a clinical finding makes a specific diagnosis come to mind), the observation presumably has some close association with the hypothesis. What might be the characteristics of that association? Perhaps the finding is almost always observed when the hypothesis turns out to be true; is that enough to explain hypothesis generation? A simple example will show that such a simple relationship is *not* enough to explain the evocation process. Consider the hypothesis that a patient is pregnant and the observation that the patient is female. Clearly, all pregnant patients are female. When a new patient is observed to be female, however, the possibility that the patient is pregnant is not immediately evoked. Thus, female gender is a highly *sensitive* indicator of pregnancy (there is a 100 percent chance that a pregnant patient is female), but it is not a good *predictor* of pregnancy (most females are not pregnant). The idea of **sensitivity**—the likelihood that a given datum will be observed in a patient with a given disease or condition—is an important one, but it will not alone account for the process of hypothesis generation in medical diagnosis.

Perhaps the clinical manifestation seldom occurs unless the hypothesis turns out to be true; is that enough to explain hypothesis generation? This idea seems to be a little closer to the mark. Suppose that a given datum is *never* seen unless a patient has a specific disease. For example, a Pap smear (a smear of cells swabbed from the cervix, at the opening to the uterus, treated with Papanicolaou's stain, and then examined under the microscope) with grossly abnormal cells (called class IV findings) is never seen unless the woman has cancer of the cervix or uterus. Such tests are called **pathognomonic**. Not only do they evoke a specific diagnosis but they also immediately prove it to be true. Unfortunately, there are few pathognomonic tests in medicine.

More commonly, a feature is seen in one disease or disease category more frequently than it is in others, but the association is not absolute. For example, there are few disease entities other than infections that elevate a patient's white-blood-cell count. Certainly it is true, for example, that leukemia can raise the white-blood-cell count, as can the use of the drug prednisone, but *most* patients who do not have infections will have normal white-blood-cell counts. An elevated white count therefore does not *prove* a patient has an infection, but it does tend to evoke or support the hypothesis that an infection is present. The word used to describe this relationship is **specificity**. An observation is highly specific for a disease if it is generally not seen in patients who do not have that disease. A pathognomonic observation is 100 percent specific for a given disease. When an observation is highly specific for a disease, it tends to evoke that disease during the diagnostic or data-gathering process.

By now, you may have realized that there is a substantial difference between a physician viewing test results that evoke a disease hypothesis and that physician being willing to act on the disease hypothesis. Yet even experienced physicians sometimes fail to recognize that, although they have made an observation that is highly specific for a given disease, it may still be more likely that the patient has other diseases (and does not have the suspected one) unless (1) the finding is pathognomonic or (2) the suspected disease is considerably more common than are the other diseases that can cause the observed abnormality. This mistake is one of the most common errors of intuition that has been identified in the medical decision-making process. To explain the basis for this confusion in more detail, we must introduce two additional terms: *prevalence* and *predictive value*.

The **prevalence** of a disease is simply a measure of the frequency with which the disease occurs in the population of interest. A given disease may have a prevalence of only 5 percent in the general population (one person in 20 will have the disease) but have a higher prevalence in a specially selected subpopulation. For example, black-lung disease has a low prevalence in the general population but has a much higher prevalence among coal miners, who develop black lung from inhaling coal dust. The task of diagnosis therefore involves *updating* the probability that a patient has a disease from the **baseline rate** (the prevalence in the population from which the patient was selected) to a post-test probability that reflects the test results. For example, the probability that any given person in the United States has lung cancer is low (i.e., the prevalence of the disease is low), but it is much higher if his chest X-ray examination shows a possible tumor. If the patient were a member of the population composed of cigarette smokers in the United States, however, then the prevalence of lung cancer would be higher. In this case, the *same* chest X-ray report would result in an even higher updated probability of lung cancer than it would had the patient been selected from the population of all people in the United States.

The **predictive value** of a test is simply the post-test (updated) *probability* that a disease is present based on the results of a test. If an observation supports the presence of a disease, the predictive value will be greater than the prevalence (also called the *pretest risk*). If the observation tends to argue against the presence of a disease, the predictive value will be lower than the prevalence. For any test and disease, then, there is one predictive value if the test result is positive and another predictive value if the test result is negative. These values are typically abbreviated PV^+ (the predictive value of a positive test) and PV^- (the predictive value of a negative test).

The process of hypothesis generation in medical diagnosis thus involves both the evocation of hypotheses *and* the assignment of a likelihood (probability) to the presence of a specific disease or disease category. The predictive value of a positive test depends on the test's sensitivity, specificity, and prevalence. The formula that describes the relationship precisely is

$$PV^+ = \frac{(\text{sensitivity})(\text{prevalence})}{(\text{sensitivity})(\text{prevalence}) + (1 - \text{specificity})\,(1 - \text{prevalence})}.$$

There is a similar formula for defining PV^- in terms of sensitivity, specificity, and prevalence. Both formulae can be derived from simple probability theory. Note that positive tests with high sensitivity and specificity may still lead to a low post-test probability of the disease (PV^+) if the prevalence of that disease is low. You should substitute values in the PV^+ formula to convince yourself that this assertion is true. It is this relationship that tends to be poorly understood by practitioners and that often is viewed as counterintuitive (which shows that your intuition can misguide you). Note also (by substitution into the formula) that test sensitivity and disease prevalence can be ignored *only* when a test is pathognomonic (i.e., when its specificity is 100 percent, which mandates that PV^+ be 100 percent). The PV^+ formula is one of many forms of Bayes' theorem, a rule for combining probabilistic data that is generally attributed to the work of Reverend Thomas Bayes in the 1700s. Bayes' theorem is discussed in greater detail in Chapter 3.

2.5.3 Methods for Selecting Questions and Comparing Tests

We have described the process of hypothesis-directed sequential data collection and have asked how an observation might evoke or refine the physician's hypotheses about what abnormalities account for the patient's illness. The complementary question is: Given a set of current hypotheses, how does the physician decide what additional data should be collected? This question also has been analyzed at length (Elstein et al., 1978; Pople, 1982) and is pertinent for computer programs that gather data efficiently to assist clinicians with diagnosis or with therapeutic decision-making (see Chapter 16). Because understanding issues of test selection and data interpretation is crucial to understanding medical data and their uses, we devote the next chapter to these and related issues of medical decision-making. In Section 3.6, for example, we shall discuss the use of decision-analytic techniques in deciding whether to treat a patient on the basis of available information or to perform additional diagnostic tests.

2.6 The Computer and Collection of Medical Data

Although this chapter has not directly discussed computer systems, the potential role of the computer in medical data storage, retrieval, and interpretation should be clear. Much of the rest of this book deals with specific applications in which the computer's primary role is data management. One question is pertinent to all such applications: How do you get the data into the computer in the first place?

The need for data entry by physicians has posed a problem for medical-computing systems since the earliest days of the field. Awkward or nonintuitive interactions at computer terminals—particularly ones requiring keyboard typing by the physician—have probably done more to inhibit the clinical use of computers than have any other factor. Doctors, and many other healthcare staff, tend simply to refuse to use computers because of the awkward interfaces that are imposed.

A variety of approaches have been used to try to finesse this problem. One is to design systems such that clerical staff can do essentially all the data entry and much of the data retrieval as well. Many clinical-research systems have taken this approach. Physicians may be asked to fill out structured paper data sheets, or such sheets may be filled out by data abstractors who review patient charts, but the actual entry of data into the database is done by paid transcriptionists.

In some applications, it is possible for data to be entered automatically into the computer by the device that measures or collects them. For example, monitors in intensive-care or coronary-care units, pulmonary-function or ECG machines, and measurement equipment in the clinical chemistry laboratory can interface directly with a computer in which a database is stored. Certain data can be entered directly by patients; there are systems, for example, that take the patient's history by presenting on a terminal multiple-choice questions that follow a branching logic. The patient's responses to the questions are used to generate hard copy reports for physicians and also may be stored directly in a computer database for subsequent use in other settings.

When physicians or other health personnel do use the machine themselves, specialized devices often allow rapid and intuitive operator-machine interaction. Most of these devices use a variant of the "point-and-select" approach—for ex-

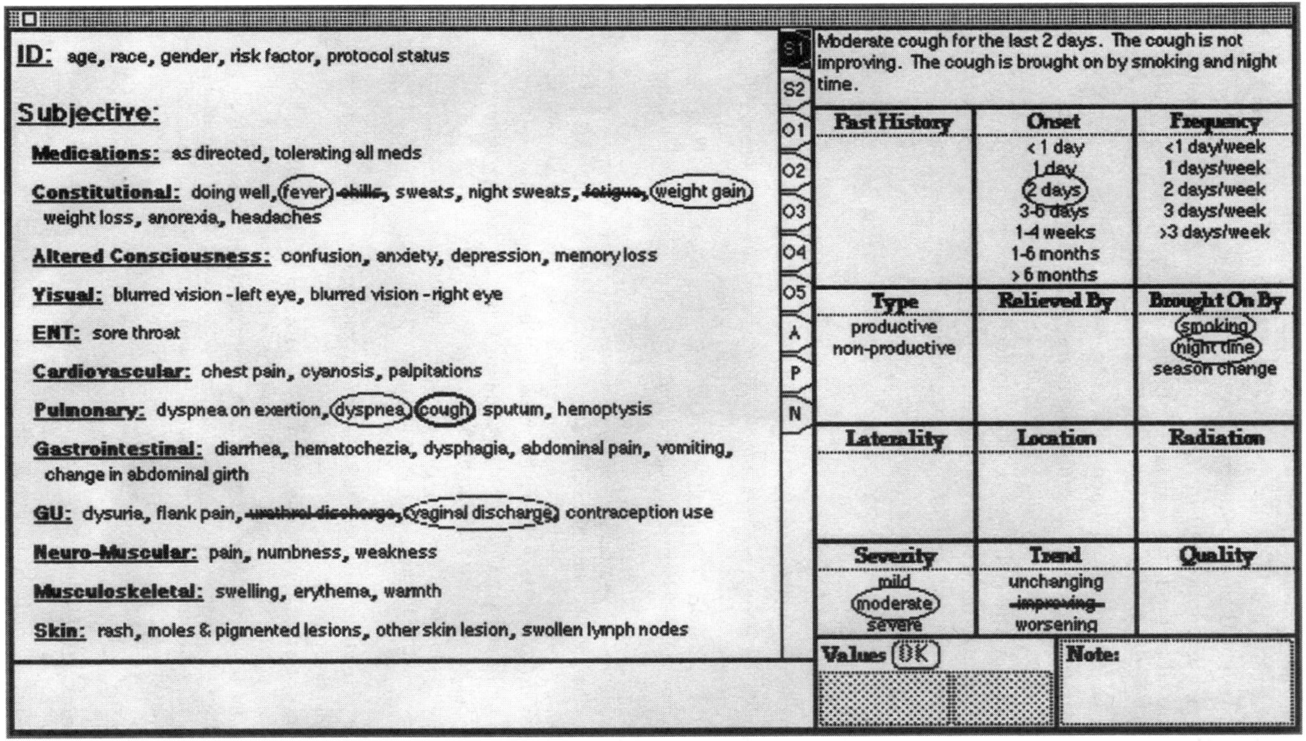

FIGURE 2.12. The user interface for PEN-Ivory, a prototype system for the entry of progress notes. The left side of the screen represents the encounter form on which the names of medical findings are listed. The right side represents the attributes palette, used to augment findings with specific modifiers (in this case, modifiers refer to "cough," the current entry, which is circled in bold on the encounter form. Users circle, line out, and scratch out words to interact with the system. A text translation of the selected finding and its attributes is displayed at the top right. The page tabs located between the encounter form and the attributes palette are used to move among the pages of the encounter form. (Example screen courtesy of Alex Poon. See also Poon A.D., Fagan L.M., Shortliffe E.H. [1996]. The PEN-Ivory project: Exploring user-interface design for the selection of items from large controlled vocabularies of medicine. *Journal of the American Medical Informatics Association,* 3(2):168–183).

ample, touch-sensitive screens, light pens, and mouse pointing devices (see Chapter 4). When conventional terminals are used, specialized keypads can be helpful. Designers frequently permit logical selection of items from menus displayed on the screen so that the user does not need to learn a set of specialized commands to enter or review data. Recently we have seen the introduction of handheld tablets with pen-based mechanisms for data entry. Some of the experimental work on pen-based methods for structured clinical data entry are particularly promising (Fig. 2.12).

These issues arise in essentially all application areas, and, because they can be crucial to the successful implementation and use of a system, they warrant particular attention in system design. As more physicians are becoming familiar with computers at home, they will find the use of computers in their practice less of a hinderance. We encourage you to consider human-computer interaction as you learn about the application areas and the specific systems described in later chapters.

Suggested Readings

Campbell J.R., Carpenter P., Sneiderman C., Cohn S., Chute C.G., Warren J. (1997). Phase II evaluation of clinical coding schemes: Completeness, taxonomy, mapping, definitions, and clarity. *Journal of the American Medical Informatics Association* 4(3):238–251; and Chute C.G., Cohn S., Campbell K.E., Oliver D., Campbell J.R. (1996). The content coverage of clinical classifications. *Journal of the American Medical Informatics Association*, 3(3):224–233.

This pair of articles reports on a detailed study of various systems for coding clinical terminology. The authors attempt to characterize each coding scheme with respect to its ability to express common clinical concepts, demonstrating that none was yet sufficiently robust to encode the complete medical record of a patient.

Patel V.L., Arocha J.F., Kaufman, D.R. (1994). Diagnostic reasoning and medical expertise. *Psychology of Learning and Motivation*, 31:187–252.

This paper illustrates the role of theory-driven psychological research and cognitive evaluation as they relate to medical decision-making and the interpretation of clinical data.

van Bemmel J.H., et al (Eds). (1988). Data, information and knowledge in medicine. *Methods of Information in Medicine*, Special issue, 27(3).

This special issue of *Methods of Information in Medicine* contains about 40 articles that were published previously in the journal. It provides a historical perspective on scientific developments in medical informatics. The first section presents 10 papers on various aspects of medical data. The remaining sections are devoted to medical systems, medical information and patterns, medical knowledge and decision-making, and medical research.

Questions for Discussion

1. You check your pulse and discover that your heart rate is 100 beats per minute. Is this rate normal or abnormal? What additional information would you use in making this judgment? How does the *context* in which data are collected influence the interpretation of those data?

2. Given the imprecision of many medical terms, why do you think that serious instances of miscommunication among healthcare professionals are not more common? Why is greater standardization of terminology necessary if computers rather than humans are to manipulate patient data?
3. Based on the discussion of coding schemes for representing medical information, discuss three challenges you foresee in attempting to construct a standardized medical terminology to be used in hospitals, physicians' offices, and research institutions throughout the United States.
4. How would medical practice change if nonphysicians were to collect all medical data?
5. To decide whether a patient has a significant urinary-tract infection, physicians commonly use a calculation of the number of bacterial organisms in a milliliter of the patient's urine. Physicians generally assume that a patient has a urinary-tract infection if there are at least 10,000 bacteria per milliliter. Although laboratories can provide such a quantification with reasonable accuracy, it is obviously unrealistic for the physician explicitly to count large numbers of bacteria by examining a milliliter of urine under the microscope. As a result, one recent article offers the following guideline to physicians: "When interpreting . . . microscopy of . . . stained centrifuged urine, a threshold of one organism per field yields a 95 percent sensitivity and five organisms per field a 95 percent specificity for bacteriuria [bacteria in the urine] at a level of at least 10,000 organisms per ml" (Senior Medical Review, 1987, p. 4).
   a. Describe an experiment that would have allowed the researchers to determine the sensitivity and specificity of the microscopy.
   b. How would you expect specificity to change as the number of bacteria per microscopic field increases from one to five?
   c. How would you expect sensitivity to change as the number of bacteria per microscopic field increases from one to five?
   d. Why does it take more organisms per microscopic field to obtain a specificity of 95 percent than it does to achieve a sensitivity of 95 percent?

3
Medical Decision-Making: Probabilistic Medical Reasoning

Douglas K. Owens and Harold C. Sox

After reading this chapter, you should know the answers to these questions:

- How is the concept of probability useful for understanding test results and for making medical decisions that involve uncertainty?
- How can we characterize the ability of a test to discriminate between disease and health?
- What information do we need to interpret test results accurately?
- What is *expected-value decision-making?* How can this methodology help us to understand particular medical problems?
- What are utilities, and how can we use them to represent patients' preferences?
- What is a *sensitivity analysis?* How can we use it to examine the robustness of a decision and to identify the important variables in a decision?
- What are influence diagrams? How do they differ from decision trees?

3.1 The Nature of Clinical Decisions: Uncertainty and the Process of Diagnosis

Because clinical data are imperfect and outcomes of treatment are uncertain, health professionals often are faced with difficult choices. In this chapter, we introduce *probabilistic medical reasoning*, an approach that can help healthcare providers to deal with the uncertainty inherent in many medical decisions. Medical decisions are made by a variety of methods; our approach is neither necessary nor appropriate for all decisions. Throughout the chapter, we provide simple clinical examples that illustrate a broad range of problems for which probabilistic medical reasoning does provide valuable insight.

As discussed in Chapter 2, medical practice *is* medical decision-making. In this chapter, we look at the *process* of medical decision-making. Together, Chapters 2 and 3 lay the groundwork for the rest of the book. In the remaining chapters, we discuss ways that computers can help clinicians with the decision-making process, and we emphasize the relationship between information needs and system design and implementation.

The material in this chapter is presented in the context of the decisions made by an individual physician. The concepts, however, are more broadly applicable.

Sensitivity and specificity are important parameters of laboratory systems that flag abnormal test results, of patient monitoring systems (Chapter 13), and of information-retrieval systems (Chapter 15). An understanding of what probability is and of how to adjust probabilities after the acquisition of new information is a foundation for our study of clinical consultation systems (Chapter 16). The importance of probability in medical decision-making was noted as long ago as 1922: "good medicine does not consist in the indiscriminate application of laboratory examinations to a patient, but rather in having so clear a comprehension of the probabilities and possibilities of a case as to know what tests may be expected to give information of value" (Peabody, 1922).

> **Example 1.** You are the director of a large urban blood bank. All potential blood donors are tested to ensure that they are not infected with the human immunodeficiency virus (HIV), the causative agent of acquired immunodeficiency syndrome (AIDS). You ask whether use of the polymerase chain reaction (PCR), a gene-amplification technique that can diagnose HIV, would be useful to identify people who have HIV. The PCR test is positive 98 percent of the time when antibody is present, and it is negative 99 percent of the time antibody is absent.[1]

If the test is positive, what is the likelihood that a donor actually has HIV? If the test is negative, how sure can you be that the person does not have HIV? On an intuitive level, these questions do not seem particularly difficult to answer. The test appears accurate, and we would expect that, if the test is positive, the donated blood specimen is likely to contain the HIV. Thus, we are shaken to find that, if only one in 1,000 donors actually is infected, the test is more often mistaken than it is correct. In fact, of 100 donors with a positive test, fewer than 10 would be infected. *There would be 10 wrong answers for each correct result.* How are we to understand this result? Before we try to find an answer, let us consider a related example.

> **Example 2.** Mr. James is a 59-year-old man with coronary artery disease (narrowing or blockage of the blood vessels that supply the heart tissue). When the heart muscle does not receive enough oxygen (hypoxia) because blood cannot reach it, the patient often experiences chest pain (angina). Mr. James has twice had coronary-artery bypass graft (CABG) surgery, a procedure in which new vessels, usually taken from the leg, are grafted onto the old ones such that blood is shunted past the blocked region. Unfortunately, he has begun to have chest pain again that becomes progressively more severe, despite medication. If the heart muscle is deprived of oxygen, the result can be a heart attack (myocardial infarction), in which a section of the muscle dies.

Should Mr. James undergo a third operation? The medications are not working; without surgery, he runs a high risk of suffering a heart attack, which may be fatal. On the other hand, the surgery is hazardous. Not only is the surgical

---

[1]The test sensitivity and specificity used in Example 1 are consistent with reported values of the sensitivity and specificity of the PCR test for diagnosis of HIV, but the accuracy of the test varies across laboratories (Owens et al., 1996b).

mortality rate for a third operation higher than that for a first or second one but also the chance that surgery will relieve the chest pain is lower than for a first operation. All choices in Example 2 entail considerable uncertainty. Furthermore, the risks are grave; an incorrect decision may substantially increase the chance that Mr. James will die. The decision will be difficult even for experienced clinicians.

These examples illustrate situations in which intuition is either misleading or inadequate. Although the test results in Example 1 are appropriate for the blood bank, a physician who uncritically reports these results would erroneously inform many people that they had the AIDS virus—a mistake with profound emotional and social consequences. In Example 2, the decision-making skill of the physician will affect a patient's quality and length of life. Similar situations are commonplace in medicine. Our goal in this chapter is to show how the use of probability and decision analysis can help to make clear the best course of action.

Decision-making is one of the quintessential activities of the healthcare professional. Some decisions are made on the basis of deductive reasoning or of physiological principles. Many decisions, however, are made on the basis of knowledge that has been gained through collective experience: The clinician often must rely on empirical knowledge of associations between symptoms and disease to evaluate a problem. A decision that is based on these usually imperfect associations will be, to some degree, uncertain. In Sections 3.1.1 through 3.1.3, we examine decisions made under uncertainty and present an overview of the diagnostic process. As Lloyd H. Smith, Jr., said, "Medical decisions based on probabilities are necessary but also perilous. Even the most astute physician will occasionally be wrong" (Smith, 1985, p. 3).

3.1.1 Decision-Making Under Uncertainty

Example 3. Mr. Kirk, a 33-year-old man with a history of a previous blood clot (thrombus) in a vein in his left leg, presents with the complaint of pain and swelling in that leg for the past 5 days. On physical examination, the leg is tender and swollen to midcalf—*signs* that suggest the possibility of deep-vein thrombosis.[2] A test (ultrasonography) is performed, and the flow of blood in the veins of Mr. Kirk's leg is evaluated. The blood flow is abnormal, but the radiologist cannot tell whether there is a new blood clot.

Should Mr. Kirk be treated for blood clots? The main diagnostic concern is the recurrence of a blood clot in his leg. A clot in the veins of the leg can dislodge, flow with the blood, and cause a blockage in the vessels of the lungs, a potentially fatal event called a *pulmonary embolus*. Of patients with a swollen

---

[2]In medicine, a *sign* is an objective physical finding (something observed by the clinician) such as a temperature of 101.2°F. A *symptom* is a subjective experience of the patient, such as feeling hot or feverish. The distinction may be blurred if the patient's experience also can be observed by the clinician.

leg, about one-half actually have a blood clot; there are numerous other causes of a swollen leg. Given a swollen leg, therefore, a physician cannot be sure that a clot is the cause. Thus, the physical findings leave considerable uncertainty. Furthermore, in Example 3, the results of the available diagnostic test are equivocal. The treatment for a blood clot is to administer anticoagulants (drugs that inhibit blood-clot formation), which pose the risk of excessive bleeding to the patient. Therefore, the physician does not want to treat the patient unless she is confident that a thrombus is present. But how much confidence *should* be required before starting treatment? We will learn that it is possible to answer this question by calculating the benefits and harms of treatment.

This example illustrates an important concept: Clinical data are imperfect. The degree of imperfection varies, but all clinical data—including the results of diagnostic tests, the history given by the patient, and the findings on physical examination—are uncertain.

3.1.2 Probability: An Alternative Method of Expressing Uncertainty

The language that physicians use to describe a patient's condition often is ambiguous—a factor that further complicates the problem of uncertainty in medical decision-making. Physicians use words such as "probable" and "highly likely" to describe their beliefs about the likelihood of disease. These words have strikingly different meanings to different individuals (Fig. 3.1). Because of the widespread disagreement about the meaning of common descriptive terms, there is ample opportunity for miscommunication.

The problem of how to express degrees of uncertainty is not unique to medicine. How is it handled in other contexts? Horse racing has its share of uncertainty. If experienced gamblers are deciding whether to place bets, they will find it unsatisfactory to be told that a given horse has a "high chance" of winning. They will demand to know the odds.

The **odds** are simply an alternate way to express a probability. The use of probability or odds as an expression of uncertainty avoids the ambiguities inherent in common descriptive terms.

3.1.3 Overview of the Diagnostic Process

In Chapter 2, we described the hypothetico-deductive approach, a diagnostic strategy comprising successive iterations of hypothesis generation, data collection, and interpretation. We discussed how observations may evoke a hypothesis and how new information subsequently may increase or decrease our belief in that hypothesis. Here, we review this process briefly in light of a specific example. For the purpose of our discussion, we separate the diagnostic process into three stages.

The first stage involves making an *initial judgment* about whether a patient is likely to have a disease. After an interview and physical examination, a physi-

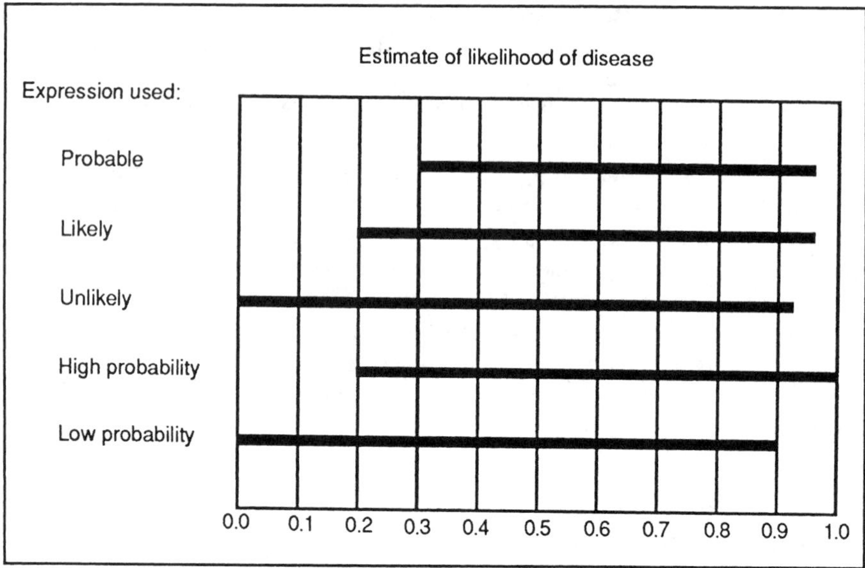

FIGURE 3.1. Probability and descriptive terms. Different physicians attach different meanings to the same terms. The bars show the wide variation in point probabilities assigned by individual physicians and other healthcare workers when they were asked to interpret these terms. (*Source:* reprinted, by permission, from Bryant G.D., Norman, G.R. [1980]. Expressions of probability: Words and numbers. *New England Journal of Medicine,* 302:411.)

cian intuitively develops a belief about the likelihood of disease. This judgment may be based on previous experience or on knowledge of the medical literature. A physician's belief about the likelihood of disease usually is implicit; she can refine it by making an explicit estimation of the probability of disease. This estimated probability, made before further information is obtained, is the **prior probability** or **pre-test probability** of disease.

Example 4. Mr. Smith, a 60-year-old man, complains to his physician that he has pressurelike chest pain that occurs when he walks quickly. After taking his history and examining him, his physician believes there is a high enough chance that he has heart disease to warrant ordering an exercise stress test. In the stress test, an electrocardiogram (ECG) is taken while Mr. Smith exercises. Because the heart must pump more blood per stroke and must beat faster (and thus requires more oxygen) during exercise, many heart conditions are evident only when the patient is physically stressed. Mr. Smith's results show abnormal changes in the ECG during exercise—a sign of heart disease.

How would the physician evaluate this patient? She would first talk to the patient about the quality, duration, and severity of his pain. Traditionally, she would then decide what to do next based on her intuition about the etiology (cause) of the chest pain. Our approach is to ask her to make her initial intuition explicit by estimating the pretest probability of disease. The clinician in this example, based on what she knows from talking with the patient, might assess the pretest or prior probability of heart disease as 0.5 (50 percent chance or 1:1 odds; see Section 3.2). We explore methods used to estimate pretest probability accurately in Section 3.2.

After the pretest probability of disease has been estimated, the second stage of the diagnostic process involves gathering more information, often by performing a diagnostic test. The physician in Example 4 ordered a test to reduce her uncertainty about the diagnosis of heart disease. The positive test result supports the diagnosis of heart disease, and this reduction in uncertainty is shown in Figure 3.2a. Although the physician in Example 4 chose the exercise stress

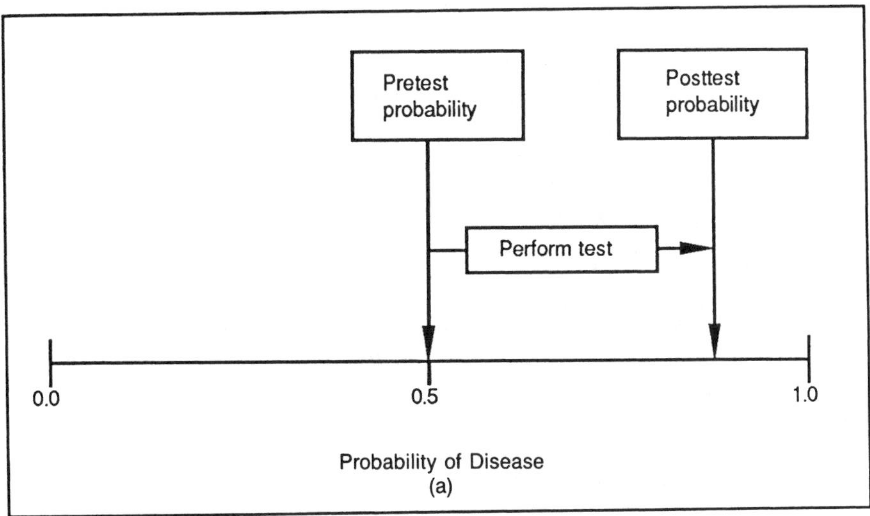

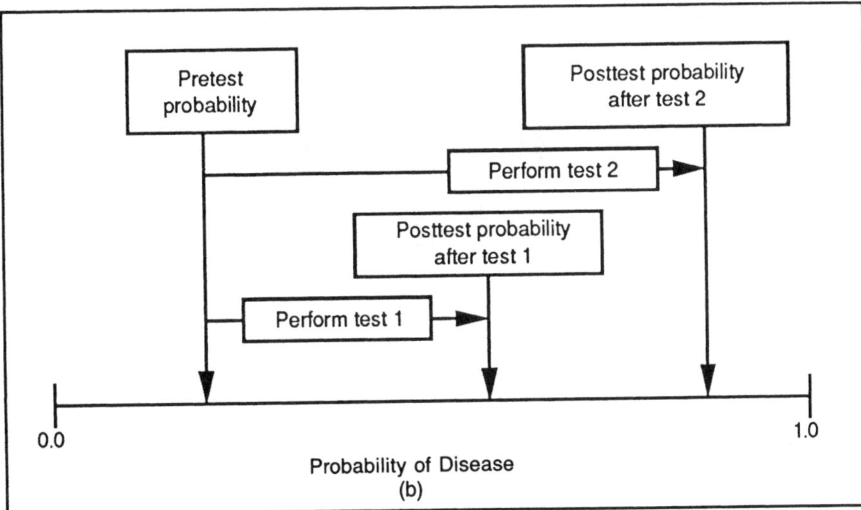

Figure 3.2. The effect of test results on the probability of disease. *(a)* A positive test result often increases the probability of disease. *(b)* Test 2 reduces uncertainty about presence of disease (increases the probability of disease) more than test 1 does.

test, there are many tests available to diagnose heart disease, and she would like to know which test she should order next. Some tests reduce uncertainty more than do others (see Fig. 3.2b), but may cost more. The more a test reduces uncertainty, the more useful it is. In Section 3.3, we explore ways to measure how well a test reduces uncertainty, expanding the concepts of test sensitivity and specificity first introduced in Chapter 2.

Given new information provided by a test, the third step is to update the initial probability estimate. The physician in Example 4 must ask, "What is the probability of disease given the abnormal stress test?" The physician wants to know the **posterior probability**, or **post-test probability**, of disease (see Fig. 3.2a). In Section 3.4, we reexamine Bayes' theorem, introduced in Chapter 2, and we discuss its use for calculating the post-test probability of disease. As we noted, to calculate post-test probability, we must know the pretest probability, as well as the sensitivity and specificity, of the test.[3]

3.2 Probability Assessment: Methods to Assess Pretest Probability

In this section, we explore the methods that physicians can use to make judgments about the probability of disease before they order tests. **Probability** is our preferred means of expressing uncertainty. In this framework, probability (p) expresses a physician's opinion about the likelihood of an event as a number between 0 and 1. An event that is certain to occur has a probability of 1; an event that is certain not to occur has a probability of 0.[4]

The probability of event A is written $p[A]$. The sum of the probabilities of all possible, collectively exhaustive outcomes of a chance event must be equal to 1. Thus, in a coin flip,

$$p[\text{heads}] + p[\text{tails}] = 1.0.$$

The probability of event A and event B occurring together is denoted by $p[A\&B]$ or by $p[A,B]$.

Events A and B are considered **independent** if the occurrence of one does not influence the probability of the occurrence of the other. The probability of two independent events A and B both occurring is given by the product of the individual probabilities:

$$p[A,B] = p[A] \times p[B].$$

[3]Note that pretest and post-test probabilities correspond to the concepts of prevalence and predictive value. The latter terms were used in Chapter 2 because the discussion was about the use of tests for screening *populations* of patients; in a population, the pretest probability of disease is simply that disease's prevalence in that population.

[4]We assume a Bayesian interpretation of probability; there are other statistical interpretations of probability.

Thus, the probability of heads on two consecutive coin tosses is $0.5 \times 0.5 = 0.25$. (Regardless of the outcome of the first toss, the probability of heads on the second toss is 0.5.)

The probability that event A will occur given that event B is known to occur is called the **conditional probability** of event A *given* event B, denoted by $p[A|B]$ and read as "the probability of A given B." Thus a post-test probability is a conditional probability predicated on the test or finding being positive. For example, if 30 percent of patients who have a swollen leg have a blood clot, we say the probability of a blood clot given a swollen leg is 0.3, denoted

$$p[\text{bloodclot}|\text{swollenleg}] = 0.3.$$

Before the swollen leg is noted, the pretest probability is simply the prevalence of blood clots in the leg in the population from which the patient was selected—a number likely to be much smaller than 0.3.

Now that we have decided to use probability to express uncertainty, how can we estimate probability? We can do so by either subjective or objective methods; each approach has advantages and limitations.

3.2.1 Subjective Probability Assessment

Most assessments that physicians make about probability are based on personal experience. The physician may compare the current problem to similar problems encountered previously and then ask, "What was the frequency of disease in similar patients whom I have seen?"

To make these subjective assessments of probability, people rely on several discrete, often unconscious mental processes that have been described and studied by cognitive psychologists (Tversky & Kahneman, 1974). These processes are termed **cognitive heuristics**.

More specifically, a cognitive heuristic is a mental process by which we learn, recall, or process information; we can think of heuristics as rules of thumb. Knowledge of heuristics is important because it helps us to understand the underpinnings of our intuitive probability assessment. Both naive and sophisticated decision-makers (including physicians and statisticians) misuse heuristics and therefore make systematic—often serious—errors when estimating probability. So, just as we may underestimate distances on a particularly clear day (Tversky & Kahneman, 1974), we may make mistakes in estimating probability in deceptive clinical situations. Three heuristics have been identified as important in estimation of probability: the representativeness heuristic, the availability heuristic, and the anchoring and adjustment heuristic.

- *Representativeness.* One way that people estimate probability is to ask themselves: What is the probability that object A belongs to class B? For instance, what is the probability that this patient who has a swollen leg belongs to the class of patients who have blood clots? To answer, we often rely on the **representativeness** heuristic in which probabilities are judged by the degree to which *A* is representative of, or similar to, *B*. The clinician will judge the probability of the development of a blood clot (thrombosis) by the degree to which the patient with a swollen leg resembles the clinician's mental image of patients with a blood clot. If the patient has all the classic findings (signs and symptoms) associated with a blood clot, the physician judges that the patient is highly likely to have a blood clot. Difficulties occur with the use of this heuristic when the disease is rare (very low prior probability, or prevalence); when the clinician's previous experience with the disease is atypical, thus giving an incorrect mental representation; when the patient's clinical profile is atypical; and when the probability of certain findings depends on whether other findings are present.

- *Availability.* Our estimate of the probability of an event is influenced by the ease with which we remember similar events. Events more easily remembered are judged more probable; this rule is the **availability** heuristic, and it is often misleading. We remember dramatic, atypical, or emotion-laden events more easily and therefore are likely to overestimate their probability. A physician who had cared for a patient who had a swollen leg and who then died from a blood clot would vividly remember thrombosis as a cause of a swollen leg. She would remember other causes of swollen legs less easily, and she would tend to overestimate the probability of a blood clot in patients with a swollen leg.
- *Anchoring and adjustment.* Another common heuristic used to judge probability is **anchoring and adjustment**. A clinician makes an initial probability estimate (the *anchor*) and then adjusts the estimate based on further information. For instance, the physician in Example 4 makes an initial estimate of the probability of heart disease as 0.5. If she then learns that all the patient's brothers had died of heart disease, the physician should raise her estimate because the patient's strong family history of heart disease increases the probability that he has heart disease, a fact she could ascertain from the literature. The usual mistake is to adjust the initial estimate (the anchor) insufficiently in light of the new information. Instead of raising her estimate of prior probability to, say, 0.8, the physician might adjust to only 0.6.

Heuristics often introduce error into our judgments about prior probability. Errors in our initial estimates of probabilities will be reflected in the posterior probabilities even if we use quantitative methods to derive those posterior probabilities. An understanding of heuristics is thus important for medical decision-making. The clinician can avoid some of these difficulties by using published research results to estimate probabilities.

3.2.2 *Objective Probability Estimates*

Published research results can serve as a guide for more objective estimates of probabilities. We can use the prevalence of disease in the population or in a subgroup of the population, or clinical prediction rules, to estimate the probability of disease.

As we discussed in Chapter 2, the **prevalence** is the frequency of an event in a population; it is a useful starting point for estimating probability. For example, if you wanted to estimate the probability of prostate cancer in a 50-year-old man, the prevalence of prostate cancer in men of that age (5 to 14 percent) would be a useful anchor point from which you could increase or decrease the probability depending on your findings. Estimates of disease prevalence in a defined population often are available in the medical literature.

Symptoms, such as difficulty with urination, or signs, such as a palpable prostate nodule, can be used to place patients into a **clinical subgroup** in which the probability of disease is known. For patients referred to a urologist for evaluation of a prostate nodule, the prevalence of cancer is about 50 percent. This approach may be limited by difficulty in placing a patient in the correct clinically defined subgroup, especially if the criteria for classifying patients are ill defined. A trend has been to develop guidelines, known as *clinical prediction rules,* to help physicians assign patients to well-defined subgroups in which the probability of disease is known.

Clinical prediction rules are developed from systematic study of patients who have a particular diagnostic problem; they define how physicians can use combinations of clinical findings to estimate probability. The symptoms or signs that make an independent contribution to the probability that a patient has a disease are identified and are assigned numerical weights based on statistical analysis of the finding's contribution. The result is a list of symptoms and signs for an individual patient, each with a corresponding numerical contribution to a total score. The total score places a patient in a subgroup with a known probability of disease.

> **Example 5.** Ms. Troy, a 65-year-old woman who had a heart attack 4 months ago, has abnormal heart rhythm (arrhythmia), is in poor medical condition, and is about to undergo elective surgery.

What is the probability that Ms. Troy will suffer a cardiac complication? Clinical prediction rules have been developed to help physicians to assess this risk (Palda & Detsky, 1997). Table 3.1 lists clinical findings and their corresponding diagnostic weights. We add the diagnostic weights for each of the patient's clinical findings to obtain the total score. The total score places the patient in a group with a defined probability of cardiac complications, as shown in Table 3.2. Ms. Troy receives a score of 20; thus, the physician can estimate that the patient has a 27 percent chance of developing a severe cardiac complication.

Objective estimates of pretest probability are subject to error because of **bias** in the studies on which the estimates are based. For instance, published prevalences may not apply directly to a particular patient. A clinical illustration is that early studies indicated that a patient found to have microscopic evidence of blood in the urine (microhematuria) should undergo extensive tests because a significant proportion of the patients would be found to have cancer or other serious diseases. The tests involve some risk, discomfort, and expense to the patient. Nonetheless, the approach of ordering tests for any patient with microhematuria

Table 3.1. Diagnostic weights for assessing risk of cardiac complications from noncardiac surgery.

Clinical finding	Diagnostic weight
Age greater than 70 years	5
Recent documented heart attack	
>6 months previously	5
<6 months previously	10
Severe angina	20
Pulmonary edema[a]	
Within 1 week	10
Ever	5
Arrhythmia on most recent ECG	5
>5 PVCs	5
Critical aortic stenosis	20
Poor medical condition	5
Emergency surgery	10

ECG = electrocardiogram; PVCs = premature ventricular contractions on preoperative electrocardiogram.
[a]Fluid in the lungs due to reduced heart function.
(*Source*: Modified from Palda V.A., Detsky A.S. [1997]. Perioperative assessment and management of risk from coronary artery disease. *Annals of Internal Medicine*, 127: 313–318.)

was widely practiced for some years. A later study, however, suggested that the probability of serious disease in asymptomatic patients with only microscopic evidence of blood was only about 2 percent (Mohr et al., 1986). In the past, many patients may have undergone unnecessary tests, at considerable financial and personal cost.

What explains the discrepancy in the estimates of disease prevalence? The initial studies that showed a high prevalence of disease in patients with microhematuria were performed on patients referred to urologists, who are specialists. The primary-care physician refers patients whom she suspects have a

Table 3.2. Clinical prediction rule for diagnostic weights in Table 3-1.

Total score	Prevalence (%) of cardiac complications[a]
0–15	5
20–30	27
>30	60

[a]Cardiac complications defined as death, heart attack, or congestive heart failure.
(*Source*: Modified from Palda V.A., Detsky A.S. [1997]. Perioperative assessment and management of risk from coronary artery disease. *Annals of Internal Medicine*, 127:313–318.)

disease in the specialist's sphere of expertise. Because of this initial screening by primary-care physicians, the specialists seldom see patients with clinical findings that imply a low probability of disease. Thus, the prevalence of disease in the patient population in a specialist's practice often is much higher than that in a primary-care practice; studies performed with the former patients therefore almost always overestimate disease probabilities. This example demonstrates **referral bias.** Referral bias is common because many published studies are performed on patients referred to specialists. Thus, you may need to adjust published estimates before you use them to estimate pretest probability in other clinical settings.

We now can use the techniques discussed in this part of the chapter to illustrate how the physician in Example 4 might estimate the pretest probability of heart disease in her patient, Mr. Smith, who has pressure-like chest pain. We begin by using the objective data that are available. The prevalence of heart disease in 60-year-old men could be our starting point. In this case, however, we can obtain a more refined estimate by placing the patient in a clinical *subgroup* in which the prevalence of disease is known. The prevalence in a clinical subgroup, such as men with symptoms typical of coronary heart disease, will predict the pretest probability more accurately than would the prevalence of heart disease in a group that is heterogeneous with respect to symptoms, such as the population at large. We assume that large studies have shown the prevalence of coronary heart disease in men with typical symptoms of angina pectoris to be about 0.9; this prevalence is useful as an initial estimate that can be adjusted based on information specific to the patient. Although the prevalence of heart disease in men with typical symptoms is high, 10 percent of patients with this history do not have heart disease.

The physician might use subjective methods to adjust her estimate further based on other specific information about the patient. For example, she might adjust her initial estimate of 0.9 upward to 0.95 or higher based on information about family history of heart disease. She should be careful, however, to avoid the mistakes that can occur when we use heuristics to make subjective probability estimates. In particular, she should be aware of the tendency to stay too close to the initial estimate when adjusting for additional information. By combining subjective and objective methods for assessing pretest probability, she can arrive at a reasonable estimate of the pretest probability of heart disease.

In this section, we summarized subjective and objective methods to determine the pretest probability, and we learned how to adjust the pretest probability after assessing the specific subpopulation of which the patient is representative. The next step in the diagnostic process is to gather further information, usually in the form of formal diagnostic tests (laboratory tests, X-ray studies, and the like). To help you to understand this step more clearly, we discuss in the next two sections how to measure the accuracy of tests and how to use probability to interpret the results of the tests.

3.3 Measurement of the Operating Characteristics of Diagnostic Tests

The first challenge in assessing any test is to determine criteria for deciding whether a result is normal or abnormal. In this section, we present the issues that you need to consider when making such a determination.

3.3.1 Classification of Test Results as Abnormal

Most biological measurements in a population of healthy people are continuous variables that assume different values for different individuals. The distribution of values often is approximated by the normal (gaussian, or bell-shaped) distribution curve (Fig. 3.3). Thus, 95 percent of the population will fall within two standard deviations of the mean. About 2.5 percent of the population will be more than two standard deviations from the mean at each end of the distribution. The distribution of values for ill individuals may be normally distributed as well. The two distributions usually overlap (see Fig. 3.3).

How is a test result classified as abnormal? Most clinical laboratories report an "upper limit of normal," which usually is defined as two standard deviations above the mean. Thus, a test result greater than two standard deviations above the mean is reported as abnormal (or positive); a test result below that cutoff is reported as normal (or negative). As an example, if the mean cholesterol con-

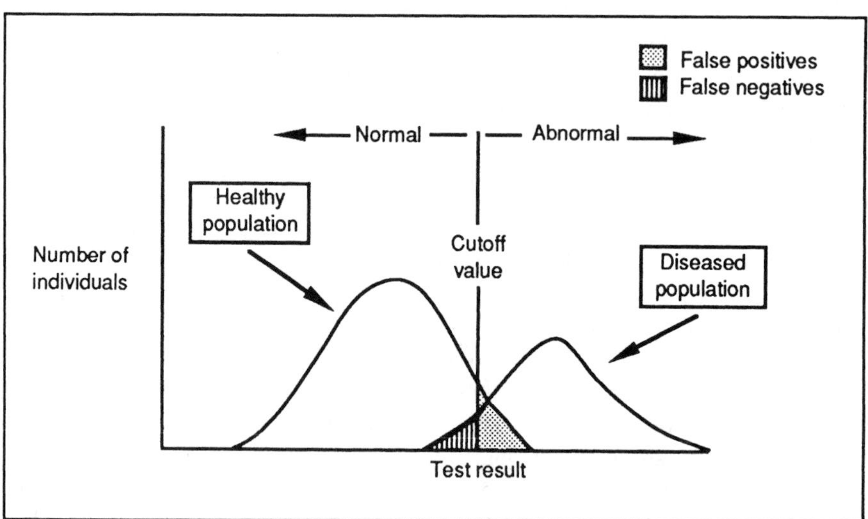

FIGURE 3.3. Distribution of test results in healthy and diseased individuals. Varying the cutoff between "normal" and "abnormal" across the continuous range of possible values changes the relative proportions of false positives and false negatives for the two populations.

centration in the blood is 220 mg/dl, a clinical laboratory might choose as the upper limit of normal 280 mg/dl because it is two standard deviations above the mean. Note that a cutoff that is based on an arbitrary statistical criterion may not have biological significance.

An ideal test would have no values at which the distribution of diseased and nondiseased people overlap. That is, if the cutoff value were set appropriately, the test would be normal in all healthy individuals and abnormal in all individuals with disease. Few tests meet this standard. If a test result is defined as abnormal by the statistical criterion, 2.5 percent of healthy individuals will have an abnormal test. If there is an overlap in the distribution of test results in healthy and diseased individuals, some diseased patients will have a normal test (see Fig. 3.3). You should be familiar with the terms used to denote these groups:

- A **true positive** (TP) is a positive test result obtained for a patient in whom the disease is present (the test result correctly classifies the patient as having the disease).
- A **true negative** (TN) is a negative test result obtained for a patient in whom the disease is absent (the test result correctly classifies the patient as not having the disease).
- A **false positive** (FP) is a positive test result obtained for a patient in whom the disease is absent (the test result incorrectly classifies the patient as having the disease).
- A **false negative** (FN) is a negative test result obtained for a patient in whom the disease is present (the test result incorrectly classifies the patient as not having the disease).

Figure 3.3 shows that varying the cutoff point (moving the vertical line in the figure) for an abnormal test will change the relative proportions of these groups. As the cutoff is moved further up from the mean of the normal values, the number of FNs increases and the number of FPs decreases. Once we have chosen a cutoff point, we can conveniently summarize test performance—the ability to discriminate disease from nondisease—in a 2×2 **contingency table**, as shown in Table 3.3. The table summarizes the number of patients in each group: TP, FP, TN, and FN. Note that the sum of the first column is the total number of diseased patients, TP + FN. The sum of the second column is the total number of nondiseased patients, FP + TN. The sum of the first row, TP + FP, is the total number of patients with a positive test result. Likewise, FN + TN gives the total number of patients with a negative test result.

Table 3.3. A 2×2 contingency table for test results.

Results of test	Disease present	Disease absent	Total
Positive result	TP	FP	TP + FP
Negative result	FN	TN	FN + TN
	TP + FN	FP + TN	

TP = true positive; TN = true negative; FP = false positive; FN = false negative.

A perfect test would have no FN or FP results. Erroneous test results do occur, however, and you can use a 2 × 2 contingency table to define the measures of test performance that reflect these errors.

3.3.2 Measures of Test Performance

Measures of test performance are of two types: measures of agreement between tests, or **measures of concordance,** and measures of disagreement, or **measures of discordance**. Two types of **concordant test results** occur in the 2 × 2 table in Table 3.3: TPs and TNs. The relative frequencies of these results form the basis of the measures of concordance. These measures correspond to the ideas of the sensitivity and specificity of a test, which we introduced in Chapter 2. We define each measure in terms of the 2 × 2 table and in terms of conditional probabilities.

The **true-positive rate** (TPR), or **sensitivity,** is the likelihood that a diseased patient has a positive test. In conditional-probability notation, sensitivity is expressed as the probability of a positive test given that disease is present:

$$p[\text{positive test}|\text{disease}].$$

Another way to think of the TPR is as a ratio. The likelihood that a diseased patient has a positive test is given by the ratio of diseased patients with a positive test to all diseased patients:

$$\text{TPR} = \frac{\text{number of diseased patients with positive test}}{\text{total number of diseased patients}}.$$

We can determine these numbers for our example from the 2 × 2 table (see Table 3.3). The number of diseased patients with a positive test is TP. The total number of diseased patients is the sum of the first column, TP + FN. So,

$$\text{TPR} = \frac{\text{TP}}{\text{TP} + \text{FN}}.$$

The **true-negative rate** (TNR), or **specificity**, is the likelihood that a nondiseased patient has a negative test result. In terms of conditional probability, specificity is the probability of a negative test given that disease is absent:

$$p[\text{negative test}|\text{no disease}].$$

Viewed as a ratio, the TNR is the number of nondiseased patients with a negative test divided by the total number of nondiseased patients:

$$\text{TNR} = \frac{\text{number of nondiseased patients with negative test}}{\text{total number of nondiseased patients}}.$$

From the 2 × 2 table (see Table 3.3),

$$\text{TNR} = \frac{\text{TN}}{\text{TN} + \text{FP}}$$

Table 3.4. A 2×2 contingency table for HIV antibody EIA.

EIA test result	Antibody present	Antibody absent	Total
Positive EIA	98	3	101
Negative EIA	2	297	299
	100	300	

EIA = enzyme-linked immunoassay.

The measures of discordance—the false-positive rate and the false-negative rate—are defined similarly. The **false-negative rate** (FNR) is the likelihood that a diseased patient has a negative test result. As a ratio,

$$\text{FNR} = \frac{\text{number of diseased patients with negative test}}{\text{total number of diseased patients}} = \frac{\text{FN}}{\text{FN} + \text{TP}}.$$

The **false-positive rate** (FPR) is the likelihood that a nondiseased patient has a positive test result:

$$\text{FPR} = \frac{\text{number of nondiseased patients with positive test}}{\text{total number of nondiseased patients}} = \frac{\text{FP}}{\text{FP} + \text{TN}}.$$

Example 6. Consider again the problem of screening blood donors for HIV. One test used to screen blood donors for HIV antibody is an enzyme-linked immunoassay (EIA). So that the performance of the EIA can be measured, the test is performed on 400 patients; the hypothetical results are shown in the 2×2 table in Table 3.4.[5]

To determine test performance, we calculate the TPR (sensitivity) and TNR (specificity) of the EIA antibody test. The TPR, as defined previously, is

$$\frac{\text{TP}}{\text{TP} + \text{FN}} = \frac{98}{98 + 2} = 0.98.$$

Thus, the likelihood that a patient with the HIV antibody will have a positive EIA test is 0.98. If the test were performed on 100 patients who truly had the antibody, we would expect the test to be positive in 98 of the patients. Conversely, we would expect two of the patients to receive incorrect, negative results, for an FNR of 2 percent. (You should convince yourself that the sum of TPR and FNR by definition must be 1: TPR + FNR = 1.)

The TNR is

$$\frac{\text{TN}}{\text{TN} + \text{FP}} = \frac{297}{297 + 3} = 0.99.$$

[5]This example assumes that we have a perfect method (different from EIA) for determining the presence or absence of antibody. We discuss the idea of *gold-standard tests* in Section 3.3.4. We have chosen the numbers in the example to simplify the calculations. In practice, the sensitivity and specificity of the HIV EIAs are greater than 99 percent.

The likelihood that a patient who has no HIV antibody will have a negative test is 0.99. Therefore, if the EIA test were performed on 100 individuals who had not been infected with HIV, it would be negative in 99 and incorrectly positive in 1. (Convince yourself that the sum of TNR and FPR also must be 1: TNR + FPR = 1.)

3.3.3 *Implications of Sensitivity and Specificity: How to Choose Among Tests*

It may be clear to you already that the calculated values of sensitivity and specificity for a continuous-valued test depend on the particular cutoff value chosen to distinguish normal and abnormal results. In Figure 3.3, note that increasing the cutoff level (moving it to the right) would decrease significantly the number of false-positive tests but also would increase the number of false-negative tests. Thus, the test would have become *more* specific but *less* sensitive. Similarly, a lower cutoff value would increase the FPs and decrease the FNs, thereby increasing sensitivity while decreasing specificity. Whenever a decision is made about what cutoff to use in calling a test abnormal, an inherent philosophic decision is being made about whether it is better to tolerate FNs (missed cases) or FPs (nondiseased people inappropriately classified as diseased). The choice of cutoff depends on the disease in question and on the purpose of testing. If the disease is serious and if life-saving therapy is available, then we should try to minimize the number of false-negative results. On the other hand, if the disease in not serious and the therapy is dangerous, we should set the cutoff value to minimize false-positive results.

We stress the point that sensitivity and specificity are characteristics not of a test per se but rather of the test *and* a criterion for when to call that test abnormal. Varying the cutoff in Figure 3.3 has no effect on the test itself (the way it is performed, or the specific values for any particular patient); instead, it trades off specificity for sensitivity. Thus, the best way to characterize a test is by the range of values of sensitivity and specificity that it can take on over a range of possible cutoffs. The typical way to show this relationship is to plot the test's sensitivity against 1 minus specificity (that is, the TPR against the FPR) as the cutoff is varied and the two test characteristics are traded off against each other (Fig. 3.4). The resulting curve, known as a **receiver operating characteristic (ROC) curve**, was originally described by researchers investigating methods of electromagnetic-signal detection and was later applied to the field of psychology (Peterson & Birdsall, 1953; Swets, 1973). Any given point along an ROC curve for a test corresponds to the test sensitivity and specificity for a given threshold of "abnormality." Similar curves can be drawn for *any* test used to associate observed clinical data with specific diseases or disease categories.

Suppose that a new test were introduced that competed with the current way of screening for the presence of a disease. For example, suppose that a new radiologic procedure for assessing the presence or absence of pneumonia became available. This new test could be assessed for trade-offs in sensitivity and speci-

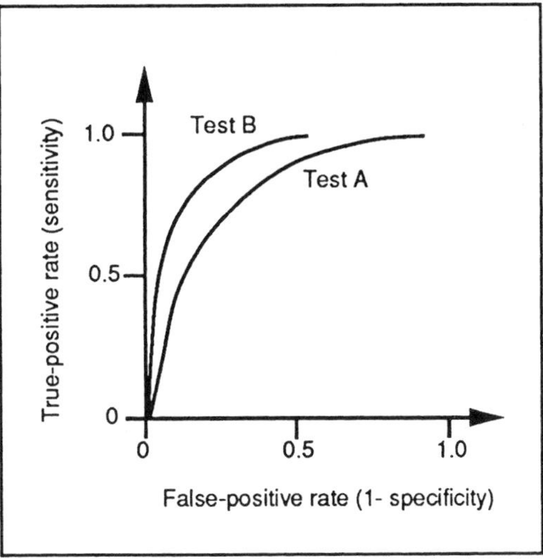

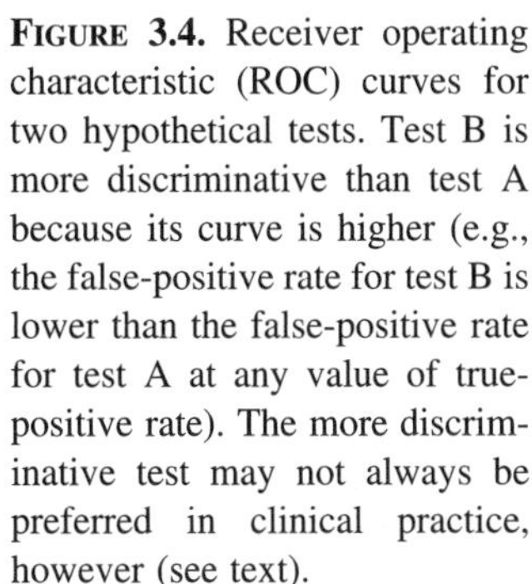
FIGURE 3.4. Receiver operating characteristic (ROC) curves for two hypothetical tests. Test B is more discriminative than test A because its curve is higher (e.g., the false-positive rate for test B is lower than the false-positive rate for test A at any value of true-positive rate). The more discriminative test may not always be preferred in clinical practice, however (see text).

ficity, and an ROC curve could be drawn. As shown in Figure 3.4, a test has better discriminating power than a competing test if its ROC curve lies above that of the other test. In other words, test B is more discriminating than test A when its specificity is greater than test A's specificity for any level of sensitivity (and when its sensitivity is greater than test A's sensitivity for any level of specificity).

Understanding ROC curves is important in understanding test selection and data interpretation. Physicians should not necessarily, however, always choose the test with the most discriminating ROC curve. Matters of cost, risk, discomfort, and delay also are important in the choice about what data to collect and what tests to perform. When you must choose among several available tests, you should select the test that has the highest sensitivity and specificity, *provided* that other factors, such as cost and risk to the patient, are equal. The higher the sensitivity and specificity of a test, the more the results of that test will reduce uncertainty about probability of disease.

3.3.4 Design of Studies of Test Performance

In Section 3.3.2, we discussed measures of test performance: a test's ability to discriminate disease from no disease. When we classify a test result as TP, TN, FP, or FN, we assume that we know with certainty whether a patient is diseased or healthy. Thus, the validity of any test's results must be measured against a gold standard: a test that reveals the patient's true disease state, such as a biopsy of diseased tissue or a surgical operation. A **gold-standard test** is a procedure that is used to define unequivocally the presence or absence of disease. The test whose discrimination is being measured is called the **index test**. The gold-standard test usually is more expensive, riskier, or more difficult to perform than is the index test (otherwise, the less precise test would not be used at all).

The performance of the index test is measured in a small, select group of patients enrolled in a study. We are interested, however, in how the test performs in the broader group of patients in which it will be used in practice. The test may perform differently in the two groups, so we make the following distinction: the **study population** comprises those patients (usually a subset of the clinically relevant population) in whom test discrimination is measured and reported; the **clinically relevant population** comprises those patients in whom a test typically is used.

3.3.5 Bias in the Measurement of Test Characteristics

We mentioned earlier the problem of *referral bias*. Published estimates of disease prevalence (derived from a study population) may differ from the prevalence in the clinically relevant population because diseased patients are more likely to be included in studies than are nondiseased patients. Similarly, published values of sensitivity and specificity are derived from study populations that may differ from the clinically relevant populations in terms of average level of health and disease prevalence. These differences may affect test performance, so the reported values may not apply to many patients in whom a test is used in clinical practice.

> **Example 7.** In the early 1970s, a blood test called the *carcinoembryonic antigen* (CEA) was touted as a screening test for colon cancer. Reports of early investigations, performed in selected patients, indicated that the test had high sensitivity and specificity. Subsequent work, however, proved the CEA to be completely valueless as a screening blood test for colon cancer. Screening tests are used in unselected populations, and the differences between the study and clinically relevant populations were partly responsible for the original miscalculations of the CEA's TPR and TNR. (Ransohoff & Feinstein, 1978)

The experience with CEA has been repeated with numerous tests. Early measures of test discrimination are overly optimistic, and subsequent test performance is disappointing. Problems arise when the TPR and TNR, as measured in the study population, do not apply to the clinically relevant population. These problems usually are the result of bias in the design of the initial studies—notably spectrum bias, test-referral bias, or test-interpretation bias.

Spectrum bias occurs when the study population includes only individuals who have advanced disease ("sickest of the sick") and healthy volunteers, as is often the case when a test is first being developed. Advanced disease may be easier to detect than early disease. For example, cancer is easier to detect when it has spread throughout the body (metastasized) than when it is localized to, say, a small portion of the colon. In contrast to the study population, the clinically relevant population will contain more cases of early disease that are more likely to be missed by the index test (FNs). Thus, the study population will have an artifactually low FNR, which produces an artifactually high TPR (TPR $= 1 -$ FNR). In addition, healthy volunteers are less likely than are patients in the clinically relevant population to have other diseases that may cause false-positive results;[6] the study population will have an artificially low FPR, and therefore the specificity will be overestimated (TNR = 1 − FPR). Inaccuracies in early estimates of the TPR and TNR of the CEA were partly due to spectrum bias.

Test referral bias occurs when a positive index test is a criterion for ordering the gold-standard test. In clinical practice, patients with negative index tests are less likely to undergo the gold-standard test than are patients with positive tests. In other words, the study population, comprising individuals with positive index-test results, has a higher percentage of patients with disease than does the clinically relevant population. Therefore, both TN and FN tests will be underrepresented in the study population. The result is overestimation of the TPR and underestimation of the TNR in the study population.

Test-interpretation bias develops when the interpretation of the index test affects that of the gold-standard test or vice versa. This bias causes an artificial concordance between the tests (the results are more likely to be the same) and spuriously increases measures of concordance—the sensitivity and specificity—in the study population. (Remember, the relative frequencies of TPs and TNs are the basis for measures of concordance). To avoid these problems, the person interpreting the index test should be unaware of the results of the gold standard test.

To counter these three biases, you may need to adjust the TPR and TNR when they are applied to a new population. All the biases result in a TPR that is higher in the study population than it is in the clinically relevant population. Thus, if you suspect bias, you should adjust the TPR (sensitivity) downward when you apply it to a new population.

Adjustment of the TNR (specificity) depends on which type of bias is present. Spectrum bias and test interpretation bias result in a TNR that is *higher* in the study population than it will be in the clinically relevant population. Thus, if these biases are present, you should adjust the specificity downward when you apply it to a new population. Test-referral bias, on the other hand, produces a measured specificity in the study population that is *lower* than it will be in the clinically relevant population. If you suspect test-referral bias, you should adjust the specificity upward when you apply it to a new population.

3.3.6 Meta-Analysis of Diagnostic Tests

Many studies evaluate the sensitivity and specificity of the same diagnostic test. If the studies come to similar conclusions about the sensitivity and specificity of

---

[6]Volunteers are often healthy, whereas patients in the clinically relevant population often have several diseases *in addition* to the disease for which a test is designed. These other diseases may cause false-positive test results. For example, patients with benign (rather than malignant) enlargement of their prostate glands are more likely than are healthy volunteers to have false-positive elevations of prostate-specific antigen (Meigs et al., 1996), a substance in the blood that is elevated in men who have prostate cancer. Measurement of prostate-specific antigen is often used to detect prostate cancer.

the test, you can have increased confidence in the results of the studies. But what if the studies disagree? For example, by 1995, over 100 studies had assessed the sensitivity and specificity of the PCR for diagnosis of HIV (Owens et al., 1996a,b); these studies estimated the sensitivity of PCR to be as low as 10 percent and to be as high as 100 percent, and they assessed the specificity of PCR to be between 40 and 100 percent. Which results should you believe? One approach that you can use is to assess the quality of the studies and to use the estimates from the highest quality studies.

For evaluation of PCR, however, even the high-quality studies did not agree. Another approach, developed recently, is to perform a **meta-analysis**: a study that combines quantitatively the estimates from individual studies to develop a **summary ROC curve** (Moses et al., 1993; Owens et al., 1996a,b). Investigators develop a summary ROC curve by using estimates from many studies, in contrast to the type of ROC curve discussed in Section 3.3.3, which is developed from the data in a single study. Summary ROC curves provide the best available approach to synthesizing data from many studies.

Section 3.3 has dealt with the second step in the diagnostic process: acquisition of further information with diagnostic tests. We have learned how to characterize the performance of a test with the sensitivity (TPR) and specificity (TNR). These measures reveal the probability of a test result given the true state of the patient. They do not, however, answer the clinically relevant question posed in the opening example: Given a positive test result, what is the probability that this patient has the disease? To answer this question, we must learn methods to calculate the post-test probability of disease.

3.4 Post-test Probability: Bayes' Theorem and Predictive Value

The third stage of the diagnostic process (see Fig. 3.2a) is to adjust our probability estimate to take into account the new information gained from diagnostic tests by calculating the post-test probability.

3.4.1 Bayes' Theorem

As we noted earlier in this chapter, a physician can use the disease prevalence in the patient population as an initial estimate of the pretest risk of disease. Once a physician begins to accumulate information about a patient, however, she revises her estimate of the probability of disease. The revised estimate (rather than the disease prevalence in the general population) becomes the pretest probability for the test that she performs. After she has gathered more information with a diagnostic test, she can calculate the post-test probability of disease with Bayes' theorem.

Bayes' theorem is a quantitative method for calculating post-test probability using the pretest probability and the sensitivity and specificity of the test. The theorem is derived from the definition of conditional probability and from the properties of probability (see the Appendix to this chapter for the derivation).

Recall that a conditional probability is the probability that event A will occur given that event B is known to occur (see Section 3.2). In general, we want to know the probability that disease is present (event A), given that the test is known to be positive (event B). We denote the presence of disease as D, its absence as −D, a test result as R, and the pretest probability of disease as $p[\text{D}]$. The probability of disease, given a test result, is written $p[\text{D}|\text{R}]$. Bayes' theorem is

$$p[\text{D}|\text{R}] = \frac{p[\text{D}] \times p[\text{R}|\text{D}]}{p[\text{D}] \times p[\text{R}|\text{D}] + p[-\text{D}] \times p[\text{R}|-\text{D}]}.$$

We can reformulate this general equation in terms of a positive test, (+), by substituting $p[\text{D}|+]$ for $p[\text{D}|\text{R}]$, $p[+|D]$ for $p[\text{R}|\text{D}]$, $p[+|-\text{D}]$ for $p[\text{R}|-\text{D}]$, and $1 - p[\text{D}]$ for $p[-\text{D}]$. From Section 3.3, recall that $p[+|\text{D}] = \text{TPR}$ and $p[+|-\text{D}] = \text{FPR}$. Substitution provides Bayes' theorem for a positive test:

$$p[\text{D}|+] = \frac{p[\text{D}] \times \text{TPR}}{p[\text{D}] \times \text{TPR} + (1 - p[\text{D}]) \times \text{FPR}}.$$

We can use a similar derivation to develop Bayes' theorem for a negative test:

$$p[\text{D}|-] = \frac{p[\text{D}] \times \text{FNR}}{p[\text{D}] \times \text{FNR} + (1 - p[\text{D}]) \times \text{TNR}}.$$

Example 8. We are now able to calculate the clinically important probability in Example 4: the post-test probability of heart disease after a positive exercise test. At the end of Section 3.2.2, we estimated the pretest probability of heart disease as 0.95, based on the prevalence of heart disease in men who have typical symptoms of heart disease and on the prevalence in people with a family history of heart disease. Assume that the TPR and FPR of the exercise stress test are 0.65 and 0.20, respectively. Substituting in Bayes' formula for a positive test, we obtain the probability of heart disease given a positive test result:

$$p[\text{D}|+] = \frac{0.95 \times 0.65}{0.95 \times 0.65 + 0.05 \times 0.20} = 0.98.$$

Thus, the positive test raised the post-test probability to 0.98 from the pretest probability of 0.95. The change in probability is modest because the pretest probability was high (0.95) and because the FPR also is high (0.20). If we repeat the calculation with a pretest probability of 0.75, the post-test probability is 0.91. If we assume the FPR of the test to be 0.05, instead of 0.20, a pretest probability of 0.95 changes to 0.996.

3.4.2 The Odds-Ratio Form of Bayes' Theorem and Likelihood Ratios

Although the formula for Bayes' theorem is straightforward, it is awkward for mental calculations. We can develop a more convenient form of Bayes' theorem by expressing probability as *odds* and by using a different measure of test discrimination.

Probability and odds are related as follows:

$$\text{odds} = \frac{p}{1 - p},$$

$$p = \frac{\text{odds}}{1 + \text{odds}}.$$

Thus, if the probability of rain today is 0.75, the odds are 3:1. Thus, on similar days, we should expect rain to occur three times for each time it does not occur.

A simple relationship exists between pretest odds and post-test odds:

$$\text{post-test odds} = \text{pretest odds} \times \text{likelihood ratio}$$

or

$$\frac{p[\mathrm{D}|\mathrm{R}]}{p[-\mathrm{D}|\mathrm{R}]} = \frac{p[\mathrm{D}]}{p[-\mathrm{D}]} \times \frac{p[\mathrm{R}|\mathrm{D}]}{p[\mathrm{R}|-\mathrm{D}]}.$$

This equation is the **odds-ratio form** of Bayes' theorem.[7] It can be derived in a straightforward fashion from the definitions of Bayes' theorem and of conditional probability that we provided earlier. Thus, to obtain the post-test odds, we simply multiply the pretest odds by the **likelihood ratio** (LR) for the test in question.

The LR of a test combines the measures of test discrimination discussed earlier to give one number that characterizes the discriminatory power of a test, defined as

$$\mathrm{LR} = \frac{p[\mathrm{R}|\mathrm{D}]}{p[\mathrm{R}|-\mathrm{D}]}$$

or

$$\mathrm{LR} = \frac{\text{probability of result in diseased people}}{\text{probability of result in nondiseased people}}.$$

The LR indicates the amount that the odds of disease change based on the test result. We can use the LR to characterize clinical findings (such as a swollen leg) or a test result. We describe either by two likelihood ratios: one corresponding to a positive test result (or the presence of a finding) and the other corresponding to a negative test (or the absence of a finding). These ratios are abbreviated LR^+ and LR^-, respectively.

$$\mathrm{LR}^+ = \frac{\text{probability that test is positive in diseased people}}{\text{probability that test is positive in nondiseased people}} = \frac{\mathrm{TPR}}{\mathrm{FPR}}.$$

[7]Some authors refer to this expression as the **odds-likelihood form** of Bayes' theorem.

In a test that discriminates well between disease and nondisease, the TPR will be high, the FPR will be low, and thus LR^+ will be much greater than 1. An LR of 1 means that the probability of a test result is the same in diseased and nondiseased individuals; the test has no value. Similarly,

$$LR^- = \frac{\text{probability that test is negative in diseased people}}{\text{probability that test is negative in nondiseased people}} = \frac{\text{FNR}}{\text{TNR}}.$$

A desirable test will have a low FNR and a high TNR; therefore, the LR^- will be much less than 1.

Example 9. We can calculate the post-test probability for a positive exercise stress test in a 60-year-old man whose pretest probability is 0.75. The pretest odds are

$$\text{odds} = \frac{p}{1-p} = \frac{0.75}{1-0.75} = \frac{0.75}{0.25} = 3, \text{ or } 3{:}1.$$

The LR for the stress test is

$$LR^+ = \frac{\text{TPR}}{\text{FPR}} = \frac{0.65}{0.20} = 3.25.$$

We can calculate the post-test odds of a positive test result using the odds-ratio form of Bayes' theorem:

$$\text{post-test odds} = 3 \times 3.25 = 9.75{:}1.$$

We can then convert the odds to a probability:

$$p = \frac{\text{odds}}{1 + \text{odds}} = \frac{9.75}{1 + 9.75} = 0.91.$$

As expected, this result agrees with our earlier answer (see the discussion of Example 8).

The odds-ratio form of Bayes' theorem allows rapid calculation, so you can determine the probability at, for example, your patient's bedside. The LR is a powerful method for characterizing the operating characteristics of a test: If you know the pretest odds, you can calculate the post-test odds in one step. The LR demonstrates that a useful test is one that changes the odds of disease. The LRs of many diagnostic tests are available (Sox et al., 1988).

3.4.3 Predictive Value of a Test

An alternative approach for estimation of the probability of disease in a person who has a positive or negative test is to calculate the predictive value of the test. The **positive predictive value** (PV^+) of a test is the likelihood that a patient who has a positive test result also has disease. Thus, PV^+ can be calculated directly from a 2×2 contingency table:

$$PV^+ = \frac{\text{number of diseased patients with a positive test}}{\text{total number of patients with a positive test}}$$

From the 2 × 2 contingency table in Table 3.3,

$$PV^{+} = \frac{TP}{TP + FP}.$$

The **negative predictive value** (PV^{-}) is the likelihood that a patient with a negative test does not have disease:

$$PV^{-} = \frac{\text{number of nondiseased patients with a negative test}}{\text{total number of patients with a negative test}}$$

From the 2 × 2 contingency table in Table 3.3,

$$PV^{-} = \frac{TN}{TN + FN}.$$

Example 10. We can calculate the PV of the EIA test from the 2 × 2 table that we constructed in Example 6 (see Table 3.4) as follows:

$$PV^{+} = \frac{98}{98 + 3} = 0.97.$$

$$PV^{-} = \frac{297}{297 + 2} = 0.99.$$

The probability that antibody is present in a patient who has a positive index test (EIA) in this study is 0.97; about 97 of 100 patients with a positive test will have antibody. The likelihood that a patient with a negative index test does *not* have antibody is about 0.99.

It is worth reemphasizing the difference between PV and sensitivity and specificity, given that both are calculated from the 2 × 2 table and they often are confused. The sensitivity and specificity give the probability of a particular test result in a patient who has a particular disease state. The PV gives the probability of true disease state once the patient's test result is known.

The PV^{+} calculated from Table 3.4 is 0.97, so we expect 97 of 100 patients with a positive index test actually to have antibody. Yet, in Example 1, we found that less than 1 of 10 patients with a positive test were expected to have antibody. What explains the discrepancy in these examples? The sensitivity and specificity (and, therefore, the LRs) in the two examples are identical. The discrepancy is due to an extremely important and often overlooked characteristic of PV: The PV of a test depends on the *prevalence* of disease in the study population (the prevalence can be calculated as TP + FN divided by the total number of patients in the 2 × 2 table). The PV cannot be generalized to a new population because the prevalence of disease may differ between the two populations.

The difference in PV of the EIA in Example 1 and in Example 6 is due to a difference in the prevalence of disease in the examples. The prevalence of antibody was given as 0.001 in Example 1 and as 0.25 in Example 6. These examples should remind us that the PV^{+} is not an intrinsic property of a test. Rather, it represents the post-test probability of disease only when the prevalence is identical to that in the 2 × 2 contingency table from which the PV^{+} was calculated.

Bayes' theorem provides a method for calculation of the post-test probability of disease for any prior probability. For that reason, we prefer the use of Bayes' theorem to calculate the post-test probability of disease.

3.4.4 Implications of Bayes' Theorem

In this section, we explore the implications of Bayes' theorem for test interpretation. These ideas are extremely important, yet they often are misunderstood.

Figure 3.5 illustrates one of the most essential concepts in this chapter: The post-test probability of disease increases as the pretest probability of disease in-

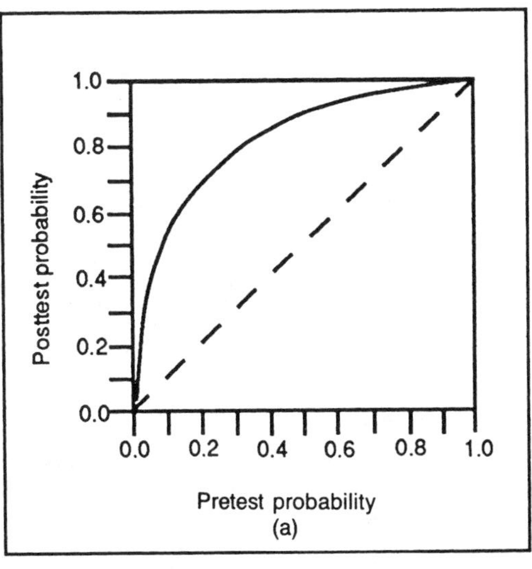

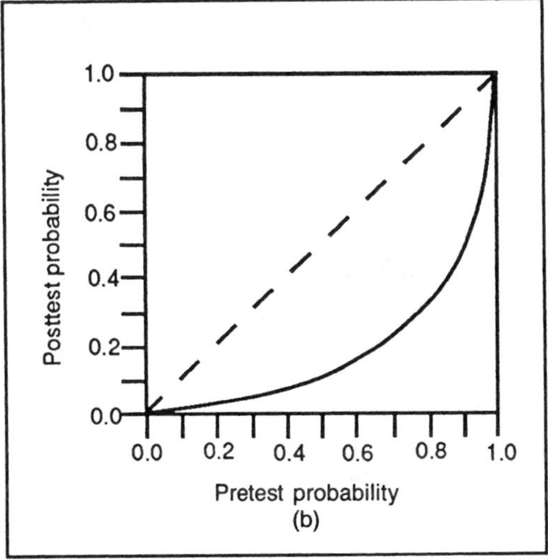

FIGURE 3.5. Relationship between pretest probability and post-test probability of disease. The dashed lines correspond to a test that has no effect on the probability of disease. Sensitivity and specificity of the test were assumed to be 0.90 for the two examples. *(a)* The post-test probability of disease corresponding to a *positive* test result (solid curve) was calculated with Bayes' theorem for all values of pretest probability. *(b)* The post-test probability of disease corresponding to a *negative* test result (solid curve) was calculated with Bayes' theorem for all values of pretest probability. (*Source:* Adapted from Sox, H.C. [1987]. Probability theory in the use of diagnostic tests: Application to critical study of the literature. In Sox H.C. [Ed.], *Common Diagnostic Tests: Use and Interpretation* [pp. 1–17]. Philadelphia: American College of Physicians. Reproduced with permission from the American College of Physicians—American Society of Internal Medicine.)

creases. We produced Figure 3.5a by calculating the post-test probability after a positive test result for all possible pretest probabilities of disease. We similarly derived Figure 3.5b for a negative test result.

The 45-degree line in each figure denotes a test in which the pretest and post-test probability are equal (LR = 1)—a test that is useless. The curve in Figure 3.5a relates pretest and post-test probabilities in a test with a sensitivity and specificity of 0.9. Note that, at low pretest probabilities, the post-test probability after a positive test result is much higher than is the pretest probability. At high pretest probabilities, the post-test probability is only slightly higher than the pretest probability.

Figure 3.5b shows the relationship between the pretest and post-test probabilities after a negative test result. At high pretest probabilities, the post-test probability after a negative test result is much lower than is the pretest probability. A negative test, however, has little effect on the post-test probability if the pretest probability is low.

This discussion emphasizes a key idea of this chapter: The interpretation of a test result depends on the pretest probability of disease. If the pretest probability is low, a positive test result has a large effect, and a negative test result has a small effect. If the pretest probability is high, a positive test result has a small effect, and a negative test result has a large effect. In other words, when the clinician is almost certain of the diagnosis before testing (pretest probability nearly 0 or nearly 1), a confirmatory test has little effect on the posterior probability (see Example 8). If the pretest probability is intermediate or if the result contradicts a strongly held clinical impression, the test result will have a large effect on the post-test probability.

Note from Figure 3.5a that, if the pretest probability is very low, a positive test result can raise the post-test probability into only the intermediate range. Assume that Figure 3.5a represents the relationship between the pretest and post-test probabilities for the exercise stress test. If the clinician believes the pretest probability of coronary artery disease is 0.1, the post-test probability will be about 0.5. Although there has been a large change in the probability, the post-test probability is in an intermediate range, which leaves considerable uncertainty about the diagnosis. Thus, if the pretest probability is low, it is unlikely that a positive test result will raise the probability of disease sufficiently for the clinician to make that diagnosis with confidence. An exception to this statement occurs when a test has a very high specificity (or a large LR^+); for example, HIV antibody tests have a specificity greater than 0.99, and therefore a positive test is convincing. Similarly, if the pretest probability is very high, it is unlikely that a negative test result will lower the post-test probability sufficiently to exclude a diagnosis.

Figure 3.6 illustrates another important concept: Test specificity affects primarily the interpretation of a positive test; test sensitivity affects primarily the interpretation of a negative test. In both parts a and b of Figure 3.6, the top family of curves corresponds to positive test results and the bottom family to negative test results. Figure 3.6a shows the post-test probabilities for tests with vary-

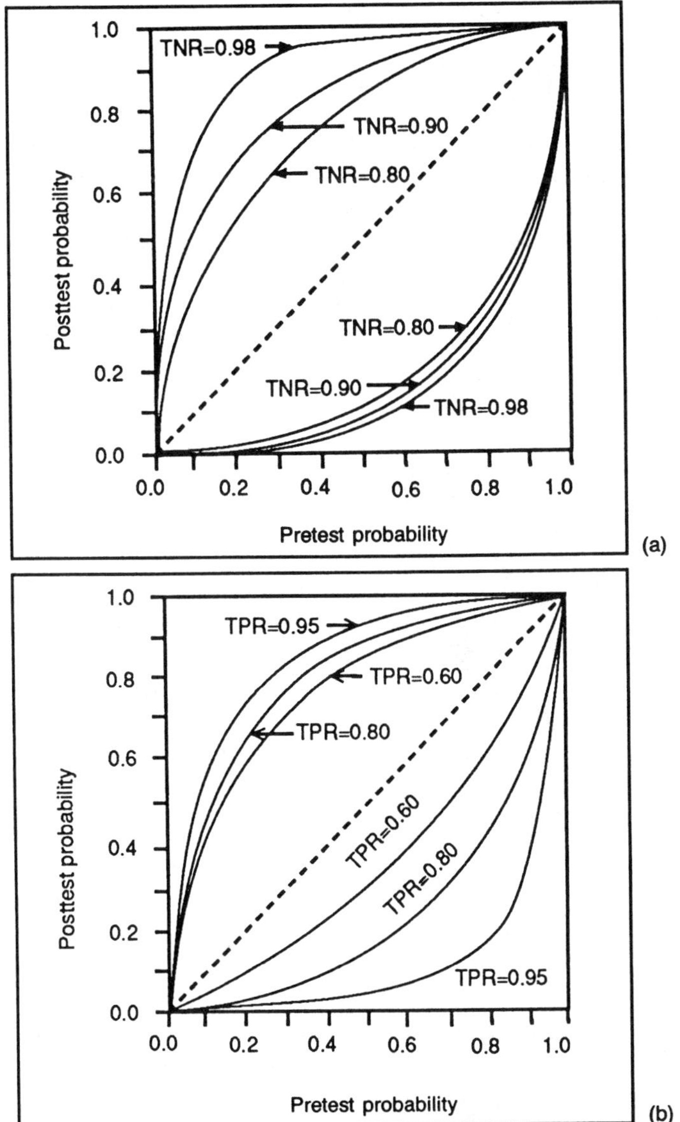

FIGURE 3.6. Effects of test sensitivity and specificity on post-test probability. The curves are similar to those shown in Figure 3.5 except that the calculations have been repeated for several values of the sensitivity (TPR = true-positive rate) and specificity (TNR = true-negative rate) of the test. *(a)* The sensitivity of the test was assumed to be 0.90, and the calculations were repeated for several values of test specificity. *(b)* The specificity of the test was assumed to be 0.90, and the calculations were repeated for several values of the sensitivity of the test. In both panels, the top family of curves corresponds to positive test results, and the bottom family of curves corresponds to negative test results. (*Source:* Adapted from Sox H.C. [1987]. Probability theory in the use of diagnostic tests: Application to critical study of the literature. In Sox H.C. [Ed.], *Common Diagnostic Tests: Use and Interpretation* [pp. 1–17]. Philadelphia: American College of Physicians. Reproduced with permission from the American College of Physicians—American Society of Internal Medicine.)

ing specificities (TNR). Note that changes in the specificity produce large changes in the top family of curves (positive test results) but have little effect on the lower family of curves (negative test results). That is, an increase in the specificity of a test markedly changes the post-test probability if the test is positive but has relatively little effect on the post-test probability if the test is negative. Thus, if you are trying to *rule in* a diagnosis,[8] you should choose a test with high specificity or a high LR^+. Figure 3.6b shows the post-test probabilities for tests with varying sensitivities. Note that changes in sensitivity produce large changes in the bottom family of curves (negative test results) but have little effect on the top family of curves. Thus, if you are trying to exclude a disease, choose a test with a high sensitivity or a high LR^-.

3.4.5 Cautions in the Application of Bayes' Theorem

Bayes' theorem provides a powerful method for calculating post-test probability. You should be aware, however, of the possible errors you can make when you use it. Common problems are inaccurate estimation of pretest probability, faulty application of test-performance measures, and violation of the assumptions of conditional independence and of mutual exclusivity.

Bayes' theorem provides a means to adjust an estimate of pretest probability to take into account new information. The accuracy of the calculated post-test probability is limited, however, by the accuracy of the estimated pretest probability. Accuracy of estimated prior probability is increased by proper use of published prevalence rates, heuristics, and clinical prediction rules. In a decision analysis, as we shall see, a *range* of prior probability often is sufficient. Nonetheless, if the pretest-probability assessment is unreliable, Bayes' theorem will be of little value.

A second potential mistake that you can make when using Bayes' theorem is to apply published values for the test sensitivity and specificity, or LRs, without paying attention to the possible effects of bias in the studies in which the test performance was measured (see Section 3.3.5). With certain tests, the LRs may differ depending on the pretest odds in part because differences in pretest odds may reflect differences in the spectrum of disease in the population.

A third potential problem arises when you use Bayes' theorem to interpret a *sequence* of tests. If a patient undergoes two tests in sequence, you can use the post-test probability after the first test result, calculated with Bayes' theorem, as the pretest probability for the second test. Then, you use Bayes' theorem a sec-

[8]In medicine, to *rule in* a disease is to confirm that the patient *does* have the disease; to *rule out* a disease is to confirm that the patient does *not* have the disease. A doctor who strongly suspects that her patient has a bacterial infection orders a culture to *rule in* her diagnosis. Another doctor is almost certain that his patient has a simple sore throat but orders a culture to *rule out* streptococcal infection (strep throat). This terminology oversimplifies a diagnostic process that is probabilistic. Diagnostic tests rarely, if ever, rule in or rule out a disease; rather, the tests raise or lower the probability of disease.

ond time to calculate the post-test probability after the second test. This approach is valid, however, only if the two tests are conditionally independent. Tests for the same disease are **conditionally independent** when the probability of a particular result on the second test does not depend on the result of the first test, *given* (conditioned on) the disease state. Expressed in conditional probability notation for the case in which the disease is present,

$$\begin{aligned} &p[\text{second test positive} \mid \text{first test positive and disease present}] \\ &\quad = p[\text{second test positive} \mid \text{first test negative and disease present}] \\ &\quad = p[\text{second test positive} \mid \text{disease present}]. \end{aligned}$$

If the conditional independence assumption is satisfied, the post-test odds = pretest odds $\times$ LR_1 $\times$ LR_2. If you apply Bayes' theorem sequentially in situations in which conditional independence is violated, you will obtain inaccurate post-test probabilities.

The fourth common problem arises when you assume that all test abnormalities result from one (and only one) disease process. The Bayesian approach, as we have described it, generally presumes that the diseases under consideration are **mutually exclusive**. If they are not, Bayesian updating must be applied with great care.

We have shown how to calculate post-test probability. In Section 3.5, we turn to the problem of decision-making when the outcomes of a physician's actions (e.g., of treatments) are uncertain.

3.5 Expected-Value Decision-Making

Medical decision-making problems often cannot be solved by reasoning based on pathophysiology. For example, clinicians need a method for choosing among treatments when the outcome of the treatments is unpredictable, as are the results of a surgical operation. You can use the ideas developed in the preceding sections to solve such difficult decision problems. Here we discuss two methods: the decision tree, a method for representing and comparing the expected outcomes of each decision alternative; and the threshold probability, a method for deciding whether new information can change a management decision. These techniques help you to clarify the decision problem and thus to choose the alternative that is most likely to help the patient.

3.5.1 Comparison of Uncertain Prospects

Like those of most biological events, the outcome of an individual's illness is unpredictable. How can a physician determine which course of action has the greatest chance of success?

Example 11. There are two available therapies for a fatal illness. The length of a patient's life after either therapy is unpredictable, as illustrated by the frequency distribution shown in Figure 3.7 and summarized in Table 3.5. Each therapy is associ-

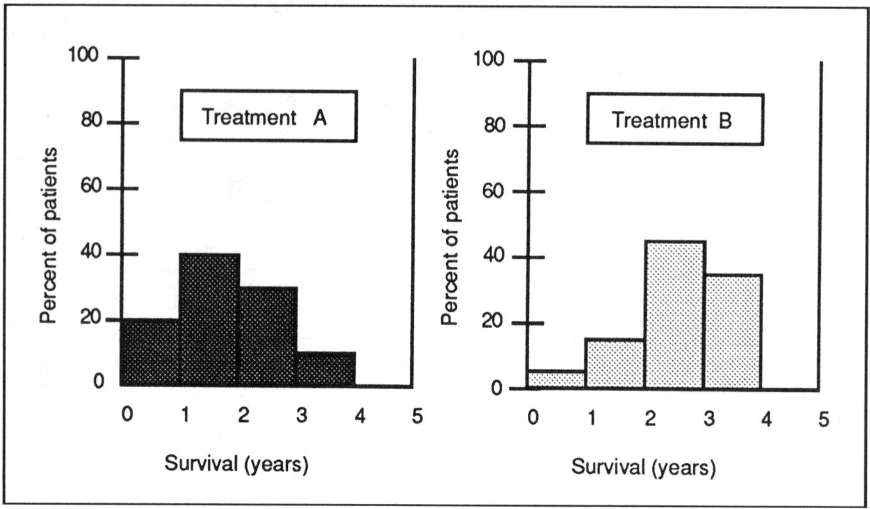

FIGURE 3.7. Survival after therapy for a fatal disease. Two therapies are available; the results of either are unpredictable.

> ated with uncertainty: Regardless of which therapy a patient receives, he will die by the end of the fourth year, but there is no way to know which year will be the patient's last. Figure 3.7 shows that survival until the fourth year is more likely with therapy B, but the patient might die in the first year with therapy B or might survive to the fourth year with therapy A.

Which of the two therapies is preferable? This example demonstrates a significant fact: A choice among therapies is a choice among gambles (i.e., situations in which chance determines the outcomes). How do we usually choose among gambles? More often than not, we rely on hunches or on a sixth sense. How *should* we choose among gambles? We propose a method for choosing called **expected-value decision-making**: We characterize each gamble by a number, and we use that number to compare the gambles.[9] In Example 11, therapy

[9]Expected-value decision-making had been used in many fields before it was first applied to medicine.

TABLE 3.5. Distribution of probabilities for the two therapies in Figure 3.7.

	Probability of death	
Years after therapy	Therapy A	Therapy B
1	0.20	0.05
2	0.40	0.15
3	0.30	0.45
4	0.10	0.35

A and therapy B are both gambles with respect to duration of life after therapy. We want to assign a measure (or number) to each therapy that summarizes the outcomes such that we can decide which therapy is preferable.

The ideal criterion for choosing a gamble should be a number that reflects preferences (in medicine, often the patient's preferences) for the outcomes of the gamble. **Utility** is the name given to a measure of preference that has a desirable property for decision-making: The gamble with the highest utility should be preferred. We shall discuss utility briefly (Section 3.5.4), but you can pursue this topic and the details of decision analysis in other textbooks (see the Suggested Readings at the end of this chapter).[10] We use the average duration of life after therapy (survival) as a criterion for choosing among therapies; remember that this model is oversimplified, used here for discussion only. Later, we consider other factors, such as the quality of life.

Because we cannot be sure of the duration of survival for any given patient, we characterize a therapy by the mean survival (average length of life) that would be observed in a large number of patients after they were given the therapy. The first step we take in calculating the mean survival for a therapy is to divide the population receiving the therapy into groups of patients who have similar survival rates. Then, we multiply the survival time in each group[11] by the fraction of the total population in that group. Finally, we sum these products over all possible survival values.

We can perform this calculation for the therapies in Example 11. Mean survival for therapy A = $(0.2 \times 1.0) + (0.4 \times 2.0) + (0.3 \times 3.0) + (0.1 \times 4.0) =$ 2.3 years. Mean survival for therapy B = $(0.05 \times 1.0) + (0.15 \times 2.0) + (0.45 \times 3.0) + (0.35 \times 4.0) = 3.1$ years.

Survival after a therapy is under the control of chance. Therapy A is a gamble characterized by an average survival equal to 2.3 years. Therapy B is a gamble characterized by an average survival of 3.1 years. If length of life is our criterion for choosing, we should select therapy B.

3.5.2 Representation of Choices with Decision Trees

The choice between therapies A and B is represented diagrammatically in Figure 3.8. Events that are under the control of chance can be represented by a **chance node**. By convention, a chance node is shown as a circle from which several lines emanate. Each line represents one of the possible outcomes. Associated with each line is the probability of the outcome occurring. For a single patient, only one outcome can occur. Some physicians object to using probability for just this reason: "You cannot rely on population data, because each patient

---

[10]A more general term for expected-value decision-making is expected *utility* decision-making. Because a full treatment of utility is beyond the scope of this chapter, we have chosen to use the term *expected value.*

[11]For this simple example, death during an interval is assumed to occur at the end of the year.

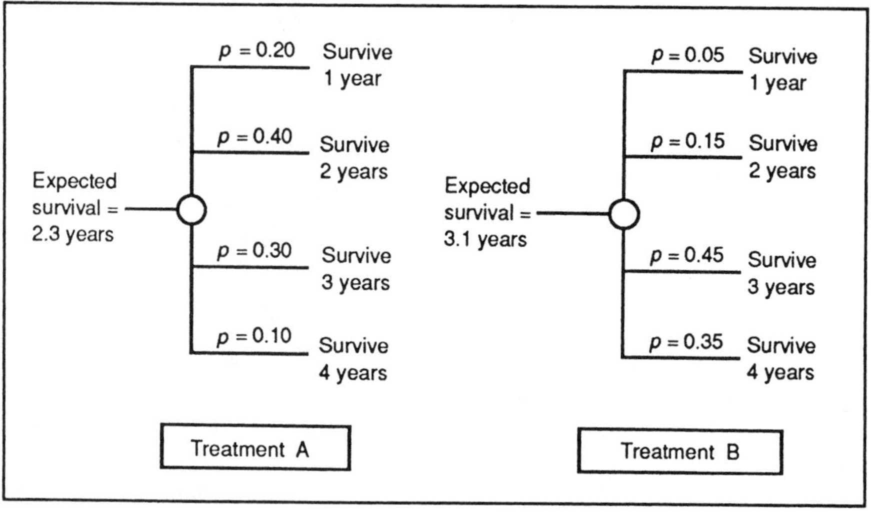

FIGURE 3.8. A chance-node representation of survival after the two therapies in Figure 3.7. The probabilities times the corresponding years of survival are summed to obtain the total expected survival.

is an individual." In fact, we often *must* use the frequency of the outcomes of many patients experiencing the same event to inform our opinion about what might happen to an individual. From these frequencies, we can make patient-specific adjustments and thus estimate the probability of each outcome at a chance node.

A chance node can represent more than just an event governed by chance. The outcome of a chance event, unknowable for the individual, can be represented by the **expected value** at the chance node. The concept of expected value is important and is easy to understand. We can calculate the mean survival that would be expected if many patients had the treatment depicted by the chance node in Figure 3.8. This average length of life is called the *expected survival* or, more generally, the *expected value of the chance node*. We calculate the expected value at a chance node by the process just described: We multiply the survival value associated with each possible outcome by the probability that that outcome will occur. We then sum the product of probability times survival over all outcomes. Thus, if several hundred patients were assigned to receive either therapy A or therapy B, the expected survival would be 2.3 years for therapy A and 3.1 years for therapy B.

We have just described the basis of expected-value decision-making. The term *expected value* is used to characterize a chance event, such as the outcome of a therapy. If the outcomes of a therapy are measured in units of duration of survival, units of sense of well-being, or dollars, the therapy is characterized by the expected duration of survival, expected sense of well-being, or expected monetary cost that it will confer on or incur for the patient, respectively.

To use expected-value decision-making, we follow this strategy when there are therapy choices with uncertain outcomes: (1) calculate the expected value of each decision alternative and then (2) pick the alternative with the highest expected value.

3.5.3 *Performance of a Decision Analysis*

We clarify the concepts of expected-value decision-making by discussing an example. There are four steps in decision analysis:

1. Create a decision tree; this step is the most difficult, because it requires formulating the decision problem, assigning probabilities, and measuring outcomes.
2. Calculate the expected value of each decision alternative.
3. Choose the decision alternative with the highest expected value.
4. Use sensitivity analysis to test the conclusions of the analysis.

Many health professionals balk when they first learn about the technique of decision analysis, because they recognize the opportunity for error in assigning values to both the probabilities and the utilities in a decision tree. They reason that the technique encourages decision-making based on small differences in expected values that are estimates at best. The defense against this concern, which also has been recognized by decision analysts, is the technique known as *sensitivity analysis*. We discuss this important fourth step in decision analysis in Section 3.5.5.

The first step in decision analysis is to create a **decision tree** that represents the decision problem. Consider the following clinical problem.

Example 12. The patient is Mr. Danby, a 66-year-old man who has been crippled with arthritis of both knees so severely that, while he can get about the house with the aid of two canes, he must otherwise use a wheelchair. His other major health problem is emphysema, a disease in which the lungs lose their ability to exchange oxygen and carbon dioxide between blood and air, which in turn causes shortness of breath (dyspnea). He is able to breathe comfortably when he is in a wheelchair, but the effort of walking with canes makes him breathe heavily and feel uncomfortable. Several years ago, he seriously considered knee-replacement surgery but decided against it, largely because his internist told him that there was a serious risk that he would not survive the operation because of his lung disease. Recently, however, Mr. Danby's wife had a stroke and was partially paralyzed; she now requires a degree of assistance that the patient cannot supply given his present state of mobility. He tells his doctor that he is reconsidering knee replacement surgery.

Mr. Danby's internist is familiar with decision analysis. She recognizes that this problem is filled with uncertainty: Mr. Danby's ability to survive the operation is in doubt, and the surgery sometimes does not restore mobility to the degree required by this patient. Furthermore, there is a small chance that the prosthesis (the artificial knee) will become infected, and Mr. Danby then would have to undergo a second risky operation to remove it. After removal of the prosthesis, Mr. Danby would never again be able to walk, even with canes. The possible outcomes of knee replacement include

> death from the first procedure and death from a second mandatory procedure if the prosthesis becomes infected (which we will assume occurs in the immediate postoperative period, if it occurs at all). Possible functional outcomes include recovery of full mobility or continued, and unchanged, poor mobility. Should Mr. Danby choose to undergo knee-replacement surgery, or should he accept the status quo?

Using the conventions of decision analysis, the internist sketches the decision tree shown in Figure 3.9. According to these conventions, a square box denotes a **decision node**, and each line emanating from a decision node represents an action that could be taken.

According to the methods of expected-value decision-making, the internist first must assign a probability to each branch of each chance node. To accomplish this task, the internist asks several orthopedic surgeons for their estimates of the chance of recovering full function after surgery (p[full recovery] = 0.60) and the chance of developing infection in the prosthetic joint (p[infection] = 0.05). She uses her subjective estimate of the probability that the patient will die during or immediately after knee surgery (p[operative death] = 0.05).

Next, she must assign a value to each outcome. To accomplish this task, she first lists the outcomes. As you can see from Table 3.6, the outcomes differ in two dimensions: length of life (survival) and quality of life (functional status). To characterize each outcome accurately, the internist must develop a measure that takes into account these two dimensions. Simply using duration of survival is inadequate because Mr. Danby values 5 years of good health more than he values 10 years of poor health. The internist can account for this trade-off factor by converting outcomes with two dimensions into outcomes with a single di-

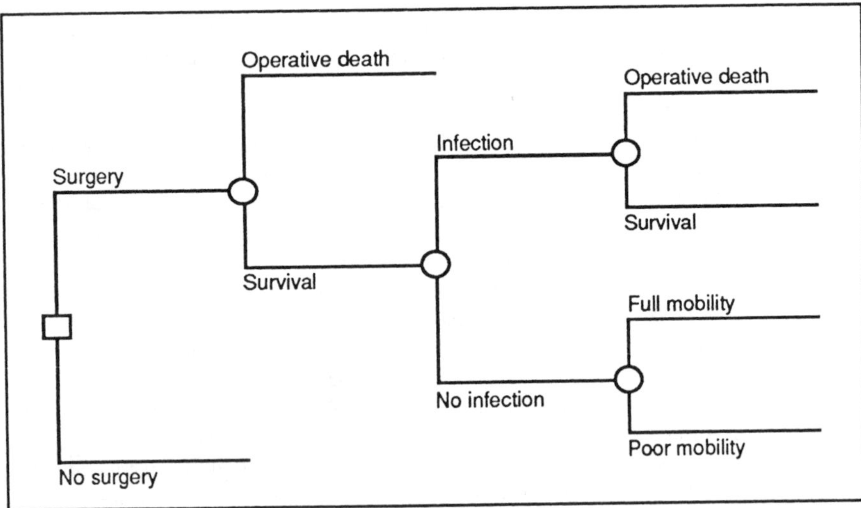

FIGURE 3.9. Decision tree for knee-replacement surgery. The box represents the decision node (whether to have surgery). The circles represent chance nodes.

TABLE 3.6. Outcomes for Example 12.

Survival (years)	Functional status	Years of full function equivalent to outcome
10	Full mobility (successful surgery)	10
10	Poor mobility (status quo or unsuccessful surgery)	6
10	Wheelchair-bound (the outcome if a second surgery is necessary)	3
0	Death	0

mension: duration of survival in good health. The resulting measure is called a **quality-adjusted life year** (QALY).[12]

She can convert years in poor health into years in good health by asking Mr. Danby to indicate the shortest period in good health (full mobility) that he would accept in return for his full expected lifetime (10 years) in a state of poor health (status quo). Thus, she asks Mr. Danby, "Many people say they would be willing to accept a shorter life in excellent health in preference to a longer life with significant disability. In your case, how many years with normal mobility do you feel is equivalent in value to 10 years in your current state of disability?" She asks him this question for each outcome. The patient's responses are shown in the third column of Table 3.6. The patient decides that 10 years of limited mobility are equivalent to 6 years of normal mobility, whereas 10 years of wheelchair confinement are equivalent to only 3 years of full function. Figure 3.10 shows the final decision tree—complete with probability estimates and utility values for each outcome.[13]

The second task that the internist must undertake is to calculate the expected value, in healthy years, of surgery and of no surgery. She calculates the expected value at each chance node, moving from right (the tips of the tree) to left (the root of the tree). Let us consider, for example, the expected value at the chance node representing the outcome of surgery to remove an infected prosthesis (Node *A* in Fig. 3.10). The calculation requires three steps:

1. Calculate the expected value of operative death after surgery to remove an infected prosthesis. Multiply the probability of operative death (0.05) by the QALY of the outcome—death (0 years): $0.05 \times 0 = 0$ QALY.
2. Calculate the expected value of surviving surgery to remove an infected knee prosthesis. Multiply the probability of surviving the operation (0.95) by the

[12]Quality-adjusted life years commonly are used as measures of utility (value) in medical decision analysis and in health-policy analysis (see, for example, the discussion of cost-effectiveness analysis in Chapter 8).

[13]In a more sophisticated decision analysis, the physician also would adjust the utility values of outcomes that require surgery to account for the pain and inconvenience associated with surgery and rehabilitation.

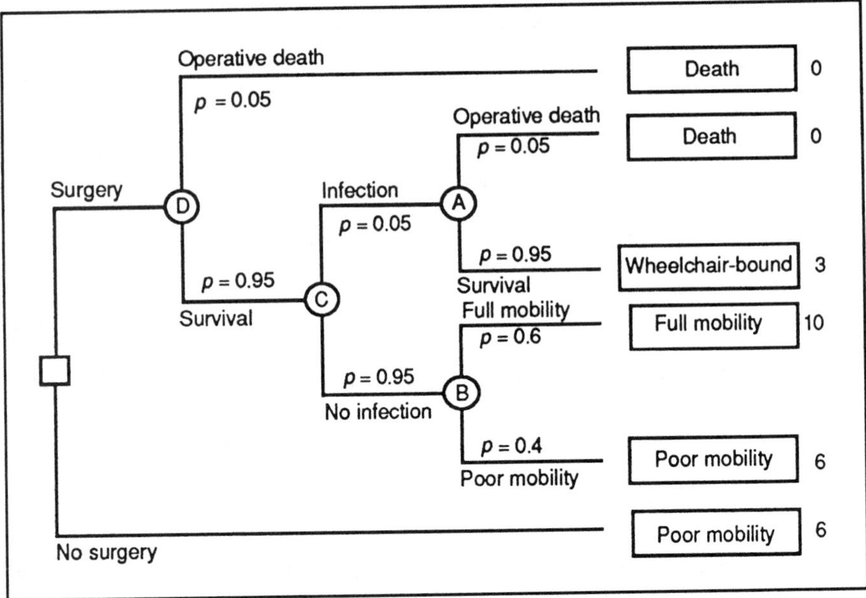

FIGURE 3.10. Decision tree for knee-replacement surgery. Probabilities have been assigned to each branch of each chance node. The patient's valuations of outcomes (measured in years of perfect mobility) are assigned to the tips of each branch of the tree.

number of healthy years equivalent to 10 years of being wheelchair bound (3 years): 0.95 × 3 = 2.85 QALYs.
3. Add the expected values calculated in step 1 (0 QALY) and step 2 (2.85 QALYs) to obtain the expected value of developing an infected prosthesis: 0 + 2.85 = 2.85 QALYs.

Similarly, the expected value at chance node *B* is calculated: (0.6 × 10) + (0.4 × 6) = 8.4 QALYs. To obtain the expected value of surviving knee-replacement surgery (Node *C*), she proceeds as follows:

1. Multiply the expected value of an infected prosthesis (already calculated as 2.85 QALYs) by the probability that the prosthesis will become infected (0.05): 2.85 × 0.05 = 0.143 QALYs.
2. Multiply the expected value of never developing an infected prosthesis (already calculated as 8.4 QALYs) by the probability that the prosthesis will not become infected (0.95): 8.4 × 0.95 = 7.98 QALYs.
3. Add the expected values calculated in step 1 (0.143 QALY) and step 2 (7.98 QALYs) to get the expected value of surviving knee replacement surgery: 0.143 + 7.98 = 8.123 QALYs.

The physician performs this process, called **averaging out at chance nodes**, for node *D* as well, working back to the root of the tree, until the expected value of surgery has been calculated. The outcome of the analysis is as follows. For surgery, Mr. Danby's average life expectancy, measured in years of normal mobility, is 7.7. What does this value mean? It does not mean that, by accepting surgery, Mr. Danby is guaranteed 7.7 years of mobile life. One look at the decision tree will show that some patients die in surgery, some develop infection, and some do not gain any improvement in mobility after surgery. Thus, an individual patient has no guarantees. If the physician had 100 similar patients who underwent the surgery, however, the *average* number of mobile years would be 7.7. We can understand what this value means for Mr. Danby only by examining the alternative: no surgery.

In the analysis for no surgery, the average length of life, measured in years of normal mobility, is 6.0, which Mr. Danby considered equivalent to 10 years of continued poor mobility. Not all patients will experience this outcome; some who have poor mobility will live longer than, and some will live less than, 10 years. The average length of life, however, expressed in years of normal mobility, will be 6. Because 6.0 is less than 7.7, *on average* the surgery will provide an outcome with higher value to the patient. Thus, the internist recommends performing the surgery.

The key insight of expected-value decision-making should be clear from this example: Given the unpredictable outcome in an individual, the best choice for the individual is the alternative that gives the best result on the average in similar patients. Decision analysis can help the physician to identify the therapy that will give the best results when averaged over many similar patients. The decision analysis is tailored to a specific patient in that both the utility functions and the probability estimates are adjusted to the individual. Nonetheless, the results of the analysis represent the outcomes that would occur *on the average* in a population of patients who have similar utilities and for whom uncertain events have similar probabilities.

3.5.4 Representation of Patients' Preferences withUtilities

In Section 3.5.3, we introduced the concept of QALYs, because length of life is not the only outcome about which patients care. Patients' preferences for a health outcome may depend on the length of life with the outcome, on the quality of life with the outcome, and on the risk involved in achieving the outcome (e.g., a cure for cancer might require a risky surgical operation). How can we incorporate these elements into a decision analysis? To do so, we can represent patients' preferences with utilities. The **utility** of a health state is a quantitative measure of the desirability of a health state from the patient's perspective. Utilities are typically expressed on a 0 to 1 scale, where 0 represents death and 1 represents ideal health. For example, a study of patients who had chest pain (angina) with exercise rated the utility of mild, moderate, and severe angina as 0.95, 0.92, and 0.82 (Nease et al., 1995). There are several methods for assessing utilities.

The **standard-gamble** technique has the strongest theoretical basis of the various approaches to utility assessment, as shown by Von Neumann and Morgenstern and described by Sox and colleagues (1988). To illustrate use of the standard gamble, suppose that we seek to assess a person's utility for the health state of asymptomatic HIV infection. To use the standard gamble, we ask our subject to compare the desirability of asymptomatic HIV infection to those of two other health states whose utility we know or can assign. Often, we use ideal health (assigned a utility of 1) and immediate death (assigned a utility of 0) for the comparison of health states. We then ask our subject to choose between asymptomatic HIV infection and a gamble with a chance of ideal health or immediate death. We vary the probability of ideal health and immediate death systematically until the subject is indifferent between asymptomatic HIV infection and the gamble. For example, a subject might be indifferent when the probability of ideal health is 0.8 and the probability of death is 0.2. At this point of indifference, the utility of the gamble and that of asymptomatic HIV infection are equal, a key relationship that allows us to calculate the utility of the gamble as the weighted average of the utilities of each outcome of the gamble $[(1 \times 0.8) + (0 \times 0.2)] = 0.8$. Thus in this example, the utility of asymptomatic HIV infection is 0.8. Use of the standard gamble enables an analyst to assess the utility of outcomes that differ in length or quality of life. Because the standard gamble involves chance events, it also assesses a person's willingness to take risks—called the person's **risk attitude**.

A second common approach to utility assessment is the **time-trade-off** technique (Sox et al., 1988; Torrance & Feeny, 1989). To assess the utility of asymptomatic HIV infection using the time-trade-off technique, we ask a person to determine the length of time in a better state of health (usually ideal health or best attainable health) that he would find equivalent to a longer period of time with asymptomatic HIV infection. For example, if our subject says that 8 months of life with ideal health was equivalent to 12 months of life with asymptomatic HIV infection, then we calculate the utility of asymptomatic HIV infection as $8 \div 12 = 0.67$. The time-trade-off technique provides a convenient method for valuing outcomes that accounts for gains (or losses) in both length and quality of life. Because the time trade-off does not include gambles, however, it does not assess a person's risk attitude. Perhaps the strongest assumption underlying the use of the time trade-off as a measure of utility is that people are risk neutral. A **risk-neutral** decision-maker is indifferent between the expected value of a gamble and the gamble itself. For example, a risk-neutral decision maker would be indifferent between the choice of living 20 years (for certain) and that of taking a gamble with a 50 percent chance of living 40 years and a 50 percent chance of immediate death (which has an expected value of 20 years). In practice, of course, few people are risk neutral. Nonetheless, the time-trade-off technique is used frequently to value health outcomes because it is relatively easy to understand.

Several other approaches are available to value health outcomes. To use the **visual-analog scale**, a person simply rates the quality of life with a health outcome (e.g., asymptomatic HIV infection) on a scale from 0 to 100. Although the visual-analog scale is easy to explain and use, it has no theoretical justification as a valid measure of utility. Ratings with the visual-analog scale, however, correlate modestly well with utilities assessed by the standard gamble and time trade-off. For a demonstration of the use of standard gambles, time-trade-offs, and the visual-analog scale to assess utilities in patients with angina, see Nease and colleagues (1995). Other approaches to valuing health outcomes include the Quality of Well Being Scale, the Health Utilities Index, and the EuroQoL (see Chapter 4 in Gold et al., 1996). Each of these instruments assesses how people value health outcomes and therefore may be appropriate for use in decision analyses or cost-effectiveness analyses.

In summary, we can use utilities to represent how patients value complicated health outcomes that differ in length and quality of life and in riskiness. Computer-based tools with an interactive format are now available for assessing utilities; they often include text and multimedia presentations that enhance patients' understanding of the assessment tasks and of the health outcomes (Lenert et al., 1995; Nease & Owens, 1994; Sumner et al., 1991).

3.5.5 Performance of Sensitivity Analysis

Sensitivity analysis is a test of the validity of the conclusions of an analysis over a wide range of assumptions about the probabilities and the values, or utilities. The probability of an outcome at a chance node may be the best estimate that is available, but there often is a wide range of reasonable probabilities that a physician could use with nearly equal confidence. We use sensitivity analysis to answer this question: Do my conclusions regarding the preferred choice change when the probability and outcome estimates are assigned values that lie within a reasonable range?

The knee-replacement decision in Example 12 illustrates the power of sensitivity analysis. If the conclusions of the analysis (surgery is preferable to no surgery) remain the same despite a wide range of assumed values for the probabilities and outcome measures, the recommendation is trustworthy. Figures 3.11 and 3.12 show the expected survival in healthy years with surgery and without surgery under varying assumptions of the probability of operative death and the probability of attaining perfect mobility, respectively. Each point (value) on these lines represents one calculation of expected survival using the tree in Figure 3.9. Figure 3.11 shows that expected survival is higher with surgery over a wide range of operative mortality rates. Expected survival is lower with surgery, however, when the operative mortality rate exceeds 25 percent. Figure 3.12 shows the effect of varying the probability that the operation will lead to perfect mobility. The expected survival, in healthy years, is higher for surgery as long as the probability of perfect mobility exceeds 20 percent, a much lower figure than is expected from previous experience with the operation. (In Example 12, the consulting orthopedic surgeons estimated the chance of full recovery at 60 percent.) Thus, the internist can proceed with confidence to recommend surgery. Mr. Danby cannot be sure of a good outcome, but he

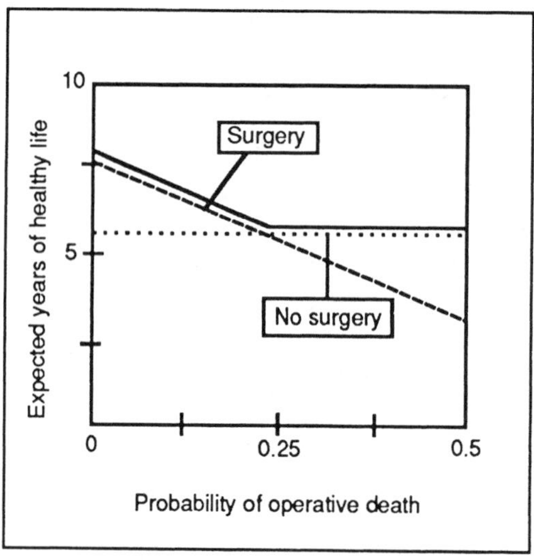

FIGURE 3.11. Sensitivity analysis of the effect of operative mortality on length of healthy life (Example 12). As the probability of operative death increases, the relative values of surgery versus no surgery change. The point at which the two lines cross represents the probability of operative death at which no surgery becomes preferable. The solid line represents the preferred option at a given probability.

has valid reasons for thinking that he is more likely to do well with surgery than he is without it.

Another way to state the conclusions of a sensitivity analysis is to indicate the range of probabilities over which the conclusions apply. The point at which the two lines in Figure 3.11 cross is the probability of operative death at which the two therapy options have the same expected survival. If expected survival is to be the basis for choosing therapy, the internist and the patient should be indifferent between surgery and no surgery when the probability of operative death

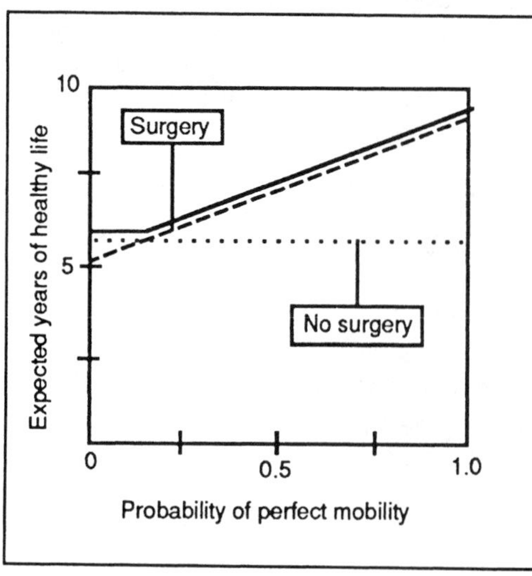

FIGURE 3.12. Sensitivity analysis of the effect of a successful operative result on length of healthy life (Example 12). As the probability of a successful surgical result increases, the relative values of surgery versus no surgery change. The point at which the two lines cross represents the probability of a successful result at which surgery becomes preferable. The solid line represents the preferred option at a given probability.

is 25 percent.[14] When the probability is lower, they should select surgery. When it is higher, they should select no surgery.

3.5.6 Representation of Long-Term Outcomes with Markov Models

In Example 12, we evaluated Mr. Danby's decision to have surgery to improve his mobility, which was compromised by arthritis. We assumed that each of the possible outcomes (full mobility, poor mobility, death, and so on) would occur shortly after Mr. Danby took action on his decision. But what if we want to model events that might occur in the distant future? For example, a patient with HIV infection might develop AIDS 10 to 15 years after infection; thus, a therapy to prevent or delay the development of AIDS could affect events that occur 10 to 15 years, or more, in the future. A similar problem arises in analyses of decisions regarding many chronic diseases: We must model events that occur over the lifetime of the patient. The decision-tree representation is convenient for decisions for which all outcomes occur during a short time horizon, but it is not always sufficient for problems that include events that could occur in the future. How can we include such events in a decision analysis? The answer is to use Markov models (Beck & Pauker, 1983; Sonnenberg & Beck, 1993).

To build a **Markov model**, we first specify the set of health states that a person could experience (e.g., Well, Cancer, and Death in Fig. 3.13). We then specify the **transition probabilities**, which are the probabilities that a person will transit from one of these health states to another during a specified time period. This period—often 1 month or 1 year—is the length of the **Markov cycle**. The

[14]An operative mortality rate of 25 percent may seem high; however, this value is correct when we use QALYs as the basis for choosing treatment. A decision-maker performing a more sophisticated analysis could use a utility function that reflects the patient's aversion to risking death.

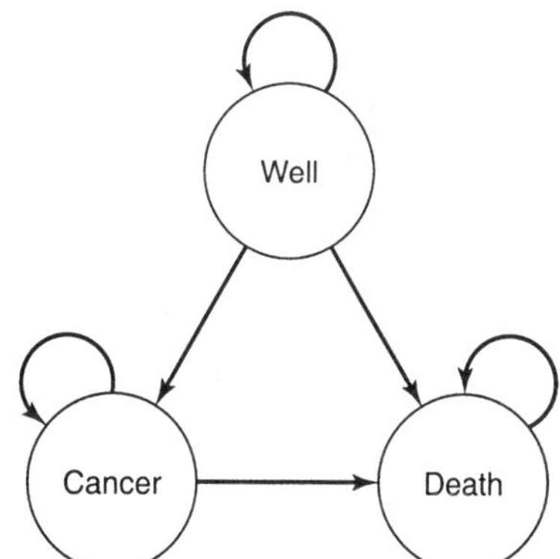

FIGURE 3.13. A simple Markov model. The states of health that a person can experience are indicated by the circles. Arrows represent allowed transitions between health states.

TABLE 3.7. Transition probabilities for the Markov model in Figure 3.13.

Health-state transition	Annual probability
Well to Well	0.9
Well to Cancer	0.06
Well to Death	0.04
Cancer to Well	0.0
Cancer to Cancer	0.4
Cancer to Death	0.6
Death to Well	0.0
Death to Cancer	0.0
Death to Death	1.0

Markov model then simulates the transitions among health states for a person (or for a hypothetical cohort of people) for a specified number of cycles; by using a Markov model, we can calculate the probability that a person will be in each of the health states at any time in the future.

As an illustration, consider a simple Markov model that has three health states, Well, Cancer, and Death (see Fig. 3.13). We have specified each of the transition probabilities in Table 3.7 for the cycle length of 1 year. Thus, we note from Table 3.7 that a person who is in the Well state will remain well with probability 0.9, will develop cancer with probability 0.06, and will die from noncancer causes with probability 0.04 during 1 year. The calculations for a Markov model are performed by computer software. Based on the transition probabilities in Table 3.7, the probabilities that a person remains well, develops cancer, or dies from noncancer causes over time is shown in Table 3.8. We can also determine from a Markov model the expected length of time that a person spends in each health state. Therefore, we can determine life expectancy, or quality-adjusted life expectancy, for any alternative represented by a Markov model.

In decision analyses that represent long-term outcomes, the analysts will often use a Markov model in conjunction with a decision tree to model the decision (Owens et al., 1995, 1997a; Salpeter et al., 1997). The analyst models the effect of an intervention as a change in the probability of going from one state to another. For example, we could model a cancer-prevention intervention (such as screening for breast cancer with mammography) as a reduction in the transition probability from Well to Cancer in Figure 3.13. For further explanation of

TABLE 3.8. Probability of future health states for the Markov model in Figure 3.13.

Health	Probability of health state at end of year						
state	Year 1	Year 2	Year 3	Year 4	Year 5	Year 6	Year 7
Well	0.9000	0.8100	0.7290	0.6561	0.5905	0.5314	0.4783
Cancer	0.0600	0.0780	0.0798	0.0757	0.0696	0.0633	0.0572
Death	0.0400	0.1120	0.1912	0.2682	0.3399	0.4053	0.4645

the use of Markov models, see the articles by Beck and Pauker (1983) and by Sonnenberg and Beck (1993).

3.6 The Decision Whether to Treat, Test, or Do Nothing

The physician who is evaluating a patient's symptoms and suspects a disease must choose among the following actions:

1. Do nothing further (neither perform additional tests nor treat the patient).
2. Obtain additional diagnostic information (test) before choosing whether to treat or do nothing.
3. Treat without obtaining more information.

When the physician knows the patient's true state, testing is unnecessary, and the doctor needs only to assess the trade-offs among therapeutic options (as in Example 12). Learning the patient's true state, however, may require costly, time-consuming, and often risky diagnostic procedures that may give misleading FP or FN results. Therefore, physicians often are willing to treat a patient even when they are not absolutely certain about a patient's true state. There are risks in this course: The physician may withhold therapy from a person who has the disease of concern, or he may administer therapy to someone who does not have the disease yet may suffer undesirable side effects of therapy.

Deciding among treating, testing, and doing nothing sounds difficult, but you have already learned all the principles that you need to solve this kind of problem. There are three steps:

1. Determine the treatment-threshold probability of disease.
2. Determine the pretest probability of disease.
3. Decide whether a test result could affect your decision to treat.

The **treatment-threshold probability** of disease is the probability of disease at which you should be indifferent between treating and not treating (Pauker & Kassirer, 1980). Below the treatment threshold, you should not treat. Above the treatment threshold, you should treat (Fig. 3.14). Whether to treat when the diagnosis is not certain is a problem that you can solve with a decision tree, such as the one shown in Figure 3.15. You can use this tree to learn the treatment-threshold probability of disease by leaving the probability of disease as an unknown, setting the expected value of surgery equal to the expected value for medical (i.e., nonsurgical, such as drugs or physical therapy) treatment, and solving for the probability of disease. (In this example, surgery corresponds to the "treat" branch of the tree in Figure 3.15, and nonsurgical intervention corresponds to the "do not treat" branch.) Because you are indifferent between medical treatment and surgery at this probability, it is the treatment-threshold probability. Using the tree completes step 1. In practice, people often determine the treatment threshold intuitively rather than analytically.

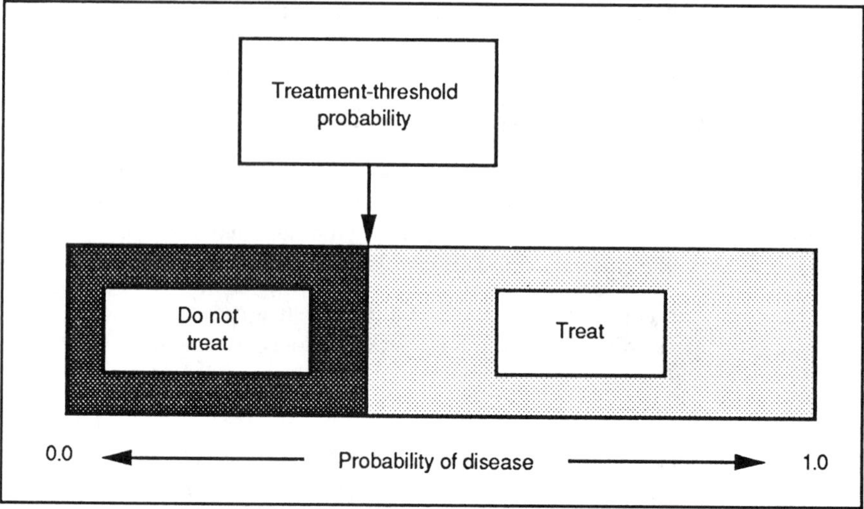

FIGURE 3.14. Depiction of the treatment-threshold probability. At probabilities of disease that are less than the treatment-threshold probability, the preferred action is to withhold therapy. At probabilities of disease that are greater than the treatment-threshold probability, the preferred action is to treat.

An alternative approach to determination of the treatment threshold probability is to use the equation

$$p^* = \frac{\mathrm{H}}{\mathrm{H} + \mathrm{B}},$$

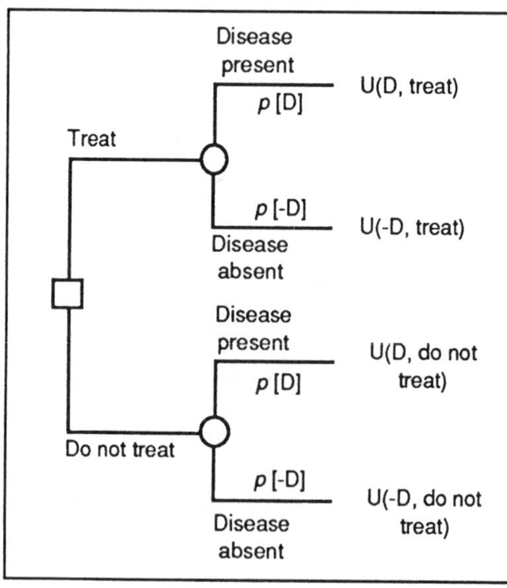

FIGURE 3.15. Decision tree with which to calculate the treatment-threshold probability of disease. By setting the utilities of the *treat* and *do not treat* choices to be equal, we can compute the probability at which the physician and patient should be indifferent to the choice. Recall that $p[-\mathrm{D}] = 1 - p[\mathrm{D}]$.

where p^* = the treatment-threshold probability, H = the harm associated with treatment of a nondiseased patient, and B = the benefit associated with treatment of a diseased patient (Pauker & Kassirer, 1980; Sox et al., 1988). We define B as the difference between the utility (U) of diseased patients who are treated and diseased patients who are not treated (U[D, treat] − U[D, do not treat], as shown in Fig. 3.15). The utility of diseased patients who are treated should be greater than that of diseased patients who are not treated; therefore, B is positive. We define H as the difference in utility of nondiseased patients who are not treated and nondiseased patients who are treated (U[−D, do not treat] − U[−D, treat], as shown in Fig. 3.15). The utility of nondiseased patients who are not treated should be greater than that of nondiseased patients who are treated; therefore, H is positive. The equation for the treatment-threshold probability fits with our intuition: If the benefit of treatment is small and the harm of treatment is large, then the treatment-threshold probability will be high. In contrast, if the benefit of treatment is large and the harm of treatment is small, the treatment threshold will be low.

Once you know the pretest probability, you know what to do in the absence of further information about the patient. If the pretest probability is below the treatment threshold, you should not treat the patient. If the pretest probability is above the threshold, you should treat the patient. Thus you have completed step 2.

One of the guiding principles of medical decision-making is this: Do not order a test unless it could change your management of the patient. In our framework for decision-making, this principle means that you should order a test only if the test result could cause the probability of disease to cross the treatment threshold. Thus, if the pretest probability is above the treatment threshold, a negative test result must lead to a post-test probability that is below the threshold. Conversely, if the pretest probability is below the threshold probability, a positive result must lead to a post-test probability that is above the threshold. In either case, the test result would alter your decision whether to treat the patient. This analysis completes step 3.

To decide whether a test could alter management, we simply use Bayes' theorem. We calculate the post-test probability after a test result that would move the probability of disease toward the treatment threshold. If the pretest probability is above the treatment threshold, we calculate the probability of disease if the test result is negative. If the pretest probability is below the treatment threshold, we calculate the probability of disease if the test result is positive.

Example 13. You are a pulmonary medicine specialist. You suspect that a patient of yours has a pulmonary embolus (blood clot lodged in the vessels of the lungs). One approach is to do a radionuclide lung scan, a test in which tiny radioactive particles are injected into a vein. These particles flow into the small vessels of the lung. A scanning device detects the radiation from the particles. The particles cannot go to a part of the lung that is supplied by a vessel that is blocked by a blood clot. Unfortunately, there are other causes of blank areas in the scan so that you cannot be sure that a blood clot is present when there is a blank area. Thus, if the scan is abnormal (shows a blank area), you must perform a definitive test to confirm the diagnosis. Such a test is a pulmonary arteriogram, in which radiopaque dye is injected into the arteries in the lung, and an X-ray image is obtained. The procedure involves further risk, discomfort, and substantial cost to the patient. If the scan is negative, you do no further tests and do not treat the patient.

To decide whether this strategy is correct, you take the following steps:

1. Determine the treatment-threshold probability of pulmonary embolus.
2. Estimate the pretest probability of pulmonary embolus.
3. Decide whether a test result could affect your decision to treat for an embolus.

First, assume you decide that the treatment threshold should be 0.10 in this patient. What does it mean to have a treatment-threshold probability equal to 0.10? If you could obtain no further information, you would treat for pulmonary embolus if the pretest probability was above 0.10 (i.e., if you believed that there was greater than a 1 in 10 chance that the patient had an embolus), and would withhold therapy if the pretest probability was below 0.10. A decision to treat when the pretest probability is at the treatment threshold means that you are willing to treat nine patients without pulmonary embolus to be sure of treating one patient who has pulmonary embolus. A relatively low treatment threshold is justifiable because treatment of a pulmonary embolism with blood-thinning medication substantially reduces the high mortality of pulmonary embolism, whereas there is only a relatively small danger (mortality of less than 1 percent) in treating someone who does not have pulmonary embolus. Because the benefit of treatment is high and the harm of treatment is low, the treatment-threshold probability will be low, as discussed earlier. You have completed step 1.

You estimate the pretest probability of pulmonary embolus to be 0.05, which is equal to a pretest odds of 0.053. Because the pretest probability is lower than the treatment threshold, you should do nothing unless a positive lung-scan result could raise the probability of pulmonary embolus to above 0.10. You have completed step 2.

To decide whether a test result could affect your decision to treat, you must decide whether a positive lung-scan result would raise the probability of pulmonary embolism to more than 0.10, the treatment threshold. Lung scans are usually reported as either negative, low probability, or high probability for pulmonary embolism. You review the literature and learn that the LR for a high probability scan is 7.0 to 8.0, and you choose to use the midpoint, 7.5.

A negative lung-scan result will move the probability of disease away from the treatment threshold and will be of no help in deciding what to do. A positive result will move the probability of disease toward the treatment threshold and could alter your management decision if the post-test probability was above the treatment threshold. You therefore use the odds-ratio form of Bayes' theorem to calculate the post-test probability of disease if the lung-scan result is reported as high probability.

$$\text{Post-test odds} = \text{pretest odds} \times \text{LR}$$
$$= 0.053 \times 7.5 = 0.40.$$

A post-test odds of 0.4 is equivalent to a probability of disease of 0.29. Because the post-test probability of pulmonary embolus is higher than the treatment threshold, a positive lung-scan result would change your management of the patient, and you should order the lung scan. You have completed step 3.

This example is especially useful for two reasons. First, it demonstrates one method for making decisions. Second, it shows how the concepts that were introduced in this chapter all fit together in a clinical example of medical decision-making.

3.7 Alternative Graphical Representations for Decision Models: Influence Diagrams and Belief Networks

In Sections 3.5 and 3.6, we used decision trees to represent decision problems. Although decision trees are the most common graphical representation for decision problems, **influence diagrams** are an important alternative representation for such problems (Nease & Owens, 1997; Owens et al., 1997b).

As shown in Figure 3.16, influence diagrams have certain features that are similar to decision trees, but they also have additional graphical elements. Influence diagrams represent decision nodes as squares and chance nodes as circles. In contrast to decision trees, however, the influence diagram also has arcs between nodes and a diamond-shaped value node. An **arc** between two chance nodes indicates that a probabilistic relationship *may* exist between the chance nodes (Owens et al., 1997b). A **probabilistic relationship** exists when the occurrence of one chance event affects the probability of the occurrence of another chance event. For example, in Figure 3.16, the probability of a positive or negative PCR test result (PCR Result) depends on whether a person has HIV infection (HIV Status); thus, these nodes have a probabilistic relationship, as indicated by the arc. The arc points from the **conditioning event** to the **conditioned event** (PCR test result is conditioned on HIV Status in Fig. 3.16). The absence of an arc between two chance nodes, however, always indicates that the nodes are independent or conditionally independent. Two events are **conditionally independent**, given a third event, if the occurrence of one of the events does not affect the probability of the other event conditioned on the occurrence of the third event.

Unlike a decision tree, in which the events usually are represented from left to right in the order in which the events are observed, influence diagrams use arcs to indicate the timing of events. An arc from a chance node to a decision node indicates that the chance event has been observed at the time the decision is made. Thus, the arc from PCR Result to Treat? in Figure 3.16 indicates that the decision-maker knows the PCR test result (positive, negative, or not obtained) when she decides whether to treat. Arcs between decision nodes indicate the timing of decisions: The arc points from an initial decision to subsequent decisions.

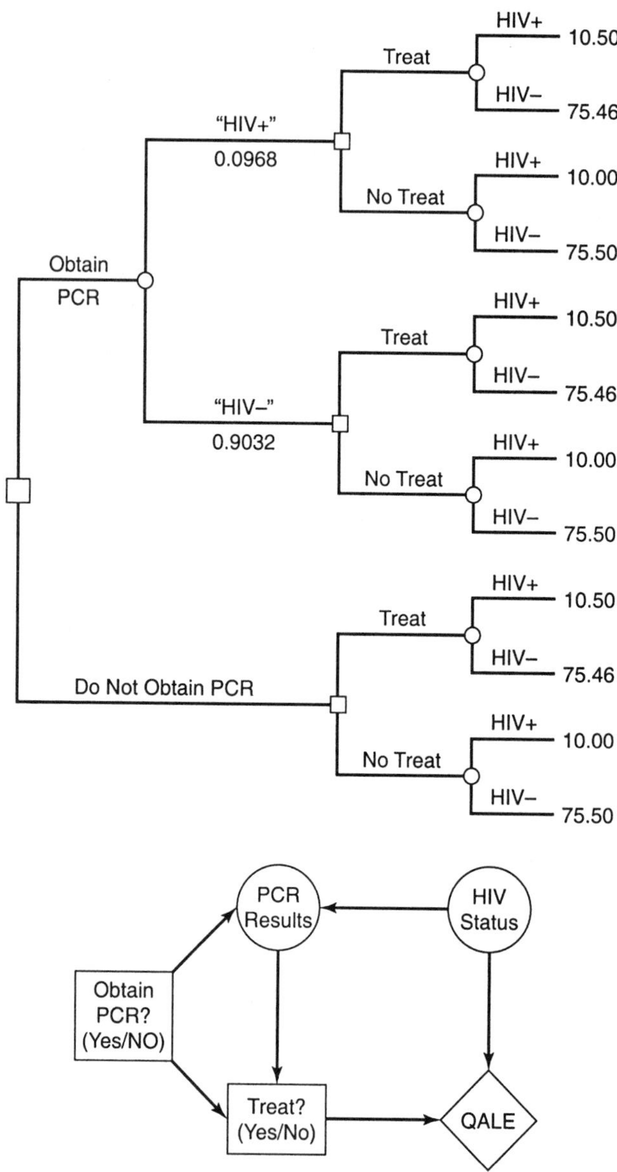

FIGURE 3.16. A decision tree (top) and an influence diagram (bottom) that represent the decisions to test for and to treat HIV infection. The structural asymmetry of the alternatives is explicit in the decision tree. The influence diagram highlights probabilistic relationships. HIV = human immunodeficiency virus; HIV+ = HIV infected; HIV− = not infected with HIV; QALE = quality-adjusted life expectancy; PCR = polymerase chain reaction. Test results are shown in quotation marks ("HIV+"), whereas the true disease state is shown without quotation marks (HIV+). (*Source:* Owens D.K., Shachter R.D., Nease R.F. [1997]. Representation and analysis of medical decision problems with influence diagrams. *Medical Decision Making,* 17(3): 241–262. Reproduced with permission.)

Thus, in Figure 3.16, the decision-maker must decide whether to obtain a PCR test before deciding whether to treat, as indicated by the arc from Obtain PCR? to Treat?

The probabilities and utilities that we need to determine the alternative with the highest expected value are contained in tables associated with chance nodes and the value node (Fig. 3.17). These tables contain the same information that we would use in a decision tree. With a decision tree, we can determine the expected value of each alternative by averaging out at chance nodes and folding back the tree (Section 3.5.3). For influence diagrams, the calculation of expected value is more complex (Owens et al., 1997b), and generally must be performed with computer software. With the appropriate software, we can use influence diagrams to perform the same analyses that we would perform with a decision tree. Diagrams that have only chance nodes are called **belief networks**; we use them to perform probabilistic inference.

Why use an influence diagram instead of a decision tree? Influence diagrams have both advantages and limitations relative to decision trees. Influence dia-

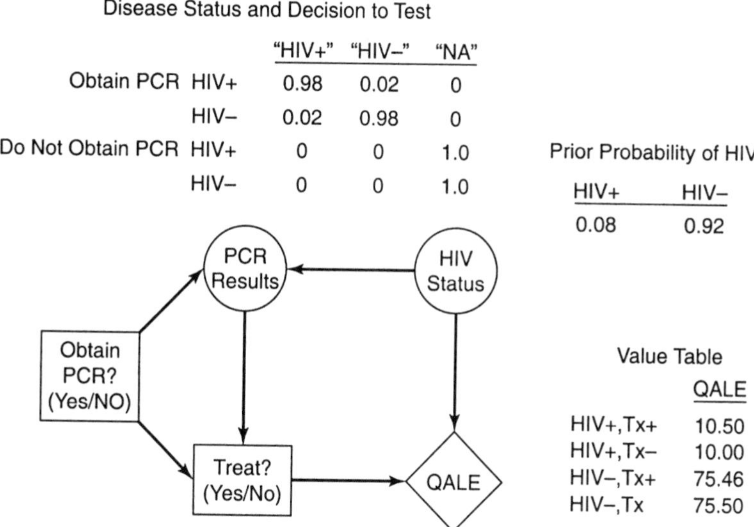

FIGURE 3.17. The influence diagram from Figure 3.16, with the probability and value tables associated with the nodes. The information in these tables is the same as that associated with the branches and endpoints of the decision tree in Figure 3.16. HIV = human immunodeficiency virus; HIV+ = HIV infected; HIV− = not infected with HIV; QALE = quality-adjusted life expectancy; PCR = polymerase chain reaction; NA = not applicable; TX+ = treated; TX− = not treated. Test results are shown in quotation marks ("HIV+"), and the true disease state is shown without quotation marks (HIV+). (*Source:* Owens D.K., Shachter R.D., Nease R.F. [1997]. Representation and analysis of medical decision problems with influence diagrams. *Medical Decision Making,* 17: 241–262. Reproduced with permission.)

grams represent graphically the probabilistic relationships among variables (Owens et al., 1997b). Such representation is advantageous for problems in which probabilistic conditioning is complex or in which communication of such conditioning is important (such as may occur in large models). In an influence diagram, probabilistic conditioning is indicated by the arcs, and thus the conditioning is apparent immediately by inspection. In a decision tree, probabilistic conditioning is revealed by the probabilities in the branches of the tree. To determine whether events are conditionally independent in a decision tree requires that the analyst compare probabilities of events between branches of the tree. Influence diagrams also are particularly useful for discussion with content experts who can help to structure a problem but who are not familiar with decision analysis. In contrast, problems that have decision alternatives that are structurally different may be easier for people to understand when represented with a decision tree, because the tree shows the structural differences explicitly, whereas the influence diagram does not. The choice of whether to use a decision tree or an influence diagram depends on the problem being analyzed, the experience of the analyst, the availability of software, and the purpose of the analysis. For selected problems, influence diagrams provide a powerful graphical alternative to decision trees.

3.8 The Role of Probability and Decision Analysis in Medicine

You may be wondering how probability and decision analysis might be integrated smoothly into medical practice. An understanding of probability and measures of test performance will prevent any number of misadventures. In Example 1, we discussed a hypothetical test that, on casual inspection, appeared to be an accurate way to screen blood donors for previous exposure to the AIDS virus. Our quantitative analysis, however, revealed that the test results were misleading more often than they were helpful because of the low prevalence of HIV in the clinically relevant population.[15]

The need for knowledgeable interpretation of test results is widespread. The federal government screens civil employees in "sensitive" positions for drug use, as do many companies. If the drug test used by an employer had a sensitivity and specificity of 0.95, and if 10 percent of the employees used drugs, one-third of the positive tests would be FPs. An understanding of these issues should be of great interest to the public, and health professionals should be prepared to answer the questions of their patients.

Although we should try to interpret every kind of test result accurately, decision analysis has a more selective role in medicine. Not all clinical decisions re-

[15]We emphasize that blood donors are screened with EIAs rather than with PCR. The sensitivity and specificity of EIAs are greater than 99%, and positive EIAs are confirmed with highly specific tests.

quire decision analysis. Some decisions depend on physiologic principles or on deductive reasoning. Other decisions involve little uncertainty. Nonetheless, many decisions must be based on imperfect data, and they will have outcomes that cannot be known with certainty at the time that the decision is made. Decision analysis provides a technique for managing these situations.

For many problems, simply drawing a tree that denotes the possible outcomes explicitly will clarify the question sufficiently to allow you to make a decision. When time is limited, even a "quick and dirty" analysis may be helpful. By using expert clinicians' subjective probability estimates and asking what the patient's utilities might be, you can perform an analysis quickly and learn which probabilities and utilities are the important determinants of the decision. You can spend time in the library or at the bedside getting accurate estimates of these important probabilities and utilities. You can solve other decision problems once and then use the decision trees as often as the need arises by changing the variables to fit the particular patient. Journals such as *Medical Decision Making* contain decision analyses that you can adapt to fit a specific patient. Once you have performed the first quantitative analysis, you often find that some of the variables in the tree have an insignificant effect on the decision. Then, in any further analyses regarding that problem, you will not need to give those variables much attention.

Healthcare professionals sometimes express reservations about decision analysis because the analysis may depend on probabilities that must be estimated, such as the pretest probability. A thoughtful decision-maker will be concerned that the estimate may be in error, particularly because the information needed to make the estimate often is difficult to obtain from the medical literature. We argue, however, that uncertainty in the clinical data is a problem for *any* decision-making method and that the effect of this uncertainty is explicit with decision analysis. The method for evaluating uncertainty is sensitivity analysis: We can examine any variable to see whether its value is critical to the final recommended decision. Thus, we can determine, for example, whether a change in pretest probability from 0.6 to 0.8 makes a difference in the final decision. In so doing, we often discover that it is necessary to estimate only a range of probabilities for a particular variable rather than a precise value. Thus, with a sensitivity analysis, we can decide whether uncertainty about a particular variable should concern us.

The growing complexity of medical decisions, coupled with the need to control costs, has led to major programs to develop clinical practice guidelines. Decision models have many advantages as aids to guideline development (Eddy, 1992): They make explicit the alternative interventions, associated uncertainties, and utilities of potential outcomes. Decision models can help guideline developers to structure guideline-development problems (Owens & Nease, 1993), to incorporate patients' preferences (Nease & Owens, 1994; Owens, 1998a), and to tailor guidelines for specific clinical populations (Owens & Nease, 1997). In addition, World Wide Web–based interfaces for decision models can provide distributed decision support for guideline developers and users by making the decision model available for analysis to anyone who has access to the Web (Sanders et al., 1999).

We have not emphasized computers in this chapter, although they can simplify many aspects of decision analysis (see Chapter 16). MEDLINE and other bibliographic-retrieval systems (see Chapter 15) make it easier to obtain published estimates of disease prevalence and test performance. Computer programs for performing statistical analyses can be used on data collected by hospital information systems. Decision-analysis software, available for personal computers, can help physicians to structure decision trees, to calculate expected values, and to perform sensitivity analyses. Researchers continue to explore methods for computer-based automated development of practice guidelines from decision models and use of computer-based systems to implement guidelines (Musen et al., 1996).

Medical decision-making often involves uncertainty for the physician and risk for the patient. Most healthcare professionals would welcome tools that help them make decisions when they are confronted with complex clinical problems with uncertain outcomes. There are important medical problems for which decision analysis offers such aid.

Appendix: Derivation of Bayes' Theorem

Bayes' theorem is derived as follows. We denote the conditional probability of disease, D, given a test result, R, $p[\mathrm{D}|\mathrm{R}]$. The prior (pretest) probability of D is $p[\mathrm{D}]$. The definition of conditional probability is

$$p[\mathrm{D}|\mathrm{R}] = \frac{p[\mathrm{R,D}]}{p[\mathrm{R}]}. \tag{3.1}$$

The probability of a test result ($p[\mathrm{R}]$) is the sum of its probability in diseased patients and its probability in nondiseased patients:

$$p[\mathrm{R}] = p[\mathrm{R,D}] + p[\mathrm{R},-\mathrm{D}].$$

Substituting into Equation 3.1, we obtain

$$p[\mathrm{D}|\mathrm{R}] = \frac{p[\mathrm{R,D}]}{p[\mathrm{R,D}] + p[\mathrm{R},-\mathrm{D}]}. \tag{3.2}$$

Again, from the definition of conditional probability,

$$p[\mathrm{R}|\mathrm{D}] = \frac{p[\mathrm{R,D}]}{p[\mathrm{D}]} \text{ and } p[\mathrm{R}|-\mathrm{D}] = \frac{p[\mathrm{R},-\mathrm{D}]}{p[-\mathrm{D}]}.$$

These expressions can be rearranged:

$$p[\mathrm{R,D}] = p[\mathrm{D}] \times p[\mathrm{R}|\mathrm{D}], \tag{3.3}$$
$$p[\mathrm{R},-\mathrm{D}] = p[-\mathrm{D}] \times p[\mathrm{R}|-\mathrm{D}]. \tag{3.4}$$

Substituting Equations 3.3 and 3.4 into Equation 3.2, we obtain Bayes' theorem:

$$p[\mathrm{D}|\mathrm{R}] = \frac{p[\mathrm{D}] \times p[\mathrm{R}|\mathrm{D}]}{p[\mathrm{D}] \times p[\mathrm{D}|\mathrm{R}] + p[-\mathrm{D}] \times p[\mathrm{R}|-\mathrm{D}]}.$$

Suggested Readings

Gold M.R., Siegel J.E., Russell L.B., Weinstein M.C. (1996). *Cost Effectiveness in Health and Medicine*. New York: Oxford University Press.

This book provides authoritative guidelines for the conduct of cost-effectiveness analyses. Chapter 4 discusses approaches for valuing health outcomes.

Nease R.F. Jr., Owens D.K. (1997). Use of influence diagrams to structure medical decisions. *Medical Decision Making,* 17(13):263–275; and Owens D.K., Schacter R.D., Nease R.F. Jr. (1997). Representation and analysis of medical decision problems with influence diagrams. *Medical Decision Making,* 17(3):241–262.

These two articles provide a comprehensive introduction to the use of influence diagrams.

Raiffa H. (1970). *Decision Analysis: Introductory Lectures on Choices Under Uncertainty*. Reading, MA: Addison-Wesley.

This book provides an advanced, nonmedical introduction to decision analysis, utility theory, and decision trees.

Sox H.C. (1986). Probability theory in the use of diagnostic tests. *Annals of Internal Medicine,* 104(1):60–66.

This article is written for physicians; it contains a summary of the concepts of probability and test interpretation.

Sox H.C., Blatt M.A., Higgins M.C., Marton K.I. (1988). *Medical Decision Making*. Boston: Butterworths.

This introductory textbook covers the subject matter of this chapter in greater detail, as well as discussing many other topics. An appendix contains the likelihood ratios of 100 common diagnostic tests.

Tversky A., Kahneman D. (1974). Judgment under uncertainty: Heuristics and biases. *Science,* 185:1124.

This now classic article provides a clear and interesting discussion of the experimental evidence for the use and misuse of heuristics in situations of uncertainty.

Weinstein M.C., Fineberg, H. (1980). *Clinical Decision Analysis*. Philadelphia: W.B. Saunders.

This textbook provides a clinical perspective of decision analysis. It addresses in detail most of the topics introduced in this chapter and covers utility assessment (including quality-adjusted life years) and cost-effectiveness analysis.

Questions for Discussion

1. Calculate the following probabilities for a patient about to undergo CABG surgery (see Example 2):
   a. The only possible, mutually exclusive outcomes of surgery are death, relief of symptoms (angina and dyspnea), and continuation of symptoms. The probability of death is 0.02, and the probability of relief of symptoms

TABLE 3.9. A 2 × 2 contingency table for the hypothetical study in problem 2.

PCR test result	Gold standard test positive	Gold standard test negative	Total
Positive PCR	2	47	49
Negative PCR	48	8	56
Total	50	55	105

PCR = polymerase chain reaction.

is 0.80. What is the probability that the patient will continue to have symptoms?

b. Two known complications of heart surgery are stroke and heart attack, with probabilities of 0.02 and 0.05, respectively. The patient asks what chance he has of having *both* complications. Assume that the complications are conditionally independent, and calculate your answer.

c. The patient wants to know the probability that he will have a stroke given that he has a heart attack as a complication of his surgery. Assume that 1 in 500 patients has *both* complications, that the probability of heart attack is 0.05, and that the events are independent. Calculate your answer.

2. The results of a hypothetical study to measure test performance of the PCR test for HIV (see Example 1) are shown in the 2 × 2 table in Table 3.9.
   a. Calculate the sensitivity, specificity, disease prevalence, PV^+, and PV^-.
   b. Use the TPR and TNR calculated in part a to fill in the 2 × 2 table in Table 3.10. Calculate the disease prevalence, PV^+, and PV^-.
3. You are asked to interpret a PCR HIV test in an asymptomatic man whose test was positive when he volunteered to donate blood. After taking his history, you learn that he is an intravenous-drug user. You know that the overall prevalence of HIV infection in your community is 1 in 500 and that the prevalence in intravenous-drug users is 20 times as high as in the community at large.
   a. Estimate the pretest probability that this man is infected with HIV.
   b. The man tells you that two people with whom he shared needles subsequently died of AIDS. Which heuristic will be useful in making a subjective adjustment to the pretest probability in part a?
   c. Use the sensitivity and specificity that you worked out in Problem 2a to calculate the post-test probability of the patient having HIV after a positive and negative test. Assume that the pretest probability is 0.10.

TABLE 3.10. A 2 × 2 contingency table to complete for problem 2b.

PCR test result	Gold standard test positive	Gold standard test negative	Total
Positive PCR	x	x	x
Negative PCR	100	99,900	x
Total	x	x	x

PCR = polymerase chain reaction.

d. If you wanted to increase the post-test probability of disease given a positive test result, would you change the TPR or TNR of the test?

4. You have a patient with cancer who has a choice between surgery or chemotherapy. If the patient chooses surgery, she has a 2 percent chance of dying from the operation (life expectancy = 0), a 50 percent chance of being cured (life expectancy = 15 years), and a 48 percent chance of not being cured (life expectancy = 1 year). If the patient chooses chemotherapy, she has a 5 percent chance of death (life expectancy = 0), a 65 percent chance of cure (life expectancy = 15 years), and a 30 percent chance that her cancer will be slowed but not cured (life expectancy = 2 years). Create a decision tree. Calculate the expected value of each option in terms of life expectancy.
5. You are concerned that a patient with a sore throat has a bacterial infection that would require antibiotic therapy (as opposed to a viral infection, for which no treatment is available). Your treatment threshold is 0.4, and based on the examination you estimate the probability of bacterial infection as 0.8. A test is available (TPR = 0.75, TNR = 0.85) that indicates the presence or absence of bacterial infection. Should you perform the test? Explain your reasoning. How would your analysis change if the test were extremely costly or involved a significant risk to the patient?
6. What are the three kinds of bias that can influence measurement of test performance? Explain what each one is, and state how you would adjust the post-test probability to compensate for each.
7. How could a computer system ease the task of performing a complex decision analysis? Look at the titles of Chapters 9 through 18 of this text. What role could each kind of system play in the medical-decision process?
8. When you search the medical literature to find probabilities for patients similar to one you are treating, what is the most important question to consider? How should you adjust probabilities in light of the answer to this question?
9. Why do you think physicians sometimes order tests even if the results will not affect their management of the patient? Do you think the reasons that you identify are valid? Are they valid in only certain situations? Explain your answers. See the January 1998 issue of *Medical Decision Making* for articles that discuss this question.
10. Explain the differences in three approaches to assessing patients' preferences for health states: the standard gamble, the time trade-off, and the visual-analog scale.

4
Essential Concepts for Medical Computing

GIO WIEDERHOLD AND THOMAS C. RINDFLEISCH

After reading this chapter, you should know the answers to these questions:

- How are medical data stored and manipulated in a computer?
- Why does a computer system have both memory and storage?
- How can data be entered into a computer accurately and efficiently?
- How can information be displayed clearly?
- What are the functions of a computer's operating system?
- What advantages does using a database-management system provide over storing and manipulating your own data directly?
- How do local-area networks facilitate data sharing and communication within healthcare institutions?
- How can the confidentiality of data stored in distributed computer systems be protected?
- How is the Internet used for medical applications?

4.1 Computer Architectures

Health professionals encounter computers in many settings. In more and more hospitals, physicians and nurses can order drugs and laboratory tests, review test results, and record medical observations using a hospital information system. Most hospitals and outpatient clinics have computers to help them manage financial and administrative information. Many physicians in private practice have purchased personal computers to allow them to access and search the medical literature, to communicate with colleagues, and to help their office staff with tasks such as billing and word processing.

Computers differ in speed, storage capacity, and cost; in the number of users that they can support; in the ways that they are interconnected; and in the types of application programs that they can run. On the surface, the differences among computers can be bewildering, and, as we discuss in Chapter 5, the selection of appropriate software and hardware is crucial to the success of a computer system. Despite these differences, however, most computers use the same basic mechanisms to store and process information and to communicate with the outside world. At the conceptual level, the similarities among machines greatly outweigh the differences. In this chapter, we discuss the fundamental concepts related to computer hardware and software, including data acquisition, security, and communications relevant to medical computing. We assume that you have already used some type of personal computer but have not been concerned with its internal workings. Our aim is to give you the background necessary for understanding the technical aspects of the applications discussed in later chapters. If you already have an understanding of how computers work, you may want to skim this chapter.

4.1.1 Hardware

Early computers were expensive to purchase and operate. Only large institutions could afford to acquire a computer and to develop its software. In the 1960s, the development of integrated circuits (ICs) on silicon chips resulted in dramatic increases in computing power per dollar. Since that time, computer hardware has become smaller, faster, and more reliable. Every year more powerful computers have cost less than weaker models from the year before. At the same time, standard software packages have been developed that remove much of the burden of writing the infrastructure of applications. The result is that computers are ubiquitous today.

General-purpose computers are classified into three types: servers, workstations, and personal computers (PCs). This distinction reflects several parameters but primarily relate to style of usage:

1. *Servers:* **Servers** are computers that share their resources with other computers and support the activities of many users simultaneously within an enterprise (e.g., admissions staff, pharmacy, and billing). Servers are often midsized or larger **mainframe** computers that are operated and maintained by professional computing personnel. A single mainframe might handle the information-processing needs of a large hospital or at least handle the large, shared databases and the data-processing tasks for activities such as billing and report generation. Smaller servers may exist in a laboratory or a group practice to carry out information-processing tasks similar to those run on mainframes. Such servers may be maintained within that unit.
2. *Personal computers:* At the other end of the spectrum are **personal computers**: relatively inexpensive single-user machines. They help users with tasks such as preparing letters and documents, creating graphics for oral presentations, and keeping track of expenses and income. They also provide access to services on the Internet—for example, sending and receiving electronic mail, searching for and displaying information, and collaborating with colleagues. The information stored on PCs is most often regarded as private and usually is not accessed by more than one user.
3. *Workstations:* **Workstations** are machines of moderate size and cost; most often, they have more processing capacity than PCs, so they can perform more demanding computing tasks, such as image processing or system modeling and simulation. They are characterized by having only a small number of users (typically only one) at any given time, by interacting effectively with servers,

by integrating information from diverse sources, and by responding to requests from other workstations. Multiple workstations in an enterprise may be connected into a network that makes integrated services available.

The boundaries between these categories of computers are not sharp. Personal computers are often powerful enough to function as workstations, and large workstations can be configured to act as servers. All types of computers can also be equipped for special tasks, such as the patient-monitoring tasks discussed in Chapter 13 and the three-dimensional modeling of anatomical regions discussed in Chapter 14. In these roles, the computers may be workstations for the specialists or servers for the larger community. **Terminals** are simple devices that have no processing capability of their own and that allow users to access servers. Terminals are quickly being replaced by PCs that, among their other functions, run programs that *emulate* terminals.

Most modern computers have similar organizations and basic **hardware** (physical equipment) structures. The most common **computer architectures** follow the principles expressed by John von Neuman in 1945. Figure 4.1 illustrates the configuration of a simple **von Neuman machine** in which the computer is composed of one or more

- **Central processing units** (CPUs) that perform computation
- **Computer memories** that store programs and data that are being used actively by a CPU
- **Storage devices**, such as disks and tapes, that provide long-term storage for programs and data

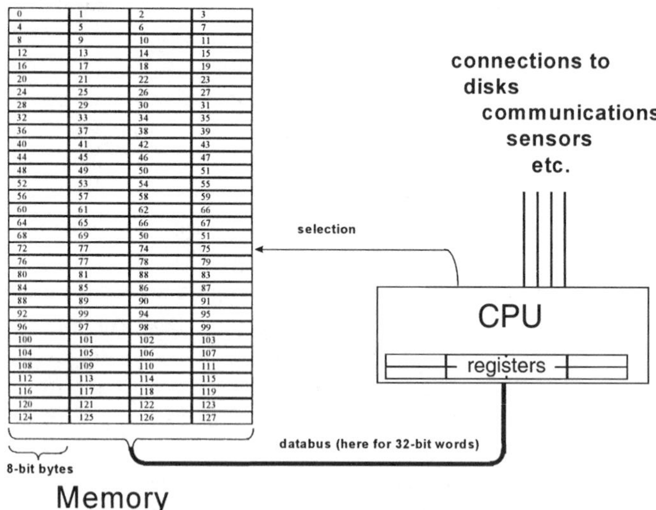

FIGURE 4.1. The von Neuman model, the basic architecture of most modern computers. The computer comprises a single central processing unit (CPU), an area for memory, and a data bus for transferring data between the two.

- **Input** and **output** devices, such as keyboards, pointing devices, video displays, and laser printers, that facilitate user interactions
- **Communication** equipment, such as modems and network interfaces, that connect computers to each other and to broader networks of computers.

Data buses are electrical pathways that transport encoded information between these subsystems.

Machines designed with other than von Neuman architectures are possible but remain relatively uncommon. Personal computers and workstations typically have only one CPU. In more sophisticated machines, when more processing power is required to solve complex problems, multiple CPUs and memories may be interconnected to support **parallel processing**. The challenge then is for the software to distribute the computation across these units to gain a proportionate benefit.

Central Processing Unit

Although complete computer systems appear to be complex, the underlying principles are simple. A prime example is a processing unit itself. Here simple components can be carefully combined to create systems with impressive capabilities. The structuring principle is that of *hierarchical organization:* Primitive units (electronic switches) are combined to form basic units that can store letters and numbers, add digits, and compare values with one another. The basic units are assembled into **registers** capable of storing and manipulating text and large numbers. These registers in turn are assembled into the larger functional units that make up the central component of a computer: the CPU.

The atomic element for all digital computers is the *binary digit* or **bit**. Each bit can assume one of two values: 0 or 1. An electronic switch that can be set to either of two states stores a single bit value. (Think of a light switch that can be either on or off.) These primitive units are the building blocks of computer systems. Sequences of bits (implemented as sequences of switches) are used to represent larger numbers and other kinds of information. For example, four switches can store 2^4, or 16, values. Because each unit can have a value of either 0 or 1, there are 16 combinations of 4-bit values: 0000, 0001, 0010, 0011, 0100, 0101, 0110, and so on, to 1111. Thus, 4 bits can represent any decimal value from 0 to 15; for instance, the sequence 0101 is the **binary** (base 2) representation of the decimal number 5—namely, $0 \times 2^3 + 1 \times 2^2 + 0 \times 2^1 + 1 \times 2^0 = 5$. A **byte** is a sequence of 8 bits; it can take on $2^8 = 256$ values.

Groups of bits and bytes can represent not only decimal integers but also fractional numbers, general characters (upper-case and lower-case letters, digits, and punctuation marks), instructions to the CPU, and more complex data types such as pictures, spoken language, and the content of a medical record. Figure 4.2 shows the **American Standard Code for Information Interchange** (ASCII), a convention for representing 95 common characters using 7 bits. These 7 bits are commonly placed into an 8-bit unit, a byte, which is the common way of transmitting and storing these characters. The eighth bit may be used for formatting

Characte	Binary code	Character	Binary code	Character	Binary code
blank	010 0000	@	100 0000	`	110 0000
!	010 0001	A	100 0001	a	110 0001
"	010 0010	B	100 0010	b	110 0010
#	010 0011	C	100 0011	c	110 0011
$	010 0100	D	100 0100	d	110 0100
%	010 0101	E	100 0101	e	110 0101
&	010 0110	F	100 0110	f	110 0110
'	010 0111	G	100 0111	g	110 0111
(	010 1000	H	100 1000	h	110 1000
)	010 1001	I	100 1001	i	110 1001
*	010 1010	J	100 1010	j	110 1010
+	010 1011	K	100 1011	k	110 1011
,	010 1100	L	100 1100	l	110 1100
-	010 1101	M	100 1101	m	110 1101
.	010 1110	N	100 1110	n	110 1110
/	010 1111	O	100 1111	o	110 1111
0	011 0000	P	101 0000	p	111 0000
1	011 0001	Q	101 0001	q	111 0001
2	011 0010	R	101 0010	r	111 0010
3	011 0011	S	101 0011	s	111 0011
4	011 0100	T	101 0100	t	111 0100
5	011 0101	U	101 0101	u	111 0101
6	011 0110	V	101 0110	v	111 0110
7	011 0111	W	101 0111	w	111 0111
8	011 1000	X	101 1000	x	111 1000
9	011 1001	Y	101 1001	y	111 1001
:	011 1010	Z	101 1010	z	111 1010
;	011 1011	[	101 1011	{	111 1011
<	011 1100	\	101 1100	|	111 1100
=	011 1101	]	101 1101	}	111 1101
>	011 1110	^	101 1110	~	111 1110
?	011 1111	_	101 1111	null	111 1111

FIGURE 4.2. The American Standard Code for Information Interchange (ASCII) is a standard scheme for representing alphanumeric characters using 7 bits. The upper-case and lower-case alphabet, the decimal digits, and common punctuation characters are shown here with their ASCII representations.

information (as in a word processor), but its use is not covered by the standard. Not all characters seen on a keyboard can be encoded and stored as ASCII. The Delete and Arrow keys are often dedicated to edit functions, and the Control, Escape, Function, and Alt keys are used to modify other keys or to interact directly with programs.

The CPU works on data that it retrieves from memory, placing them in working registers. By manipulating the contents of its registers, the CPU performs the mathematical and logical functions that are basic to information processing: addition, subtraction, and comparison ("is greater than," "is equal to," "is less than"). In addition to registers that perform computation, the CPU also has registers that it uses to store instructions—a **computer program** is a set of such instructions—and to control processing. In essence, a computer is an instruction follower: It fetches an instruction from memory and then executes the instruction, which usually is an operation that requires the retrieval, manipulation, and storage of data into memory or registers. The processor performs a simple loop, fetching and executing each instruction of a program in sequence. Some instructions can direct the processor to begin fetching instructions from a different place in memory or point in the program. Such a transfer of control provides flexibility in program execution.

Memory

The computer's working memory stores the programs and data currently being used by the CPU. Working memory has two parts: **read-only memory** (ROM) and **random-access memory** (RAM).

Read-only memory, or fixed memory, is permanent and unchanging. It can be read, but it cannot be altered or erased. It is used to store a few crucial programs that do not change and that must be available at all times. One such predefined program is the **bootstrap** sequence, a set of initial instructions that is executed each time the computer is started. ROM also is used to store programs that must run quickly—for example, the graphics programs that run the Macintosh interface.

More familiar to computer users is RAM, often just called **memory**. Random-access memory can be both read and written into. It is used to store the programs, control values, and data that are in current use. It also holds the intermediate results of computations and the images to be displayed on the screen. RAM is much larger than ROM. Its size is one of the primary parameters used to describe a computer. For example, we might speak of a 32-megabyte personal computer. A 32-megabyte memory can store 33,554,432 bytes of information; a **megabyte** is 2^{20} or 1,048,576 bytes. (A **kilobyte** is 2^{10} or 1024 bytes, and a **gigabyte** is 2^{30} or 1,073,741,824 bytes.)

The bytes of memory are numbered—say from 0 to 33,554,431 for a 32-megabyte computer. The CPU accesses each word in memory by specifying this number or **address**. A sequence of bits that can be accessed by the CPU as a unit is called a **word**. The **word size** is a function of the computer's design; it typically is an even number of bytes. Early personal computers had word sizes of 8 or 16 bits; newer, faster computers have 32-bit or 64-bit word sizes that allow processing of larger chunks of information at a time.

The computer's memory is relatively expensive, especially for fast read-write access; therefore, it is limited in size. It is also **volatile**: Its contents are changed when the next program runs and are not retained when power is turned off. For many medical applications we need to store more information than can be held in memory, and we want to save all that information for a long time. To save valuable programs, data, or results we place them into storage.

Long-Term Storage

Programs and data that must persist over long periods are stored on peripheral storage devices, which provide storage less costly per unit than that provided by memory. The needed information is loaded from such storage into working memory whenever it is used. Conceptually, storage can be divided into two types. **Active storage** is used to store data that have long-term validity and that may need to be retrieved with little delay (in a few seconds or less); an example is the medical record of a patient who currently is being treated within the hospital. **Archival storage** is used to store data for documentary or legal purposes; an example is the medical record of a patient who has been discharged.

Computer storage also provides a basis for the sharing of information. Whereas memory is volatile, data written on storage in **databases** is available to other users who can access the computer's storage devices. Databases complement direct communication among computer users and have the advantage that the writers and readers need not be present at the same time in order to share information.

Magnetic disks are the most common medium for active storage. A disk storage unit, like the one shown in Figure 4.3, consists of one or more disks (either

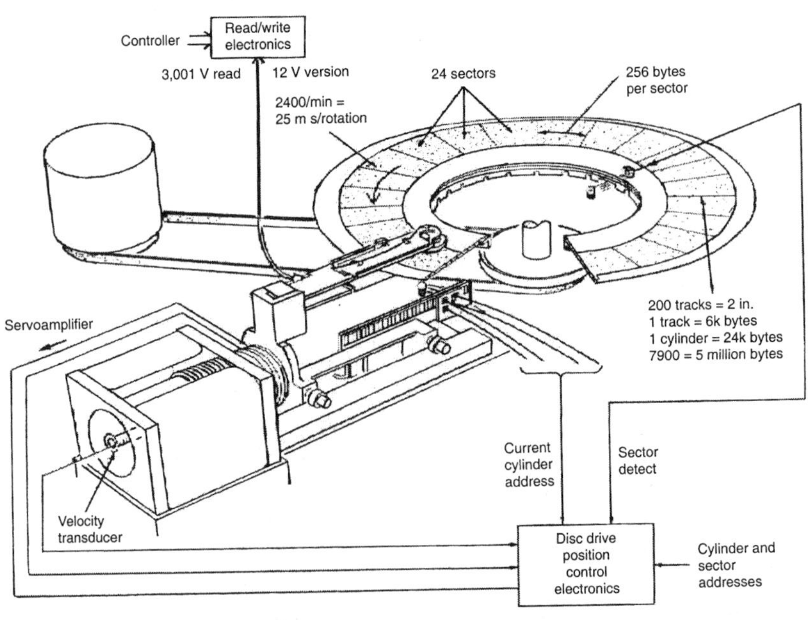

FIGURE 4.3. A typical magnetic disk drive. Drive parameters—such as number of tracks, data density along the tracks, rotation speed, and seek time across tracks—improve continually with technology advances. (*Source:* Drawing courtesy of Hewlett-Packard.)

fixed or removable), a drive system to rotate the disk, moveable read-write heads to access the data, a mechanism to position the read-write head over the disk's surface, and associated electronics. Several disks may be stacked in a disk drive, and typically both surfaces of a disk can be written on. The read-write heads are mounted on arms so that they can access most of the surface. Each magnetic disk is a round, flat plate of magnetizable material. The disk spins beneath its read-write head; as it spins, data can be copied from or to the disk surface by the read-write head. Writing places a sequence of magnetized domains on the disk's surface along circular tracks. Reading detects the presence or absence of magnetization along those tracks.

Magnetic disks are less expensive per unit stored than memory, but data retrieval is much slower. Whereas the CPU can quickly access any data element in RAM by addressing the memory location directly, it must access externally stored data in two time-consuming steps. First, it must mechanically position the read-write head over the track that stores the data. Then, it must search through that track sequentially, following the track as the disk rotates. Once the read-write head has been positioned correctly, blocks of data can be transferred rapidly. Whereas data in memory can be accessed in microseconds or less, access times for data stored on disk are typically on the order of 0.1 second.

Disks can be either **hard disks** or **floppy disks**. Floppy disks can be removed from their drive units and are inexpensive relative to hard disks. They are useful for local archiving of data and for shipping of data through the mail. Floppy disks may hold one megabyte or more. Hard disks are typically fixed in the units and often hold 1 or more gigabytes.

A common medium for archival storage is **magnetic tape**, which is a ribbon of plastic covered with magnetizable material. Like the disk drive, a tape drive has a read-write head that places or detects magnetized domains along the tracks of the tape. Magnetic tape is still the least expensive medium for storing information, but retrieval of data archived on tape is slow. An operator (either human or robotic) must locate the tape and physically mount it on a tape drive, a procedure that can take minutes or hours. The tape then must be scanned linearly from the beginning until the information of interest is located.

A wide variety of tape formats exists. Early tapes were mounted on reels. Now there are various cartridges available that are based on video-recording technologies and have much higher recording densities. Tape cartridges that hold tens of gigabytes of data fit in the palm of your hand. Archiving data on tape has the risk that the contents may become corrupted over the years unless they are refreshed regularly. Also, older tape formats may become obsolete, and the devices needed for retrieval from those formats may disappear. Converting large archives to newer formats is a major undertaking.

Optical **compact disk** (CD) storage has grown rapidly in popularity. A large quantity of data can be stored on optical disks—currently somewhat under 1 gigabyte per disk. The short wavelength of light permits a much higher density of data-carrying spots on the surface than can be placed by magnetic techniques. A semiconductor laser reads data by detecting reflections from the disk; data are written by the laser that is set at a higher intensity to alter the reflectivity. Most common is **compact disk read-only memory** (CD-ROM), used for prerecorded information, such as large programs to be distributed. Optical storage has also become attractive for applications such as distributing full-text literature, storing permanent medical records, and archiving digitized X-ray images (see Chapter 14). Another example of a medical application of CD-ROM technology is in the storage and distribution of portions of the MEDLINE collection of medical literature (see Chapter 15) and the Unified Medical Language System Metathesaurus (see Chapter 6).

Hardware for writing onto CDs is becoming less expensive, to the point that systems are practical even for PCs. Such systems are limited to recording data once but allow reading of those data as often as desired. Such a disk is called a **WORM** (write once, read many [times]). Rewritable CDs are also available. Their slow access time and slow writing speed limit their use mainly to archiving, in place of tape cartridges. A major obstacle to overcome is the lack of a fast and economical means for indexing and searching the huge amount of information that can be stored. The newest format that has become available is **digital video disks** (DVDs), which can hold enormous volumes of information. If these devices become established in the marketplace, given that they are also used for entertainment, they may be available longer than devices used exclusively for computers.

The choices of storage devices and media have major effects on the performance and cost of a computer system. Data that are needed rapidly must be kept in more expensive active storage—typically hard disks. Less time-critical data can be archived on less expensive media, which have longer access times. Because data are often shared, the designer must also consider who will want to read the data and how the data will be read. People can share by copying the data and physically transporting the copy to a destination with a compatible drive unit. Tapes, floppy disks, or DVDs are all convenient for transport. An alternative to physical transport is remote access to persistent storage by means of communication networks; the practice of sending files using file transfer programs or as attachments to electronic mail messages is rapidly replacing physical exchange of files on disks. Compatibility of storage devices becomes less important, but the capabilities of the communication networks and their protocols are crucial (see later discussion of Internet communication).

Input Devices

Data and user-command entry remain the most costly and awkward aspects of medical data processing. Certain data can be acquired automatically; for example, many laboratory instruments provide electronic signals that can be transmitted to computers directly, and many diagnostic radiology instruments produce output in digital form. Furthermore, redundant data entry can be minimized if data are shared among computers over networks or across direct interfaces. For example, if a clinic's computer can acquire data from a laboratory computer directly, clinic personnel will not have to reenter into the computer-based medical record the information displayed on printed reports of laboratory-test results. Many types of data are, however, still entered into the medical record manually by data-entry clerks or by other healthcare personnel. The most common instrument for data entry is the typewriter-style **keyboard** associated with a **video display terminal** (VDT). As an operator types characters on the keyboard, they are echoed back for viewing on the **display monitor**. A **cursor** indicates the current position on the screen. Most programs allow the cursor to be moved with Arrow keys or with a mouse so that insertions and corrections are convenient to make. Although clerical personnel often are comfortable with this mode of data entry, many health professionals lack typing skills and are not motivated to learn them. Thus, systems developers have experimented with a variety of alternative input devices that minimize or eliminate the need to type.

With a **mouse**, a user can *select* an item displayed on the screen by moving the mouse on the desktop to position the cursor on the screen and then clicking on a mouse button. With a **touch screen**, a user can select items simply by pointing—when the user's finger touches the screen, it uniquely identifies a position in the grid that crosses the screen, indicating the item of interest. Alternatively, a **light pen**, a **track ball**, or a **joystick** can be used to mark positions on a screen, but these devices are mainly used in specialized settings. There are also three-dimensional pointing devices, where the indicator is held in front of the screen, and a three-dimensional display provides feedback to the user.

Often, these pointing devices are used in conjunction with **menus**, which are lists of items that users can select among (Fig. 4.4). Thus, users can enter data simply by clicking on relevant items rather than by typing characters. By listing or highlighting only valid options, menus also facilitate coding and can enforce the use of a standardized vocabulary. To deal with a large number of choices, menus are arranged hierarchically; for example, to order a treatment, a physician might first select *drug order* from a menu of alternative actions, then the appropriate *drug class* from a submenu, and finally an individual drug from the next submenu. If there are still many alternatives, the drug list might be divided further; for example, the drugs might be grouped alphabetically by name. Menu selection is efficient; an experienced user can select several screens per second. Typing, for example, a drug name, is more time consuming and carries the risk of misspelling. Menu design is still an art. An excess of displayed choices slows down the user—more than seven entries require careful reading. Also, if the system designer's concepts do not match those of the user, then the user can get lost in the hierarchy and be frustrated. Finally, there is evidence that users who use a mouse for extensive periods may be subject to repetitive-stress wrist injury.

Graphical displays provide system developers with great flexibility to create interesting and attractive interfaces to programs. For example, the input screens of the ONCOCIN system, intended to provide physicians with advice on cancer-treatment protocols, look just like the paper flowcharts that physicians have used for years. Physicians enter patient data into the database directly by using a mouse to select values from menus (Fig. 4.5). In addition, graphics open the door for

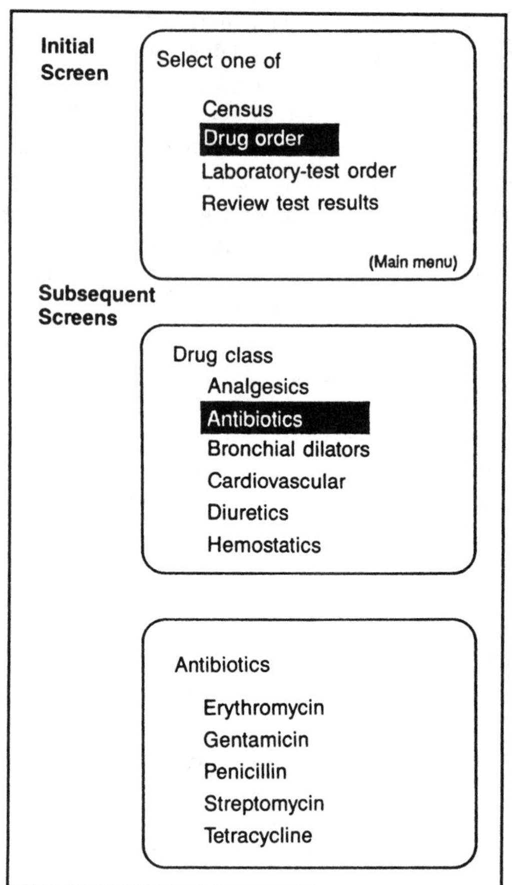

FIGURE 4.4. Initial and subsequent screens of a menu-driven order-entry system. The highlighted entry indicates which item was selected (with a mouse, light pen, or finger) to display the subsequent screen.

intuitive data entry—for instance, the use of images to record information and of **icons** to specify commands. Physicians can use images to indicate the location of an injury, the size of a tumor, the area to be covered by radiation therapy, and so on (Fig. 4.6). Because of the imprecision of medical language, a graphical indication of the affected body parts can be a valuable supplement to coded or textual descriptions. Graphical interfaces and flowsheets are now commonplace in commercial clinical information systems, and image libraries are being incorporated to support the documentation process.

Using icons for selection again requires designing the interface carefully. Icons must be distinctive and intuitive. Having hundreds of icons on a screen is not helpful, and having many similar icons is even less so. Icons are often labeled with brief texts and may also show longer explanations when selected. Techniques suitable for occasional users are typically inefficient for frequent users, but users often move from familiar tasks to unfamiliar ones and vice versa, and switching modes is awkward.

Lymphoma Flow Sheet

Mass / X-ray

Disease Activity

Hematology									
WBC x 1000	8.6	9.0	1.5	4.2	9.0	3.6	5.6	3.3	?
% polys	71	93	29						
% lymphs			43						
PCV	29.6	32.9	33.7	33.6	30.9	31.6	28.4	29.3	
Hemoglobin	10.1	11.1	11.3	11.6	10.4	10.5	9.4	9.9	?
Platelets x 1000	562	511	516	592	436	255	500	345	?
Sed. Rate	100								
% total granulocytes	75	93	39	82.6	83.4	90.3	80.3	70.1	?
Granulocytes	6.45		.585		7.506		4.4968		

326

7	8	9	erase
4	5	6	n/a
1	2	3	clear
			abort
	0		done

Chemotherapy

Radiotherapy

Symptom Review

Toxicity ?

Physical Examination

Chemistry ?

To order: Labs and Procedures

To order: Nuclear Medicine and Tomography

Scheduling

Time									
Day	28	03	10	17	24	30	7	14	21
Month	May	Jun	Jun	Jun	Jun	Jun	Jul	Jul	Jul
Year	87	87	87	87	87	87	87	87	87

FIGURE 4.5. The data-entry screen of the ONCOCIN consultation system. The screen is a computer-based representation of the familiar paper flowchart on which physicians normally record information regarding their cancer patients. The physician can enter the platelet count into the database by selecting digits from the numerical menu displayed in the upper-right corner of the figure. Only the hematology section of the flowchart currently is visible. The physician can view data on disease activity, chemotherapies, and so on by selecting from the alternative section headings. (*Source:* Courtesy of Stanford Medical Informatics, Stanford University.)

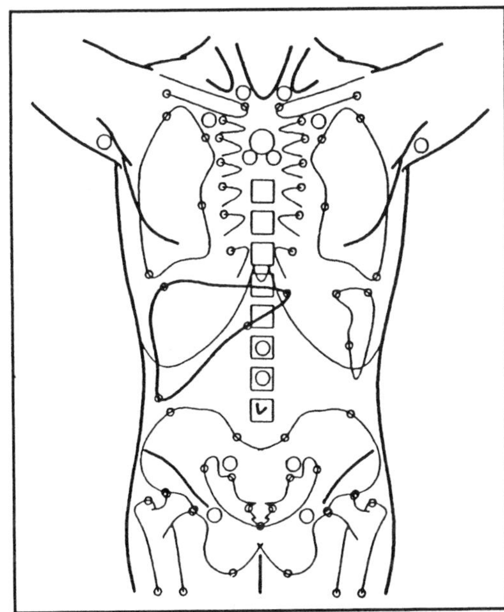

FIGURE 4.6. Images can be used to provide an alternate means of entering data. Rather than describing the location of a tumor in words, a physician using the ONCOCIN consultation system can indicate the location of a lesion by selecting regions on a torso. In this figure, the physician has indicated involvement of the patient's liver. (*Source:* Courtesy of Stanford Medical Informatics, Stanford University.)

Much medical information is available as narrative text—for example, physician-transcribed visit notes, hospital discharge summaries, and all the medical literature. **Text-scanning devices** can scan lines or entire pages of typeset text and convert each character into its ASCII-coded binary format. These devices reduce the need to retype information that previously was typed, but they cannot adequately capture handwritten information. Even with typed material, scanners often have error rates of several percent, so the entered material must be reviewed carefully if it is important.

Most physicians are comfortable dictating their notes; therefore, researchers have investigated the possibility of using voice input for data entry. The simplest method for capturing voice data is to record messages directly from a microphone. The voice signal then is encoded in digital form (see Section 4.2), identified as a voice message, and stored and transmitted with the other computer data. When the data are retrieved, the message is simply played back through a speaker. Search and indexing is, however, not enabled in that case. With automatic speech recognition, the digitized voice signals are matched to the patterns of a vocabulary of known words. The speech input is then stored as ASCII-coded text. Currently, systems exist that can interpret sequences of discrete words, and there are successful systems that can recognize continuous speech in which the sounds run together. This technology is improving in flexibility and reliability, but error rates are sufficiently high that review of recognized passages is still advisable.

In neither case does the computer *understand* the content of the messages. This same lack of understanding applies to most textual data, which are entered, stored, retrieved, and printed without any analysis of their meaning.

Output Devices

The *presentation* of results, or of the **output**, is the complementary step in the processing of medical data. Many systems compute information that is transmitted to healthcare providers and is displayed immediately on VDTs so that action can be taken. Another large volume of output consists of reports, which are printed or simply are kept available to document the actions taken. Chapter 9 describes various reports and messages that are commonly used to present patient information. Here we describe the devices that are used to convey these outputs.

Most immediate output appears at its destination on a display screen, such as the **cathode-ray tube** (CRT) display of a VDT, often in color. Many VDTs often also include at least rudimentary sound capability as well, so if results require urgent attention, a signal such as a ringing bell may alert personnel to the data's arrival. More routinely, results are placed in storage and are automatically retrieved when an appropriate provider accesses the patient's record. Important findings may also be highlighted on the screen in boldface type or a special color.

When entering or reviewing data, users can edit the data displayed on the screen before releasing them for persistent storage. Graphical output is essential for summarizing and presenting the information derived from voluminous data.

Most computers have the ability to produce graphical output, but specific health-care information systems differ greatly in their capabilities to display trend lines, images, and other graphics.

A graphics screen is divided into a grid of picture elements called **pixels**. One or more bits in memory represent the output for each pixel. In a black and white monitor, the value of each pixel on the screen is associated with the level of intensity, or **gray scale**. For example, 2 bits can distinguish $2^2 = 4$ display values per pixel: black, white, and two intermediate shades of gray. For color displays, the number of bits per pixel determines the **contrast** and **color resolution** of an image. Three sets of multiple bits are necessary to specify the color of pixels on color graphics monitors, giving the intensity for red, green, and blue components of each pixel color, respectively. For instance, three sets of 2 bits per pixel provides $2^6 = 64$ color mixtures. The number of pixels per square inch determines the **spatial resolution** of the image (Fig. 4.7). As we discuss in Chapter 14, both parameters determine the requirements for storing images. A display with high spatial resolution requires an array of about 2,000 × 2,000 pixels, whereas a 640 × 480 array is a typical minimum needed for a textual display. Liquid-crystal-display (LCD) color projectors are readily available so the video output of a workstation can also be projected onto a screen for group presentations.

Much diagnostic information is produced in image formats that can be transmitted to and clearly shown on graphics terminals. Examples are ultrasound observations, magnetic resonance images (MRIs), computed tomography (CT) scans, and the like. High-resolution displays can even be adequate for display of digitally encoded X-ray images. Computer processing can add value to such image output, as described in Chapter 14.

For portability and traditional filing, output is *printed* on paper. Printing information is slower than is displaying it on a screen, so printing is best done in advance of need. In a clinic, relevant portions of various patient records may be printed on high-volume printers the night before scheduled visits. For presentations, the ease of printing has allowed viewgraph transparencies to replace traditional slides (which are made from film that must be exposed and developed). Subsequently, the availability of high-quality LCD projectors has begun to replace use of static viewgraphs, allowing production of more dynamic presentations.

Laser printers use an electromechanically controlled laser beam to generate an image on a xerographic surface, which then is used to produce paper copies, just as is done in a copier. Laser printers permit the user to select from a variety of fonts and to produce graphics that match closely the look of visual displays. Their resolution is often better than that of displays, allowing up to 600 dots (pixels) per inch (commercial typesetting equipment may have a resolution of 1,200 dots per inch).[1] Whenever the resolution of printers and visual termi-

[1]Whereas printer resolution is typically measured in dots (or pixels) *per inch,* CRT resolution is measured for the *entire* screen (e.g., a large high-quality monitor may have an array of 1,200 × 1,600 pixels).

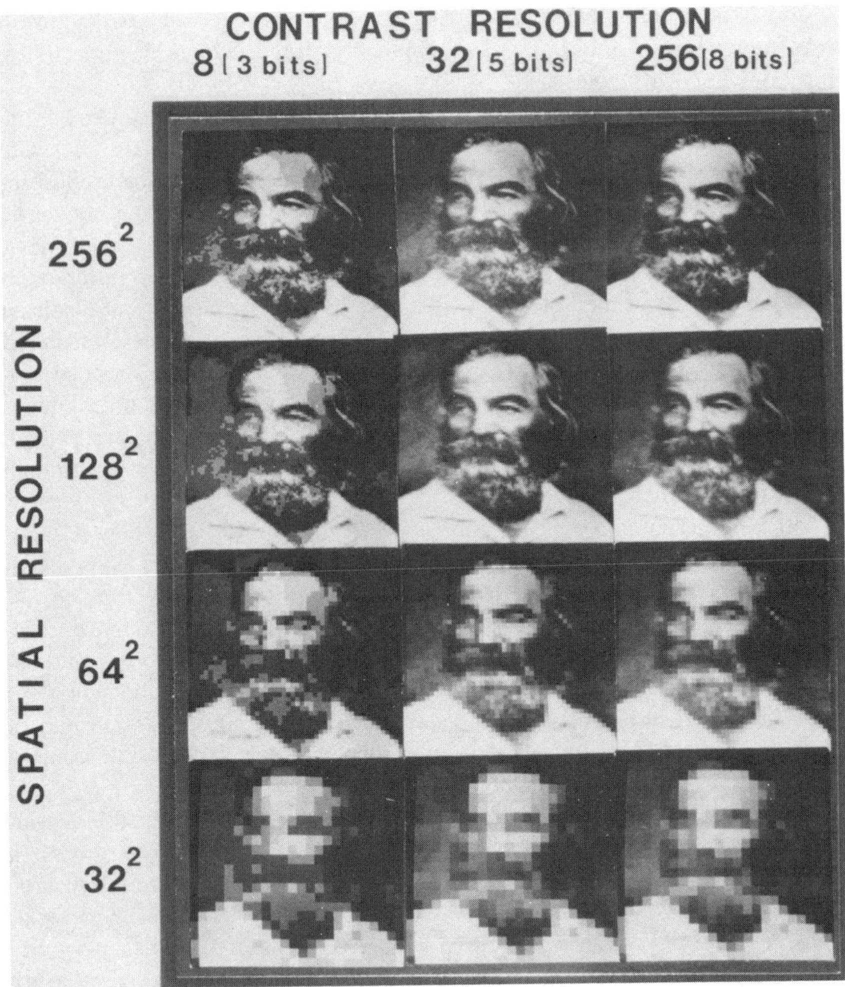

Figure 4.7. Demonstration of how varying the number of pixels and the number of bits per pixel affects the spatial and contract resolution of a digital image. The image in the upper-right corner was displayed using a 256 × 256 array of pixels, 8 bits per pixel; the subject (Walt Whitman) is easily discernible. (*Source:* Reproduced, with permission, from Price R.R., James A.E. [1982]. Basic principles and instrumentation of digital radiography. In Price R.R., et al. (Eds.), *Digital Radiography: A Focus on Clinical Utility*. Orlando, FL: WB Saunders.)

nals differs, output displays should be designed with care to make both forms of output equally acceptable.

Color printing with laser technology is still relatively costly, but prices are dropping. Color **ink-jet printers** are less expensive and still dominate the market. Liquid ink is sprayed on paper by a head that moves back and forth for each line of pixels. Ink-jet printers have lower resolution than that of laser printers and are relatively slow, especially at high resolution. To avoid blotting of the ink droplets, coated paper is used for output at more than 200 pixels per inch. Special absorbent stock is needed for transparencies. Because they are inexpensive, color ink-jet printers can be easily placed close to personal computers, and the color can be used effectively to enhance readers' comprehension of clinical results. Ink-jet printers that produce images of photographic quality are also becoming available. Here the base colors are merged while being sprayed so that true color mixes are placed on the paper.

Multiple-sheet forms require **impact printers** to produce the duplicate copies. Inexpensive impact printers are based on typewriter technology; more expensive, high-volume ones are based on print chain or drum technologies. **Dot-matrix printers** print small dots on paper similar to the way VDTs form characters on a screen from small dots. Impact printers are slow and noisy so that the use of multipart forms is becoming less common. Instead, multiple copies of a form are printed on laser or ink-jet printers, sometimes requiring extra work in obtaining signatures on each of the copies.

Local Data Communications

Information can be shared most effectively by allowing access for all authorized participants whenever and wherever they need it. Transmitting data electronically among applications and computer systems facilitates such sharing by minimizing delays and by supporting more interactive collaborations. Using paper for this purpose results in a much more passive type of information sharing. As we describe in Chapter 10, data communication and integration are critical functions of healthcare information systems. Modern computing and communications are deeply intertwined.

Computer systems used in health care are specialized to fulfill the diverse needs of health professionals in various areas, such as physicians' offices, laboratories, pharmacies, intensive-care units, and business offices. Even if their hardware is identical, their content will differ, and some of that content must be shared with other applications in the healthcare organization. Over time, the hardware in the various areas will also diverge—for example, imaging departments will require more storage, other areas will use more power, and still others will serve more users. Demand for growth and funding to accommodate it occur at different times. Communication among diverse systems bridges the differences in computing environments.

Communication can occur via telephone lines, dedicated or shared wires, fiberoptic cables, or radio waves. In each case different communication interfaces must be attached to the computer, different conventions or communication protocols must be obeyed, and a different balance of performance and reliability can be expected.

A traditional and economical method for communicating computer information is to use the existing dial-up telephone system. A sending computer dials a receiving computer, and, when the connection is established, a **modem** (modulator-demodulator) converts the digital data from a computer to analog signals in the voice range. The tones are transmitted over the telephone lines. At the receiver, the tones are reconverted to the original digital form by another modem and are placed into the computer memory. The receiver can return responses to the sender, sending results or requests for more data. Thus, a conversation takes place between computers. When the conversation is complete, the modems disconnect and the telephone line is released.

As technologies improve, modems can support increasing transmission speeds, or **bit rates**. The overall bit rate of a communication link is a combination of the rate at which signals (or symbols) can be transmitted and the efficiency with which digital information (in the form of bits) is encoded in the symbols. Frequently the term **baud** is used to indicate the signal transmission speed—one baud corresponds to one signal per second. At lower speeds, bits are encoded one per signal, so the baud rate and bit rate are similar. At higher speeds, more complex methods are used to encode bits in the channel signals. Thus, a 56,000 bit per second (bps) modem may use a signal rate of only 8,000 baud and an encoding that transmits up to 8 bits per signal. A rate of 2,400 bps is the minimum for useful text-only transmission. For graphics information speeds of 28,000 bps or 56,000 bps are desirable. The net rate is actually less, and current Federal Communication Commission (FCC) regulations actually limit dial-up telephone-line transmission to 53,000 bps (about 5,000 characters equivalent per second).

Dedicated analog telephone lines can handle higher rates, but their main advantage is that no time is wasted in dialing. The absence of switching also reduces the error rate and the losses that accrue from retransmission to compensate for such errors. Long-range dedicated telephone lines are expensive and are mainly used for high-traffic connections and limited distances—say, from a medical center to a nearby ambulatory-care clinic.

Digital telephone services are becoming widely available now and can be expected to become commonplace in the next few years. **Integrated Services Digital Network** (ISDN) and **Digital Subscriber Line** (DSL) services allow relatively high-speed network communications using conventional telephone wiring (twisted pairs). Currently, they allow sharing of data and voice transmission up to a total rate of 1.5 megabits per second (Mbps). Their error rate, and the cost of dealing with errors, is lower as well, because no transformations to and from tones occur. No modem is needed, but an interface unit is still required, at a cost similar to a capable modem. The rates charged by the telephone companies for ISDN/DSL lines also differ from those for analog lines. In remote areas digital services may be unavailable, but it appears that the telephone companies will soon have such services in most areas, including over wireless telephone channels. Transmission also can occur via cable modems using television cable or direct satellite broadcast. These alternatives have a very high capacity, but that capacity is then shared by all subscribers, and the practical limits for intensive two-way transmission are not yet clear. Also, because television service is designed to deliver information at high speed to the end user's site, but not in the other direction, these services are most often asymmetrical, with relatively low-speed telephone service used to communicate back to the data source.

Frame Relay is a network protocol designed for sending digital information over shared, **wide-area networks** (WANs). It transmits variable-length messages or packets of information efficiently and inexpensively over dedicated lines that may handle aggregate speeds up to 45 Mbps. **Asynchronous Transfer Mode** (ATM) is a protocol designed for sending streams of small, fixed-length cells of information (each 53 bytes long) over very high-speed dedicated connections—most often digital optical circuits. The underlying optical transmission circuit sends cells synchronously and supports multiple ATM circuits. The cells associated with a given ATM circuit are queued and processed asynchronously with respect to each other in gaining access to the multiplexed (optical) transport medium. Because ATM is designed to be implemented by hardware switches, information bit rates up to 600 Mbps are possible today, and speeds up to 10 gigabits per second (Gbps) are expected in the future.

For communication needs in an office, a building, or a campus, installation of a **local-area network** (LAN) allows local data communication without involving the telephone company. Such a network is dedicated to linking multiple computer **nodes** together at high speeds to facilitate the sharing of resources—data, software, and equipment—among multiple users. Users working at individual workstations can retrieve data and programs from network **file servers**: computers dedicated to storing files, both shared and private. The users can process information locally and then save the results over the network to the file server or send output to a fast, shared printer.

There are a variety of **protocols** and technologies for implementing LANs, although the differences should not be apparent to the customer. Typically data are transmitted as messages or **packets** of data; each packet contains the data to be sent, the network addresses of the sending and receiving nodes, and other control information. LANs are limited to operating within a geographical area of at most a few miles and often are restricted to a specific building or a single department. Separate remote LANs may be connected via telephone lines or dedicated digital service, providing convenient communication between machines on different networks. The telecommunication department of a healthcare organization often takes responsibility for implementating and linking multiple LANs to form an enterprise network. An important service provided by the network administrators is integrated access to WANs, specifically to the Internet (see later discussion of Internet communication).

In the beginning, most LANs used coaxial cables as the communication medium because they could deliver reliable, high-speed communications. With improved communication signal processing technologies, however, **twisted-pair wires** have become the standard. Twisted-pair wiring is inexpensive and has a high **bandwidth** (capacity for information transmission)—at least 100 Mbps. Twisted-pair wiring is susceptible to electrical interference, although less so than telephone connections. An alternate medium, **fiberoptic cable**, offers the highest bandwidth (over 1 billion bps [or 1 Gbps]) and a high degree of reliability because it uses light waves to transmit information signals and is not susceptible to interference. Fiberoptic cable is used in LANs to increase transmission speeds and distances by at least 1 order of magnitude over twisted-pair wire. In addition, fiberoptic cable is lightweight and easy to install. Splicing and connecting into optical cable is more difficult than into twisted-pair wire, however, so inhouse delivery of networking services to the desktop is still easier using twisted-pair wires. Fiberoptic cable and twisted-pair wires are often used in a complementary fashion—fiberoptic cable for the high-speed, shared backbone of an enterprise network or LAN and twisted-pair wires extending out from side-branch hubs to bring service to the workplace.

When costs of network cabling are high, a LAN service can be piggy backed onto a **private branch exchange** (PBX), the organization's internal telephone system. Now the telephone wires are used to transfer both voice signals and data. Digital data are converted to analog signals and can be transmitted to any location where the telephones are connected. But speeds are limited, perhaps to 9,600 bps, so PBX use focuses on textual interaction and excludes most graphics. When coaxial cable installations are in place (e.g., in closed circuit television or in cable television services), LANs using coaxial cable can transmit signals using either broadband or baseband technology. **Broadband** is adapted from the technology for transmitting cable television. A broadband LAN can transmit multiple signals simultaneously, providing a unified environment for sending computer data, voice messages, and images. Cable modems provide the means for encoding and decoding the data, and each signal is sent within an assigned frequency range (channel). **Baseband** is simpler and is used in most LAN installations. It transmits digital signals over a single set of wires, one packet at a time, without special encoding as a television signal.

Messages also can be transmitted through the air by microwave, satellite signal, or line-of-sight laser-beam transmission, but these modes have limited application. Users in a hospital or clinic can use radio signals from portable devices to communicate with their workstations or with servers that contain clinical data and thus can gain entry to the LANs and associated services. Hospitals have many instruments that generate electronic interference, and often have reinforced concrete walls, so that radio transmission may not be fully reliable.

Rapid data transmission is supported by LANs. Most LANs today operate at 10 Mbps, but standards for 100-Mbps networks are in place, and cost-effective commercial technology is available to install 100-Mbps service. At 10 Mbps, the entire contents of this book could be transmitted in a few seconds. Multiple users and high-volume data transmissions such as video congest a LAN, however, so the effective transmission speed seen by each user may be much lower. When demand is high, multiple LANs can be installed. Gateways and routers shuttle packets among these networks to allow sharing of data between computers as though the machines were on the same LAN. A **router** is a special computer that is connected to more than one network and is equipped to forward packets that originate on one network to machines that have addresses on another network.

Gateways perform routing and can also translate packet formats if the two connected networks run different protocols.

Internet Communication

External routers can also link the users on a LAN to a **regional network** and then to the **Internet**. The Internet is a WAN that is composed of many regional and local networks interconnected by long-range **backbone links**. The Internet and the regional networks, begun by the National Science Foundation in the mid-1980s, included a regional network system to provide coverage for metropolitan or larger areas—for instance, in the San Francisco Bay area (BARRnet), in the New York area (NYSERnet), in Texas (SesquiNet), and so on (Quarterman, 1990). Regional networking service is now provided by commercial communications companies, and users get access to the regional networks through their institutions or privately by paying an **Internet service provider** (ISP). There are other WANs, some operated by demanding commercial users, and others by parts of the federal government, such as the Department of Defense, the National Aeronautics and Space Administration, and the Department of Energy. Nearly all countries have their own networks so that information can be transmitted to most computers in the world. Gateways of various types connect all these networks, whose protocols and capabilities may differ (Fig. 4.8).

All Internet participants agree on many conventions called **Internet standards**. The most fundamental is the protocol suite referred to as the **Transmission Control Protocol/Internet Protocol** (TCP/IP). Data transmission is always by structured packets, and all machines are identified by a standard for 32-bit IP addresses. **Internet protocol addresses** consist of a sequence of four 8-bit numbers, each ranging from 0 to 255—most often written as a dotted sequence of numbers: a.b.c.d. Although IP addresses are not assigned geographically (the way that ZIP codes are), the first number identifies a region, the second a local area, the third a local net, and the fourth a specific computer. Computers that are permanently linked into the Internet have a *fixed* IP address assigned, whereas users that reach the Internet by dialing into an ISP get a temporary address that persists just during a session.

Because 32-bit numbers are difficult to remember, computers on the Internet also have names assigned. Multiple names may be used for a given computer that performs distinct services. The names can be translated to IP addresses—for example, when they are used to designate a remote machine—by means of a hierarchical name-management system called the **Domain Name System** (DNS). Designated computers, called **name-servers**, convert a name into an IP address before the message is placed on the network; routing takes place based on only the numeric IP address. Names are also most often expressed as dotted sequences of name segments, but there is no correspondence between the four numbers of an IP address and the parts of a name. The Internet is growing rapidly; therefore, periodic reorganizations of parts of the network are common. Numeric IP addresses may have to change, but the logical name for a resource can stay the

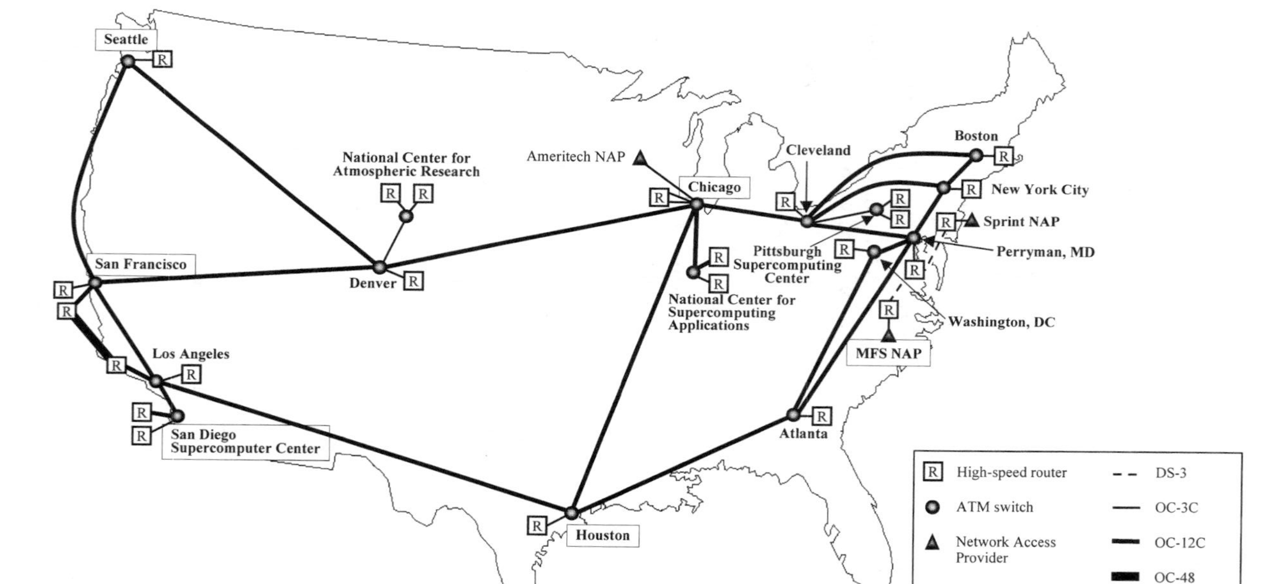

FIGURE 4.8. The vBNS (very high-speed Backbone Network Service) network developed by the National Science Foundation since 1995 as a successor to the NSFNet. The NSFNet in turn replaced the Advanced Research Projects Agency Network (ARPAnet) and established the network architecture in general use today—cross-country backbones connected to gateways into regional network providers. The vBNS network is itself a transitional experimental network that is establishing the engineering and applications principles for practical very high-speed communications services in support of research and education institutions throughout the United States. The circles at junctions of cross-country lines are high-speed ATM switches. The routers are Network Access Providers, which supply network connectivity for regional Internet Service Providers and connections to other networks. DC-3 = Digital Signal level 3 (T3) line at 44.736 Mbps; OC-3C = Optical Carrier 3 synchronous optical transmission line at 155.52 Mbps; OC-12C = Optical Carrier 12 synchronous optical transmission line at 622.08 Mbps; OC-48 = Optical Carrier 48 synchronous optical transmission line at 2.488 Gbps. (*Source:* MCI-Worldcom.)

same and the (updated) DNS can take care of keeping the translation up to date. Three conventions are in use for composing Internet names from segments:

1. *Hierarchical convention:* Under the most common convention for the United States, names are composed of hierarchical segments increasing in specificity from right to left, beginning with one of the top-level domain-class identifiers—for example, *computer.institution.class* (smi.stanford.edu) or *institution.class* (whitehouse.gov). Currently the defined top-level domain classes are .com, .edu, .gov, .mil, .org, and .net (for commercial, educational, government, military, nonprofit, and ISP organizations, respectively). More classes are likely to be defined in the future. Name hierarchies can be as deep as desired, but simplicity helps users to remember the names. Other conventions have evolved as well: *www* is often used to name the **World Wide Web (WWW)** services on a computer (e.g., www.nlm.nih.gov) (see Section 4.1.2, Software for Network Communications).
2. *Geographic convention:* Names are composed of hierarchical segments increasing in specificity from right to left and beginning with a top-level country domain identifier—for example, institution.town.state.country (NRI.reston.va.us or city.palo-alto.ca.us). Many countries outside of the United States use a combination of these conventions, such as using csd.Abdn.ac.UK, for the Computer Science department at the University of Aberdeen (an academic institution in the United Kingdom). Note that the case of an IP address is ignored, although additional fields, such as those used to locate World Wide Web resources, may be case sensitive.
3. *Attribute list address (X.400) convention:* Names are composed of a sequence of attribute-value pairs that specifies the components needed to resolve the address—for example, /C=GB/ADMD=BT/PRMD=AC/O=Abdn/OU=csd/, which is equivalent to the address csd.Abdn.ac.UK. This convention derives from the X.400 address standard that is used mainly in the European community. It has the advantage that the address elements (for example, /C for Country name, /ADMD for Administrative Management Domain name, /PRMD for Private Management Domain name, and so on) are explicitly labeled and may come in any order. Country designations differ as well. However, this type of address is generally more difficult for humans to understand and has not been adopted broadly in the Internet community.

An institution that has many computers may provide a service whereby all its communications (e.g., incoming electronic mail) go to a single address, for example, stanford.edu, and then local tables are used to direct each message to the right computer or individual. Such a scheme insulates outsiders from internal naming conventions and changes.

The routing of packets of information between computers on the Internet is the basis for a rich array of information services. Each such service—be it resource naming, electronic mail, file transfer, remote computer log in, World Wide Web, or another service—is defined in terms of a set of protocols that governs how computers speak to each other. These worldwide intercomputer-linkage conventions allow global sharing of information resources, as well as personal and group communications. The Web's popularity is changing how we deal with people, form communities, entertain ourselves, and perform research. The scope of all these activities is more than we can cover in this book, so we restrict ourselves to topics important to health care. Even with this limitation, we can only scratch the surface of many topics.

4.1.2 Software

All the functions performed by the hardware of a computer system—data acquisition from input devices, transfer of data and programs to and from working memory, computation and information processing by the CPU, formatting and presentation of results—are directed by computer programs, or **software**.

Programming Languages

In our discussion of the CPU in Section 4.1, we explained that a computer processes information by manipulating words of information in registers. Instructions that tell the processor which operations to perform also are sequences of 0s and 1s, a binary representation called **machine language** or **machine code.** Machine-code instructions are the only instructions that a computer can process directly. These binary patterns, however, are difficult for people to understand and manipulate. People think best symbolically. Thus, a first step toward making programming easier and less error prone was the creation of an assembly language. **Assembly language** replaces the sequences of bits of machine-language programs with words and abbreviations meaningful to humans; a programmer instructs the computer to LOAD a word from memory, ADD an amount to the contents of a register, STORE it back into memory, and so on. A program called an **assembler** translates these instructions into binary machine-language representation before execution of the code. There is a one-to-one correspondence between instructions in assembly and machine languages. To increase efficiency, we can combine sets of assembly instructions into **macros** and thus reuse them. An assembly-language programmer must consider problems on a hardware-specific level, instructing the computer to transfer data between registers and memory and to perform primitive operations, such as incrementing registers and comparing characters (Fig. 4.9).

On the other hand, the problems that the users of a computer wish to solve are real-world problems on a higher conceptual level. They want to be able to instruct the computer to perform tasks such as to retrieve the latest serum creatinine test result, to monitor the status of hypertensive patients, or to compute a patient's current account balance. To make communication with computers more understandable and less tedious, computer scientists developed higher-level, user-oriented **symbolic-programming languages**.

Using a higher-level language, such as one of those listed in Table 4.1, a programmer defines variables to represent higher-level entities and specifies arithmetic and symbolic operations without worrying about the details of how the hardware performs these operations. The details of managing the hardware are hidden from the programmer, who can specify with a single statement an operation that may translate to tens or hundreds of machine instructions. A **compiler** is used to translate automatically a high-level program into machine code. Some languages are *interpreted* instead of compiled. An **interpreter** converts and executes each statement before moving to the next statement, whereas a compiler translates all the statements at one time, creating a binary program, which can subsequently be executed many times. MUMPS (M) is an interpreted language, LISP may either be interpreted or compiled, and FORTRAN routinely is compiled before execution. Hundreds of languages have been developed—we discuss here only a few that are important from a practical or conceptual level.

Each statement of a language is characterized by **syntax** and **semantics**. The syntactic rules describe how the statements, declarations, and other language constructs are written—they define the language's grammatical structure. Semantics is the meaning given to the various syntactic constructs. The following sets of

Assembly-language program:

```
        ORG 0          /Origin of program is location 0
        LDA A          /Load operand from location A
        ADD B          /Add operand from location B
        STA C          /Store sum in location C
        HLT            /Halt
A,      DEC 3          /Location A contains decimal 3
B,      DEC 15         /Location B contains decimal 15
C,      DEC 0          /Location C contains decimal 0
        END            /End of program
```

Machine-language program:

Location	Instruction code
0	0010 0000 0000 0100
1	0001 0000 0000 0101
10	0011 0000 0000 0110
11	0111 0000 0000 0001
100	0000 0000 0000 0011
101	0000 0000 0000 1111
110	0000 0000 0000 0000

FIGURE 4.9. An assembly-language program and a corresponding machine-language program to add two numbers and to store the result.

TABLE 4.1. Distinguishing features of 12 common programming languages.

Programming language	First year	Primary application domain	Type	Operation	Type checks	Procedure call method	Data management method
FORTRAN	1957	Mathematics	Procedural	Compiled	Little	By reference	Simple files
COBOL	1962	Business	Procedural	Compiled	Yes	By name	Formatted files
Pascal	1978	Education	Procedural	Compiled	Strong	By name	Record files
Smalltalk	1976	Education	Object	Interpreted	Yes	By defined methods	Object persistence
PL/1	1965	Math, business	Procedural	Compiled	Coercion	By reference	Formatted files
Ada	1980	Math, business	Procedural	Compiled	Strong	By name	Formatted files
Standard ML	1989	Logic, math	Functional	Compiled	Yes	By value	Stream files
MUMPS (M)	1962	Data handling	Procedural	Interpreted	No	By reference	Hierarchical files
LISP	1964	Logic	Functional	Either	No	By value	Data persistence
C	1976	Data handling	Procedural	Compiled	Little	By reference	Stream files
C++	1986	Data handling	Hybrid	Compiled	Yes	By reference	Object files
JAVA	1995	Data display	Object	Either	Strong	By value	Object classes

statements (written in Pascal, FORTRAN, COBOL, and LISP) all have the same semantics:

Pascal	FORTRAN	COBOL	LISP
`C:= A + B;`	`C:= A + B`	`LN IS "The value is NNN.FFF"`	`(SETQ C (PLUS A B))`
`PRINTF (c)`	`WRITE 10, 6 C`	`ADD A TO B, GIVING C`	`(format file6`
`no layout choice`	`10 FORMAT ("The value is" F5.2")`	`MOVE C TO LN`	`"The value is ~5,2F C)`
		`WRITE LN`	

They instruct the computer to add the values of variables A and B, to assign the result to variable C, and to write the result onto a file. Each language has a distinct syntax for indicating which operations to perform. Regardless of the particular language in which a program is written, in the end, the computer manipulates sequences of 0s and 1s within its registers.

Computer languages are tailored to handle specific types of computing problems, as shown in Table 4.1, although all these languages are sufficiently flexible to deal with nearly any type of problem. Languages that were intended to apply to a broader range of problems, such as PL/1, tend to be more complex. Languages that focus on a simple, general computational infrastructure, such as C, have to be augmented with large collections of libraries of procedures, and learning the specific libraries takes more time than does learning the language itself. Languages also differ in usability. A language meant for education and highly reliable programs will include features to make it foolproof, such as a way of checking that the types of values, such as integers, decimal numbers, and strings of characters, match throughout their use. Many languages provide for some **coercion**—the automatic conversion of data types when a mismatch occurs—but strong coercion can fool programmers into thinking that programs are correct when they really have unintended mismatches. Without **type checking**, smart programmers can instruct the computers to perform some operations more efficiently than is possible in a more constraining language.

Sequences of statements are grouped into *procedures*. Procedures enhance the clarity of larger programs and also provide a basis for reuse of the work of other programmers. Large programs are in turn mainly sequences of invocations to such procedures, some coming from libraries (such as format in LISP) and others written for the specific application. These procedures are called with *arguments*—for example, the medical record number of a patient—for a procedure to retrieve a value, such as the patient's age: age(number). An important distinction among languages is how those arguments are transmitted. Just giving the value is the safest method. Giving the name provides the most information to the procedure, and giving the reference (a pointer to where the value is stored) allows the procedure to go back to the source, which can be efficient but also allows changes that may not be wanted. Discussions about languages often emphasize these various features, but the underlying concern is nearly always the trade-off of protection versus power.

Programmers work in successively higher levels of abstraction by writing, and later invoking, standard procedures in the form of functions and subroutines. Built-in functions and subroutines create an environment in which users can perform complex operations by specifying single commands. Tools exist to combine related functions for specific tasks—for instance, to build a forms interface that displays retrieved data in a certain presentation format.

Specialized languages can be used directly by nonprogrammers for well-understood tasks, because such languages define additional procedures for specialized tasks and hide yet more detail. For example, users can search for and retrieve data from large databases using the Structured Query Language (SQL) of database-management systems (discussed later in this section). With the help of statistical languages, such as SAS or SPSS, users can perform extensive statistical calculations, such as regression analysis and correlation. Other users may use a spreadsheet program, such as Lotus 1-2-3 or Excel, to record and manipulate data with formulas in the cells of a spreadsheet. In each case, the physical details of the data-storage structures and the access mechanisms are hidden from the user. Each of these programs provides it own specialized language for instructing a computer to perform desired high-level functions.

The end users of a computer may not even be aware that they are programming if the language is so natural that it matches their needs in an intuitive manner. Moving icons on a screen and dragging and dropping them into boxes or onto other icons is a form of programming supported by many layers of interpreters and compiler-generated code. If the user saves a **script** (a keystroke-by-keystroke record) of the actions performed for later reuse, then she has created a program. Some systems allow such scripts to be viewed and edited for later updates and changes; for example, there is a macro function available in the Microsoft Excel spreadsheet and in the Microsoft Word text editor.

Even though many powerful languages and packages handle these diverse tasks, we still face the challenge of incorporating multiple functions into a larger system. It is easy to envision a system where a Web browser provides access to statistical results of data collected from two related databases. Such interoperation is not yet simple, however, and people must have programming expertise to resolve the details of incompatibilities among the specialized tools.

Data Management

Data provide the infrastructure for recording and sharing information. Data become information when they are organized to affect decisions and actions (see Chapter 2). Accessing and moving data from the points of collection to the points of use are among the primary functions of computing in medicine. These applications must deal with large volumes of varied data and manage them, for *persistence,* on external storage. The mathematical facilities of computer languages are based on common principles and are, strictly speaking, equivalent. The same conceptual basis is not available for data management facilities. Some languages allow only internal structures to be made persistent; in that case, external library programs are used for handling storage.

Handling data is made easier if the language supports moving structured data from internal memory to external, persistent storage. Data can, for instance, be viewed as a *stream,* a model that matches well with data produced by some instruments, by TCP connections over the Internet, or by a ticker tape. Data can also be viewed as *records,* matching well with the rows of a table (Fig. 4.10); or data can be viewed as a *hierarchy,* matching well with the structure of a medical record, including patients, their visits, and their findings during a visit.

If the language does not directly support the best data structure to deal with an application, then people must do additional programming to construct the desired structure out of the available facilities. The resulting extra layer, however, typically costs money and introduces inconsistencies among applications trying to share information.

Operating Systems

Users interact with the computer through an **operating system** (OS): a program that supervises and controls the execution of all other programs and that directs the operation of the hardware. The OS is software that is included with a computer system and manages the resources, such as memory, storage, and devices, for the user. Once started, the **kernel** of the OS resides in memory at all times and runs in the background. It manages memory, assigns the CPU to specific tasks, supervises other programs running in the computer, controls communication among hardware components, manages the transfer of data from input devices and to output devices, and handles the details of file management such as the creation, opening, reading, writing, and closing of data files. In shared systems, it allocates the resources of the system among the competing users. The OS insulates users from much of the complexity of handling these processes. Thus, users are able to concentrate on higher-level problems of information management. They do get involved in specifying which programs to run and in giving names to the directory structures and files that are to be made persistent. These names provide the links to the user's work from one session to another. Deleting files that are no longer needed and archiving those that should be kept securely are other interactions that users have with the OS.

Programmers can write **application programs** to automate routine operations that store and organize data, to perform analyses, to facilitate the integration and communication of information, to perform bookkeeping functions, to monitor pa-

Record-Number	Name	Sex	Date-of-Birth
22-546-998	Adams, Clare	F	11Nov1998
62-847-991	Barnes, Tanner	F	07Dec1997
47-882-365	Clark, Laurel	F	10May1998
55-202-187	Davidson, Travis	M	10Apr2000

FIGURE 4.10. A simple patient data file containing records for four pediatric patients. The key field of each record contains the medical-record number that uniquely identifies the patient. The other fields of the record contain demographic information.

tient status, to aid in education—in short, to perform all the functions provided by medical computing systems (see Chapter 5). These programs are then filed by the OS and are available to its users when needed.

Personal computers typically operate as **single-user systems,** whereas servers are **multiuser systems**. Workstations can handle either approach, although they often give a single user preference. For a *multiuser* system, in which many users share a single processor, two primary modes of operation are available. Large mainframe servers may operate in **batch mode**, where users communicate with the computer only to initiate processing and to obtain results upon completion. In **time-sharing mode**, all users have simultaneous access to their **jobs**; users interact through the OS, which switches resources rapidly among all the jobs that are running. Because people work slowly compared with computer CPUs, the computer can respond to multiple users, seemingly at the same time. Thus, all users have the illusion that they have the full attention of the machine, as long as they do not make very heavy demands. Such shared resource access is important where databases must be shared, as we discuss below in Database-Management Systems. When it is managing sharing, the OS spends resources for queuing, switching, and requeuing jobs. If the total demand is too high, the overhead increases disproportionately and slows the service for everyone. High individual demands are best allocated to workstations, which can be nearly as powerful as mainframes and which dedicate all resources to a primary user.

Because nearly all computers need to perform a variety of services, all systems except the simplest PC OSs support **multiprogramming**. In a multiprogramming system, several application programs reside in main memory simultaneously. Multiprogramming permits the effective use of multiple devices; while the CPU is executing one program, another program may be receiving input from external storage, and another may be generating results on the laser printer. In **multiprocessing** systems, several processors (CPUs) are used by the OS within a single computer system, thus increasing the overall processing power. Note, however, that multiprogramming does not imply having multiple processors.

Memory is still often a scarce resource, especially under multiprogramming. When many programs and their data are active simultaneously, they may not fit in the physical memory on the machine. To solve this problem, the OS will partition users' programs and data into **pages**, which can be kept in temporary storage and are brought into main memory as needed. Such a storage allocation is called **virtual memory**. Virtual memory can be several times the size of real memory, so users can allocate many more pages than main memory can hold. Also individual programs and their data can use more memory than is available on a specific computer. Under virtual memory management, each address referenced by the CPU goes through an address mapping from the **virtual address** of the program to a physical address in main memory (Fig. 4.11). When a memory page is referenced that is not in physical storage, the CPU creates space for it by swapping out a little-used page to secondary storage and bringing in the needed page from storage. This mapping is handled automatically by the hardware but still creates significant delays, so the total use of virtual memory must be limited to a level that permits the system to run efficiently.

A large collection of **system programs** is generally associated with the kernel of an OS. These programs include utility programs, such as **graphical user interface** (GUI) routines; **text** and **graphic editors**; compilers to handle programs written in higher-level languages; **debuggers** for newly created programs; communication software; diagnostic programs to help maintain the computer system; and substantial libraries of standard routines (such as for listing and viewing files, starting and stopping programs, and checking on system status). Modern libraries include tools such as sorting programs and programs to perform complex mathematical functions and routines to present and manipulate windows that access a variety of application programs, handle their point-and-click functions, allow a variety of fonts, and the like. The storage demands of these libraries is increasing—a few hundred megabytes for system programs is not unusual on PCs, and workstations and mainframes have several times those requirements. Not all system programs will ever be used by a user, but determining what is needed and deleting the rest is more work than most users want to undertake.

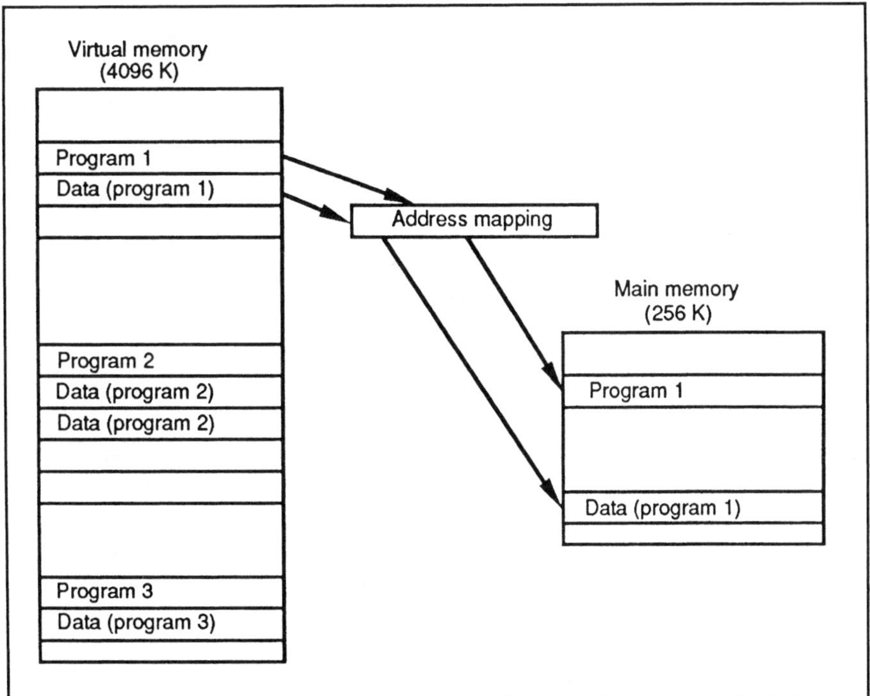

FIGURE 4.11. Virtual-memory system. Virtual memory provides users with the illusion that they have many more addressable memory locations than there are in real memory—in this case, more than five times as much. Programs and data stored on peripheral disks are swapped into main memory when they are referenced; logical addresses are translated automatically to physical addresses by the hardware.

Database-Management Systems

Throughout this book, we emphasize the importance to good medical decision-making of timely access to relevant and complete data from diverse sources. Computers provide the primary means for organizing and accessing these data; however, the programs to manage the data are complex and are difficult to write. Database technology supports the integration and organization of data and assists users with data entry, long-term storage, and retrieval. Programming data-management software is particularly difficult when multiple users share data (and thus may try to access data simultaneously), when they must search through voluminous data rapidly and at unpredictable times, and when the relationships among data elements are complex. For healthcare applications, it is important that the data be complete and virtually error free. Furthermore, the need for long-term reliability makes it unwise to entrust a medical database to locally written programs. The programmers tend to move from project to project, computers will be replaced, and the organizational units that maintain the data will be reorganized.

Not only the individual data values but also their meanings and their relationships to other data must be stored. For example, an isolated data element (e.g., the number 99.7) is useless unless we know that that number represents a human's body temperature in degrees Fahrenheit and is linked to other data necessary to interpret its value—the value pertains to a particular patient who is identified by a unique medical record number, the observation was taken at a certain time (02:35, 7Feb2000) in a certain way (orally), and so on. To avoid loss of descriptive information, we must keep together clusters of related data throughout processing. These relationships can be complex; for example, an observation may be linked not only to the patient, but also to the person recording the observation, to the instrument that he used to acquire the values, and to the physical state of the patient (refer to Chapter 2).

The meaning of data elements and the relationships among those elements are captured in the structure of the database. **Databases** are collections of data, typically organized into fields, records, and files (see Fig. 4.10). The **field** is the most primitive element; each field represents one data element. For example, the database of a hospital's registration system typically has fields such as the patient's identification number, name, date of birth, gender, admission date, and admitting diagnosis. Fields are usually grouped together to form **records**. A record is uniquely identified by one or more **key fields**—for example, patient-identification number and observation time. Records that contain similar information are grouped in **files**. In addition to files about patients and their diagnoses, treatments, and drug therapies, the database of a healthcare information system will have separate files containing information about charges and payments, personnel and payroll, inventory, and many other topics. All these files relate to one another: They may refer to the same patients, to the same personnel, to the same services, to the same set of accounts, and so on.

Once programmers know the structure and format of a data file, they can write programs to access the data directly. For example, if they know that a patient's identification number is stored in the first field of each record as a string of 10 alphanumeric characters, they can write programs to read each record, to extract the contents of the first field by its relative address, and to store the value in a variable, PATIENT-ID. If, however, the structure of the database changes—for example, because new fields are added to a record—programmers will have to modify all such existing programs. When data are to be shared, there will be continuing requirements for additions and reorganizations to the files. The desire for **data independence**—that is, keeping the applications of one set of users independent from changes made to applications by another group—is the key reason for using a database management system for shared data.

A **database-management system** (DBMS) is an integrated set of programs that helps users to store and manipulate data easily and efficiently. The conceptual (logical) view of a database provided by a DBMS allows users to specify *what* the results should be without worrying too much about *how* they will be obtained; the DBMS handles the details of managing and accessing data. A crucial part of a database kept in a DBMS is the **schema**, a machine-readable definition of the contents and organization of the records of all the data files. Programs are insulated by the DBMS from changes in the way that data are stored, because the programs access data by field name rather than by address. The schema file of the DBMS must be modified to reflect changes in record format, but the application programs that use the data do not need to be altered. A DBMS also provides facilities for entering, editing, and retrieving data. Often, fields are associated with lists or ranges of valid values; thus, the DBMS can detect and request correction of some data-entry errors, thereby improving database integrity.

Users retrieve data from a database in either of two ways. Users can query the database directly using a *query language* to extract information in an ad hoc fashion—for example, to retrieve the records of all male hypertensive patients aged 45 to 64 years for inclusion in a retrospective study. Figure 4.12 shows the syntax for such a query using SQL. Query formulation can be difficult, however; users must understand the contents and underlying structure of the database to construct a query correctly. Often, database programmers formulate the requests for health professionals.

To support occasional use, **front-end applications** to database systems can help a user retrieve information using a menu based on the schema. Certain applications, such as a drug order–entry system, will use a database system without the pharmacist or ordering physician being aware of the latter's presence. The medication-order records placed in the database create communication transactions with the pharmacy; then, the pharmacy application creates the daily drug lists for the patient-care units.

Some database queries are routine requests—for example, the resource-utilization reports used by healthcare administrators and the end-of-month financial reports generated for business offices. Thus, DBMSs often also provide an alternative, simpler means for formulating such queries, called **report generation.** Users specify their data requests on the input screen of the report-

```
SELECT    Patient-ID, Name, Age, Systolic

FROM      Patients

WHERE     Sex = 'M' and
          Age >= 45 and
          Age <= 64 and
          Systolic > 140
```

Figure 4.12. An example of a simple database query written in Structured Query Language (SQL). The program will retrieve the records of males whose age is between 45 and 64 years and whose systolic blood pressure is greater than 140 mm Hg.

generator program. The report generator then produces the actual query program using information stored in the schema, often at predetermined intervals. The reports are formatted such that they can be distributed without modification. The report-generation programs can extract header information from the schema. Routine report generation should, however, be periodically reviewed in terms of its benefits. Reports that are not read are a waste of computer, natural, and people resources. A reliable database will be able to provide needed and up-to-date information when that information is required.

Many DBMSs support multiple **views**, or models, of the data. The data stored in a database have a single physical organization, yet different user groups can have different perspectives on the contents and structure of a database. For example, the clinical laboratory and the finance department might use the same underlying database, but only the data relevant to the individual application area are available to each group. Basic patient information will be shared; the existence of other data is hidden from groups that do not need them. Application-specific descriptions of a database are stored in such **view schemas**. Through the views, a DBMS controls access to data, as discussed in Section 4.3. Thus, a DBMS facilitates the integration of data from multiple sources and avoids the expense of creating and maintaining multiple files containing redundant information. At the same time, it accommodates the differing needs of multiple users. The use of database technology, combined with communications technology (see the following discussion of Software for Network Communications), will enable healthcare institutions to attain the benefits both of independent, specialized applications and of large integrated databases.

Database design and implementation has become a highly specialized field. Most medical applications use standard products from established vendors. An introduction to the topic is provided by Ullman and Widom (1997). Wiederhold's book (1981) discusses the organization and use of databases in healthcare settings.

Software for Network Communications

The ability of computers to communicate with each other over local and remote networks brings tremendous power to computer users. Internet communications make it possible to share data and resources among diverse users and institutions around the world. Network users can access shared patient data (such as a hospital's medical records) or nationwide databases (such as bibliographic databases of scientific literature or genomics databases describing what is known about the biomolecular basis of life and disease). Networks make it possible for remote users to communicate with one another and to collaborate. In this section, we introduce the important concepts that allow you to understand network technology.

Network power is realized by means of a large body of communications software. This software handles the physical connection of each computer to the network, the internal preparation of data to be sent or received over the network, and the interfaces between the network data flow and applications programs. There are now tens of millions of computers of different kinds on the Internet and hundreds of programs in each machine that service network communications. Two key ideas make it possible to manage the complexity of network software: *network service stacks* and *network protocols*. These strategies allow communication to take place between any two machines on the Internet, ensure that application programs are insulated from changes in the network infrastructure, and make it possible for users to take advantage easily of the rapidly growing set of information resources and services. The **network stack** serves to organize software *within* a machine. Because the responsibilities for network communications are divided into different levels, with clear interfaces between the levels, network software is made more modular. The four-level network stack for TCP/IP is shown in Figure 4.13, which also compares that stack to the seven-level stack defined by the International Standards Organization.

At the lowest level—the Data Link and Physical Transport level—programs manage the physical connection of the machine to the network, the physical-medium packet formats, and the means for detecting and correcting errors. The Network level implements the IP method of addressing packets, routing packets, and controlling the timing and sequencing of transmissions. The Transport level converts packet-level communications into several services for the Application level, including a reliable serial byte stream (TCP), a transaction-oriented User Datagram Protocol (UDP), and newer services such as real-time video.

The Application level is where programs run that support electronic mail, file sharing and transfer, World Wide Web posting, downloading, browsing, and many other services. Each layer communicates with only the layers directly above

ISO Level	TCP/IP Service Level
5–7	Applications: SMTP, FPT, TELNET, DNS, ...
4	Transport: TCP and UDP
3	Network: IP (including ICMP, ARP, and RARP)
1–2	Data Link and Physical Transport: (Ethernet, Token Rings, Wireless, ...)

Figure 4.13. TCP/IP network service level stack and corresponding levels of the Open Systems Interconnection (OSI) Reference model developed by the International Standards Organization (ISO). Each level of the stack specifies a progressively higher level of abstraction. Each level serves the level above and expects particular functions or services from the level below it. SMTP = Simple Mail Transport Protocol; FTP = File Transfer Protocol; DNS = Domain Name System; TCP = Transmission Control Protocol; UDP = User Datagram Protocol; IP = Internet Protocol; ICMP = Internet Control Message Protocol; ARP = Address Resolution Protocol; RARP = Reverse Address Resolution Protocol.

and below it and does so through specific interface conventions. The network stack is machine and OS dependent—because it has to run on particular hardware and to deal with the OS on that machine (filing, input–output, memory access, and so on). But its layered design serves the function of modularization. Applications see a standard set of data-communication services and do not each have to worry about details such as how to form proper packets of an acceptable size for the network, how to route packets to the desired machine, how to detect and correct errors, or how to manage the particular network hardware on the computer. If a computer changes its network connection from a **Token Ring** to an **Ethernet** network, or if the **topology** of the network changes, the applications are unaffected. Only the lower level Data Link and Network layers need to be updated.

Internet protocols are shared conventions that serve to standardize communications *between* machines—much as, for two people to communicate effectively, they must agree on the meaning of the words they are using, the style of the interaction (lecture versus conversation), a procedure for handling interruptions, and so on. Protocols are defined for every Internet service (such as routing, electronic mail, and World Wide Web access) and establish the conventions for representing data, for requesting an action, and for replying to a requested action. For example, protocols define the format conventions for electronic mail addresses and text messages (RFC822), the attachment of multimedia content

(Multipurpose Internet Mail Extensions—MIME), the delivery of electronic mail messages (Simple Mail Transport Protocol—SMTP), the transfer of files (File Transfer Protocol—FTP), connections to remote computers (Telnet), the formatting of Web pages (Hypertext Markup Language—HTML), the exchange of routing information, and many more. By observing these protocols, machines of different types can communicate openly and can interoperate with each other. When requesting a Web page from a server using the Hypertext Transfer Protocol (HTTP), the client does not have to know whether the server is a UNIX machine, a Windows NT machine, or a mainframe running VMS—they all appear the same over the network if they adhere to the HTTP protocol. The layering of the network stack is also supported by protocols. As we said, within a machine, each layer communicates with only the layer directly above or below. Between machines, each layer communicates with only its peer layer on the other machine, using a defined protocol. For example, the SMTP application on one machine communicates with only an SMTP application on a remote machine. Similarly, the Network layer communicates with only peer Network layers—for example, to exchange routing information or control information using the Internet Control Message Protocol (ICMP).

We briefly describe four of the basic services available on the Internet: electronic mail, FTP, Telnet, and access to the World Wide Web.

1. *Electronic mail:* Users send and receive messages from other users via electronic mail, mimicking use of the postal service. The messages travel rapidly: Except for queuing delays at gateways and receiving computers, their transmission is nearly instantaneous. Electronic mail was one of the first protocols invented for the Internet (around 1970, when what was to become the Internet was still called the ARPAnet). A simple electronic mail message consists of a **header** and a **body**. The header contains information formatted according to the RFC822 protocol, which controls the appearance of the date and time of the message, the address of the sender, addresses of the recipients, the subject line, and other optional header lines. The body of the message contains free text. The user addresses electronic mail directly to the intended reader by giving the reader's account name or a personal alias followed by the IP address of the machine on which the reader receives mail—for example, JohnSmith@IP.address. The body of the electronic mail message may contain arbitrary multimedia information, such as drawings, pictures, sound, or video, if it is encoded according to the MIME standard. Mail is sent to the recipient using the SMTP standard. It may either be read on the machine holding the addressee's account or it may be downloaded to the addressee's personal computer for reading using either the Post Office Protocol (POP) or the Internet Mail Access Protocol (IMAP). There is, of course, no guarantee that the reader will be able or willing to read the electronic mail when a message arrives. Some mail protocols allow the sender to specify an acknowledgment to be returned when the mail has been deposited or has been read. Electronic mail has become an important communication path in health care, allowing *asynchro-*

nous (one-way) communications between participants. Requests for services, papers, meetings, and even collaborative exchanges are largely handled by electronic mail (Lederberg, 1978).

It is easy to broadcast electronic mail by sending it to a **mailing list** or specific **listserve**, but electronic mail etiquette conventions dictate that such communications be focused and relevant. **Spamming**, which is sending electronic mail solicitations or announcements to broad lists, is generally annoying to recipients, but it is difficult to prevent. Conventional electronic mail is sent in clear text over the network so that anyone observing network traffic can read its contents. Protocols for encrypted electronic mail, such as Privacy Enhanced Mail (PEM), are also available, but are not yet widely deployed; they ensure that the contents are readable by only the intended recipients.

2. *File Transfer Protocol (FTP):* FTP facilitates sending and retrieving large amounts of information—of a size that is uncomfortably large for electronic mail. For instance, programs and updates to programs, complete medical records, papers for review, and the like are best transferred via FTP. File Transfer Protocol access requires several steps: (1) accessing the remote computer using the IP address, (2) providing user identification to authorize access, (3) specifying the name of a file to be sent or fetched using the file-naming convention at the destination site, and (4) transferring the data. For open sharing of information by means of FTP sites, the user identification is by convention "anonymous" and with the requestor's electronic mail address as the password.
3. *Telnet:* Telnet allows a user to login on a remote computer. If the log in is successful, the user becomes a fully qualified user of the remote system, and the user's own machine becomes a relatively passive terminal. The smoothness of such a terminal emulation varies depending on the differences between the local and remote computers. Many Telnet programs emulate well-known terminal types, such as the VT100 or 3270, which are widely supported and minimize awkward mismatches of character-use conventions. Modest amounts of information can be brought into the user's machine by copying data displayed in the terminal window into a local text editor or other program (pasting).
4. *World Wide Web (WWW):* World Wide Web **browsing** facilitates user access to remote information resources made available by Web servers. The user interface is typically a **Web browser** that understands the basic World Wide Web protocols. The **Universal Resource Locator** (URL) is used to specify *where a resource is located* in terms of the protocol to be used, the domain name of the machine it is on, and the name of the information resource within the remote machine. The Hypertext Markup Language describes *what the information should look like when displayed.* These formats are oriented toward graphic displays, and greatly exceed the capabilities associated with Telnet. The Hypertext Markup Language supports conventional text, font settings, headings, lists, tables, and other display specifications. Within HTML documents, highlighted **buttons** can be defined that point to other HTML documents or services. This **hypertext** facility makes it possible to create a web of cross-referenced works that can be navigated by the user. The Hypertext

Markup Language can also refer to subsidiary documents that contain other types of information—for example, graphics, equations, images, video, speech—that can be seen or heard if the browser has been augmented with **helpers** or **plug-ins** for the particular format used. Capable browsers, such as Netscape or Internet Explorer, also provide choices for downloading the presented information so that no separate FTP tasks need to be initiated. The Hypertext Transfer Protocol is used to communicate between browser clients and servers and to retrieve HTML documents.

Hypertext Markup Language documents can also include small programs written in the Java language, called **applets**, which will execute on the user's computer when referenced. Applets can provide animations and also can compute summaries, merge information, and interact with selected files on the user's computer. The Java language is designed such that operations that might be destructive to the user's machine environment are blocked, but downloading remote and untested software still represents a substantial security risk (see Section 4.3).

A **client-server** interaction is a generalization of the four interactions we have just discussed, involving interactions between a client (requesting) machine and a server (responding) machine. A client–server interaction, in general, supports collaboration between the user of a local machine and a remote computer. The server provides information and computational services according to some protocol, and the user's computer—the client—does complementary processing. A common function provided by servers is database access. Retrieved information is transferred to the client in response to requests, and then the client may perform specialized analyses on the data. The final results can be stored locally, printed, or mailed to other users.

4.2 Data Acquisition and Signal Processing

A prominent theme of this book is that capturing and entering data into a computer manually is difficult, time consuming, error prone, and expensive. **Real-time acquisition** of data from the source by direct electrical connections to instruments can overcome these problems. Direct acquisition of data avoids the need for people to measure, encode, and enter the data manually. Sensors attached to a patient convert biological signals—such as blood pressure, pulse rate, mechanical movement, and electrocardiogram (ECG)—into electrical signals, which are transmitted to the computer. Tissue density can be obtained by scanning of an X-ray transmission. The signals are sampled periodically and are converted to digital representation for storage and processing. Automated data-acquisition and signal-processing techniques are particularly important in patient-monitoring settings (see Chapter 13). Similar techniques also apply to the acquisition and processing of human voice input.

Most naturally occurring signals are **analog signals**—signals that vary continuously. The first bedside monitors, for example, were wholly analog devices.

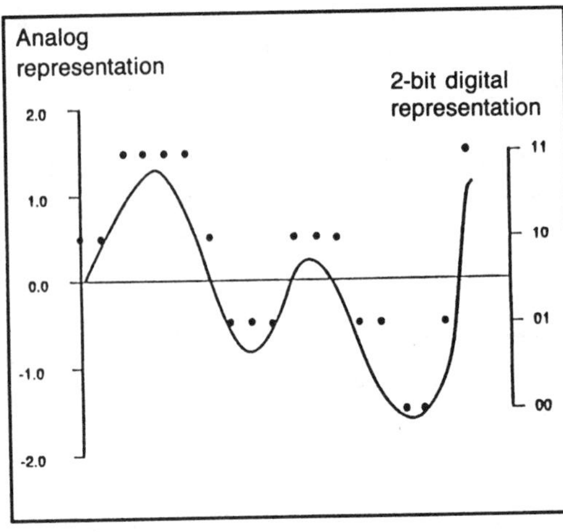

FIGURE 4.14. Analog-to-digital conversion (ADC). ADC is a technique for transforming continuous-valued signals to discrete values. In this example, each sampled value is converted to one of four discrete levels (represented by 2 bits).

Typically, they acquired an analog signal (such as that measured by the ECG) and displayed its level on a dial or other continuous display (see, e.g., the continuous signal recorded on the ECG strip shown in Fig. 13.10).

The computers with which we work are digital computers. A **digital computer** stores and processes values in discrete values taken at discrete points and at discrete times. Before computer processing is possible, analog signals must be converted to digital units. The conversion process is called **analog-to-digital conversion** (ADC). You can think of ADC as *sampling and rounding*—the continuous value is observed (sampled) at some instant and is rounded to the nearest discrete unit (Fig. 4.14). You need 1 bit to distinguish between two levels (e.g., on or off); if you wish to discriminate among four levels, you need 2 bits (because $2^2 = 4$), and so on.

Two parameters determine how closely the digital data represent the original analog signal: the precision with which the signal is recorded and the frequency with which the signal is sampled. The **precision** is the degree to which a digital estimate of a signal matches the actual value. The number of bits used to encode the digital estimate and their correctness determines precision; the more bits, the greater the number of levels that can be distinguished. Precision also is limited by the accuracy of the equipment that converts and transmits the signal. Ranging and calibration of the instruments, either manually or automatically, is necessary for signals to be represented with as much precision as possible. Improper ranging will result in loss of information. For example, a change in a signal that varies between 0.1 and 0.2 volts will be undetectable if the instrument has been set to record changes between -2.0 and 2.0 in 0.5-volt increments (Fig. 4.15 shows another example of improper ranging).

The **sampling rate** is the second parameter that affects the correspondence between an analog signal and its digital representation. A sampling rate that is too low relative to the rate with which a signal changes value will produce a poor representation (Fig. 4.16). On the other hand, oversampling increases the expense of processing and storing the data. As a general rule, you need to sample at least

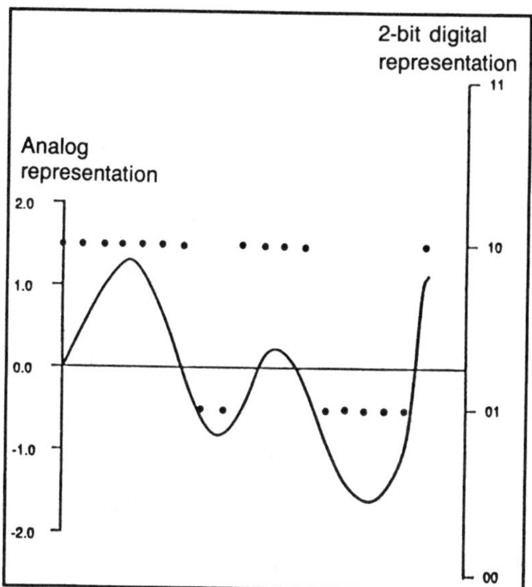

FIGURE 4.15. Effect on precision of ranging. The amplitude of signals from sensors must be ranged to account, for example, for individual patient variation. As illustrated here, the details of the signal may be lost if the signal is insufficiently amplified. On the other hand, overamplification will produce clipped peaks and troughs.

twice as frequently as the highest-frequency component that you need from a signal. For instance, looking at an ECG, we find that the basic repetition frequency is at most a few per second, but that the QRS wave (see Section 13.3) contains useful frequency components on the order of 150 cycles per second. Thus, the data-sampling rate should be at least 300 measurements per second. The rate calculated by doubling the highest frequency is called the **Nyquist frequency.**

Another aspect of signal quality is the amount of **noise** in the signal—the component of the acquired data that is *not* due to the specific phenomenon being measured. Primary sources of noise include random fluctuations in a signal detector or electrical or magnetic signals picked up from nearby devices and power lines. Once the signal has been obtained from a sensor, it must be transmitted to the computer. Often, the signal is sent through lines that pass near other equipment. En route, the analog signals are susceptible to electromagnetic interference. Inaccuracies in the sensors, poor contact between sensor and source (e.g., the patient), and disturbances from signals produced by processes other than the one being studied (e.g., respiration interferes with the ECG) are other common sources of noise.

Three techniques, often used in combination, minimize the amount of noise in a signal before its arrival in the computer:

1. *Shielding, isolation, and grounding* of cables and instruments carrying analog signals all reduce electrical interference. Often, two twisted wires are used to transmit the signal—one to carry the actual signal and the other to transmit the ground voltage at the sensor. At the destination, a differential amplifier measures the difference. Most types of interference affect both wires equally; thus, the difference should reflect the true signal. The use of glass fiberoptic

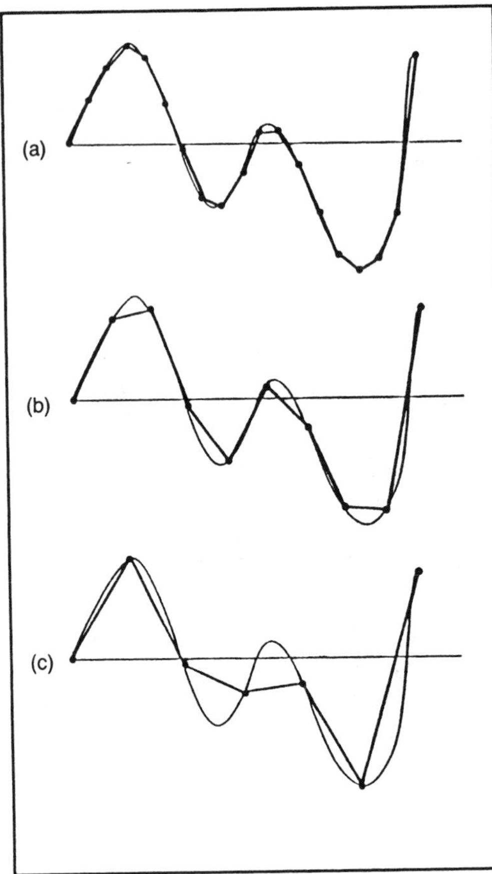

Figure 4.16. The greater the sampling rate, the more closely the sampled observations will correspond to the underlying analog signal. The sampling rate in *a* is highest; that in *b* is lower; and that in *c* is the lowest. When the sampling rate is very low (as in *c*), the results of the analog-to-digital conversion can be misleading. Note the degradation of the quality of the signal from *a* to *c*. (Figure 13.7 illustrates the effects of varying sampling rate on the quality of an ECG signal.)

cables, instead of copper wires, for signal transmission eliminates interference from electrical machinery, because optical signals are not affected by electrical or magnetic fields.

2. For robust transmission over long distances, analog signals can be *converted* into a **frequency-modulated** (FM) representation. An FM signal represents changes of the signal as changes of frequency rather than of amplitude. Frequency modulation reduces noise greatly, because interference directly disturbs only the amplitude of the signal. As long as the interference does not create amplitude changes near the high carrier frequency, no loss of data will occur during transmission.

Conversion of analog signals to digital form provides the most robust transmission. The nearer to the source the conversion occurs, the more effective this technique is. Digital transmission of signals is inherently less noise sensitive than is analog transmission: Interference rarely is great enough to change a 1 value to a 0 value or vice versa. Furthermore, digital signals can be coded, permitting detection and correction of faults. Placing a microprocessor near the signal source is now the most common way to achieve such a conversion. The development of **digital signal processing (DSP) chips**—also used for computer voice mail and other applications—will accelerate this trend.

3. **Filtering algorithms** can be used to reduce the effect of noise. Usually, these algorithms are applied to the data once the latter have been stored in memory. A characteristic of noise is its relatively random pattern. Repetitive signals, such as an ECG, can be integrated over several cycles, thus reducing the effects of random noise. When the noise pattern differs from the signal pattern, *Fourier analysis* can be used to filter the signal; a signal is decomposed into its individual components, each with a distinct period and amplitude. (Wiederhold and Clayton's article in the Suggested Readings explains Fourier analysis in greater detail.) Unwanted components of the signal are assumed to be noise and are eliminated. Some noise (such as the 60-cycle interference caused by a building's electrical circuitry) has a regular pattern. In this case, the portion of the signal that is known to be caused by interference can be filtered out.

Once the data have been acquired and cleaned up, they typically are processed to reduce their volume and to abstract information for use by interpretation programs. Often, the data are analyzed to extract important parameters, or *features,* of the signal—for example, the duration or intensity of the ST segment of an ECG. The computer also can analyze the shape of the waveform by comparing the signal to models of known patterns, or templates. In speech recognition, the voice signals can be compared with stored profiles of spoken words. Further analysis is necessary to determine the meaning or importance of the signals—for example, to allow automated ECG-based cardiac diagnosis or **speech understanding**.

4.3 Data and System Security

Medical records contain much information about us. These documents and databases include data ranging from height and weight measurements, blood pressures, and notes regarding bouts with the flu, cuts, or broken bones to information about topics such as fertility and abortions, emotional problems and psychiatric care, sexual behaviors, sexually transmitted diseases, human immunodeficiency virus (HIV) status, substance abuse, physical abuse, and genetic predisposition to diseases. Some data are generally considered to be mundane, others highly sensitive. Within the medical record, there is much information about which any given person may feel sensitive. As discussed in Chapter 7, health information is considered to be confidential, and access to such information must be controlled because disclosure could harm us, for example, by causing social embarrassment or prejudice, by affecting our insurability, or by limiting our ability to get and hold a job. Medical data also must be protected against loss. If we are to depend on electronic medical records for care, they must be available whenever and wherever we need care, and the information that they contain must be accurate and up to date. Orders for tests or treatments must be validated to ensure that they are issued by authorized providers. The records must also support administrative review and provide a basis for legal accountability. These requirements touch on three separate concepts involved in protecting healthcare information.

Privacy refers to the desire of a person to control disclosure of personal health and other information. **Confidentiality** applies to information—in this context, the ability of a person to control the release of her personal health information to a care provider or information custodian under an agreement that limits the further release of that information. **Security** is the protection of privacy and confidentiality through a collection of policies, procedures, and safeguards. Security measures enable an organization to maintain the integrity and availability of information systems and to control access to these systems' contents. Health privacy and confidentiality are discussed further in Chapter 7.

Concerns about and methods to provide security are part of most computer systems, but healthcare systems are distinguished by having especially complex considerations for the use and release of information. In general, the security steps taken in a healthcare information system serve five key functions (National Research Council, 1997):

1. **Availability** ensures that accurate and up-to-date information is available when needed at appropriate places.
2. **Accountability** helps to ensure that users are responsible for their access to and use of information based on a documented need and right to know.
3. **Perimeter definition** allows the system to control the boundaries of trusted access to an information system, both physically and logically.
4. **Role-limited access** enables access for personnel to only that information essential to the performance of their jobs and limits the real or perceived temptation to access information beyond a legitimate need.
5. **Comprehensibility and control** ensures that record owners, data stewards, and patients can understand and have effective control over appropriate aspects of information confidentiality and access.

The primary approach to ensuring *availability* is to protect against loss of data by performing regular system backups. Because hardware and software systems will never be perfectly reliable, information of long-term value is copied onto archival storage, and copies are kept at remote sites to protect the data in case of disaster. For short-term protection, data can be written on duplicate storage devices. If one of the storage devices is attached to a remote processor, then additional protection is conferred. Critical medical systems must be prepared to operate even during environmental disasters. Therefore, it is also important to provide secure housing and alternative power sources for CPUs, storage devices, network equipment, and so on. It is also essential to maintain the integrity of the information-system software to ensure availability. Backup copies provide a degree of protection against software failures; if a new version of a program damages the system's database, the backups allow operators to rollback to the earlier version of the software and database contents.

Unauthorized software changes—for example, in the form of viruses—are also a threat. A **virus** may be attached to an innocuous program or data file, and, when that program is executed or data file is opened, several actions take place:

1. The viral code copies itself into other files residing in the computer.
2. It attaches these files to outgoing messages, to spread itself to other computers.
3. The virus may collect email addresses for mailout of its copies.
4. The virus may destroy or modify other files, often to escape detection.

A software virus causes havoc with computer operations, even if it does not do violent damage, by disturbing operations and system access. To protect against viruses, all programs loaded onto the system should be checked against known viral codes and for unexpected changes in size or configuration. It is not always obvious that a virus program has been imported. For example, a word-processing document may include macros that help in formatting the document. Such a macro can also include viral codes, however, so the document can be infected. Spreadsheets, graphical presentations, and so on are also subject to infection by viruses.

Accountability for use of medical data can be promoted both by surveillance and by technical controls. Most people working in a medical environment are highly ethical. In addition, knowledge that access to and use of data records are being watched, through scanning of access **audit trails,** serves as a strong impediment to abuse. Technical means to ensure accountability include two additional functions: *authentication* and *authorization.*

1. The user is **authenticated** through a positive and unique identification process, such as name and password combination.
2. The authenticated user is **authorized** within the system to perform only certain actions appropriate to her role in the healthcare system—for example, to search through certain medical records of only patients under her care.

Authentication and authorization can be performed most easily within an individual computer system, but, because most institutions operate multiple computers, it is necessary to coordinate these access controls consistently across all the systems. Enterprise-wide access-control standards and systems are available but have been deployed to only a limited extent.

Perimeter definition requires that you know who your users are and how they are accessing the information system. For healthcare providers within a small physician practice, physical access can be provided with a minimum of hassle using simple name and password combinations. If a clinician is traveling or at home and needs remote access to a medical record, however, greater care must be taken to ensure that the person is who he claims to be and that communications containing sensitive information are not observed inappropriately. But where is the boundary for being considered a trusted insider? Careful control of where the network runs and how users get outside access is necessary. Most organizations install a **firewall** to define the boundary: All sharable computers of the institution are located within the firewall. Anyone who attempts to access a shared system from the outside must first pass through the firewall, where strong authentication controls are in place. Having passed this authentication step, the user can then access services within the firewall (still limited by the applicable authorization controls). Even with a firewall in place, it is important for enterprise system administrators to monitor to ensure that the firewall is not bypassed—for example, a malicious intruder could install a modem on an inside telephone line or load unauthorized software.

Strong authentication and authorization controls depend on cryptographic technologies. **Cryptographic encoding** is a primary tool for protecting data that are stored and are transmitted over communication lines. Two kinds of cryptography are in common use—secret-key cryptography and public-key cryptography. In **secret-key cryptography**, the same key is used to encrypt and to decrypt information. Thus, the key must be kept secret, known to only the sender and intended receiver of information. In **public-key cryptography**, two keys are used, one to encrypt the information and a second to decrypt it. Because two keys are involved, only one need be kept secret. The other one can be made publicly available. This arrangement leads to important services in addition to exchange of sensitive information, such as provision of digital signatures (certifies authorship), content validation (indicates the contents of a message have not been changed), and nonrepudiation (indicates that an order or payment for goods received cannot be repudiated). Under either scheme, once data are encrypted, a key is needed to decode and make the information legible and suitable for processing.

Keys of longer length provide more security, because they are harder to guess. Because powerful computers can help intruders to test millions of candidate keys rapidly, keys of 56-bit length are no longer considered secure, and keys of 128 bits are entering service. If a key is lost, then the information encrypted with the key is effectively lost as well. If a key is stolen, or if too many copies of the key exist for them to be tracked, then unauthorized people may gain access to information. Holding the keys in **escrow** by a trusted party can provide some protection against loss.

Cryptographic tools can be used to control authorization as well. The authorization information may be encoded as digital **certificates**, which then can be validated with a certification authority and checked by the services so that the services do not need to check the authorizations themselves. Centralizing authentication and authorization functions simplifies the coordination of access control, allows for rapid revocation of privileges as needed, and reduces the possibility of an intruder finding holes in the system.

Role-limited access control is based on extensions of authorization schemes. Even when overall system access has been authorized and is protected, further checks must be made to control access to specific data within the record. A medical record is not partitioned according to external access criteria, and the many different collaborators in health care all have diverse needs for, and thus rights to, the information collected in the medical record. Examples include the following:

- *Patients:* the contents of their own medical records
- *Community physicians:* records of their patients
- *Specialty physicians:* records of patients referred for consultations
- *Public health agencies:* incidences of communicable diseases
- *Medical researchers:* anonymous records or summarization of data for patient groups
- *Billing clerks:* records of services, with supporting clinical documentation as required by insurance companies
- *Insurance payers:* justifications of charges

Different types of information kept in the medical records have different rules for release, as determined by state and federal law and as set by institutional policy following legal and ethical considerations. For instance, the medical record of a patient who has heart problems might include notations that the patient also had a positive HIV test result, which should not be revealed to health services researchers conducting an unrelated outcomes study. Based on institutional policy, such notations might be masked before release of records for research purposes. Depending on the study design, the patients' names and other identifying information might also be masked.

To protect the confidentiality of medical records against inappropriate release to collaborators, the records should be inspected before release, but such checking requires more resources than most healthcare institutions are able to devote. To date, relatively few resources have been devoted to system security and ensuring confidentiality of healthcare data; most such resources are used to resolve problems after a violation is reported (National Research Council, 1997). Even minimal encryption is rarely used because of the awkwardness created in handling the keys and accessing the data. Concerns over privacy protection are increasing, however, and such concerns are beginning to be supported by legal requirements of responsible trusteeship by collectors and holders of medical records. To respond to these new requirements, we need better tools to protect privacy and the confidentiality of health information (Sweeney, 1996; Wiederhold et al., 1996).

4.4 Summary

As we have discussed in this chapter, the synthesis of large-scale information systems is accomplished through the careful construction of hierarchies of hardware and software. Each successive layer is more abstract and hides many of the details of the preceding layer. Simple methods for storing and manipulating data ultimately produce complex information systems that have powerful capabilities. Communication links that connect local and remote computers in arbitrary configurations, and the security mechanisms that span these systems, transcend the basic hardware and software hierarchies. Thus, without worrying about the technical details, users can access a wealth of computational resources and can perform complex information-management tasks, such as storing and retrieving, communicating, and processing information.

Suggested Readings

Hennessy J.L., Patterson D.A. (1996). *Computer Architecture: A Quantitative Approach* (2nd ed.). San Francisco: Morgan Kaufmann.

This technical book provides an in-depth explanation of the physical and conceptual underpinnings of computer hardware and its operation. It is suitable for technically oriented readers who want to understand the details of computer architecture.

McDonald C.J. (Ed.). (1987). *Images, Signals, and Devices (M.D. Computing: Benchmark Papers).* New York: Springer-Verlag.

The second in a series of Benchmark Papers from M.D. Computing, this volume introduces the use of computers in bioengineering. It contains articles on imaging and monitoring, including overviews of technologies such as computed tomography.

McDonald C.J. (Ed.). (1987). *Tutorials (M.D. Computing: Benchmark Papers).* New York: Springer-Verlag.

The third in a series of Benchmark Papers, this volume contains 17 tutorials originally published in *M.D. Computing,* including articles on computer hardware, local-area networks, operating systems, and programming languages. The collection will be of interest to computing novices who wish to understand how computers work or who would like to learn elementary programming skills.

National Research Council. (1997). *For the Record: Protecting Electronic Health Information.* Washington, D.C.: National Academy Press.

This report documents an extensive study of current security practices in U.S. healthcare settings and recommends significant changes. It sets guidelines for policies, technical protections, and legal standards for acceptable access to and use of healthcare information. It is well suited for lay, medical, and technical readers who are interested in an overview of this complex topic.

Tanenbaum A. (1996). *Computer Networks* (3rd ed.). Englewood Cliffs, NJ: Prentice-Hall.

The heavily revised edition of a classic textbook on computer communications, this book is well organized, clearly written, and easy to understand. The introductory chapter describes network architectures and the International Standards Organization's OSI reference model. Each of the remaining chapters discusses in detail a layer of the OSI model.

Ullman J.D., Widom J. (1997). *A First Course in Database Systems.* Englewood Cliffs, NJ: Prentice Hall.

This introductory-level book covers databases from the points of view of the database designer, user, and application programmer. It includes comprehensive coverage of SQL programming and of the design of databases using both the entity-relationship model and the object-oriented model.

Wiederhold G. (1981). *Databases for Health Care.* New York: Springer-Verlag.

This book uses a healthcare perspective to introduce the concepts of database technology. Although dated in some respects, the book describes the structures and functions of databases and discusses the scientific and operational issues associated with their use, including the problems of missing data and the conflict between data sharing and data confidentiality.

Wiederhold G., Clayton P.D. (1985). Processing biological data in real time. *M.D. Computing,* 2(6):16–25.

This article discusses the principles and problems of acquiring and processing biological data in real time. It covers much of the material discussed in the signal-processing section of this chapter and it provides more detailed explanations of analog-to-digital conversion and Fourier analysis.

Questions for Discussion

1. Why do computer systems use magnetic disks to store data and programs rather than keeping the latter in main memory where they could be accessed much more quickly?
2. What are four considerations in deciding whether to keep data in active versus archival storage?
3. Explain how an operating system insulates users from hardware changes.
4. Discuss the advantages and disadvantages of individual workstations linked in a LAN versus shared access to mainframe computers.
5. Define the terms *data independence* and *database schema*. How do database management systems facilitate data independence?
6. Why have so many different computer languages been developed?

5
System Design and Engineering

GIO WIEDERHOLD AND EDWARD H. SHORTLIFFE

After reading this chapter, you should know the answers to these questions:

- What key functions do medical computer systems perform?
- Why is communication between medical personnel and computing personnel crucial to the successful design and implementation of a medical information system?
- What are the trade-offs between purchasing a turnkey system and developing a custom-designed system?
- What resources are available remotely for medical computer systems?
- What design features most heavily affect a system's acceptance by health professionals?
- Why do systems in health care, once implemented and installed successfully, have a long lifetime?

5.1 How Can a Computer System Help in Health Care?

In Chapter 4, we introduced basic concepts related to computer and communications hardware and software. In this chapter, we see how information systems created from these components can be used by health professionals to support healthcare delivery. We describe the basic functions performed by health information systems and discuss important considerations in system design, implementation, and evaluation. You should keep these concepts in mind as you read about the various medical computing applications in the chapters that follow. Think about how each system meets (or fails to meet) the needs of its users and about the practical reasons why certain systems have been accepted for routine use in patient care whereas other systems have failed to make the transition from the research environment to the real world.

At a minimum, a system's success depends on the selection of appropriate hardware and on the implementation of efficient data-storage, data-transmission, and data-processing methods. We do not discuss, however, the technical issues related to specific hardware and software choices—those determinations are beyond the scope of this book. Instead, we provide a general introduction to practical issues in the design and implementation of systems. In particular, we stress the importance of designing systems that not only meet users' requirements for information but also fit smoothly into users' everyday routines. There are many types of users of a healthcare information system, and often it is necessary to consider each, one at a time.

There are *healthcare professionals*, for whom the quality of the results is paramount, but who are invariably pressed for time. There are *administrators*, who have to make personnel and financial decisions crucial to institutional well-being. There are *clerks*, who may enter and retrieve much of the data. Some systems also provide for direct interaction by *patients*. In addition, there are *operational personnel* who maintain the system and ensure its reliability. Initially there are professional system *designers* and *implementers*, but their numbers and availability decrease as the systems move into routine operation. Before they depart, designers and implementers must provide adequate documentation and training. For instance, clerks require clear procedures for their interaction with the system so that errors are minimized. A central theme of this chapter is the importance of communication between healthcare and computing professionals in defining problems and developing solutions that can be implemented within an institution. With this perspective, we explore the factors that create a need for automation and discuss important considerations in the design, development, and evaluation of medical information systems.

5.1.1 What Is a System?

Until now, we have referred freely to *medical information systems* and *computer systems*. What do we mean when we refer to a *system*? In the most general sense, a **system** is an organized set of procedures for accomplishing a task. It can be described in terms of (1) the problem to be solved, (2) the data and knowledge required to address the problem, and (3) the internal process for transforming the available **input** into the desired **output** (Fig. 5.1). When we talk about systems in this book, we usually mean *computer-based* (or just *computer*) systems. A

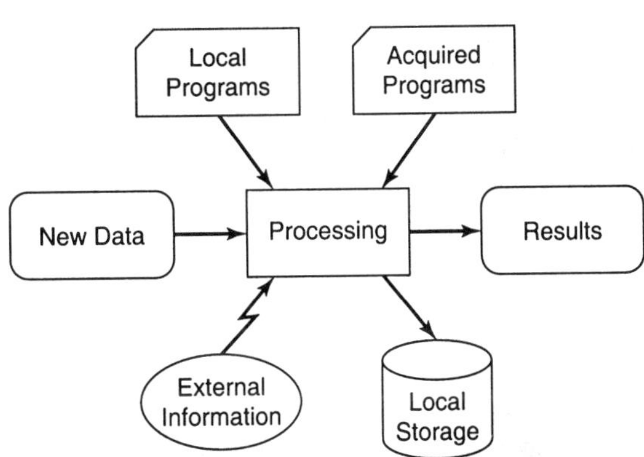

FIGURE 5.1. A computer system applies locally defined and general procedures to produce results from new input data, from stored data, and from information obtained from remote external sources.

computer system combines both manual and automated processes; people and machines work in concert to manage and use information. A computer system has these components:

- **Hardware:** The physical equipment, including the central processing unit (CPU), data-storage devices, terminals, and printers
- **Software:** The computer programs that direct the hardware to carry out the automated processes—that is, to process input data and stored information and perhaps to prompt the users regarding manual processes
- **Customers:** The users who interact with the software and hardware of the system and use the results or forward them to others. There will be other users who are concerned with system operations, backup, and maintenance

The role of a computer is, broadly speaking, the conversion of data into information. Every piece of data must be supplied by a person, by another computer system, or by data-collection equipment, as seen in patient monitoring (see Chapter 13). Output information is delivered to healthcare professionals or becomes input to another computer system. In other words, a medical computer system is a module of the overall healthcare delivery system.

The overall healthcare system not only determines the need for the computer system (e.g., which data must be processed and which reports must be generated) but also the requirements for the system's operation (e.g., the necessary degree of reliability and timeliness of access to information). Acquisition of a computer system has implications for the organization of an institution. Who controls the information? Who is responsible for the accuracy of the data? How will the system be financed?

The installation of a computer system may have sociological consequences as well. The introduction of a new system alters the work routines of healthcare workers. Furthermore, it may affect the traditional roles of healthcare workers and the existing relationships among groups of individuals—for example, between physicians and nurses, between nurses and patients, and between physicians and patients. Important ethical and legal questions that arise include the confidentiality of patient information, the appropriate role of computers in patient care (especially in medical decision-making), and the responsibility of developers and users for ensuring the correct operation of the system (see Chapter 7). Although the technical challenges in system development must be met, organizational factors are often crucial determinants of the success of a computer system within the initial institution. These factors can differ greatly among institutions and can make the transfer of a well-functioning system to another site difficult.

5.1.2 Functions of a Computer System

Computers have been used in every aspect of healthcare delivery, from the simple processing of business data, to the collection and interpretation of physiological data, to the education of physicians and nurses. Each chapter in Unit II of this book describes an important area for the application of computers in biomedicine. The unique characteristics of each problem area create special requirements for system builders to address. The motivation for investing in these applications, however, is the computer's ability to help health professionals in some aspect of information management. We identify eight topics that define the range of basic functions that may be provided by medical computer systems:

1. Data acquisition and presentation
2. Record keeping and access
3. Communication and integration of information
4. Surveillance
5. Information storage and retrieval
6. Data analysis
7. Decision support
8. Education

These functions recur in the discussions of each of the types of systems addressed in Chapters 9 through 18. You will note that most systems assist their users with several tasks. In addition, although decision support is a primary function for only two categories of applications, essentially all uses of computers in medicine can be viewed as supporting decision-making.

Data Acquisition

Health professionals require assistance with data acquisition when the number of data that must be collected and processed overwhelms human capabilities. One of the first uses of computers in a medical setting was the automatic analysis of specimens of blood and other body fluids by instruments that measure chemical concentrations or that count cells and organisms and the presentation of the results in a clear form. Marking results that are outside the expected range can alert the healthcare staff. Computer-based patient-monitoring systems that collect physiological data directly from patients were another early application of computing technology (see Chapter 13). Such systems ensure that vital signs, electrocardiograms (ECGs), and other indicators of patient status are measured frequently and consistently. More recently, researchers have developed medical imaging applications as described in Chapter 14, including computed tomography, magnetic-resonance imaging, and digital-subtraction angiography. The calculations for these computationally intensive applications cannot be performed manually; the computers collect and manipulate millions of individual bits of information.

Early computer-based medical instruments and measurement devices that perform data acquisition were self-contained. Today, most systems can supply data directly into the patient record, although the interfaces are often awkward and poorly standardized (see Chapter 6). We can also consider computer-based history-taking systems to be data-acquisition systems because they free health professionals from the need to collect and enter routine demographic and history information.

Record Keeping

Given the data-intensive nature of healthcare delivery, it is no surprise that record keeping is a primary function of many medical computer systems. Computers are well suited to performing tedious and repetitive data-processing tasks, such as collecting and tabulating data, transcribing data from one form to another, and formatting and producing reports. They are particularly useful for processing large volumes of data. Thus, an automated billing system is a natural application of computers in healthcare settings; typically it was the first component installed when a hospital, clinic, or private practice decided to use computer technology.

Individual departments within a hospital also have their own computer systems and maintain their own records. For instance, clinical laboratories use computer-based information systems to keep track of orders and specimens and to report test results; most pharmacy and radiology departments also have acquired computers to perform analogous functions. Their systems may connect to outside services (e.g., pharmacy systems are typically connected to one or more drug distributors) so that ordering and delivery are rapid and local inventories can be kept small. By automating processing in areas such as these, healthcare facilities are able to speed up services, reduce direct labor costs, and minimize the number of errors.

Computer systems acquired by departments in hospitals are often obtained from specialized vendors. Such vendors contribute their experience in serving clinical laboratories, pharmacy operations, or other areas. They will supply their customers with updates when capabilities improve or regulations change. Some of the services may actually be provided remotely at a vendor's site. Unfortunately, this diversity makes it difficult to integrate the information from the disparate systems into a coherent whole, a problem addressed in Chapter 10.

Communication and Integration

In hospitals and other distributed healthcare environments, myriad data are collected by multiple health professionals who work in a variety of settings; each patient receives care from a host of providers—nurses, physicians, technicians, pharmacists, and so on. Communication among the members of the team is essential for effective healthcare delivery. Data must be available to decision-makers when and where they are needed; computers help by storing, transmitting, and displaying those data. As we describe in Chapters 2 and 9, the patient record is the primary vehicle for communication of clinical information. A critical limitation of the traditional paper-based patient record, however, is the concentration of information in a single location, which prohibits simultaneous access by multiple people. Hospital information systems (HISs) (Chapter 10) and automated patient-record systems (Chapter 9) allow decentralization of many activities, such as admission, appointment, and resource scheduling; review of laboratory-test results; and inspection of patient records.

Often the information necessary for decision-making is not available within a single computer system. Clinical systems are often diverse for technical and historical reasons. Furthermore, in many institutions, clinical and financial activities are supported by separate organizational units. Hospital administrators must integrate clinical and financial information to analyze costs and to evaluate the efficiency of healthcare delivery. Similarly, clinicians may need to review data collected at other healthcare institutions, or they may wish to consult online databases of biomedical information. Local-area networks that permit sharing of information among independent computers and wide-area networks that permit exchange of information among geographically distributed sites provide good communication infrastructures. Actual integration of information requires additional software, adherence to standards, and operational staff to keep it all working as technology and systems evolve.

Surveillance

Timely reactions to data are crucial for quality in health care especially when a patient has unexpected problems. Data overload, created by the growth of information technology, is as detrimental to good decision-making as is data insufficiency. Data indicating a need for action may be available but are easily overlooked by overloaded health professionals. Surveillance and monitoring systems can help people cope with all the data relevant to patient management by calling attention to significant events or situations—for example, by reminding doctors of the need to order screening tests and other preventive measures (see Chapter 9) or by warning them when a dangerous event or constellation of events has occurred.

Laboratory systems routinely identify and flag abnormal test results. Similarly, when patient-monitoring systems in intensive-care units detect abnormalities in patient status, they sound alarms to alert nurses and physicians to potentially dangerous changes. A pharmacy system that maintains computer-based drug-profile records for patients can screen incoming drug orders and warn physicians who order a drug that interacts with another drug that the patient is receiving or a drug to which the patient has a known allergy or sensitivity. By correlating data from multiple sources, an integrated HIS can monitor for complex events, such as interactions among patient diagnosis, drug regimen, and physiological status (indicated by laboratory-test results). For instance, a change in cholesterol level can be due to prednisone given to an arthritic patient and may not indicate a dietary problem.

Information Storage and Retrieval

Storage and retrieval of information is essential to all computer systems. Storing information permits sharing of information with people who are not available at the same time. Storage must be well organized and indexed so that information recorded in a patient-record system allows effective retrieval. Here the variety of users must be considered. Getting cogent recent information about a patient entering the office differs from the needs that a researcher will have in accessing the same data. The query languages provided by many automated patient-record and clinical research systems assist researchers in retrieving pertinent records from among the many saved in the large databases of patient information. As we discuss in Chapter 15, bibliographic-retrieval systems now are essential to effective searching of the medical literature.

Data Analysis

Raw data as acquired by computer systems are often excessively voluminous. Data analysis systems can aid decision-makers by presenting information in a clear and understandable form. Presentations of data can use graphs to facilitate trend analysis or compute secondary parameters (means, standard deviations, rates of change, and so on) to help spot abnormalities. Effective clinical research systems have modules for performing powerful statistical analyses of large sets of patient data. The researcher, however, should have some insight into the methods being used. For clinicians graphics are essential for interpretation of data and results.

Decision Support

In a sense, all the functions described here support decision-making by health professionals. The distinction between decision-support systems and systems that monitor events and issue alerts is not clearcut; the two differ primarily in the degree to which they interpret data and recommend patient-specific action. The best-known examples of decision-support systems are the clinical consultation systems that use population statistics or encode expert knowledge to assist physicians in diagnosis and treatment planning. Similarly, some nursing information systems help nurses to evaluate the needs of individual patients and thus assist their users in allocating nursing resources. In Chapter 16, we discuss computer-based systems that use algorithmic, statistical, or artificial-intelligence techniques to provide advice about patient care.

Education

Rapid growth in biomedical knowledge and in the complexity of therapy management has produced an environment in which students cannot learn all they need to know during training—they must learn how to learn and must make a lifelong educational commitment. Today, physicians and nurses have available a broad selection of computer programs designed to help them acquire and maintain the knowledge and skills they need to care for their patients. The simplest programs are of the drill-and-practice variety; more sophisticated programs can help students to learn complex problem-solving skills, such as diagnosis and therapy management (see Chapter 17). Computer-aided instruction provides a valuable means by which health professionals can gain experience and learn from mistakes without endangering real patients. Clinical decision-support systems and other systems that can explain their recommendations also perform an educational function. In the context of real patient cases, they can suggest actions and explain the reasons for those actions.

5.1.3 *Identifying and Analyzing the Need for a Computer System*

The first step in the introduction of computers into healthcare settings is to identify a clinical, administrative, or research need—an inadequacy or inefficiency in the delivery of health care. The decision to acquire a computer system may be motivated by a desire to improve the *quality* of care, to lower the *cost* of care, to improve *access* to care, or to collect the information needed to document and evaluate the healthcare delivery process itself. Some computer-based systems correct defects in the old system; for example, more accurate record keeping can reduce the level of drug-administration errors. Other computer systems can provide functions not possible with a manual system—for example, allow integrated access to patient records. In some cases, a computer system simply duplicates the capabilities of the prior system but at lower cost.

The sophistication of medical computer systems has increased substantially since the late 1950s and early 1960s, when computers were first applied to the problems of healthcare delivery. The developers of new systems make progress by building on lessons learned from past experiments, emulating the successes and trying to avoid the mistakes of earlier systems. As the discipline has matured, researchers and users have gained a better understanding of both the types of problems computer systems can solve and the requirements for system success.

Clearly, computers facilitate many aspects of healthcare delivery. Installing a computer system, however, is not a panacea; an information system cannot aid in decision-making, for example, if critical information does not exist or if health professionals do not know how to apply the information once they have it. Similarly, a computer will not transform a poorly organized system into one that operates smoothly—automating a defective system can make matters worse, not better. Replacing a computer system in a unit of the hospital with one that performs local tasks better but does not communicate smoothly with other units will often make the overall situation worse. A careful analysis before attempting computer-based improvements allows system developers and healthcare personnel to clarify the requirements for change and may identify correctable deficiencies in current systems.

Ideally, we first recognize a *need*, and then search for techniques to address it. At times, this logical sequence has been inverted; the development of new hardware or computing methodologies may motivate system developers to apply state-of-the-art technology in a medical context. Development that is driven by technology, however, often fails. The adoption of any new system requires users to learn and to adjust to a new routine, and, given the time constraints under which health professionals operate, users may be unwilling to discard a working system unless they perceive a clear reason to change.

Once health professionals have recognized a need for a computer system, the next step is to identify the function or combination of functions that fulfills that need. There usually are many possible solutions to a broadly defined problem.

A precise definition of the problem narrows the range of alternative solutions. Is the problem one of access to data? Do health professionals have the data they need to make informed decisions? Is the problem an inability to analyze and interpret data? As we explained in the previous section, computer systems perform a variety of functions, ranging from simply displaying relevant information to aiding actively in complex decision-making.

The natural temptation is to minimize this important first step of problem definition and to move directly to the solution phase. This approach is dangerous, however, and it may result in the development of an unacceptable system. Consider, for example, a situation in which physicians desire improved access to patient data. Healthcare personnel may seek assistance from technologists to implement a specific technical solution to the perceived problem. They may request that each patient's complete medical history be stored in a computer. When that is achieved, however, they may find that the relevant information is hidden among the many irrelevant data and is more tedious to access than before. If the system developers had analyzed the problem carefully, they might have realized that the raw medical data simply were too voluminous to be informative. A more appropriate solution also might include filtering or other data processing so that only essential information or easy-to-read summaries are displayed.

The development of information systems requires a substantial commitment in terms of labor, money, and time. Once health professionals have clearly defined the need for a system, the question of worth inevitably arises. Scarce resources devoted to this project are unavailable for other potential projects. The administrator of a healthcare institution who works within a fixed budget must decide whether to invest in a computer system or to spend the money in other ways—for example, an institutional decision-maker may prefer to purchase new laboratory equipment or to expand the neonatal intensive-care unit.

To assess the value of a medical information system relative to competing needs, the administrator must estimate the costs and the benefits attributable to the system. Some benefits are relatively easy to quantify. If admission clerks can process each admission twice as fast using the new system as they could using the old one, an institution needs fewer clerks to perform the same amount of work—a measurable savings in labor costs. Many benefits, however, are less easily quantified. For example, how can we quantify the benefits due to reduced patient mortality, increased patient satisfaction, or reduced stress and fatigue among the staff? In Chapter 8 we introduce cost-benefit and cost-effectiveness analyses—two methodologies that can help decision-makers to assess the worth of a computer system relative to alternative investments.

5.2 Understanding Medical Information Systems

Whether they aim to produce a comprehensive information system for a 500-bed hospital, a patient-record system for a small clinic, or a simple billing program for a physician in private practice, system developers should follow the same basic process. In the initial phase of system development, the primary task is to define the problem. The goal is to produce a clear and detailed statement of the system's objectives—that is, what the system will do and what conditions it must meet if it is to be accepted by its users. The systems analysts also must establish the relative priorities of multiple, sometimes conflicting, goals—for example, low cost, high efficiency, easy maintenance, and high reliability.

Once analysts have clearly specified the goals of the system, they must choose among alternative approaches for meeting those goals. Ideally, a commercial system exists that provides all the desired functions, but it may be necessary to design a system to handle new requirements and novel functions. After acquisition or development of a system, the next step is to establish the system within the organization. Major activities at this stage include training users, installing and testing the system, and, finally, evaluating and maintaining the operational system on an ongoing basis.

We frame the discussion of this section in terms of institutional system planning and development. Many of the same issues, however, apply to the development of smaller systems as well, albeit on a correspondingly smaller scale of complexity.

5.2.1 An Illustrative Case Study

In addition to identifying functional requirements, a **requirements analysis** must be sensitive to the varying needs and probable concerns of the system's intended users. These *human* aspects of computer-system design often have been overlooked, and the results can be devastating. Consider, for example, the following hypothetical case, which embodies many of the issues that are the subject of this chapter.[1]

This example, although hypothetical, does not exaggerate the kinds of reactions that computer systems sometimes have evoked in clinical settings. Developers of real-world systems have encountered similar problems after introducing their systems into real clinical settings. This example was inspired in part by the experience of one of the authors with a pharmacy system that was implemented in several teaching wards of the hospital where he served his medical internship. The initial version of the system failed to account for key aspects of the way in which health professionals practiced medicine. All drug orders had to be entered into the computer, and, because the terminals were located at the nursing stations, physicians could no longer complete their orders at the bedside. They either had to return to the nursing station after seeing each patient or had to enter all the orders after completing patient rounds. Furthermore, physicians personally had to enter the orders. The system did not allow them to countersign or-

---

[1]This case study is adapted from one written by E.H. Shortliffe and appeared in "Coming to terms with the computer," in Reiser S.J., Anbar M. (Eds), *The Machine at the Bedside: Strategies for Using Technology in Patient Care*. (pp. 235–239). Cambridge, England: Cambridge University Press, 1984. It is used here with permission from Cambridge University Press.

A major teaching hospital purchased and installed a large computer system that assists physicians with ordering drugs and laboratory tests, the clinical laboratories with reporting laboratory test results, head nurses with creating nursing schedules, and the admissions staff with monitoring hospital occupancy. Personnel access the system using the PCs located in each nursing unit. There also are printers associated with each unit so that the computer can generate reports for the patient charts and worksheets used by the hospital staff. This information system depends on a large, dedicated computer, which is housed in the hospital complex and is supported by several full-time personnel. It has modules to assist hospital staff with both administrative and clinical duties. The following four modules are the primary subsystems used in patient care.

1. *The pharmacy system:* With this component of the information system, physicians order drugs for their patients; the requests are displayed immediately in the hospital pharmacy. Pharmacists then fill the prescriptions and affix computer-printed labels to each bottle. The drugs are delivered to the ward by a pneumatic-tube system. The computer keeps a record of all drugs administered to each patient and warns physicians about possible drug interactions at the time that new prescriptions are ordered.
2. *The laboratory system:* With this component, physicians order laboratory tests for their patients. The requests are displayed in the clinical laboratory, and worksheets are created to assist laboratory personnel in planning blood-drawing schedules and performing tests. As soon as test results are available, health professionals can display them on the screen of any workstation, and paper summaries are printed on the wards for inclusion in the patients' charts.
3. *The bed-control system:* The admissions office of the hospital, in conjunction with the various ward administrators, uses this component to keep track of the location of patients within the hospital. When patients are transferred to another ward, the computer is notified so that physicians, telephone operators, and other personnel can locate them easily. The system also is used to identify patients whose discharge has been ordered; thus, the system aids the admissions office in planning bed assignments for new patients.
4. *The diagnosis system:* To help physicians reach correct diagnoses for their patients, this component provides a clinical consultation program. Physicians enter their patient's signs and symptoms and can combine them with laboratory-test results and X-ray examination results. The system then suggests a list of likely diagnoses.

Despite the new capabilities provided by the system, after 3 months of use it received mixed reviews about its effectiveness. Most of the people who raised concerns were involved in patient care. A consulting expert was called in to assess the computer system's strengths and weaknesses. She interviewed members of the hospital staff and noted their responses.

One nurse said, "I like the system a lot. I found it hard to get used to at first (I never have been a very good typist), but once I got the hang of it, I found that it simplified much of my work. The worst problem has turned out to be dealing with doctors who don't like the system; when they get annoyed, they tend to take it out on us, even though we're using the system exactly as we've been trained to do.

For instance, I can't log onto the computer as a physician to log verbal orders in someone else's name, and that makes some of the doctors furious. The only time I personally get annoyed with the computer is when I need to get some work done and the other nurses are using all the ward workstations. They ought to have a few more machines available."

One medical resident was less than enthusiastic about the new clinical system. "I wish they'd rip the darn thing out! It is totally unrealistic in terms of the kinds of things it asks us to do or won't allow us to do. Did the guys who built it have any idea what it is like to practice medicine in a hospital like this? For example, the only way we used to be able to keep our morning ward rounds efficient was to bring the chart rack with us and to write orders at the bedside. With the new system, we have to keep sending someone back to the ward workstation to log orders for a patient. What's worse, they won't let the medical student order drugs, so we have to send an intern. Even the nurses aren't allowed to log orders in our name—something to do with the 'legality' of having all orders entered by a licensed physician—but that was never a problem with paper order sheets as long as we eventually countersigned the orders. Some of the nursing staff are doing everything by the book now, and sometimes they seem to be obstructing efficiency rather than aiding it. And the designers were so hung up on patient confidentiality that we have a heck of a time cross-covering patients on other services at night. The computer won't let me write orders on any patient who isn't 'known' to be mine, so I have to get the other physicians' passwords from them when they sign out to me at night. And things really fall apart when the machine goes down unexpectedly. Everything grinds to a halt, and we have to save our management plant on paper and transcribe them into the system when it finally comes up. I should add that the system always seems to be about three hours late in figuring out about patient transfers. I'm forever finding that the computer still thinks a patient is on the first floor when I know he's been transferred to the intensive care unit.

"In addition, the 'diagnosis system' is a joke. Sure, it can generate lists of diseases, but it doesn't really understand what the disease processes are, can't explain why it thinks one disease is more likely than another, and is totally unable to handle patients who have more than one simultaneous disease. I suppose the lists are useful as memory joggers, but I no longer even bother to use that part of the system.

"And by the way, I still don't really know what all those options on the screen mean. We had a brief training session when they first installed the system, but now we're left to fend for ourselves. Only a couple of the house staff seem to know how to make the system do what they want reliably. What's the best part of the system? I guess it is the decrease in errors in orders for drugs and lab tests and the improved turnaround time on those orders—but I'm not sure the improvement is worth the hassle. How often do I use the system? As rarely as possible!"

A hospital pharmacist said, "The system has been a real boon to our pharmacy operation. Not only can we fill new orders promptly because of the improved communication but also the system prints labels for the bottles and has saved us the step of typing them ourselves. Our inventory control also is much improved; the system produces several useful reports that help us to anticipate shortages and to keep track of drugs that are about to expire. The worst thing about the system, from my point of view, is the effect it has had on our interaction with the medical staff. We used to spend some of our time consulting with the ward teams about drug interactions, for example. You know, we'd look up the relevant articles and report back at ward rounds the next day. Now our role as members of the ward teams has been reduced by the system's knowledge about drugs. Currently, a house officer finds out about a potential drug interaction at the moment she is ordering a treatment, and the machine even gives references to support the reported incompatibility."

One member of the hospital's computing staff expressed frustration, "Frankly, It think the doctors have been too quick to complain about this system. It has been here for only three months, and we're still discovering problems that will take some time to address. What bothers me is the gut reaction many of them seem to have; they don't even *want* to give the system a chance. Every hospital is a little different, and it is unrealistic to expect any clinical system to be right for a new institution on the first day. There has to be a breaking-in period. We're trying hard to respond to the complaints we've heard through the grapevine. We hope that the doctors will be pleased when they see that their complaints are being attended to and new features are being introduced."

ders entered by nurses or medical students. The inflexibility of the system forced physicians to alter their practice patterns. The physicians objected loudly, and the system was subsequently removed. Although the system was later redesigned to remedy the earlier problems, it was never reimplemented at least in part because of persistent negative bias caused by the failure of the earlier version.

In another instance, the introduction of a new blood bank system at a large institution instigated disputes between physicians and nurses over responsibility for the entry of blood orders. In this case, the system was designed to encourage direct order entry but also allowed nurses to enter orders. Given the option, physicians continued to write paper orders and relied on nurses for order entry. Nurses, however, balked at performing this task, which they perceived as being the physicians' responsibility. Even seemingly trivial matters potentially can cause problems. At the same institution, for example, objection by surgeons was one factor in the decision to use passwords rather than machine-readable identification cards to control system access; surgeons typically do not carry personal belongings when wearing surgical garb and thus would have been unable to log onto the system (Gardner, 1989).

These cases help to emphasize the importance of responsiveness to needs as they are perceived by the intended *users* and of awareness of different users' varying perspectives when a system is intended to meet both clinical and administrative goals. The key considerations suggested by the scenario include (1) analyzing where the system is to fit into the existing information flow, (2) deciding what to purchase from a commercial system vendor and what to develop internally, (3) designing for the actual customers, (4) involving those customers throughout the development, and (5) planning for subsequent changes. We discuss these topics in detail in Section 5.3.

5.2.2 *Involving Future Users During Development*

Although the central focus of this chapter is *computer*-based information systems, it is important to realize that people are a critical component of these systems. People identify the need for systems; people develop, implement, and evaluate the systems; and, eventually, people operate the systems. A successful system must take into account both the needs of the intended users and the constraints under which these users function.

Even the most perceptive and empathetic developer cannot anticipate all the needs of all types of users. Thus, the success of a system depends on interaction between health and technical personnel as well as among the heathcare professionals. Effective communication among the participants, however, is potentially difficult because these people are likely to have widely varying background, education, experience, and styles of interaction. Appointing a wide variety of personnel to a large design committee is likely to be ineffective as well, because committees are best suited for forging compromise solutions, whereas computer systems can and should serve a precise set of objectives.

A major barrier to communication is attributable to a difference between the healthcare and general scientific paradigms. In Chapter 1, we discussed the ways in which clinical information differs from the information used in the basic sciences (recall the difference between low-level and high-level sciences discussed in Section 1.3), and we examined reasons why medical computing differs from basic computer science. In medical practice, as in other human tasks, we expect that a person who can deal with a certain type of problem can, with little incremental effort, extrapolate to handle similar and related problems. In the formal mathematical sciences, however, the ability to solve problems can depend critically on what appear to be small, but fundamental differences in basic assumptions.

The rigor of the mathematical approach also is reflected in computer systems so that computer systems will never be as flexible as people are. Although it is easy to imagine that a computer program that deals with one class of problems embodies sufficient concepts to deal with other (seemingly) similar problems, the work required to adapt or extend the program often costs as much as the original development and sometimes costs much more. Occasionally, adaptation is impossible. For healthcare professionals the difficulty of altering some aspects of software is hard to appreciate, because these people interact mainly with humans rather than with seemingly smart machines.

Empathy for the differences in the two approaches to problem-solving can minimize certain problems. Medical information specialists—people trained in both computer science and health science—can facilitate communication and mediate discussions. They can ease the process of specifying accurately and realistically the need for a system and of designing workable solutions to satisfy those needs. One objective of this book is to provide basic material for people who serve in this intermediary role.

5.3 Developing and Implementing Systems in Health Care

The initial task is to circumscribe what a new system in a healthcare setting should encompass. Will the new system replace all existing computing capabilities, or will it provide new functions, or will it replace some existing system? If it replaces an existing system, the current functions being provided can be enumerated and the data requirements specified. For new functions additional data will be needed, and if some older functions can be omitted, the input requirements might actually be less. Sometimes a new system may replace parts of multiple existing processes, making the task of defining its functions and data requirements yet harder. In Section 5.3.2 methods to chart those considerations are presented.

5.3.1 System Acquisition Alternatives

There are vendors willing to sell systems for any task that a healthcare institution may require. For most tasks some vendor will have a system already designed and ready to be adapted to your specifications. The actual functions and data requirements of a system acquired from a vendor may, however, differ from what was envisaged. The manner in which desired functions are provided will also differ among vendors. Demonstrations by vendors to customers can provide insights, and the feedback obtained may well change the expectations that were specified initially. Some desired features may turn out to be costly, and compromises are likely.

Some required services can be obtained by contracting for them remotely. Searches for published information are best performed over the Internet (Chapter 15). Some services, such as managing supply inventories, may be jointly supported by in-house staff and external contractors. We address remote operations in Section 5.3.4.

For essential operations, a healthcare institution must obtain or develop its own systems. We focus on the software requirements because the selection of hardware is primarily determined by the requirements that software imposes.

Commercial Off-the-Shelf Software

Much software is available off the shelf from commercial companies. The selection is widest for the more general needs, such as financial management—general ledger, accounts payable, and general accounts receivable. For healthcare institutions the selection is more limited or may require adaptation to the institution. For instance, financial receivables in health care—largely based on mixes of insurance, government, and private payments—have more complexity than standard business systems allow. Software companies that serve the healthcare industry can provide appropriate software. Even for specific healthcare functions multiple products will be available. The major concern becomes ensuring smooth interaction among software packages obtained from different vendors. The emerging standards for remote services may be helpful.

Once an organization has decided to acquire a new computer system, it faces the choice of buying a commercial system or building a system in-house. The primary trade-off between purchasing a **turnkey system**—a vendor-supplied system that requires only installation and "the turn of a key" to make it operational—and developing a **custom-designed system** is one of compatibility with the conventions in the institution versus expense and delay. Substantial new systems take years to design and develop. A vendor-supplied system usually is less expensive than is a custom-designed system, because the vendor can spread the costs of development and subsequent maintenance over multiple clients. A compromise is to customize a vendor system to the needs that are particular to one's institution, but the costs for changes not foreseen by the vendor will be disproportionally high. The maintenance costs for computer systems is on the order of 10 to 25 percent per year, and customization greatly increases those costs. If an institution can find a commercial system that approximately meets its needs, then it should purchase that system, even it has to change its own methods somewhat.

If no available commercial system for some function is adequate, then the institution may choose to build its own system or to make do with the current system; the option of keeping the current system should always be considered as one of the possible alternatives. Building an entire system for all functions in a healthcare institution is never a viable option. Before embarking on in-house development of any software system, administrators must assess whether the institution possesses the resources necessary for long-term success. For example, do in-house staff have the knowledge and experience to manage development and implementation of a new system? Can subsystems and components be obtained so that the local effort is minimized? Can outside consultants and technical staff be hired to assist? Who will maintain the system if it is installed successfully? In Section 5.3.3, we describe the development process, mainly to show its complexity.

Turnkey systems include all the hardware, software, and technical support necessary to operate the system. They should become operational rapidly, and most delays will be due to integration of the system with existing services. Unfortunately, the functions supplied by a turnkey system rarely match an institution's information-management needs. The system may not perform all the desired functions, may provide superfluous features, or may require some reorganization and modification of responsibilities and established flows of information within the institution. It is also important to consider carefully the reputation of the vendor and the terms of the contract and to answer questions such as, "What is the extent of the support and maintenance?" and "To what extent can the system be parameterized to the institution (e.g., selecting interchange standards to other systems in the institution, handling local billing policies, and dealing with multiple pharmacies)?"

Technology Transfer

Attractive innovations are often demonstrated in a research setting; however, developers should not underestimate the difficulty of transferring the technology to a working environment. One rule of thumb we accept is that the work needed to develop an academically successful demonstration of a new computing technology is one-seventh of the work required to transform the demonstration into a practical system. Professional experience is needed to validate that the new system works under all conditions encountered in a clinical practice and that the system can recover from mechanical failures. If new linkages are needed to other systems, more work is needed, and if those systems have to be adapted, even slightly, arrangements with their owners and vendors have to be made. Even though changes required for integration may be minor, understanding and validating changes to other systems incur a high cost. During integration, computing personnel must modify the existing system, develop and check interfaces, and retrain the various types of users. The effect is that the time and cost already estimated must be multiplied by a further factor of three or four. The difficulty of technology transfer has been a significant obstacle to the growth of medical computing.

5.3.2 Specifying Information Processes

In the healthcare environment, the major portion of computing deals with data rather than complex algorithms. Most data are obtained from patients, laboratories, healthcare personnel, and insurance providers and then are transmitted, stored, transformed, summarized, and analyzed to help health professionals, managers, and patients to plan actions and interventions. Certain data must be archived for legal purposes. To understand the task that a system, or subsystem, performs, it is best to consider the **data flow**.

Data Flow

A graphical representation called the **data-flow diagram** (DFD) provides a succinct way to understand the objectives of a system. It represents the sources of data, the processes for transforming the data, and the points in the system where long-term or short-term data storage is required, and the destinations where reports are generated or where results from queries are presented. The DFD in Figure 5.2a is a model of a simple laboratory information system. It illustrates the flow of laboratory-test orders and results, as well as the basic functions of the proposed system: (1) creation of specimen collection schedules, (2) analysis of results, (3) reporting of test results, and (4) performance of quality-assurance activities. The designer can describe each higher-level process in the DFD by creating a more detailed DFD (Fig. 5.2b).

The initial DFD is often based on an analysis of current activities and processes. That approach helps people to identify outputs that are not obvious or that are needed only for rare cases—for example, for investigation of infrequent infec-

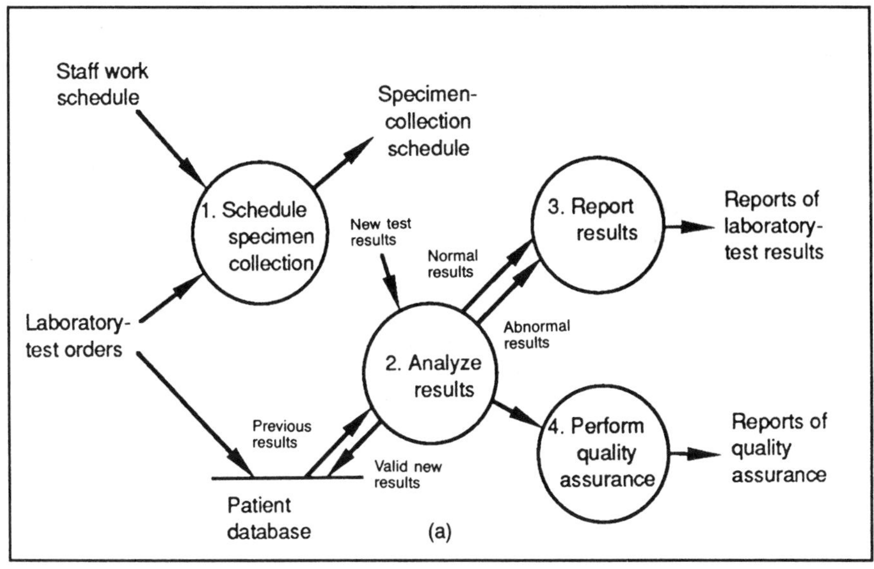

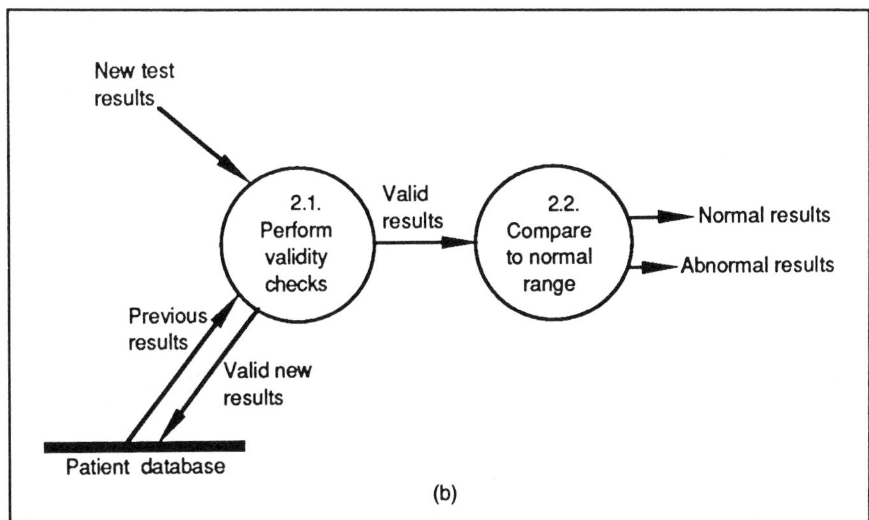

FIGURE 5.2. A data-flow diagram (DFD) that graphically represents the processes and data flows within a laboratory information system. *(a) Bubbles* depict processes (or functions), *vectors* depict data flows, and *straight lines* depict databases. *(b)* Often, DFDs are layered to show greater detail within higher-level processes. This second-level DFD decomposes the process of analyzing test results into two lower-level processes. Note that the net inputs and outputs of this DFD match the inputs and outputs of the higher-level process shown in part *a*.

tions. It is easy to overlook information that is informally obtained. Many informal mechanisms for communication and storage disappear when computers are used to collect and store data. Health professionals trade much valuable information in hallways and at nursing stations; for example, they will discuss a baffling case to help develop new insights and approaches. Some crucial information never enters the formal record but is noted on scraps of paper or stored in people's memories. System designers must take care to identify and replace such mechanisms. Once all needed outputs are indicated on the DFD, analysts can trace back to ensure that all required inputs are available in the flow. The absence of even minor functions can produce errors in healthcare delivery and will be perceived as a failure of the system, leading to resistance by the users. Recall from the hypothetical case, for example, the friction between physicians and nurses that arose when the new system failed to allow for verbal orders. Often, technologists discount resistance as an unwillingness to keep up with progress, but they should interpret it as a signal that something is wrong with the new system.

Using the clear graphical representation of the DFD helps the intended users to recognize aberrations and provide feedback to the system designers. A DFD in which everything seems to connect to everything else is not helpful for analysis or implementation. Complex data flows should first be simplified so that the implementation is straightforward. If the result is still complex, a good layout can help. Major data flows should go left to right, minor flows should be shown in lighter colors, and special cases can use overlays. The final DFD can differ greatly from the initial one.

Data Storage

Most of the data and information that is documented in a DFD is stored in databases. For most systems a central decision is the choice of database software. Database software is large and crucial to reliable operations. There are several off-the-shelf database-management systems, and there are vendors who provide software to process the stored data. Existing systems may already have made commitments to some database system vendor. It is best to limit the variety of such complex software and to share its maintenance costs. It is hence wise to ensure that the databases that come with commercial software are *open*—that is, documented, set up, and maintained in a stable manner so that *foreign* applications can extract and contribute data to them.

Most business software today depends on relational databases. Such databases provide a means for exchanging information among software components that are otherwise independent. A schema must be adopted, expanded, or designed that specifies all the data that the software will exchange. Of course, once healthcare databases are open, serious issues about access to and release of private medical data arise, as discussed in Chapter 7.

Software components may need to be written to interact with an open database, but a database schema constrains the design of the programs and simplifies the implementation choices. The standards associated with the relational approach also simplify exchange of data over communication links, so redundancy in both data entry and result reporting can be avoided.

For medical-records systems, off-the-shelf software has not been easy to adapt. Clinical patient information is too complex to be easily and efficiently mapped into relational databases, so the benefits of open databases and component-based transaction services have not yet been realized in the core of medical applications. This means that many healthcare institutions have to deal with databases for medical functions that are not open. For those systems even minor changes may require contractual negotiations with a vendor.

5.3.3 Building a New Software System

If the institution is prepared to build a computer system to meet some specific needs, system developers can employ a variety of software-engineering tools to organize and manage the development process. Although major efforts are rare in today's healthcare settings, it is useful to understand this process for interacting with vendors or enthusiastic innovators. Software system-development tools include formal techniques for system analysis, methodologies of **structured programming,** and testing methods. They are supplemented by methods for managing the project and metrics for assessing the performance of the product and of the software-development process itself. The field of **software engineering** had its beginnings in the late 1960s and early 1970s. As the systems being developed grew more complex, teams of programmers, analysts, and managers replaced individual programmers who had worked in isolation. Many software prototypes are still developed individually but must be moved to a managed setting before they can be marketed and distributed.

In the 1980s, the costs of hardware (which previously had dominated the total cost of a system) declined rapidly. The largest system cost now is software maintenance, an aspect rarely considered when building prototypes. More recently, standard software components have become available so that new approaches to the creation of systems are opening up. There is no single right way to implement computer systems in health care.

Software Lifecycle

Figure 5.3 depicts the classic waterfall model of any engineering development process from requirements analysis through specification, design, implementation, testing, and maintenance. Specialists may be engaged for each of the phases. The tasks of one phase should be completed and documented before the next phase is tackled so that the specialists for the next phase are presented with a complete specification. As Figure 5.3 suggests, however, problems found in a later phase require feedback to earlier phases and can cause expensive rework. If the work delegated to future phases is well understood, the waterfall model can work well. If the specifications challenge later phases, the risk of cost over-

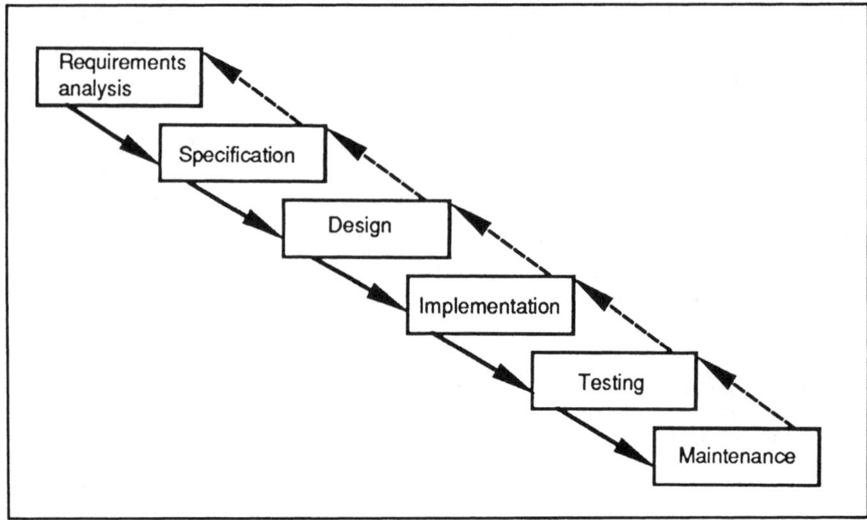

FIGURE 5.3. The waterfall model represents the traditional system-development process. It recognizes six sequential phases, each with feedback to the earlier phase.

runs and even failure is great. For instance, specifying X-ray images to be displayed at every terminal within 1/10 of a second requires extensive resources, and, if their cost becomes intolerable, the entire design might have to be revised.

Although the *waterfall* model conveys a clear view of the software life cycle, the delays inherent in such a phased development process make this methodology inappropriate for innovative applications. It is hard to obtain adequate specifications when you are developing an application for inexperienced customers. The customers will not see the product until the testing phase and cannot provide feedback until that time. If it takes years to complete the first four phases of the process, even good specifications are likely to have become obsolete—the organizations and their information sources and needs will have changed.

Requirements for some healthcare systems are presented in Section 5.1.2, but just listing the requirements is insufficient for phase 2. The requirements have to be quantified: Where is the information needed, how fast, how often, and how reliable should it be? High reliability can mean that more processing and integration has to be included in the design. A single program for a single user is often built without explicit attention to phases 2 and 3, but a large project requires a different approach.

In the **specification phase,** the general system requirements are analyzed and formalized. Systems analysts specify the intended behavior precisely and concisely—the specific functions the system must accomplish, the data it will require, the results it will produce, the performance requirements for speed and reliability, and so on. They specify the answers to questions such as, "What are the sources of necessary information?" and "What are the existing mechanisms for communication in the current system?" Here the DFD becomes an important tool, and the choice made about the database system, as discussed in Section 5.3.2, will often constrain this phase.

Once the functional specification has been produced and validated against the requirements specified by the prospective users, it is expanded into a design that can be implemented. The initial task is to partition the system into manageable modules. All but the smallest systems are partitioned into subsystems, subsystems into smaller components, and so on, until the whole has been decomposed into manageable components (Fig. 5.4). A single module should not require more than a few implementors and not take more than a few months. Any subsystem should also have few data flows into and out of it, as determined by the DFD. Simplicity allows subsequent testing to cover all cases. Notice in Figure 5.4, for example, that a centralized HIS can be viewed as a hierarchy of nested and interrelated subsystems. In general, a system has strong internal linkages relative to its linkages with the external world.

As part of the design, the hardware needed now and in the future is determined; there may be trade-offs in which more hardware can simplify the design and its implementation. For instance, copying data to locations close to a critical customer can improve response time and availability in case of communication problems.

In the **implementation phase**, the subsystems are created in-house or are obtained from public or commercial sources. Even good design specifications cannot cover all the details at the module level. For a good implementation, the module programmers must still understand the healthcare setting. If the system does

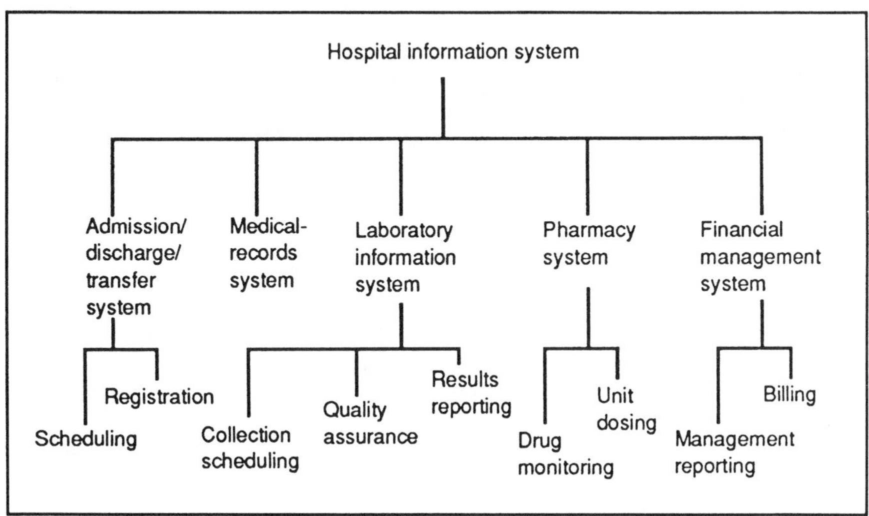

FIGURE 5.4. A hospital information system comprises interrelated subsystems that serve individual departments. In turn, each subsystem comprises multiple functional components.

not function suitably for users, namely, if they find the output wrong or not sufficiently helpful, then costly rework will be needed after the testing phase. Such problems might be caused because the implementation was wrong, the design did not foresee performance problems, the specification was imprecise, or requirements were incomplete or became obsolete. If the errors are due to earlier phases, making the corrections becomes more costly.

An alternative to the implementation phase is to acquire as many readymade components as can be found and put them together into a system. The components are selected to match the specifications, and less design and little implementation takes place. Analysts can visit sites where the components are used, and customers can see sample results early on. Early feedback to the design phase can occur. Because available components will rarely match requirements precisely, compromises will have to be made, although many vendors will try to create powerful components that match the needs of many institutions. If some components fail to meet the needs of the customer, the vendor may be induced to improve them, the specifications may be reduced, or staff may decide to build some components in-house, raising the subsequent maintenance costs.

When all the components are ready, **system integration** takes place. Mistakes in partitioning, missing data flows, and incomplete interface specification become apparent. For large systems, built by many people, this is the riskiest phase. Even competent people may interpret specifications and design documents differently; some differences make integration impossible without redesign.

Testing of the system has to be planned carefully. Subsystems are tested by their developers, because customers probably will not be able to test incomplete functions. Because testing implies the discovery of failure points, this phase has to start slowly to allow for repair of errors so as to avoid frustration by the testers—especially when real customers begin to do testing. It is in this phase that we find out whether the hypothetical requirements, stated initially, are adequate. If they are not, major rework may be needed. More than 50 percent of systems are abandoned at this point.

If the system, after testing by builders and customers, is accepted for routine use, the **maintenance phase** starts. Ongoing changes in requirements will necessitate changes in the system. In theory, the same cycle should be followed for any substantial changes, but the original large staff rarely remains available, and thus the adjustments may be made haphazardly. Because software-based systems often remain in place for 10 to 20 years, the maintenance phase, costing perhaps 20 percent per year, requires more financial commitment than the original development phases required.

Alternative Methodologies

To obtain early results and reduce the risk of failure, a software-development group may follow alternative methodologies. In the **spiral model**, the group generates a simple prototype system by performing the four initial phases rapidly.

The result is presented to the customers, who assess it and expand and modify the requirements. Then a second cycle ensues (Fig. 5.5). After a few cycles, the prototype is made operational; the operational prototype will require some maintenance, but any significant changes have to wait for yet another iteration of the spiral. Ideally, each cycle takes 3 to 6 months, so the patience of the customers is not exhausted. In the spiral model, the staff is expected to remain intact for many iterations so that essential knowledge is not lost, because little time is spent on documentation.

The spiral model methodology also entails substantial risks:

1. The initial prototype is so minimal that the result is not of sufficient interest to the users, and no meaningful feedback ensues; for instance, a system may not permit access to actual patient data.
2. The system has not attained sufficient functionality after several cycles, so it cannot be placed into service; for instance, laboratory results are not yet automatically included in a patient's record.
3. An acceptable small system cannot be scaled to the next level on a standard cycle because of an overly simplified initial design decision, so major rework is needed; for example, no means exist for out-of-queue processing, so stat (emergency) laboratory tests cannot be given priority.

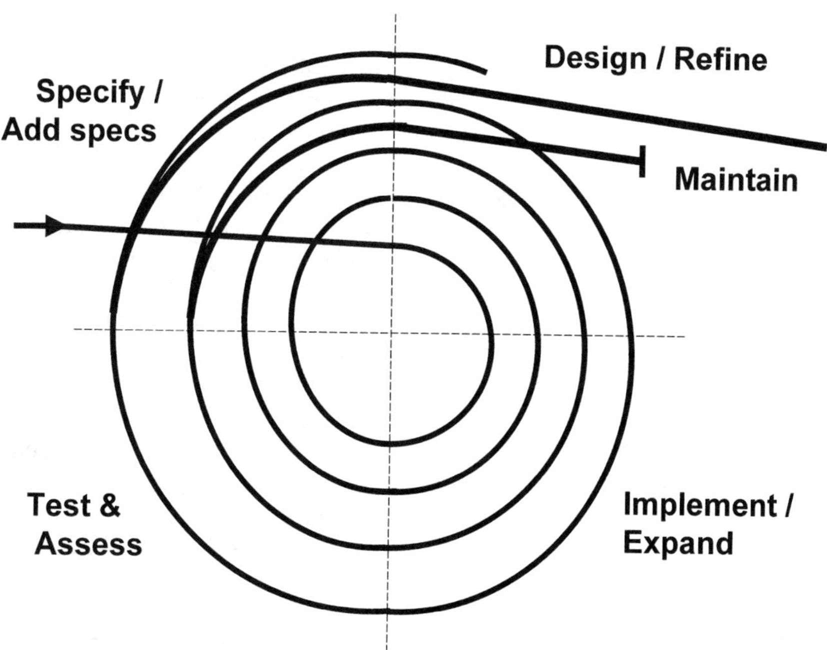

FIGURE 5.5. The spiral model of implementation. Rapid iterations lead to system cycles that can be assessed incrementally by the customers.

Developers have experimented with other software engineering methodologies, but all require that developers and customers perform similar tasks. For instance, by assessing what components are likely to be hard to build and giving them more attention, the team can reduce implementation risks while accelerating delivery. This *water sluice* methodology avoids a problem of the spiral model in which, to satisfy the cyclic time constraints, the easy processes are done first. Making correct assessments requires considerable experience.

Business Objects

Object-oriented programming focuses on the specification of small, reusable data structures and associated methods, called *objects*. For instance, a *visit object* may be defined as a component of a patient record with methods as *schedule, check-in, record findings, issue orders*, and so on. The visit object must have well-defined interactions with other objects of concern to the system, such as *patient, doctor, nurse, clinic*, or *pharmacy*. Given a suite of suitable objects, this approach allows rapid composition of software modules. Programmers must have substantial experience to define objects of sufficient competence and generality while allowing for their many interactions, as required in healthcare systems.

For complex data, the object-oriented approach may be best. All the data related to major concepts in the information systems is brought together and is accessed via methods that isolate the complexity of the data structures from the programs that use the data. Programming languages that enable object-oriented programming are listed in Table 4.1. The design of object classes to support a specific business domain is a complex task, but there are standard libraries of defined objects. If these libraries are used, the programming task is reduced to prescribing the sequence and content of the interactions among these objects—for example, patients, their problems, and their visits.

Standard libraries for some domains are now available—for example, presentation graphics, telecommunications, and business finance. Many organizations are defining and implementing collections of business objects for a variety of other areas. However, if multiple groups enter a single topic area, their products will not interoperate, and it will take some time before dominant library products emerge. If multiple libraries are needed for a project, an interchange format for data is needed as well. Having a standard database can provide the required storage, but such a database could not hold the data as organized with the objects. As of this writing, no significant business-object libraries addressing clinical information have matured, but the Object Management Group (OMG), a not-for-profit consortium, is actively developing standards.

Summary

As we indicated in Section 5.3.1, few healthcare organizations have the resources to see major software-system developments through to a successful completion. If a modest computer system can address problems specific to some healthcare setting, however, it may be worthwhile to undertake a local effort. There are still problems that require novel solutions and technology not available from most vendors of healthcare systems. Many problems in health care are poorly structured and may require methods based on artificial intelligence. Such an effort will typically be established as a subsystem in the institutional network and be initially isolated from daily operational responsibilities. The subsystem will depend on available complementary system resources, such as an existing patient-admitting system. Using the spiral approach, experience can be gathered from local customers that outsiders would not be able to supply. It is still essential to ensure reliability, security, and data confidentiality, as discussed in Chapter 7. A new subsystem, no matter how beneficial, is likely to be rejected if it entails risks to the routine services of healthcare delivery, patients' confidence, or cost accounting.

5.3.4 Incorporating Remote Services

Our healthcare systems do not operate in isolation. Within the institution, there may be several distinct computer systems, such as in the laboratory, in physician offices, and in account billing. Outside of the institution, there are other organizations that use computer systems, such as drug and linen suppliers, laboratories that do outsourced work, insurance companies, public-health-service agencies, and the National Institutes of Health, including the National Library of Medicine. The capabilities of modern networks, as introduced in Chapter 4, enable direct linkages to all these systems, with the potential to reduce greatly paper copies and manual transcription of information. The interfaces are diverse, however, without widely adopted standards, as discussed in Chapter 6. Even when standard interfaces are agreed on at one point, technology makes them obsolete eventually. Nonetheless, the ability to interact with remote services is essential, and the cost of maintaining interfaces is less than that of transcribing the information by hand or of entering it manually into the home system (see Section 5.3.5). The external services require different interfaces depending on whether they are **informational services** (informal, broad public access) or **business services** (contractual, user access only).

Information on the World Wide Web

For informational systems accessed via the World Wide Web, the HyperText Markup Language (HTML) dominates Web services. A **markup language** identifies items of the contents. The term *hyper* refers to the capability of references in an HTML document to link to other documents through a Universal Resource Locator (URL), which identifies files at remote locations, such as http://www.dlib.org. The Hypertext Markup Language focuses on the presentation of information and allows the definition of text, headings, tables, images, or even program fragments that provide dynamic displays, using the Java language (see Chapter 4.1.2). This information is interpreted by a **browser**, which provides the most suitable display. When a browser finds inconsistencies, errors, or novel specifications, it provides the most reasonable presentation. The utility of these tools for healthcare information is presented in Chapter 15.

For business services, the inherent flexibility of the web and HTML is also a liability. There is no guarantee of completeness of the information or of consistency of content. Many standards have been developed for data interchange; each typically is created for a specific domain, as discussed in Chapter 6. To allow data-quality interchange on the web, an HTML-like format XML is being promulgated; it contains basic definitions but allows domain-specific extensions, which are intended to be sufficiently rigorous that conformance can be validated (Connolly, 1997). Moving the capabilities of existing standards into new web technologies will take some time, although a common infrastructure will enable easier integration of remote services.

5.3.5 Designing for Effectiveness

A system's success depends not only on whether it meets the users' informational needs but also on how it interacts with those users. There are many types of users, ranging from technical specialists to people who simply require services. The resident's complaints in the hypothetical example illustrated an important point: The disruption of effective and established routines and the inconvenience often associated with computer information systems can cause users to work around the system and thus to fail to use its features. Studies of the attitudes of healthcare personnel regarding computer-based clinical consultation systems have shown that successful programs not only must provide expert-level advice but also must be integrated into the daily routines of physicians and other users [Friedman and Gustafson, 1977; Teach and Shortliffe, 1981; Detmer and Friedman, 1994). Computer-based information systems should acknowledge the hectic schedules of health professionals and should demystify and simplify the mechanics of the human–computer interface. By involving users in system design, developers can avoid many of the impediments to widespread success.

The following parameters of computer systems are among the most important to consider during system design:

- *Quality and style of interface:* From a customer's point of view, a system's interface *is* the system. In the past, developers of medical computer systems have paid insufficient attention to the quality of the interface between people and computers. To be effective, interfaces must have clear presentations, avoid unnecessary detail, and provide a consistent interaction. A growing body of research related to the psychology of the human–machine interaction joins taste and common sense in making computer use acceptable. Menus, graphics, and the use of color all help to make systems more attractive and simpler to learn and use. Today, mouse pointing devices are ubiquitous, but they require that users settle down in front of the screen. Physicians are often reluctant to type at a keyboard; furthermore, sitting down and starting an interaction is awkward in many healthcare settings. Thus, system developers have experimented with a number of alternative devices for interaction, including light pens and touch screens. Researchers are investigating speech recognition and natural-language understanding with the hope that someday talking with computers will be as natural and easy as talking with humans. In systems that perform decision support and offer advice about patient care, the style of communication is particularly important. Is the system too terse or too verbose? Does it project a helpful attitude or does it seem pedantic or judgmental? Can it justify its recommendations?

- *Convenience:* Users must have convenient access to the system. The number and placement of workstations and printers are important considerations if the system is to be assimilated into users' routines. For example, if a patient-record system is intended to replace the traditional patient record, it must be accessible wherever and whenever health professionals need to look up patient data—in the physician's office, in the nursing station, possibly at the bedside, and so on. Sufficient workstations should be available that users do not have to wait to use the system, even during times of peak use.
- *Speed and response:* System developers must choose hardware and communication lines that have sufficient capacity to handle customers' demands for information during peak hours. The software must allow users timely access to the data in the form they need. Minor errors in formulating information requests must be easily undone. Health professionals are understandably reluctant to use systems that are hostile, tedious, or unduly time consuming.
- *Reliability:* Health personnel must resort to manual procedures if they are to continue to work in the event of hardware or software failure. Frequent data back up and redundant hardware can minimize the loss of data and the amount of time that the system is unavailable.
- *Security:* The confidentiality of sensitive medical data is an important issue in the design of medical information systems (see Chapter 7). The system should be easily accessible to authorized personnel, yet it should not release information to unauthorized users. These conflicting goals are difficult to achieve. The most common compromise solution is to assign an account with a password to each user. Variable access to the data then can be controlled for individual users or for classes of users. Certain operations may be restricted to particular workstations. For example, the ability to modify patient charges is best restricted to financial personnel working from workstations located in the accounting office.
- *Integration:* The integration of independent systems eliminates some of the difficulties and enhances the benefits of using computer systems. If, for example, a laboratory system and a pharmacy system are independent and incompatible, health professionals must access two separate systems (possibly from different terminals) to view a single patient's data. If the two systems need to share data, people will have to collect output from the first and reenter it into the second system. The development of local-area networks has provided the infrastructure to allow exchange of information among independent systems and has reduced the need for redundant entry and storage of critical information (a waste of time and a source of errors).

5.3.6 *Planning for Change*

Many medical information systems—particularly custom-designed systems—take a long time to develop. This delay is risky; it is hard for the medical establishment to perceive what is being done by the system-development staff, and the development staff receives no feedback on the correctness of the assumptions on which they are basing their design. The involvement of users through demonstrations and training sessions and the incremental installation of the system can build the enthusiasm and support of users and can provide computing personnel an invaluable means for evaluating progress.

Prototype systems—working models that exhibit the essential features of the system under development—facilitate communication between computing personnel and users. Users develop a realistic idea of what the system will look like, how it will work, and what it will do. Developers receive feedback and can modify the system in response to users' comments, thus improving the likelihood that the final system will be deemed acceptable. A good prototype provides a realistic demonstration of the method of interaction with the system and should be able to deal with most of the common varieties of data input. Much simplification, however, is possible when reliability and data permanence can be ignored, as they can be in a prototype system that is intended only for demonstration and discussion.

Formal training courses also can help to dispel the mystery of a new system. Without adequate reinforcement, however, people are apt to forget what they learn. A training program for a new system should start slowly and extend over the period of its implementation so that surprises are minimized. When some subsystem installation is imminent, health professionals should receive specific and intensive training in its use. Experience with windows and mouse interfaces suggests that the development of intuitive metaphors allows users to experiment and explore their capabilities and will reduce the need for formal training. The feedback provided to the developers during successive phases helps to ensure that problems will not be repeated or multiplied as the system nears completion.

Training is simplified if part of the system is operational. Customers can see real examples of the system in action and thus are less likely to develop overly ambitious expectations. Because those parts of the system that are installed first usually are less problematic, the initial phase is likely to be a success. The attitude generated by initial success can enhance the acceptance of the system in other areas, including those areas that inherently are more difficult to address using computer-based techniques. In hospitals, for instance, computer systems often are used first in the admissions office, where the applications are relatively straightforward, and later are expanded for use on medical wards, where the user community is particularly diverse and demanding.

5.4 Summary

A variety of software and information services is available for healthcare applications, ranging from turnkey systems ,covering many of the needs of an institutions, through major subsystems for hospital departments and large Web-based services that require only remote access to databases and to object libraries that are helpful for building local applications. Unfortunately, composing an effective and economical system that is fully sufficient for the financial, clinical, and ancillary needs in health care is nearly impossible. Today, most healthcare institutions are faced with the choice of either committing to a major vendor, and accepting that vendor's complete system or a subset thereof, or dealing with a variety of purchased, adapted, and in-house developed subsystems that overlap and have gaps. Gaps often require human transcription and replicated data input. The maintenance of the systems requires ongoing efforts to keep them up-to-date as operational and clinical requirements and processes change.

Information-systems development is a political as well as a technical process. Health institutions, just like all other organizations, are composed of different groups of individuals, and often these groups have conflicting priorities, objectives, and values. The technical issues are generally complex and difficult; careful implementation processes can conflict with urgent needs. Risks are rife in internal software development, in acquiring vendors' software, and in their integration. Health administrators, physicians, nurses, ancillary personnel, and patients have diverse needs that the computer system must accommodate. Information systems can alter relationships among these people—they affect patterns of communication, perceived influence, authority, and control. A strategy for implementation must recognize and deal with these political forces. A new system should disrupt the organizational infrastructure as little as possible. Keen's article (listed in the Suggested Readings) discusses the political aspects of system development and implementation in greater detail.

Suggested Readings

Anderson J.G., Jay S.J. (Eds.). (1987). *Use and Impact of Computers in Clinical Medicine.* New York: Springer-Verlag.

This collection of papers presents research on the factors that affect the adoption, diffusion, and utilization of clinical information systems in hospitals. It includes chapters on the attitudes of health professionals toward computers and the probable effects of clinical systems on aspects of medical practice, such as the role of physicians, relations between doctors and patients, and the organization of the healthcare-delivery system.

Blum B. (1992). *Software Engineering, A Holistic Approach.* New York: Oxford University Press.

This philosophical but unbiased textbook on software engineering was written by a practioner who has had substantial experience developing clinical applications. It covers the system-development process, data-flow diagrams, and structured coding technique

Boehm B., Egyed A., Kwan J., Port D., Shah A., Madachy, R. (1998). Using the WinWin Spiral Model: A case study. *IEEE Computer*, 31(7):33–44.

This brief note introduces the WinWin Spiral Model, mainly in relation to student projects. The WinWin Spiral Model has two add-ons to the classic spiral model: (1) analysis at the beginning of each spiral cycle and (2) process anchor points.

Booch G. (1994). *Object-Oriented Design with Applications* (2nd ed.). Redwood City, CA: Benjamin-Cummings.

This is an introduction to object-oriented programming, by one of its chief proponents and tool builders.

Keen P.G.W. (1981). Information systems and organizational change. *Communications of the ACM*, 24:24.

This paper emphasizes the pluralistic nature of organizations. It discusses the changes in patterns of communication, influence, and control that often occur when new information systems are implemented, and it suggests strategies for minimizing social inertia and resistance.

Monson-Haefel, R. (1999). *Enterprise JavaBeans*. Cambridge, MA: O'Reilly & Associates.

JavaBeans is a technology to define business objects that can be composed to assemble rapidly an analyzable and maintainable data-processing system.

Reiser S.J., Anbar M. (Eds.). (1984). *The Machine at the Bedside: Strategies for Using Technology in Patient Care.* Cambridge: Cambridge University Press.

This book discusses the theory and use of healthcare technologies—such as intensive care, diagnostic imaging, and electronic fetal monitoring—in the context of legal, ethical, economic, and social concerns. It contains 23 case studies that depict the benefits and limitations of using these technologies.

Shlaer S., Mellor S.J. (1992). *Object Life Cycles, Modeling the World in States.* Englewood Cliffs, NJ: Prentice-Hall.

This influential textbook was developed by protagonists of the object-oriented software development approach.

Questions for Discussion

1. Reread the hypothetical case in Section 5.2.1.
   a. What are three primary benefits of the clinical system? What are three primary disadvantages?
   b. Do you think that the benefits of the system outweigh the disadvantages? Are there adequate noncomputer-based solutions to the problems with which the system was designed to help? If so, what are they?
   c. How would you change the system in your institution or in one you have read about? Among the topics you might address are the effects of the system on hospital routine, computer reliability, and terminal availability and the adequacy of user training programs.
2. Describe an outpatient clinic's billing system in terms of inputs, outputs, and processes. Sketch a simple data-flow diagram that represents your model of the system.
3. Discuss the inherent tension between protecting the confidentiality of patient records and providing health professionals with rapid and convenient access to clinical information. What level of system security do you think provides an appropriate balance between these conflicting goals?
4. Discuss three barriers to technology transfer among healthcare institutions.
5. Explain the difference between *outcome* and *process* measures of system performance. Identify two outcome and two process parameters that you might

use to evaluate the performance of a clinical consultation system that assists physicians in diagnosing disease. Describe an experiment that you could perform to evaluate the effect of the system on one of these parameters. What potential difficulties can you foresee in conducting your experiment? What can you do to compensate for these difficulties?

6. In what three ways is the use of a clinical consultation system similar to the use of human consultants or static sources of medical information such as textbooks? In what three ways is it different?

6
Standards in Medical Informatics

W. EDWARD HAMMOND AND JAMES J. CIMINO

After reading this chapter, you should know the answers to these questions:

- Why are standards important in medical informatics?
- What organizations are active in standards development?
- What aspects of medical information management are supported today by standards?
- What is the process for creating consensus standards?
- What factors and organizations influence the creation of standards?

6.1 The Idea of Standards

Ever since Eli Whitney developed interchangeable parts for rifle assembly, standards have been created and used to make things or processes work more easily and economically—or, sometimes, to work at all. A standard can be defined in many physical forms, but essentially it comprises a set of rules and definitions that specify how to carry out a process or produce a product. Sometimes, a standard is useful because it provides a way to solve a problem that other people can use without having to start from scratch. Generally, though, a standard is useful because it permits two or more disassociated people to work in some cooperative way. Every time you screw in a light bulb or play a music cassette, you are taking advantage of a standard. Some standards evolve over time[1]; others are developed deliberately.

The first computers were built without standards, but hardware and software standards quickly became a necessity. Although computers work with values such as 1 or 0, and with "words" such as 10101100, humans need a more readable language (see Chapter 4). Thus, standard character sets, such as ASCII and

[1]The current standard for railroad-track gauge originated with Roman chariot builders, who set the axle length based on the width of two horses. This axle length became a standard as road ruts developed, requiring that the wheels of chariots—and all subsequent carriages—be the right distance apart to drive in the ruts. When carriage makers were called on to develop railway rolling stock, they continued to use the same axle standard.

EBCDIC, were developed. The first standard computer language, COBOL, was written originally to simplify program development but was soon adopted as a way to allow sharing of code and development of software components that could be integrated. As a result, COBOL was given official standard status by the American National Standards Institute (ANSI).[2] In like manner, hardware components depend on standards for exchanging information to make them as interchangeable as were Whitney's gun barrels.

A 1987 technical report from the International Standards Organization (ISO) states that "Any meaningful exchange of utterances depends upon the prior existence of an agreed upon set of semantic and syntactic rules" (International Standards Organization, 1987). In medical informatics, where the emphasis is on collection, manipulation, and transmission of information, standards are greatly needed but have only recently begun to be available. At present, the standards scene is evolving so rapidly that any description is inevitably outdated within a few months. In this chapter we therefore emphasize the need for standards in general, standards-development processes, current active areas of standards development, and key participating organizations that are making progress in the development of usable standards.

6.2 The Need for Health-Informatics Standards

Standards are generally required when excessive diversity creates inefficiencies or impedes effectiveness. The healthcare environment has traditionally consisted of a set of loosely connected, organizationally independent units. Patients receive care across primary, secondary, and tertiary care settings, with little bidirectional communication and coordination among the services. Patients are cared for by one or more primary physicians, as well as by specialists. There is little coordination and sharing of data between inpatient care and outpatient care. Both the system and patients, by choice, create this diversity in care. Within the inpatient setting, the clinical environment is divided into clinical specialties that frequently treat the patient without regard to what other specialities have done. Ancillary departments function as detached units, performing their tasks as separate service units, reporting results without follow-up about how those results are used or whether they are even seen by the ordering physician. Reimbursement requires patient information that is often derived through a totally separate process, based on the fragmented data collected in the patient's medical record and abstracted specifically for billing purposes. The resulting set of diagnosis and procedure codes often correlates poorly with the patient's original information (Jollis et al., 1993).

Early hospital information systems (HISs) for billing and accounting purposes were developed on large, monolithic mainframe computers (see Chapter 10); they

[2]Interestingly, medical informaticians were responsible for the second ANSI standard language: MUMPS (now known as M).

followed a pattern of diversity similar to that seen in the healthcare system itself. As new functions were added in the 1970s, they were implemented on mainframe computers and were managed by a data-processing staff that usually was independent of the clinical, and even of the administrative, staff. The advent of the minicomputer supported the development of departmental systems, such as those for the clinical laboratory, radiology department, or pharmacy. This model of the central mainframe coupled with independent minicomputer-based departmental systems is still common in installed systems today. Clinical systems, as they have developed, continue to focus on dedicated departmental operations, and clinical-specialty systems thus do not permit the practicing physician to see a unified view of the patient.

There are many pressures on healthcare information systems to change the status quo such that data collected for a primary purpose can be reused in a multitude of ways. Newer models for healthcare delivery, such as integrated delivery networks, health-maintenance organizations (HMOs), and preferred provider organizations (PPOs), have increased the need for coordinated, integrated, and consolidated information (see Chapters 10 and 19) even though the information comes from disparate departments and institutions. Various management techniques, such as continuous quality improvement and case management, require up-to-date, accurate abstracts of patient data. Post-hoc analyses for clinical and outcomes research require comprehensive summaries across patient populations. Advanced tools, such as clinical workstations (Chapter 9) and decision-support systems (Chapter 16), require ways to translate raw patient data into generic forms for tasks as simple as summary reporting and as complex as automated medical diagnosis. All these needs must be met in the existing setting of diverse, interconnected information systems—an environment that cries out for implementation of standards.

One obvious need is for standardized identifiers for individuals, healthcare providers, health plans, and employers so that such participants can be recognized across systems. Choosing such an identifier is much more complicated than simply deciding how many digits the identifier should have. Ideal attributes for these sets of identifiers have been described in a publication from the American Society for Testing and Materials (ASTM) (American Society for Testing and Materials, 1999). The identifier must include a check digit to ensure accuracy when the identifier is entered by a human being into a system. A standardized solution must also determine mechanisms for issuing identifiers to individuals, facilities, and organizations; for maintaining databases of identifying information; and for authorizing access to such information (also see Chapter 10).

The Health Care Financing Administration (HCFA) has defined a National Provider Identifier (NPI) that will likely become the national standard. This number is a seven-character alphanumeric base identifier plus a one-character check digit. No meaning is built into the number, each number is unique and is never reissued, and alpha characters that might be confused with numeric characters (for example, 0, 1, 2, 4, and 5 can be confused with O, I or L, Z , Y, and S) have been eliminated. HCFA has also defined a Payor ID for identifying healthcare plans. A proposal has been made to use the Internal Revenue Service's employer-identification number for employers.

The most controversial issue is identifying each individual or patient. Many people consider assignment and use of such a number to be an invasion of privacy and are concerned that it could be easily linked to other databases. Public Law 104-191, passed in August 1996 (see Section 6.3.3), requires that Congress formally define suitable identifiers. The Department of Health and Human Services has recommended the identifiers discussed above, except for the person identifier. The decision was made to postpone that recommendation until privacy legislation is in place (see Chapter 7).

We also need standards for encoding data about the patient that are collected by one system and used by another. A hospital-admissions system records that a patient has the diagnosis of diabetes mellitus, a pharmacy system records that the patient has been given gentamicin, a laboratory system records that the patient had certain results on kidney-function tests, and a radiology system records that a doctor has ordered an X-ray examination for the patient that requires intravenous iodine dye. Other systems need ways to store these data, to present the data to clinical users, to send warnings about possible disease–drug interactions, to recommend dosage changes, and to follow the patient's outcome. A standard for coding patient data is nontrivial when one considers the need for agreed-on definitions, use of qualifiers, differing (application-specific) levels of granularity in the data, and synonymy, not to mention the breadth and depth that such a standard would need to have.

The inclusion of medical knowledge in clinical systems is becoming increasingly important and commonplace. Sometimes, the knowledge is in the form of simple facts, such as the maximum safe dose of a medication or the normal range of results for a laboratory test. Much medical knowledge is more complex, however. It is challenging to encode such knowledge in ways that computer systems can use (see Chapter 2), especially if one needs to avoid ambiguity and to express logical relations consistently. Thus the encoding of clinical knowledge using an accepted standard would allow many people and institutions to share the work done by others. One standard designed for this purpose is the Arden Syntax, discussed in Chapter 16.

Because the tasks we have described require coordination of systems, methods are needed for transferring information from one system to another. Such transfers were traditionally accomplished through custom-tailored point-to-point interfaces, but this technique has become unworkable as the number of systems and the resulting permutations of necessary connections have grown. A current approach to solving the multiple-interface problem is through the development of messaging standards. Such messages must depend on the preexistence of standards for patient identification and data encoding.

Although the technical challenges are daunting, methods for encoding patient data and shipping those data from system to system are not sufficient for developing practical systems. Security must also be addressed before such exchanges can be allowed to take place. Before a system can divulge patient information, it must ensure that requesters are who they say they are and that they are permitted access to the requested information (see Chapter 4). Although each clinical system can have its own security features, system builders would rather draw on available standards and avoid reinventing the wheel. Besides, the secure exchange of information requires that interacting systems use standard technologies. Fortunately, many researchers are busy developing such standards.

6.3 Standards Undertakings and Organizations

It is helpful to separate our discussion of the general process by which standards are created from our discussion of the specific organizations and the standards that they produce. The process is relatively constant, whereas the organizations form, evolve, merge, and are disbanded. Let us consider, for purposes of illustration, how a standard might be developed for sending laboratory data, in electronic form, from one computer system to another in the form of a message.

6.3.1 *The Standards-Development Process*

There are four ways in which a standard can be produced:

1. *Ad hoc method:* A group of interested people and organizations (e.g., laboratory-system and hospital-system vendors) agree on a standard specification. These specifications are informal and are accepted as standards through mutual agreement of the participating groups. An example produced by this method is the American College of Radiology/National Electrical Manufacturers Association (ACR/NEMA) DICOM standard for medical imaging.
2. *De facto method:* A single vendor controls a large enough portion of the market to make its product the market standard. An example is Microsoft's Windows.
3. *Government-mandate method:* A government agency, such as the HCFA or the National Institute for Standards and Technology (NIST) creates a standard and legislates its use. An example is HCFA's UB92 insurance-claim form.
4. *Consensus method:* A group of volunteers representing interested parties works in an open process to create a standard. Most healthcare standards are produced by this method. An example is the Health Level 7 (HL7) standard for clinical-data interchange (Fig. 6.1).

The process of creating a standard proceeds through several stages (Libicki, 1995). It begins with an *identification stage*, during which someone becomes aware that there exists a need for a standard in some area and that technology has reached a level that can support such a standard. In our example, suppose there are several laboratory systems sending data to several central hospital systems—a standard message format would allow each laboratory system to talk to all the hospital systems without specific point-to-point interface programs being developed for each possible laboratory-to-laboratory or laboratory-to-hospital

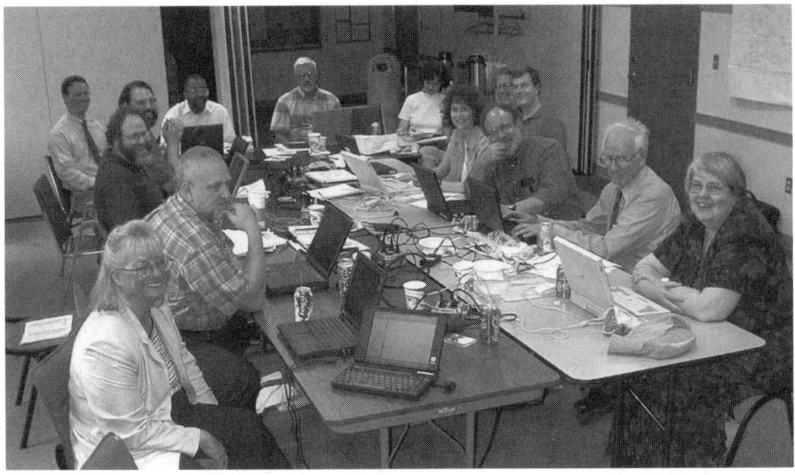

FIGURE 6.1. A Standards-Development Meeting. The development of effective standards often requires numerous group meetings over many years. Volunteers bring varying expertise and perspectives to the meetings so that consensus can gradually be achieved. Here an HL7 group is shown at one of their meetings (see Section 6.5.2). (*Source:* Courtesy of HL7, photograph by George Beeler.)

combination. If the time for a standard is ripe, then several individuals can be identified and organized to help with the *conceptualization stage*, in which the characteristics of the standard are defined. What must the standard do? What is the scope of the standard? What will be its format?

In the laboratory system example above, one key discussion would be on the scope of the standard. Should the standard deal only with the exchange of laboratory data, or should the scope be expanded to include other types of data exchange? Should the data elements being exchanged be sent with a tag identifying the data element, or should the data be defined positionally? In the ensuing *discussion stage*, the participants will begin to create an outline that defines content, to identify critical issues, and to produce a time line. In the discussion, the pros and cons of the various concepts are discussed. What will be the specific form for the standard? For example, will it be message based? Will the data exchange be based on a query or on a trigger event? Will the standard define the message content, the message syntax, the vocabulary, and the network protocol, or will the standard deal with a subset of these issues?

The participants are generally well informed in the domain of the standard, so they appreciate the needs and problems that the standard must address. Basic concepts are usually topics for heated discussion; subsequent details may follow at an accelerated pace. Many of the participants will have experience in solving problems to be addressed by the standard and will protect their own approaches. The meanings of words are often debated. Compromises and loosely defined terms are often accepted to permit the process to move forward. In our example, the likely participants would be vendors of competing laboratory systems and vendors of competing hospital systems. All participants would be familiar with the general problems but would have their own proprietary approach to solving them. Definitions of basic concepts normally taken for granted, such as what constitutes a test or a result, would need to be clearly stated and agreed on.

The writing of the draft standard is usually the work of a few, dedicated individuals—typically people who represent the vendors in the field. Other people then review that draft; controversial points are discussed in detail, and solutions are proposed and finally accepted. Writing and refining the standard is further complicated by the introduction of people new to the process who have not been privy to the original discussions and who want to revisit points that have been resolved earlier. The balance between moving forward and being open is a delicate one. Most standards-writing groups have adopted an **open policy**: Anyone can join the process and can be heard. Most standards-development organizations—certainly those by accredited groups—support an open balloting process. A draft standard is made available to all interested parties, inviting comments and recommendations. All comments are considered. Negative ballots must be addressed specifically. If the negative comments are persuasive, the standard is modified. If they are not, the issues are discussed with the submitter in an attempt to convince the person to remove the negative ballot. If neither of these efforts is successful, the comments are sent to the entire balloting group to see whether the group is persuaded to change its vote. The resulting vote then determines the content of the standard. Issues might be general, such as deciding what types of laboratory data to include (pathology? blood bank?), or specific, such as deciding the specific meanings of specific fields (do we include the time the test was ordered? specimen drawn? test performed?).

A standard will generally go through several versions on its path to maturity. The first attempts at implementation are frequently met with frustration as participating vendors interpret the standard differently and as areas not addressed by the standard are encountered. These problems may be dealt with in subsequent versions of the standard. Backward compatibility is a major concern as the standard evolves. How can the standard evolve, over time, and still be economically responsible to both vendors and users? An implementation guide is usually produced to help new vendors profit from the experience of the early implementers.

A critical stage in the life of a standard is *early implementation*, when acceptance and rate of implemention are important to success. This process is influenced by accredited standards bodies, by the federal government, by major vendors, and the marketplace. The maintenance and promulgation of the standard are also important to ensure widespread availability and continued value of the standard. Some form of conformance testing is ultimately necessary to ensure that vendors adhere to the standard and to protect its integrity.

Producing a standard is an expensive process in terms of both time and money. Vendors and users must be willing to support the many hours of work, usually on company time; the travel expense; and the costs of documentation and distribution. In the United States, the production of a consensus standard is voluntary, in contrast to in Europe, where most standards development is funded by governments.

An important aspect of standards is *conformance*, a concept that covers compliance with the standard and also usually includes specific agreements among users of the standard who affirm that specific rules will be followed. An example of a group that has defined a conformance specification for HL7 is the Andover Working Group, a consortium of vendors and healthcare-provider organizations, which is using HL7 (see Section 6.5.2) and other standards. The conformance document identifies specifically what data elements will be sent, when, and in what form.

A second important concept is *certification*. The use of most standards is enhanced by a certification process in which a neutral body certifies that a vendor's product in fact does comply and conform with the standard.

6.3.2 Information-Standards Organizations

Sometimes, standards are developed by organizations that need the standard to carry out their principal functions; in other cases, coalitions are formed for the express purpose of developing a particular standard. The latter organizations are discussed later, when we examine the particular standards developed in this way. There are also *standards organizations* that exist for the sole purpose of fostering and promulgating standards. In some cases, they include a membership with expertise in the area where the standard is needed. In other cases, the organization provides the rules and framework for standard development but does not offer the expertise needed to make specific decisions for specific standards, relying instead on participation by knowledgeable experts when a new standard is being studied.

In this section we describe in some detail several of the best-known **standards development organizations** (SDOs). Our goal has been to familiarize you with the names or organizational and historical aspects of the most influential health-related standards groups. For a detailed understanding of an organization or the standards it has developed, you will need to refer to current primary resources. Many of the organizations maintain web sites with excellent current information on their status.

American National Standards Institute

ANSI is a private, nonprofit membership organization founded in 1918. It originally served to coordinate the U.S. voluntary census standards systems. Today, it is responsible for approving official *American National Standards*. ANSI membership includes over 1,100 companies; 30 government agencies; and 250 professional, technical, trade, labor, and consumer organizations.

ANSI does not write standards; rather, it assists standards developers and users from the private sector and from government to reach consensus on the need for standards. It helps them to avoid duplication of work, and it provides a forum for resolution of differences. ANSI administers the only government-recognized system for establishing American National Standards. ANSI also represents U.S. interests in international standardization. ANSI is the U.S. voting representative in the ISO and the International Electrotechnical Commission (IEC). There are three routes for a standards development body to become ANSI approved so as to produce an American National Standard: Accredited Organization, Accredited Standards Committee, and Accredited Canvass.

An organization that has existing organizational structure and procedures for standards development may be directly accredited by ANSI to publish American National Standards, provided that it can meet the requirements for due process, openness, and consensus. HL7 (discussed in Section 6.5.2) is an example of an ANSI Accredited Organization.

ANSI may also create internal Accredited Standards Committees (ASCs) to meet a need not filled by an existing Accredited Organization. ASC X12 (discussed in Section 6.5.2) is an example of such a committee.

The final route, Accredited Canvass, is available when an organization does not have the formal structure required by ANSI: Through a canvass method that meets the criterion of balanced representation of all interested parties, a standard may be approved as an American National Standard. For example, ACR/NEMA (see Section 6.5.2) could choose to use this method to publish its imaging standard as an American National Standard.

CEN Technical Committee 251

The European Committee for Standardization (Comité Europeén de Normalisation—CEN), established Technical Committee 251 (TC 251) in 1991 for the development of standards for healthcare informatics. The major goal of TC 251 is to develop standards for communication among independent medical information systems so that clinical and management data produced by one system can be transmitted to another system. The organization of TC 251 parallels work in the United States through various Working Groups. These groups similarly deal with a data-interchange standard; medical-record standards; code and vocabulary standards; imaging standards; and security, privacy, and confidentiality. People in both Europe and the United States are working to coordinate all areas of standardization. Draft standards are being shared. Common solutions are being accepted as desirable. Groups are working together at various levels toward a common goal. Standards of interest include EUCLIDES, for interfacing reference laboratory systems to healthcare settings; EDIFACT, for transmission of electronic documents; and a message standard developed by Project Team 007 (PT 007) for transmitting content of electrocardiogram (ECG) carts to computers (EUCLIDES, EDIFACT, and PT 007 are further discussed at the end of Section 6.5.2).

ISO Technical Committee 215

In January 1998, the ISO created a new technical committee (TC 215) for medical informatics. The scope of this TC is standardization in the field of information for health and health information and communications technology to achieve compatibility and interoperability between independent systems. The TC will also address issues required to ensure compatibility of data for comparative statistical purposes and to reduce duplication of effort and redundancies. The United States has been assigned the duties of Secretariat, and those duties have been specifically assigned to ASTM (see below). ASTM will also serve as the Technical Advisory Group Administrator.

American Society for Testing and Materials

ASTM was founded in 1898 and chartered in 1902 as a scientific and technical organization for the development of standards for characteristics and performance of materials. The original focus of ASTM was standard test methods. The charter was subsequently broadened in 1961 to include products, systems, and services, as well as materials. ASTM is the largest nongovernment source of standards in the United States. It has over 30,000 members who reside in over 90 different countries. ASTM is a charter member of ANSI. ASTM technical committees are assigned 12 ISO committee and subcommittee secretariats and have over 50 assignments to serve as Technical Advisory Groups (TAGs) for developing U.S. positions on international standards. ASTM Committee E31 on Computerized Systems is responsible for the development of the medical-information standards. Table 6.1 shows the domains of its various subcommittees.

Healthcare Informatics Standards Board

Responding to a request by CEN TC 251 to identify a single American organization that represents the standards work in the United States, ANSI formed a Healthcare Informatics Standards Planning Panel (HISPP) in January 1992. This panel had a balanced representation from standards-development groups, healthcare vendors, government agencies, and healthcare providers.

Table 6.1. ASTM E31 subcommittees.

Subcommittee	Medical-information standard
E31.01	Controlled Vocabularies for Healthcare Informatics
E31.10	Pharmaco-Informatics Standards
E31.11	Electronic Health Record Portability
E31.13	Clinical Laboratory Information Management Systems
E31.14	Clinical Laboratory Instrument Interface
E31.16	Interchange of Electrophysiological Waveforms and Signals
E31.17	Access, Privacy, and Confidentiality of Medical Records
E31.19	Electronic Health Record Content and Structure
E31.20	Data and System Security for Health Information
E31.21	Health Information Networks
E31.22	Health Information Transcription and Documentation
E31.23	Modeling for Health Informatics
E31.24	Electronic Health Record System Functionality
E31.25	XML for Document Type Definitions in Healthcare

One of the charter goals of the HISPP was to coordinate the work of the message-standards group for healthcare data interchange and healthcare informatics to achieve the evolution of a unified set of nonredundant, nonconflicting standards that is compatible with ISO and non-ISO communications environments. In addition, a balanced subcommittee of the planning panel was formed to interact with and to provide input to CEN TC 251 in a coordinated fashion and to explore avenues of international standards development. A second subcommittee, with the specific objective of coordinating HISPP activities with TC 251, met in November 1992 and agreed to basic rules in the distribution of working documents (once approved by HISPP) to TC 251.

As work progressed and more organizations became actively interested in healthcare standards, ANSI and the members of HISPP recognized the need for a permanent body to coordinate the healthcare standards activities. The ANSI Board was petitioned to form a Healthcare Informatics Board. In December 1995, the HISPP was dissolved and the Healthcare Informatics Standards Board (HISB) was created.

The scope of the HISB includes standards for

1. Healthcare models and electronic healthcare records
2. Interchange of healthcare data, images, sounds, and signals within and between organizations and practices
3. Healthcare codes and terminology
4. Communication with diagnostic instruments and healthcare devices
5. Representation and communication of healthcare protocols, knowledge, and statistical databases
6. Privacy, confidentiality, and security of medical information
7. Additional areas of concern or interest with regard to healthcare information

A major contribution of the HISB has been the creation and maintenance of an Inventory of Health Care Information Standards pertaining to the Health Insurance Portability and Accountability Act of 1996 (discussed in Section 6.3.3).

Computer-Based Patient Record Institute

The Computer-Based Patient Record Institute (CPRI) has been an active proponent of standards activities since its inception in 1992. Although not a standards developer, CPRI has made major contributions in the area of content of the computer-based patient record; security, privacy, and confidentiality; the universal health identifier; and vocabulary and terminology.

6.3.3 Health Insurance Portability and Accountability Act of 1996

The Health Insurance Portability and Accountability Act of 1996 (HIPAA) was signed into law on August 21, 1996. The administrative-simplification portion of HIPAA requires that the Secretary of Health and Human Services (HHS) adopt

1. The Secretary must adopt standards for transactions, and data elements for such transactions, to enable health information to be exchanged electronically that are appropriate for financial and administrative transactions consistent with the goals of improving the operation of the health care system and reducing costs, including:
   a. Health Claims or equivalent encounter information
   b. Health Claims Attachments
   c. Enrollment and Disenrollment in a Health Plan
   d. Eligibility For a Health Plan
   e. Health Care Payment and Remittance Advice
   f. Health Plan Premium Payments
   g. First Report of Injury
   h. Health Claim Status
   i. Referral Certification and Authorization
   j. Coordination of Benefits
2. The Secretary shall adopt standards providing for a unique health identifier for each individual, employer, health plan, and health care provider for use in the health care system.
3. The Secretary shall adopt standards for code sets for appropriate data elements for financial and administrative transactions.
4. The Secretary shall adopt security standards that . . . specify procedures for the electronic transmission and authentication of signatures.

Figure 6.2. Requirements of the Health Insurance Portability and Accountability Act of 1996. These requirements define the first round of standards required to meet the immediate needs of the healthcare community.

standards for the electronic transmission of specific administrative transactions. These standards will apply to health plans, healthcare clearinghouses, and healthcare providers who transmit any health information in electronic form; Figure 6.2 shows the kinds of transactions covered. Recommendations made thus far include the use of X12N standards for health claims.

6.4 Coded Terminologies, Vocabularies, and Nomenclatures

As we discussed in Chapter 2, the capture, storage, and use of clinical data in computer systems is complicated by lack of agreement on terms and meanings. The many terminologies discussed in this section have been developed to ease the communication of coded medical information.

6.4.1 Motivation for Controlled Terminologies

The encoding of medical information is a basic function of most clinical systems. Standards for such encoding can serve two purposes. First, they can save system developers from reinventing the wheel. For example, if an application allows caregivers to compile problem lists about their patients, using a standard vocabulary saves developers from having to create their own. Second, using commonly accepted standards can facilitate exchange of data among systems. For example, if a central database is accepting clinical data from many sources, the task is greatly simplified if each source is using the same coding scheme. System developers often ignore available standards and continue to develop their own solutions. It is easy to believe that the developers have resisted adoption of standards because it is too much work to understand and adapt to any system that was "not invented here." The reality, however, is that the available standards are often inadequate for the needs of the users (in this case, system developers). As a result, no standard terminology enjoys the wide acceptance sufficient to facilitate the second function: exchange of coded clinical information.

In discussing coding systems, the first step is to clarify the differences among a **terminology**, a **vocabulary**, and a **nomenclature**. These terms are often used interchangeably by creators of coding systems and by authors discussing the subject. Fortunately, although there are few accepted standard terminologies, there is a generally accepted standard *about* terminology: ISO Standard 1087 (Terminology—Vocabulary). Figure 6.3 lists the various definitions for these terms. For our purposes, we consider the currently available standards from the viewpoint of their being terminologies.

The next step in the discussion is to determine the basic use of the terminology. In general, there are two different levels relevant to medical data encoding: abstraction and representation. **Abstraction** entails examination of the recorded data and then selection of items from a terminology with which to label the data. For example, a patient might be admitted to the hospital and have a long and complex course; for the purposes of billing, however, it might be relevant only

- **Object:** Any part of the perceivable or conceivable world
- **Name:** Designation of an object by a linguistic expression
- **Concept:** A unit of thought constituted through abstraction on the basis of properties common to a set of objects
- **Term:** Designation of a defined concept in a special language by a linguistic expression
- **Terminology:** Set of terms representing the system of concepts of a particular subject field
- **Nomenclature:** System of terms that is elaborated according to preestablished naming rules
- **Dictionary:** Structured collection of lexical units, with linguistic information about each of them
- **Vocabulary:** Dictionary containing the terminology of a subject field

FIGURE 6.3. Terminologic terms, adapted from ISO Standard 1087. Terms not defined here—such as *definition*, *lexical unit*, and *linguistic expression*—are assumed by the Standard to have common meanings.

that the patient was diagnosed as having had a myocardial infarction. Someone charged with abstracting the record to generate a bill might then reduce the entire set of information to a single code. **Representation**, on the other hand, is the process by which as much detail as possible is coded. Thus, for our medical-record example, the representation might include codes for each physical finding noted, laboratory test performed, and medication administered.

When we discuss a controlled terminology, we should consider the domain of discourse. Virtually any subject matter can be coded, but there must be a good match with any standard selected for the purpose. For example, a terminology used to code disease information might be a poor choice for coding entries on a problem list because it might lack items such as "Abdominal Pain," "Cigarette Smoker," or "Health Maintenance."

The next consideration is the content of the standard itself. There are many issues, including the degree to which the standard covers the terminology of the intended domain; the degree to which data are coded by assembly of terms into descriptive phrases (postcoordination) versus selection of a single, precoordinated term; and the overall structure of the terminology (list, strict hierarchy, multiple hierarchy, semantic network, and so on). There are also many qualitative issues to consider, including the availability of synonyms and the possibility of redundant terms (i.e., more than one way to encode the same information).

Finally, we should consider the methods by which the terminology is maintained. Every standard terminology must have an ongoing maintenance process, or it will become obsolete rapidly. The process must be timely and must not be disruptive to people using an older version of the terminology. For example, if the creators of the terminology choose to rename a code, what happens to the data previously recorded with that code?

6.4.2 Specific Terminologies

With these considerations in mind, let us survey some of the several popular, available controlled terminologies. People often say, tongue in cheek, that the best thing about standards is that there are so many from which to choose. We give introductory descriptions of a few current and common terminologies. New terminologies appear annually, and existing proprietary terminologies often become publicly available. When reviewing the following descriptions, try to keep in mind the background motivation for a development effort. All these standards are evolving rapidly, and you should consult the websites or other primary sources for the most recent information.

International Classification of Diseases and Its Clinical Modifications

One of the best-known terminologies is the *International Classification of Diseases* (ICD). First published in 1893, it has been revised at roughly 10-year intervals, first by the Statistical International Institute and later by the World Health Organization (WHO). The *Ninth Edition* (ICD-9) was published in 1977 (World

481 Pneumococcal Pneumonia

482 Other Bacterial Pneumonia
482.0 Pneumonia due to Klebsiella Pneumoniae
482.1 Pneumonia due to Pseudomonas
482.2 Pneumonia due to Haemophilus Influenzae
482.3 Pneumonia due to Streptococcus
482.4 Pneumonia due to Staphylococcus
482.8 Pneumonia due to Other Specified Bacteria
482.9 Bacterial pneumonia unspecified

484 Pneumonia in Infectious Disease Classified Elsewhere
484.3 Pneumonia in Whooping Cough
484.4 Pneumonia in Tularemia
484.5 Pneumonia in Anthrax

FIGURE 6.4. Bacterial pneumonias coded in ICD-9. The extensive set of codes for mycobacterial disease has been omitted for simplicity.

Health Organization, 1977) and the *Tenth Edition* (ICD-10) in 1992 (World Health Organization, 1992). The coding system consists of a *core classification* of three-digit codes that are the minimum required for reporting mortality statistics to WHO. A fourth digit (in the first decimal place) provides an additional level of detail; usually .0 to .7 are used for more specific forms of the core term, .8 is usually "other," and .9 is "unspecified." Terms are arranged in a strict hierarchy, based on the digits in the code. For example, bacterial pneumonias are classified as shown in Figure 6.4. In addition to diseases, ICD also includes several "families" of terms for medical-specialty diagnoses, health status, disablements, procedures, and reasons for contact with healthcare providers.

ICD-9 has generally been perceived as inadequate for the level of detail desired for statistical reporting in the United States (Kurtzke, 1979). In response, the U.S. National Center for Health Statistics published a set of **clinical modifications** (Commission on Professional and Hospital Activites, 1978). **ICD-9-CM**, as it is known, is compatible with ICD-9 and provides extra levels of detail in many places by adding fourth-digit and fifth-digit codes. Figure 6.5 shows a sample additional detail. Most of the diagnoses assigned in the United States are coded in ICD-9-CM, allowing compliance with international treaty (by conversion to ICD-9) and supporting billing requirements (by conversion to *diagnosis-related groups*, or DRGs). A clinical modification for ICD-10 has not yet been released.

Diagnosis-Related Groups

Another U.S. creation for the purpose of abstracting medical records is the DRGs, developed initially at Yale University for use in prospective payment in the Medicare program (3M Health Information System, updated annually). In this

003 Other Salmonella Infections
- 003.0 Salmonella Gastroenteritis
- 003.1 Salmonella Septicemia
- 003.2 Localized Salmonella Infections
  - 003.20 Localized Salmonella Infection, Unspecified
  - 003.21 Salmonella Meningitis
  - 003.22 Salmonella Pneumonia
  - 003.23 Salmonella Arthritis
  - 003.24 Salmonella Osteomyelitis
  - 003.29 Other Localized Salmonella Infection
- 003.8 Other specified salmonella infections
- 003.9 Salmonella infection, unspecified

FIGURE 6.5. Example of fifth-digit codes in the Clinical Modifications of ICD-9 (ICD-9-CM). The four-digit codes are identical to those in ICD-9; the five-digit codes were introduced in ICD-9-CM. Note that Salmonella Pneumonia has been added as a child in the 003 section; it is not included under 482 (Other Bacterial Pneumonia) or 484 (Pneumonia in Infectious Disease Classified Elsewhere).

case, the coding system is an abstraction of an abstraction: It is applied to lists of ICD-9-CM codes that are themselves derived from medical records. The purpose of DRG coding is to provide a relatively small number of codes for classifying patient hospitalizations while also providing some separation of cases based on severity of illness. The principal bases for the groupings are factors that affect cost and length of stay. Thus, a medical record containing the ICD-9-CM *primary* diagnosis of Pneumococcal Pneumonia (481) might be coded with one of 18 codes (Fig. 6.6), depending on associated conditions and procedures; additional codes are possible if the pneumonia is a secondary diagnosis.

International Classification of Primary Care

The World Organization of National Colleges, Academies and Academic Associations of General Practitioners/Family Physicians publishes the International Classification of Primary Care (ICPC) with the WHO. ICPC is a classification of some 800 diagnostic concepts that are partially mapped into ICD-9. ICPC contains all 380 concepts of the *International Classification of Health Problems in Primary Care (ICHPPC), Third Edition,* including reasons for an encounter. ICPC provides seven axes of terms and a structure to combine them to represent clinical encounters. Although the granularity of the terms is generally larger than that of other classification schemes (e.g., all pneumonias are coded as R81), the ability to represent the interactions of the concepts found in a medical record is much greater through the *postcoordination* of atomic terms. In postcoordination, the coding is accomplished through the use of multiple codes as needed to describe the data. Thus, for example, a case of bacterial pneumonia would be coded in ICPC as a combination of the code R81 and the code for the particular test

Respiratory disease w/ major chest operating room procedure, no major complication or comorbidity	75
Respiratory disease w/ major chest operating room procedure, minor complication or comorbidity	76
Respiratory disease w/ other respiratory system operating procedure, no complication or comorbidity	77
Respiratory infection w/ minor complication, age greater than 17	79
Respiratory infection w/ no minor complication, age greater than 17	80
Simple Pneumonia w/ minor complication, age greater than 17	89
Simple Pneumonia w/ no minor complication, age greater than 17	90
Respiratory disease w/ ventilator support	475
Respiratory disease w/ major chest operating room procedure and major complication or comorbidity	538
Respiratory disease, other respiratory system operating procedure and major complication	539
Respiratory infection w/ major complication or comorbidity	540
Respiratory infection w/ secondary diagnosis of bronchopulmonary dysplasia	631
Respiratory infection w/ secondary diagnosis of cystic fibrosis	740
Respiratory infection w/ minor complication, age not greater than 17	770
Respiratory infection w/ no minor complication, age not greater than 17	771
Simple Pneumonia w/ minor complication, age not greater than 17	772
Simple Pneumonia w/ no minor complication, age not greater than 17	773
Respiratory infection w/ primary diagnosis of tuberculosis	798

FIGURE 6.6. Diagnosis-related group codes assigned to cases of bacterial pneumonia depending on co-occurring conditions or procedures (mycobacterial disease is not shown here except as a co-occurring condition). "Simple Pneumonia" codes are used when the primary bacterial pneumonia corresponds to ICD-9 code 481, 482.2, 482.3, or 482.9 (refer to Figs. 6.4 and 6.5) and when there are only minor or no complications. The remaining ICD-9 bacterial pneumonias (482.0, 482.1, 482.2, 482.4, 482.8, 484, and various other codes such as 003.22; refer to Fig. 6.4) are coded as "Respiratory Disease" or "Respiratory Infection." Cases in which pneumonia is a secondary diagnosis may also be assigned other codes (such as 798), depending on the primary condition.

result that identifies the causative agent. This method is in contrast to the *precoordination* approach in which every type of pneumonia is assigned its own code.

Current Procedural Terminology

The American Medical Association developed the *Current Procedural Terminology* (CPT) in 1966 (American Medical Association, updated annually) to provide a precoordinated coding scheme for diagnostic and therapeutic procedures that has since been adopted in the United States for billing and reimbursement. Like the DRG codes, CPT codes specify information that differentiates the codes based on cost. For example, there are different codes for pacemaker insertions, depending on whether the leads are "epicardial, by thoracotomy" (33200), "epicardial, by xiphoid approach" (33201), "transvenous, atrial" (33206), "transvenous, ventricular" (33207), or "transvenous, AV sequential" (33208). CPT also provides information about the reasons for a procedure. For example, there are codes for arterial punctures for "withdrawal of blood for diagnosis" (36600), "monitoring" (36620), "infusion therapy" (36640), and "occlusion therapy" (75894). Although limited in scope and depth, the CPT-4 is the most widely accepted nomenclature in the United States for reporting physician procedures and services for federal and private insurance third-party reimbursement.

Diagnostic and Statistical Manual of Mental Disorders

The American Psychiatric Association published its *Diagnostic and Statistical Manual of Mental Disorders, Revised Third Edition* (DSM-III-R) in 1987 (American Psychiatric Association, 1987) and the *Fourth Edition* (DSM-IV) in 1994 (American Psychiatric Association, 1994), revised in 1996 (DSM-IV-R). The DSM nomenclature provides definitions of psychiatric disorders and includes specific diagnostic criteria. Thus, it is used not only for coding patient data but also as a tool for assigning diagnoses. Each edition of DSM has been coordinated with corresponding editions of ICD; DSM-IV is coordinated with ICD-10.

Systematized Nomenclature of Medicine and Its Predecessors

Drawing from the New York Academy of Medicine's *Standard Nomenclature of Diseases and Operations* (SNDO) (New York Academy of Medicine, 1961), the College of American Pathologists developed the *Standard Nomenclature of Pathology* (SNOP) as a multiaxial system for describing pathologic findings (College of American Pathologists, 1971) through postcoordination of topographic (anatomic), morphologic, etiologic, and functional terms. SNOP has been used widely in pathology systems in the United States; its successor, the *Systematized Nomenclature of Medicine* (SNOMED) has evolved beyond an abstracting scheme to become a comprehensive coding system.

Largely the work of Roger Côté and David Rothwell, SNOMED was first published in 1975 and then was revised as SNOMED II in 1979. SNOMED III is a greatly expanded version: the *Systematized Nomenclature of Human and Veterinary Medicine—SNOMED International* (Côté et al., 1993). SNOMED consists of a set of axes (now 11), each of which serves as a taxonomy for a specific set of concepts (organisms, diseases, procedures, and so on), containing a total of over 130,000 terms. Coding of patient information is accomplished through the postcoordination of terms from multiple axes to represent complex terms that may be desired but do not exist in SNOMED. For example, although many of the various bacterial pneumonia terms seen in other terminologies are in SNOMED (Fig. 6.7), a user can construct additional terms by pairing a generic pneumonia term with a bacteria term taken from the Living Organism axis.

Despite its long history and extensive efforts to provide the codes needed for coding in electronic medical records, SNOMED has not been widely embraced.

DE-10000	Bacterial infectious disease, NOS	(L-10000)
DE-10100	Bacterial pneumonia, NOS	(T-28000)(M-40000)(L-10000)
DE-11205	Pneumonia in anthrax	(T-28000)(M-40000)
DE-13212	Pneumonia in pertussis	(T-28000)(M-40000)
DE-13430	Pneumonic plague, NOS	(T-28000)(L-1E401)(DE-01750)
DE-13431	Primary pneumonic plague	(T-28000)(L-1E401)(DE-01750)
DE-13432	Secondary pneumonic plague	(T-28000)(L-1E401)(DE-01750)
DE-13510	Pneumococcal pneumonia	(T-28000)(M-40000)(L-25116)
DE-13934	Salmonella pneumonia	(T-28000)(L-17100)
DE-14120	Staphylococcal pneumonia	(T-28000)(L-24800)
DE-14213	Pneumonia due to Streptococcus	(T-28000)(M-40000)(L-25100)
DE-14817	Tuberculous pneumonia	(T-28000)(M-40000)(L-21801)
DE-15104	Pneumonia in typhoid fever	(T-28000)(M-40000)
DE-15613	Haemophilus influenzae pneumonia	(T-28000)(L-1F701)
DE-15710	Legionella pneumonia, NOS	(L-20401)
DE-15716	Pittsburg pneumonia	(L-20402)
DE-15810	Mycoplasma pneumonia	(T-28000)(L-22018)
DE-19110	Bacterial infection due to Klebsiella pneumoniae	(L-16001)
DE-19111	Pneumonia due to Klebsiella pneumoniae	(T-28000)(M-40000)(L-16001)
DE-19134	Achromobacter pneumonia	
DE-19151	Pneumonia due to Pseudomonas	(T-28000)(M-40000)(L-23400)
DE-19162	Pneumonia due to Proteus mirabilis	(T-28000)(M-40000)(L-16802)
DE-19204	Pneumonia due to E. coli	(T-28000)(M-40000)(L-15602)
DE-21611	Ornithosis with pneumonia	(T-28000)(M-40000)(L-2A902)
DE-21704	Pneumonia in Q fever	(T-28000)(M-40000)
DE-3632A	AIDS with bacterial pneumonia	(T-28000)(L-34800)(L-10000)
DE-3632B	AIDS with pneumococcal pneumonia	(T-28000)(L-34800)(L-25100)
DE-36333	AIDS with pneumonia, NOS	(T-28000)(M-40000)(L-34800)
D2-50100	Bronchopneumonia, NOS	(T-26000)(M-40000)
D2-50104	Peribronchial pneumonia	(T-26090)(M-40000)
D2-50110	Hemorrhagic bronchopneumonia	(T-26000)(M-40790)
D2-50120	Terminal bronchopneumonia	(T-26000)(M-40000)
D2-50130	Pleurobronchopneumonia	(T-26000)(M-40000)
D2-50130	Pleuropneumonia	(T-26000)(M-40000)
D2-50140	Pneumonia, NOS	(T-28000)(M-40000)
D2-50142	Catarrhal pneumonia	(T-28000)(M-40000)
D2-50150	Unresolved pneumonia	(T-28000)(M-40000)
D2-50152	Unresolved lobar pneumonia	(T-28770)(M-40000)
D2-50154	Organized pneumonia	
D2-50160	Granulomatous pneumonia, NOS	(T-28000)(M-44000)
D2-50300	Aspiration pneumonia, NOS	(T-28000)(M-40000)(G-C001) (F-29200)
D2-61020	Gangrenous pneumonia	(T-28000)(M-40700)
D8-72532	Infective pneumonia acquired prenatally, NOS	

FIGURE 6.7. SNOMED International codes for pneumonia. The first set of terms are those from the Disease axis, which are included under the Bacterial Infectious Disease hierarchy (excluding several veterinary diseases). NOS-not otherwise specified. The codes shown on the right are the SNOMED codes that, when taken together, are the equivalent of the precoordinated bacterial pneumonia terms. For example, "Pneumococcal pneumonia" (DE-13510) is the precoordination of the terms "Lung, NOS" (T-28000), "Inflammation, NOS" (M-40000), and "Streptococcus pneumoniae" (L-25116). The second set of terms shows some of the other pneumonia terms in SNOMED that could be coupled with specific Living Organism terms to allow postcoordinated coding of concepts not coded explicitly in SNOMED.

The latest version goes a long way toward addressing past complaints about missing terms; however, the structure of previous versions, also found to be an impediment to use, has persisted in SNOMED International. The main problem with using SNOMED for coding patient information is that it is *too* expressive. Because there are few rules about how the postcoordination coding should be done, the same expression might end up being represented differently by different coders. For example, "acute appendicitis" can be coded as a single disease term, as a combination of a modifier ("acute") and a disease term ("appendicitis"), or as a combination of a modifier ("acute"), a morphology term ("inflammation") and a topography term ("vermiform appendix"). Each of these codings is correct, yet there is no formal way, in SNOMED, to know that they have equivalent meaning. Such freedom of expression may be welcome to people who must encode human utterances, but it is frustrating to system developers who must make sure that their applications can recognize medical concepts.

A recent development in the evolution of SNOMED is the creation of a "reference terminology" (SNOMED-RT) that is designed to encourage consistent use of the terms by defining explicitly the relationships among them. Some of the problems with earlier versions of SNOMED are being resolved in this process (Campbell et al., 1998).

Read Clinical Codes

The *Read Clinical Codes* comprise a set of codes designed specifically for use in coding electronic medical records. Developed by James Read in the 1980s (Read, 1990; Read & Benson, 1986), the first version was adopted by the British National Health Service (NHS) in 1990. Version 2 was developed to meet the needs of hospitals for cross-mapping their data to ICD-9. Version 3 (NHS Centre for Coding and Classification, 1994a) was developed to support not only medical record summarization but also patient-care applications directly. Whereas previous versions of the Read Codes were organized in a strict hierarchy, Version 3 took an important step by allowing terms to have multiple parents in the hierarchy; that is, the hierarchy became that of a directed acyclic graph. Figure 6.8 shows the hierarchy for bacterial pneumonia. Version 3.1 added the ability to make use of term modifiers through a set of templates for combining terms in specific, controlled ways so that both precoordination and postcoordination are used. Finally, the NHS has undertaken a series of *terms projects* that are expanding the content of the Read Codes to ensure that the terms needed by practitioners are represented in the Codes (NHS Centre for Coding and Classification, 1994b).[3]

---

[3]In 1999, the developers and maintainers of SNOMED and the Read Codes announced that they had reached an agreement to merge their efforts and to produce a single joint clinical terminology. This promising development suggests that a single terminology suitable for clinical patient records may be in sight.

- Respiratory Disorder
  - Infection of the Lower Respiratory Tract and Mediastinum
    - Acute Lower Respiratory Tract Infection
      - Pneumonia
        - Bacterial Pneumonia
          - Actinomycotic Pneumonia
          - Haemophilus Influenzae Pneumonia
          - Legionella pneumonia
          - Pneumococcal Pneumonia
          - Pneumonic Plague
            - Primary Pneumonic Plague
            - Secondary Pneumonic Plague
            - Pneumonic plague, unspecified
          - Salmonella Pneumonia
            - Typhoid Pneumonia
          - Staphylococcal Pneumonia
          - Meningococcal Pneumonia
          - Pneumonia due to Klebsiella pneumoniae
          - Pseudomonal pneumonia
          - Escherichia coli pneumona
          - Proteus pneumonia
          - Tularemia pneumonia
          - Pertussis pneumonia
          - Anthrax pneumonia
          - Nocardial pneumonia
          - Toxoplasma pneumonia
          - Streptococcal pneumonia
            - Group B streptococcal pneumonia
          - Secondary bacterial pneumonia *
          - Other bacterial pneumonia *
            - Pneumonia due to other specified bacteria *
              - Pneumonia due to bacteria NOS *
            - Bacterial pneumonia NOS *
          - Pneumonia due to other aerobic gram-negative bacteria *
          - Pneumonia in bacterial disease classified elsewhere *

FIGURE 6.8. Bacterial pneumonias in the Read Clinical Codes. A user can code additional infections by using Bacterial Pneumonia with one of the prescribed modifiers (Bacteria). Some of these terms also appear in other hierarchy locations; for example, Meningococcal Pneumonia also appears under Meningococcal Infection (which is under Bacterial Disease). The asterisk (*) denotes optional terms that are included for use in classification by epidemiologists or coders but would not be included in a clinical record. (NOS = not otherwise specified.)

Gabrieli Medical Nomenclature

Also in the 1980s, Elmer Gabrieli developed the *Gabrieli Medical Nomenclature* (Gabrieli, 1989) at the University of Buffalo. The system was then adopted for use in a proprietary system. It consists of a single, large hierarchy that contains successively more complex expressions as you move down through the hierarchy. The aim of this system is to take precoordination to the extreme, providing a code for every utterance that might be found in a medical record (Fig. 6.9). Although initially available as a commercial product, the developers have used it as the basis for nomenclature work under the ASTM (American Society for Testing and Materials, 1989). The ASTM is currently working to move this nomenclature through the standards development process.

Nursing Terminologies

Nursing organizations have been extremely active in the development of standard coding systems for abstracting patient records. One review counted a total of 13 separate projects worldwide (Wake et al., 1993). These projects have arisen because general medical terminologies fail to represent the kind of clinical concepts needed in nursing care. For example, the kinds of problems that appear in a physician's problem list (such as "myocardial infarction" and "diabetes mellitus") are relatively well represented in many of the terminologies that we have described, but the kinds of problems that appear in a nurse's assessment (such as "activity intolerance" and "knowledge deficit related to myocardial infarction") are not (also see Chapter 12). Preeminent nursing terminologies include the *North American Nursing Diagnosis Association* (NANDA) codes, the *Nursing Outcomes Classification* (NOC), the *Georgetown Home Health Care Classification* (HHCC), and the Omaha System (which covers problems, interventions, and outcomes). Despite the proliferation of standards for nursing terminologies, gaps remain in the coverage of this domain (Henry & Mead, 1997).

GALEN

In Europe, a consortium of universities, agencies, and vendors, with funding from the Advanced Informatics in Medicine initiative (AIM), has formed the GALEN project to develop standards for representing coded patient information (Rector et al., 1995). GALEN is developing a reference model for medical concepts using a formalism called Structured Meta Knowledge (SMK). In SMK, terms are defined through relationships to other terms, and grammars are provided to allow combinations of terms into sensible phrases. The reference model is intended to allow representation of patient information in a way that is independent of the language being recorded and of the data model used by an electronic medical record system. The GALEN developers are working closely with CEN TC 251 (see Section 6.2.2) to develop the content that will populate the reference model with actual terms.

Logical Observations, Identifiers, Names, and Codes

An independent consortium, led by Clement J. McDonald and Stanley M. Huff, has created a naming system for tests and observations. Originally called *Laboratory Observations, Identifiers, Names and Codes* (LOINC), the system is being extended to include nonlaboratory observations (vital signs, electrocardio-

4-3-3-2-1-7-1 Pneumonia
4-3-3-2-1-7-1-3 Causes of Pneumonia
4-3-3-2-1-7-1-3-1 Bacterial Pneumonia
4-3-3-2-1-7-1-3-1-1 Presumed Bacterial Pneumonia
4-3-3-2-1-7-1-3-1-2 Streptococcus Pneumonia
4-3-3-2-1-7-1-3-1-3 Staphylococcus Aureus Pneumonia
4-3-3-2-1-7-1-3-1-3-1 Staphylococcal Pneumonia
4-3-3-2-1-7-1-3-1-4 Streptococcus Pyogenes Pneumonia
4-3-3-2-1-7-1-3-1-5 Neisseria Meningitidis Pneumonia
4-3-3-2-1-7-1-3-1-6 Branhamella Catarrhalis Pneumonia
4-3-3-2-1-7-1-3-1-7 Hemophilus Influenzae Pneumonia
4-3-3-2-1-7-1-3-1-8 Klebsiella Pneumonia
4-3-3-2-1-7-1-3-1-9 Escherichia Coli Pneumonia
4-3-3-2-1-7-1-3-1-10 Serratia Species Pneumonia
4-3-3-2-1-7-1-3-1-11 Enterobacteria Species Pneumonia
4-3-3-2-1-7-1-3-1-12 Proteus Species Pneumonia
4-3-3-2-1-7-1-3-1-13 Pseudomonas Aeruginosa Pneumonia
4-3-3-2-1-7-1-3-1-14 Pseudomonas Capacia Pneumonia
4-3-3-2-1-7-1-3-1-15 Pseudomonas Multiphilia Pneumonia
4-3-3-2-1-7-1-3-1-16 Pseudomonas Pseudoalcaligenes Pneumonia
4-3-3-2-1-7-1-3-1-17 Actinobacter Species Pneumonia
4-3-3-2-1-7-1-3-1-18 Legionella Species Pneumonia
4-3-3-2-1-7-1-3-1-19 Anaerobic Microbial Pneumonia
4-3-3-2-1-7-1-3-1-19-1 Fusobacterium Species Pneumonia
4-3-3-2-1-7-1-3-1-19-2 Bacteroides Species Pneumonia
4-3-3-2-1-7-1-3-1-19-3 Peptostreptococcus Species Pneumonia
4-3-3-2-1-7-1-3-1-19-4 Microaerophilic Streptococcus Pneumonia
4-3-3-2-1-7-1-3-1-20 Actinomyces Pneumonia
4-3-3-2-1-7-1-3-1-21 Nocardia Species Pneumonia
4-3-3-2-1-7-1-3-1-22 Mycoplasma Pneumonia
4-3-3-2-1-7-1-3-1-23 Coxiella Burnetti Pneumonia
4-3-3-2-1-7-1-3-1-24 Chlamydia Psittaci Pneumonia
4-3-3-2-1-7-1-3-1-25 Chlamydia Trachomatis Pneumonia
4-3-3-2-1-7-1-3-1-26 Pseudomonas Pseudomallei Pneumonia
4-3-3-2-1-7-1-3-1-27 Pasteurella Pneumonia
4-3-3-2-1-7-1-3-1-28 Francisella Pneumonia
4-3-3-2-1-7-1-3-1-29 Yersinia Pestis Pneumonia
4-3-3-2-1-7-1-3-1-30 Bacillis Anthracis Pneumonia
4-3-3-2-1-7-1-3-1-31 Brucella Species Pneumonia
4-3-3-2-1-7-1-3-1-32 Chlamydial Pneumonia
4-3-3-2-1-7-1-3-1-33 Mycobacterial Pneumonia
4-3-22-1 Bacterial Disease
4-3-22-1-1 Bacteriogenic Pneumonia
4-3-22-1-1-2 Pneumococcus Pneumonia
4-3-22-1-1-3 Staphylococcal Pneumonia
4-3-22-1-1-3-1 Primary Staphylococcal Pneumonia
4-3-22-1-1-3-2 Secondary Staphylococcal Pneumonia
4-3-22-1-1-4 Streptococcal Pneumonia

grams, and so on), so *Logical* has replaced *Laboratory* to reflect the change (Huff, 1998). Figure 6.10 shows some typical *fully specified names* for common laboratory tests. The standard specifies structured coded semantic information about each test, such as the substance measured and the analytical method used. Using this system, a person can code new names for new tests, which can be recognized by other users of the coded information; however, officially recognized names (such as those in the Fig. 6.10) are given more compact LOINC codes. The LOINC committee is collaborating with CEN to coordinate their work with the similar EUCLIDES work in Europe (EUCLIDES Foundation International, 1994).

National Drug Codes

The *National Drug Codes* (NDC), produced by the Food and Drug Administration (FDA), is applied to all drug packages. It is widely used in the United States, but it is not as comprehensive as the WHO codes described below. The FDA designates part of the code based on drug manufacturer, and each manufacturer defines the specific codes for their own products. As a result, there is no uniform class hierarchy for the codes, and codes may be reused at the manufacturer's discretion.

World Health Organization Drug Dictionary and the Anatomical-Therapeutic-Chemical Index

The WHO Drug Dictionary is an international classification of drugs that provides proprietary drug names used in different countries, as well as all active ingredients and the chemical substances, with Chemical Abstract numbers. Drugs are classified according to the Anatomical-Therapeutic-Chemical (ATC) classification, with cross-references to manufacturers and reference sources. The current dictionary contains 24,300 proprietary drug names, 14,700 single ingredient drugs, 9,500 multiple ingredient drugs, and 6,900 chemical substances. The dictionary now covers drugs from 34 countries and grows at a rate of about 2,000 new entries per year.

FIGURE 6.9. Bacterial pneumonias coded in the Gabrieli (ASTM) Medical Nomenclature. (Sixteen descendants of Mycobacterial pneumonia are not shown.) Some terms appear in multiple locations (e.g., Staphylococcal Pneumonia, which has additional descendants in one context). Note that Bacterial Pneumonia and Bacteriogenic Pneumonia are not considered synonymous and have different descendants. Similarly, Streptococcus Pneumonia (4-3-3-2-1-7-1-3-1-2) and Streptococcal Pneumonia (4-3-22-1-1-4) are not considered synonymous. Additional bacterial pneumonias can be found elsewhere in the hierarchy, such as Listerial Pneumonia (4-3-22-1-29-6-1), Staphylococcus Aureus Pneumonia in a Granulocytopenic Host (4-3-3-2-1-7-1-1-1-2), its child Staphylococcus Epidermidis Pneumonia in a Granulocytopenic Host, and Staphylococcus Pneumonia in Children (16-10-5-7-2-14-1-3).

Blood glucose	GLUCOSE:MCNC:PT:BLD:QN:
Plasma glucose	GLUCOSE:MCNC:PT:PLAS:QN:
Serum glucose	GLUCOSE:MCNC:PT:SER:QN:
Urine glucose concentration	GLUCOSE:MCNC:PT:UR:QN:
Urine glucose by dip stick	GLUCOSE:MCNC:PT:UR:SQ:TEST STRIP
Glucose tolerance test at 2 hours	GLUCOSE^2H POST 100 G GLUCOSE PO: MCNC:PT:PLAS:QN:
Ionized whole blood calcium	CALCIUM.FREE:SCNC:PT:BLD:QN:
Serum or plasma ionized calcium	CALCIUM.FREE:SCNC:PT:SER/PLAS:QN:
24 hour calcium excretion	CALCIUM.TOTAL:MRAT:24H:UR:QN:
Whole blood total calcium	CALCIUM.TOTAL:SCNC:PT:BLD:QN:
Serum or plasma total calcium	CALCIUM.TOTAL:SCNC:PT:SER/PLAS:QN:
Automated hematocrit	HEMATOCRIT:NFR:PT:BLD:QN: AUTOMATED COUNT
Manual spun hematocrit	HEMATOCRIT:NFR:PT:BLD:QN:SPUN
Urine erythrocyte casts	ERYTHROCYTE CASTS:ACNC:PT:URNS:SQ: MICROSCOPY.LIGHT
Erythrocyte MCHC	ERYTHROCYTE MEAN CORPUSCULAR HEMOGLOBIN CONCENTRATION:MCNC:PT:RBC:QN:AUTOMATED COUNT
Erythrocyte MCH	ERYTHROCYTE MEAN CORPUSCULAR HEMOGLOBIN:MCNC:PT:RBC:QN: AUTOMATED COUNT
Erythrocyte MCV	ERYTHROCYTE MEAN CORPUSCULAR VOLUME:ENTVOL:PT:RBC:QN:AUTOMATED COUNT
Automated Blood RBC	ERYTHROCYTES:NCNC:PT:BLD:QN: AUTOMATED COUNT
Manual blood RBC	ERYTHROCYTES:NCNC:PT:BLD:QN: MANUAL COUNT
ESR by Westergren method	ERYTHROCYTE SEDIMENTATION RATE:VEL:PT:BLD:QN:WESTERGREN
ESR by Wintrobe method	ERYTHROCYTE SEDIMENTATION RATE:VEL:PT:BLD:QN:WINTROBE

Figure 6.10. Examples of common laboratory test terms as they are encoded in LOINC. The major components of the fully specified name are separated here by ":" and consist of the substance measured, the property (e.g., MCNC = mass concentration; SCNC = substance concentration; NFR = numeric fraction; and NCNC = number concentration), the time (PT = point in time), the specimen, and the method (SQ = semiquantitative; QN = quantitative; QL = qualitative).

Medical Subject Headings

The *Medical Subject Headings* (MeSH), maintained by the United States' National Library of Medicine (NLM) (National Library of Medicine, updated annually), is the vocabulary by which the world medical literature is indexed. MeSH arranges terms in a structure that breaks from the strict hierarchy used by most other coding schemes. Terms are organized into hierarchies and may appear in multiple places in the hierarchy (Fig. 6.11). Although it is not generally used as

- Respiratory Tract Diseases
  - Lung Diseases
    - Pneumonia
      - Bronchopneumonia
      - Pneumonia, Aspiration
        - Pneumonia, Lipid
      - Pneumonia, Lobar
      - Pneumonia, Mycoplasma
      - Pneumonia, Pneumocystis Carinii
      - Pneumonia, Rickettsial
      - Pneumonia, Staphylococcal
      - Pneumonia, Viral
    - Lung Diseases, Fungal
      - Pneumonia, Pneumocystis Carinii
  - Respiratory Tract Infections
    - Pneumonia
      - Pneumonia, Lobar
      - Pneumonia, Mycoplasma
      - Pneumonia, Pneumocystis Carinii
      - Pneumonia, Rickettsial
      - Pneumonia, Staphylococcal
      - Pneumonia, Viral
    - Lung Diseases, Fungal
      - Pneumonia, Pneumocystis Carinii

FIGURE 6.11. Partial tree structure for the Medical Subject Headings showing pneumonia terms. Note that terms can appear in multiple locations, although they may not always have the same children, implying that they have somewhat different meanings in different contexts. For example, Pneumonia means "lung inflammation" in one context (line 3) and "lung infection" in another (line 16).

a direct coding scheme for patient information, it plays a central role in the Unified Medical Language System.

Unified Medical Language System

In 1986, Donald Lindberg and Betsy Humphreys, at the NLM, began consulting contractors to identify ways to construct a resource that would bring together and disseminate controlled medical vocabularies. An experimental version of the *Unified Medical Language System* (UMLS) was first published in 1989 (Humphreys, 1990); the UMLS has been updated annually since then. Its principal component is the Metathesaurus, which contains over 331,000 terms collected from over 40 different sources (including many of those that we have discussed), and attempts to relate synonymous and similar terms from across the different sources (Fig. 6.12). Figure 6.13 lists the preferred names for all pneumonia concepts in the Metathesaurus; Figure 6.14 shows how like terms are grouped into concepts and are tied to other concepts through semantic relationships.

Interchange Registration of Coding Schemes

To accommodate the many coding schemes that are in use (and are likely to persist) in healthcare applications today, the CEN Project Team PT 005 has defined

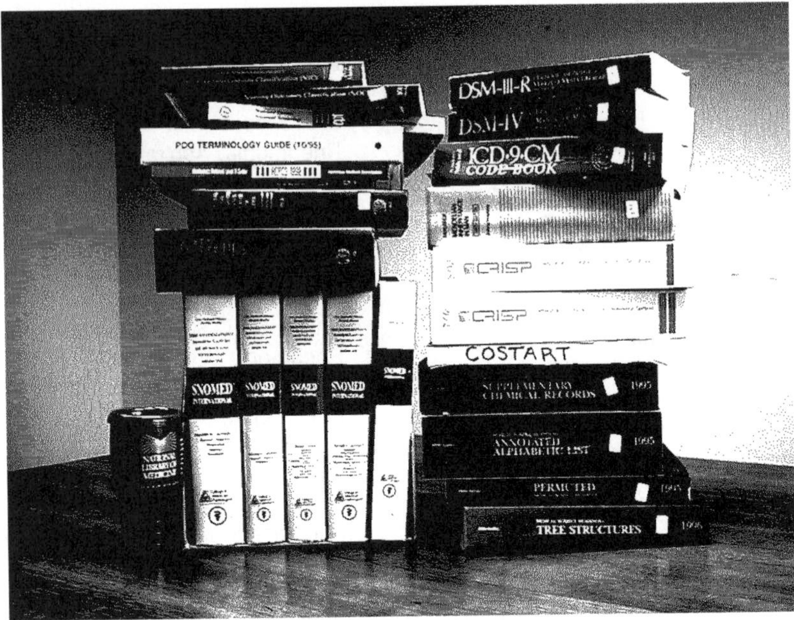

FIGURE 6.12. Sources for the UMLS. The Unified Medical Language System, comprises contributed terminologies from a large number of sources, including all the text compendia shown here. (*Source:* Courtesy National Library of Medicine and Lexical Technolgoy, Inc.)

a draft standard that describes procedures for international registration of coding schemes used in health care (Health Care Financial Management Association, 1992). The protocol specifies the allocation of a unique six-character Health Care Coding Scheme Designator (HCD) to each registered coding scheme. A code value can then be assigned an unambiguous meaning in association with an HCD.

6.5 Data-Interchange Standards

The recognition of the need to interconnect healthcare applications led to the development and enforcement of **data-interchange standards**. The conceptualization stage began in 1980 with discussions among individuals in an organization called the American Association for Medical Systems and Informatics (AAMSI). In 1983, an AAMSI task force was established to pursue those interests in developing standards. The discussions were far ranging in topics and focus. Some members wanted to write standards for everything, including a standard medical vocabulary, standards for hospital information systems, standards for the computer-based patient record, and standards for data interchange. Citing the need for data interchange between commercial laboratories and health-

C0004626: Pneumonia, Bacterial
C0023241: Legionnaires' Disease
C0032286: Pneumonia due to other specified bacteria
C0032308: Pneumonia, Staphylococcal
C0152489: Salmonella pneumonia
C0155858: Other bacterial pneumonia
C0155859: Pneumonia due to Klebsiella pneumoniae
C0155860: Pneumonia due to Pseudomonas
C0155862: Pneumonia due to Streptococcus
C0155865: Pneumonia in pertussis
C0155866: Pneumonia in anthrax
C0238380: PNEUMONIA, KLEBSIELLA AND OTHER GRAM NEGATIVE BACILLI
C0238381: PNEUMONIA, TULAREMIC
C0242056: PNEUMONIA, CLASSIC PNEUMOCOCCAL LOBAR
C0242057: PNEUMONIA, FRIEDLAENDER BACILLUS
C0275977: Pneumonia in typhoid fever
C0276026: Haemophilus influenzae pneumonia
C0276039: Pittsburgh pneumonia
C0276071: Achromobacter pneumonia
C0276080: Pneumonia due to Proteus mirabilis
C0276089: Pneumonia due to E. Coli
C0276523: AIDS with bacterial pneumonia
C0276524: AIDS with pneumococcal pneumonia
C0339946: Pneumonia with tularemia
C0339947: Pneumonia with anthrax
C0339952: Secondary bacterial pneumonia
C0339953: Pneumonia due to escherichia coli
C0339954: Pneumonia due to proteus
C0339956: Typhoid pneumonia
C0339957: Meningococcal pneumonia
C0343320: Congenital pneumonia due to staphylococcus
C0343321: Congenital pneumonia due to group A hemolytic streptococcus
C0343322: Congenital pneumonia due to group B hemolytic streptococcus
C0343323: Congenital pneumonia due to Escherichia coli
C0343324: Congenital pneumonia due to pseudomonas
C0348678: Pneumonia due to other aerobic gram-negative bacteria
C0348680: Pneumonia in bacterial diseases classified elsewhere
C0348801: Pneumonia due to streptococcus, group B
C0349495: Congenital bacterial pneumonia
C0349692: Lobar (pneumococcal) pneumonia
C0375322: Pneumococcal pneumonia {Streptococcus pneumoniae pneumonia}
C0375323: Pneumonia due to Streptococcus, unspecified
C0375324: Pneumonia due to Streptococcus Group A
C0375326: Pneumonia due to other Streptococcus
C0375327: Pneumonia due to anaerobes
C0375328: Pneumonia due to escherichia coli {E. Coli}
C0375329: Pneumonia due to other gram-negative bacteria
C0375330: Bacterial pneumonia, unspecified

FIGURE 6.13. Some of the bacterial pneumonia concepts in the Unified Medical Language System Metathesaurus.

Bacterial pneumonia
Source: CSP93/PT/2596-5280; DOR27/DT/U000523; ICD91/PT/482.9; ICD91/IT/482.9
Parent: *Bacterial Infections; Pneumonia; Influenza with Pneumonia*
Child: *Pneumonia, Mycoplasma*
Narrower: *Pneumonia, Lobar; Pneumonia, Rickettsial; Pneumonia, Staphylococcal; Pneumonia due to Klebsiella Pneumoniae; Pneumonia due to Pseudomonas; Pneumonia due to Hemophilus influenzae (H. influenzae)*
Other: *Klebsiella Pneumoniae, Streptococcus Pneumoniae*

Pneumonia, Lobar
Source: ICD91/IT/481; MSH94/PM/D011018; MSH94/MH/D011018; SNM2/RT/M-40000; ICD91/PT/481; SNM2/PT/D-0164; DXP92/PT/U000473; MSH94/EP/D011018; INS94/MH/D011018;INS94/SY/D011018
Synonym: Pneumonia, diplococcal
Parent: *Bacterial Infections; Influenza with Pneumonia*
Broader: *Bacterial Pneumonia; Inflammation*
Other: *Streptococcus Pneumoniae*
Semantic: inverse-is-a: *Pneumonia*
has-result: *Pneumococcal Infections Pneumonia, Staphylococcal*
Source: ICD91/PT/482.4; ICD91/IT/482.4; MSH94/MH/D011023; MSH94/PM/D011023; MSH94/EP/D011023; SNM2/PT/D-017X; INS94/MH/D011023; INS94/SY/D011023
Parent: *Bacterial Infections; Influenza with Pneumonia*
Broader: *Bacterial Pneumonia*
Semantic inverse-is-a: *Pneumonia; Staphylococcal Infections Pneumonia, Streptococcal*
Source: ICD91/IT/482.3
Other: *Streptococcus Pneumoniae Pneumonia due to Streptococcus*
Source: ICD91/PT/482.3
ATX: Pneumonia AND Streptococcal Infections AND NOT Pneumonia, Lobar
Parent: *Influenza with Pneumonia*

Pneumonia in Anthrax
Source: ICD91/PT/484.5; ICD91/IT/022.1; ICD91/IT/484.5
Parent: *Influenza with Pneumonia*
Broader: *Pneumonia in other infectious diseases classified elsewhere*
Other: *Pneumonia, Anthrax*

Pneumonia, Anthrax
Source: ICD91/IT/022.1; ICD91/IT/484.5
Other: *Pneumonia in Anthrax*

FIGURE 6.14. Some of the information available in the Unified Medical Language System about selected pneumonia concepts. Concept's preferred names are shown in italics. Sources are identifiers for the concept in other vocabularies. Synonyms are names other than the preferred name. ATX is an associated Medical Subject Heading expression that can be used for Medline searches. The remaining fields (Parent, Child, Broader, Narrower, Other, and Semantic) show relationships among concepts in the Metathesaurus. Note that concepts may or may not have hierarchical relations to each other through Parent–Child, Broader–Narrower, and Semantic (is-a and inverse-is-a) relations. Note also that *Pneumonia, Streptococcal* and *Pneumonia due to Streptococcus* are treated as separate concepts, as are *Pneumonia in Anthrax* and *Pneumonia, Anthrax*.

care providers, the task force agreed to focus on data-interchange standards for clinical laboratory data. Early activities were directed mainly toward increasing interest of AAMSI members in working to create healthcare standards.

The development phase was multifaceted. The AAMSI task force became subcommittee E31.11 of the ASTM and developed and published ASTM standard 1238 for the exchange of clinical-laboratory data. Two other groups—many members of which had participated in the earlier AAMSI task force—were formed to develop standards, each with a slightly different emphasis: HL7 and MEDIX. The American College of Radiology (ACR) joined with the National Electronic Manufacturers Association (NEMA) to develop a standard for the transfer of image data. Two other groups developed related standards independent of the medical informatics community: ANSI X12 for the transmission of commonly used business transactions, including healthcare claims and benefit data, and the National Council for Prescription Drug Programs (NCPDP) for the transmission of third-party drug claims. Development was further complicated by the independent creation of standards by several groups in Europe, including EUCLIDES and EDIFACT.

6.5.1 General Concepts and Requirements

The purpose of a data-interchange standard is to permit one system, the **sender**, to transmit to another system, the **receiver**, all the data required to accomplish a specific communication, or **transaction set**, in a precise, unambiguous fashion. To complete this task successfully, both systems must know what format and content is being sent and must understand the words or vocabulary, as well as the delivery mode. When you order merchandise, you fill out a form that includes your name and address, desired items, quantities, colors, sizes, and so on. You might put the order form in an envelope and mail it to the supplier at a specified address. There are standard requirements, such as where and how to write the receiver's (supplier's) address, your (the sender's) address, and the payment for delivery (the postage stamp). The receiver must have a mailroom, a post-office box, or a mailbox to receive the mail.

A communications model, called the Open Systems Interconnection (OSI) reference model (ISO 7498-1), has been defined by the ISO (see Section 4.1.2 and the discussion of software for network communications). It describes seven levels of requirements or specifications for a communications exchange: Physical, Data Link, Network, Transport, Session, Presentation, and Application (Rose, 1989; Stallings, 1987a; Tanenbaum, 1987). Level 7, the application level, deals primarily with the semantics or data-content specification of the transaction set or message. For the data-interchange standard, HL7 requires the definition of all the data elements to be sent in response to a specific task, such as the admission of a patient to a hospital. In many cases, the data content requires a specific vocabulary that can be understood by both sender and receiver. For example, if a physician orders a laboratory test that is to be processed by a commercial laboratory, the ordering system must ensure that the name of the test on the order is the same as the name that the laboratory uses. When a panel of tests is ordered, both systems must share a common understanding of the panel composition. This vocabulary understanding is best ensured through use of a vocabulary table that contains both the test name and a unique code. Unfortunately, several code sets exist for each data group, and none are complete. An immediate challenge to the medical-informatics community is to generate one complete set. In other cases, the vocabulary requires a definition of the domain of the set, such as what are the possible answers to the data parameter "ethnic origin."

The sixth level, Presentation, deals with what the syntax of the message is, or how the data are formatted. There are both similarities and differences at this level across the various standards bodies. Two philosophies are used for defining syntax: one proposes a *position-dependent* format; the other uses a *tagged-field* format. In the position-dependent format, the data content is specified and defined by position. For example, the sixth field, delimited by "|", is the gender of the patient and contains an M, F, or U or is empty. A tagged field representation is "SEX = M."

The remaining OSI levels—Session, Transport, Network, Data Link, and Physical—govern the communications and networking protocols and the physical connections made to the system. Obviously, some understanding at these lower levels is necessary before a linkage between two systems can be successful. Increasingly, standards groups are defining scenarios and rules for using various protocols at these levels, such as TCP/IP (see Section 4.1.2). Much of the labor in making existing standards work lies in these lower levels.

Typically, a transaction set or message is defined for a particular event, called a **trigger event**. The message is composed of several data segments; each data segment consists of one or more data fields. Data fields, in turn, consist of data elements that may be one of several data types. The message must identify the sender and the receiver, the message number for subsequent referral, the type of message, special rules or flags, and any security requirements. If a patient is involved, a data segment must identify the patient, the circumstances of the encounter, and additional information as required. A reply from the receiving system to the sending system is mandatory in most circumstances and completes the communications set.

It is important to understand that the sole purpose of the data-interchange standard is to allow data to be sent from the sending system to the receiving system; the standard does not in any manner constrain the application system that uses those data. Application independence permits the data-interchange standard to be used for a wide variety of applications. However, the standard must ensure that it accommodates all data elements required by the complete application set.

6.5.2 *Specific Data-Interchange Standards*

As health care increasingly depends on the connectivity within an institution, an enterprise, an integrated delivery system, a geographical system, or even a national integrated system, the ability to interchange data in a seamless manner becomes critically important. The economic benefits of data-interchange standards are immediate and obvious. Consequently, it is in this area of healthcare standards that most effort has been expended. All of the Standards Development Organizations in health care have some development activity in data-interchange standards.

In the following sections we summarize many of the current standards for data-interchange. Examples are provided to give you a sense of the technical issues that arise in defining a data-exchange standard, but details are beyond the scope of this book. For more information, consult the primary resources or the websites for the relevant organizations.

American College of Radiology/National Electronic Manufacturers Association

With the introduction of computed tomography and other digital diagnostic imaging modalities, people needed a standard method for transferring images and associated information between devices, manufactured by different vendors, that display a variety of digital image formats. The American College of Radiology (ACR) formed a relationship with the National Electronic Manufacturers Association (NEMA) in 1983 to develop such a standard for exchanging radiographic images, creating a unique professional/vendor group. The purposes of the ACR/NEMA standard were to promote a generic digital-image communication format, to facilitate the development and expansion of picture-archiving and communication systems (PACSs; see Chapter 14), to allow the creation of diagnostic databases for remote access, and to enhance the ability to integrate new equipment with existing systems.

Version 1 of the ACR/NEMA standard, published in 1985, specified a hardware interface, a data dictionary, and a set of commands. This standard supported only point-to-point communications. Version 2, published in 1988, introduced a message structure that consisted of a command segment for display devices, a new hierarchy scheme to identify an image, and a data segment for increased specificity in the description of an image (e.g., the details of how the image was made and of the settings).

In the ACR/NEMA standard, individual units of information, called *data elements*, are organized within the data dictionary into related groups. Groups and elements are numbered. Each individual data element, as contained within a message, consists of its group-element tag, its length, and its value. Groups include Command, Identifying, Patient, Acquisition, Relationship, Image Presentation, Text, Overlay, and Pixel Data.

The latest version of the ACR/NEMA Standard is the Digital Imaging and Communications in Medicine (DICOM) Version 3.0. It incorporates an object-oriented data model and adds support for ISO standard communications. DICOM provides full networking capability; specifies levels of conformance; is structured as a nine-part document to accommodate evolution of the standard; introduces explicit information objects for images, graphics, and text reports; introduces service classes to specify well-defined operations across the network; and specifies an established technique for identifying uniquely any information object. DICOM also specifies image-related management-information exchange, with the potential to interface to hospital information systems and radiology information systems.

The general syntax used by DICOM in representing data elements includes a data tag, a data-length specification, and the data value. That syntax is preserved over a hierarchical nested data structure of items, elements, and groups. Data elements are defined in a data dictionary and are organized into groups. A data set consists of the structured set of attributes or data elements and the values related to an information object. Data-set types include images, graphics, and text. A multivendor demonstration of DICOM Version 3.0 was first demonstrated at the Radiological Society of North America (RSNA) meeting in Chicago in November 1992.

The protocol architecture for DICOM Version 3.0 is shown in Figure 6.15. The bold line indicates the OSI upper-layer service boundary. Figure 6.15, which illustrates the communication services for a point-to-point environment and for a networked environment, identifies the communication services and the upper-

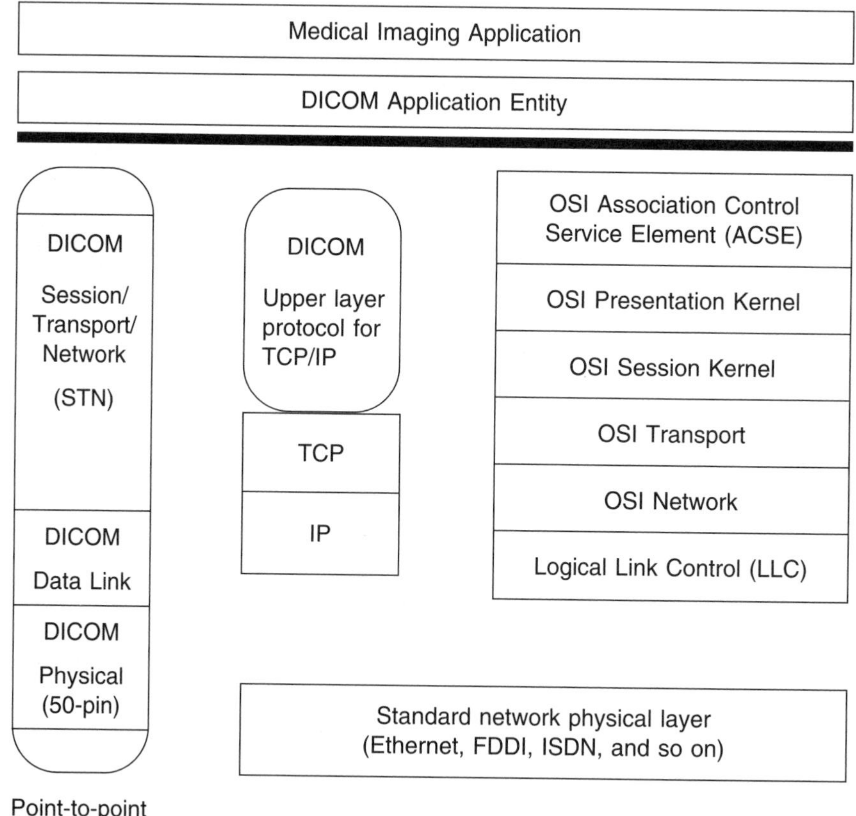

FIGURE 6.15. DICOM communications-protocol architecture illustrating the different approaches to dealing with the OSI reference model communication levels.

level protocols necessary to support communication between DICOM Application Entities. The upper-layer service supports the use of a fully conformant stack of OSI protocols to achieve effective communication. It supports a wide variety of international standards-based network technologies using a choice of physical networks such as Ethernet, FDDI, ISDN, X.25, dedicated digital circuits, and other local area network (LAN) and wide area network (WAN) technologies. In addition, the same upper-layer service can be used in conjunction with TCP/IP transport protocols.

American Society for Testing Materials E31

In 1984, the first ASTM healthcare data-interchange standard was published: E1238, Standard Specification for Transferring Clinical Observations Between Independent Systems. This standard is used in large commercial and reference clinical laboratories in the United States and has been adopted by a consortium of French laboratory system vendors who serve 95 percent of the laboratory volume in France. The ASTM E1238 standard is message based; it uses position-defined syntax and is similar to the HL7 standard (see next section). Related data-interchange standards include E1394 (from Subcommittee E31.13), Standard Specification for Transferring Information Between Clinical Instruments and Computer Systems, and E1467 (from Subcommittee E31.16), Specification for Transferring Digital Neurophysiological Data Between Independent Computer Systems. Another important ASTM standard is E1460 (from Subcommittee E31.15), Defining and Sharing Modular Health Knowledge Bases (Arden Syntax for Medical Logic Modules; see Chapter 16). In 1998, ownership of the Arden Syntax was transferred to HL7, where it will be developed by the Arden Syntax and Clinical Decision Support Technical Committee. An example of the ASTM 1238 standard describing a message transmitted between a clinic and a commercial clinical laboratory is shown in Figure 6.16.

```
H|~^\&|95243|HAMMO001|COMMUNITY AND FAMILY MEDICINE|BOX 2914^DUKE
UNIVERSITY MEDICAL CENTER^DURHAM^NC|919-684-6721||SMITHKLINE
CLINICAL LABS|TEST MESSAGE|D|2|199401170932<cr>

P|1|999-99-9999|||GUNCH^MODINE^SUE||19430704|F|<cr>

RT 1, BOX 97^ZIRCONIA^NC^27401||704-982-
1234||DOCTOR^PRIMARY^A^^DR.<cr>

OBR|1|101||80018^CHEM 18|R||||N|||||M D&PRIMARY&A&DR.<cr>

OBR|2|102||85025^AUTO CBC|R||||N||||| MD&PRIMARY&A&DR.
```

FIGURE 6.16. An example of a message in the ASTM 1238 format. The message consists of the header segment, H, the patient segment, P, and general order segments, OBR. Primary delimiters are the vertical bars (|); secondary delimiters are the carets (^). Note the similarities of this message to the HL7 message in Figure 6.17.

Health Level 7

An ad hoc standards group was formed in March 1987 as a result of efforts to develop an integrated hospital information system by interconnecting function-specific systems. That group adopted the name **HL7** to reflect the applications (seventh) level of the OSI reference model.[4] The original primary goal of HL7 was to provide a standard for the exchange of data among hospital-computer applications that eliminated, or substantially reduced, the hospital-specific interface programming and program maintenance that was required at that time. The standard was designed to support single, as well as batch, exchanges of transactions among the systems implemented in a wide variety of technical environments. Today, HL7 has over 500 organizational members and over 1,800 individual members; HL7 is the most widely implemented healthcare data-messaging standard and is in use at over 1,500 healthcare facilities.

The standard was built on existing production protocols—particularly ASTM 1238. The HL7 standard is message based and uses an event trigger model that causes the sending system to transmit a specified message to the receiving unit, with a subsequent response by the receiving unit. Messages are defined for various trigger events. Version 1.0 was published in September 1987 and served mainly to define the scope and format of standards. Version 2.0, September 1988, was the basis for several data-interchange demonstrations involving more than 10 vendors. Version 2.1, June 1990, was widely implemented in the United States and abroad. In 1991, HL7 became a charter member of ANSI; on June 12, 1994, it became an ANSI-accredited Standards Development Organization. Version 2.2 was published in December 1994; on February 8, 1996, it was approved by ANSI as the first healthcare data-interchange American National Standard. Version 2.3, March 1997, considerably expanded the scope by providing standards for the interchange of data relating to patient administration (admission, discharge, transfer, and outpatient registration), patient accounting (billing), order entry, clinical-observation data, medical information management, patient and resource scheduling, patient-referral messages, patient-care messages that support communication for problem-oriented records, adverse-event reporting, immunization reporting, and clinical trials, as well as a generalized interface for synchronizing common reference files.

Figure 6.17 illustrates the exchange that occurs when a patient is transferred from the operating room (which uses a system called DHIS) to the surgical intensive-care unit (which uses a system called TMR). Note the similarity between these messages and the ASTM example.

Version 3 of the standard (1999) is object oriented and based on a Reference Information Model (RIM) being developed by HL7. The RIM has evolved from a number of commercial and academic healthcare data models, and it accommodates the data elements defined in the current (Version 2.3) HL7 standard.

---

[4]See http://www.hl7.org/ for current information about HL7 and its evolution.

```
MSH|^~&\|DHIS|OR|TMR|SICU|199212071425|password|ADT|16603529|P|2.1<cr>

EVN|A02|199212071425||<cr>

PID|||Z99999^5^M11||GUNCH^MODINE^SUE|RILEY|19430704 |F||C|RT. 1, BOX
97^ZIRCONIA^NC^27401 |HEND|(704)982-1234|(704)983-1822||S|C||245-33-
9999<cr>

PV1|1|I|N22^2204|||OR^03|0940^DOCTOR^HOSPITAL^A||| SUR|||||A3<cr>

OBR|7|||93000^EKG REPORT|R|199401111000|199401111330|||RMT||||19940111
11330|?|P030||||||199401120930||||||88-126666|A111|VIRANYI^ANDREW<cr>

OBX|1|ST|93000.1^VENTRICULAR RATE(EKG)||91|/MIN|60-100<cr>

OBX|2|ST|93000.2[carot]ATRIAL RATE(EKG)||150|/MIN|60-100<cr>

. . .

OBX|8|ST|93000&IMP^EKG DIAGNOSIS|1|^ATRIAL FIBRILATION<cr>
```

FIGURE 6.17. An example of an HL7 ADT transaction message. This message includes the Medical Subject Heading header segment, the EVN trigger definition segment, the PID patient-identification segment, the PV1 patient-visit segment, the OBR general-order segment, and several OBX results segments.

This RIM is a collection of subject areas, scenarios, classes, attributes, use cases, actors, trigger events, interactions, and so on that depict the information needed to specify HL7 messages. In this sense it is more than a data-interchange standard, seeking to merge standards notions that include terminology and representation as well as data exchange. The stated purpose of the RIM is to provide a model for the creation of message specifications and messages for HL7. The RIM is not intended as a general purpose healthcare data model, although it might become that in time.

IEEE MEDIX

The Institute of Electrical and Electronics Engineers (IEEE) is an international organization that is a member of both ANSI and ISO. Through IEEE, many of the world's standards in telecommunications, electronics, electrical applications, and computers have been developed. There are two major IEEE standards projects in health care. IEEE P1157, Medical Data Interchange Standard (MEDIX), was organized in November 1987 to draft a standard for the exchange of data between hospital computer systems. The MEDIX committee, in formation, was committed to developing a standard set of hospital-system interface transactions based on the ISO standards for all seven layers of the OSI reference model. Its work has produced a family of documents that defines the communications models for medical data interchange among diverse systems.

IEEE 1073, Standard for Medical Device Communications, has produced a family of documents that defines the entire seven-layer communications requirements for the **medical information bus** (MIB). The MIB is a robust, reliable communication service designed for bedside devices in the intensive-care unit, operating room, and emergency room (see Chapter 13 for further discussion of the MIB in patient-monitoring settings).

The National Council for Prescription Drug Programs

The National Council for Prescription Drug Programs (NCPDP) is a trade organization. The Standardization Committee within the NCPDP has developed a standard format for the electronic submission of third-party drug claims. The standard was developed to accommodate the eligibility verification process at the point of sale and to provide a consistent format for electronic claims processing. Primarily pharmacy providers, insurance carriers, third-party administrators, and other responsible parties use the standard. This standard addresses the data format and content, transmission protocol, and other appropriate telecommunication requirements.

Version 1, released in 1988, used formats with fixed fields only. Version 2 added only typographical corrections to the Version 1 standard. The major thrust of the changes in Versions 3.0 and 3.1, in 1989, was the change from fixed-field transactions to a hybrid or variable format in which the fields can be tailored to the required content of the message. The current release is Version 3.2 (February 1992): It introduces the fixed-length Recommended Transaction Data Sets (RTDS), which define three different message types, and a separate Data Dictionary format. The Data Dictionary defines permissible values and default values for fields contained in the specification.

The standard uses defined separator characters at a group and a field level. The telecommunications specifications for sending two prescriptions includes three required sections (Transaction Header; Group Separator, First-Claim Information; and Group Separator, Second-Claim Information [R]) and three optional sections (Header Information, First-Claim Information, and Second-Claim Information [O]). The NCPDP communication standard is used in more than 60 percent of the nation's total prescription volume.

ANSI X12

Accredited Standards Committee (ASC) X12, an independent organization accredited by ANSI, has developed message standards for purchase-order data, invoice data, and other commonly used business documents. The subcommittee X12N has developed a group of standards related to providing claim, benefits, and claim payment or advice. The specific standards that strongly relate to the healthcare industry are shown in Table 6.2.

The X12 standards define commonly used business transactions in a formal, structured manner called *transaction sets*. A transaction set is composed of a transaction-set header control segment, one or more data segments, and a transaction-set trailer control segment. Each segment is composed of a unique segment ID; one or more logically related simple data elements or composite

TABLE 6.2. ANSI X12 standards.

Code	Title	Purpose
148	First Report of Injury, Illness or Incident	Facilitates the first report of an injury, incident, or illness
270	Health-Care Eligibility/Benefit Inquiry	Provide for the exchange of eligibility information and for response to individuals in a healthcare plan
271	Health-Care Eligibility/Benefit Information	
275	Patient Information	Supports the exchange of demographic, clinical, and other patient information to support administrative reimbursement processing as it relates to the submission of health-care claims for both health-care products and services
276	Health-Care Claim Status Request	Queries the status of a submitted claim and reports the status of a submitted claim
277	Health-Care Claim Status Notification	
278	Health-Care Service Review Information	Provides referral certification and authorization information
811	Consolidated Service Invoice/Statement	Facilitate health-plan premium billing and payment
820	Payment Order/Remittance Advice	
IHCLME	Interactive Health-Care Claim/Encounter	Supports administrative reimbursement processing as it relates to the submission of health-care claims for both health-care products and services in an interactive environment
IHCE/BI	Interactive Health-Care Eligibility/Benefit Inquiry	Provide for the exchange of eligibility information and for response to individuals within a health plan
IHCE/BR	Interactive Health-Care Eligibility/Benefit Response	

data structures, each preceded by a data element separator; and a segment terminator. Data segments are defined in a data-segment directory; data elements are defined in a data-element directory; composite data structures are defined in a composite data structure directory; control segments and the binary segment are defined in a data-segment directory.

A sample 835 Interchange Document is shown in Figure 6.18. This standard is similar to ASTM and HL7 in that it uses labeled segments with positionally defined components.

There are several additional organizations that either create standards related to health care or have influence on the creation of standards.

American Dental Association

In 1983, the American Dental Association (ADA) committee MD 156, became an ANSI-accredited committee responsible for all specifications for dental materials, instruments, and equipment. In 1992, a Task Group of the ASC MD 156 was es-

```
ST*835*0001<n/l>
BPR*X*3685*C*ACH*CTX*01*122000065*DA*296006596*IDNUMBER*
SUPPLECODE*01*134999883*DA*867869899*940116<n/l>
TRN*1*45166*IDNUMBER<n/l>
DTM*009*940104<n/l>
N1*PR*HEALTHY INSURANCE COMPANY<n/l>
N3*1002 WEST MAIN STREET<n/l>
N4*DURHAM*NC*27001<n/l>
N1*PE*DUKE MEDICAL CENTER<n/l>
N3*2001 ERWIN ROAD<n/l>
N4*DURHAM*NC*27710<n/l>
CLP*078189203*1*6530*4895*CIN<n/l>
CAS*PR*1*150<n/l>
CAS*PR*2*550<n/l>
NM1*15*IAM*A*PATIENT<n/l>
REF*1K*942238493<n/l>
DTM*232*940101<n/l>
DTM*233*940131<n/l>
SE*22*0001<n/l>
```

Figure 6.18. An example of ANSI X12 Interchange Document (Standard 835). This message is derived from a batch process, business-document orientation to a data-interchange model. The example does not include the control header or the functional-group header. The first line identifies the segment as a transaction-set header (ST). The last line is the transaction-set trailer (SE).The leading alphanumeric characters are tags that identify data content. For example, DTM is a date/time reference; N3 is address information; and BPR is the beginning segment for payment order/remittance advice.

tablished to initiate the development of technical reports, guidelines, and standards on electronic technologies used in dental practice. Five working groups promote the concept of a dental computer-based clinical workstation and allow the integration of different software and hardware components into one system. Areas of interest include digital radiography, digital intraoral video cameras, digital voice-text-image transfer, periodontal probing devices, and CAD/CAM. Proposed standards include Digital Image Capture in Dentistry, Infection Control in Dental Informatics, Digital Data Formats for Dentistry, Construction and Safety for Dental Informatics, Periodontal Probe Standard Interface, Computer Oral Health Record, and Specification for the Structure and Content of the Computer-Based Patient Record.

Uniform Code Council

The Uniform Code Council (UCC) is an ANSI-approved organization that defines the universal product code. Standards include specifications for the printing of machine-readable representations (bar codes).

Health Industry Business Communications Council

The Health Industry Business Communications Council (HIBCC) has developed the Health Industry Bar Code (HIBC) Standard, composed of two parts. The

HIBC Supplier Labeling Standard describes the data structures and bar-code symbols for bar coding of healthcare products. The HIBCC Provider Applications Standard describes data structures and bar code symbols for bar coding of identification data in a healthcare provider setting. HIBCC also issues and maintains Labeler Identification Codes that identify individual manufacturers. The HIBCC administers the Health Industry Number System, which provides a unique identifier number and location information for every healthcare facility and provider in the United States The HIBCC also administers the Universal Product Number Repository, which identifies specific products and is recognized internationally.

Workgroup for Electronic Data Interchange

The Workgroup for Electronic Data Interchange (WEDI) was formed in 1991 as a broad healthcare coalition to promote greater healthcare electronic commerce and connectivity in response to a challenge by then-Secretary of Health and Human Services Louis Sullivan, MD. The challenge was to bring together industry leaders to identify ways to reduce administrative costs in health care through thoughtful implementation of Electronic Data Interchange (EDI).

Specifically, the goals of WEDI are

- To define, prioritize, and reach consensus on critical issues affecting the acceptance of electronic commerce by the healthcare community
- To serve as a primary resource for identifying and removing obstacles that impede implementation of electronic commerce
- To educate and promote action by providing information resources on the benefits and effective use of electronic commerce, and on the implementation products and services available

WEDI incorporated as a formal organization in 1995. It has developed action plans to promote EDI standards, architectures, confidentiality, identifiers, health cards, legislation, and publicity. WEDI is one of four organizations named specifically in the HIPAA law to be consulted in the development of healthcare standards that would be selected to meet HIPAA requirements.

The European Clinical Data Exchange Standard

The European Clinical Data Exchange Standard (EUCLIDES) provides a standard for clinical laboratory data interchange between independent and heterogeneous medical information systems (NCPDP Telecommunication, 1992; Draft Application Protocol, 1993; Standard for Health Care Interchange, 1993). EUCLIDES is being supported by the Commission of the European Communities within the framework of the Advanced Informatics in Medicine (AIM) program.

A three-pronged approach to standardizing data interchange was adopted by EUCLIDES: semantics (nomenclature and coding), syntax, and message transfer. EUCLIDES has made a significant contribution to data-interchange standards through the development of the EUCLIDES Coding System. This coding system provides a multilingual, multiaxial, coded nomenclature designed for the unambiguous transfer of laboratory data between sites that does not disturb local usage of terminology at different sites. Coding lists contain all terms, including synonyms, that are in routine use in Europe in all branches of laboratory medicine.

The Electronic Data Interchange for Administration, Commerce, and Transport

The Electronic Data Interchange for Administration, Commerce and Transport (EDIFACT) is a set of international standards, projects, and guidelines for the electronic interchange of structured data related to trade in goods and services between independent computer-based information systems (NCPDP Data Dictionary, 1994). The standard includes application-level syntax rules, message-design guidelines, syntax-implementation guidelines, data-element dictionary, code list, composite data-elements dictionary, standard message dictionary, uniform rules of conduct for the interchange of trade data by transmission, and explanatory material.

The basic EDIFACT (ISO 9735) syntax standard was formally adopted in September 1987 and has undergone several updates. In addition to the common syntax, EDIFACT specifies standard messages (identified and structured sets of statements covering the requirements of specific transactions), segments (the groupings of functionally related data elements), data elements (the smallest items in a message that can convey data), and code sets (lists of codes for data elements). The ANSI ASC X12 standard is similar in purpose to EDIFACT, and work is underway to coordinate and merge the two standards.

EDIFACT is concerned not with the actual communications protocol but rather with the structuring of the data that are sent. EDIFACT is independent of the machine, media, system, and application and can be used with any communications protocol or with physical magnetic tape.

Standard Communications Protocol for Computer-Assisted Electrocardiography

Project Team PT 007 of TC 251 produced a prestandard for electrocardiogram (ECG) cart-to-host communication (Health Care Financial Management Association, 1993). The primary aim of this Standard Communications Protocol for Computer-Assisted Electrocardiography (SCP-ECG) is to ensure that ECG reports and data from any vendor's computer-based ECG recorder can be transmitted on a direct connected serial line to any other vendor's central ECG management system. The same standard would also allow standardized transmission of digitized ECG data and results between various computer systems. The standard supports the conventional 12-lead ECG and the vectorcardiogram. The current version does not accommodate body-surface mapping potentials, recordings of intracardiac potentials, Holter monitoring, or exercise ECG recordings.

The SPC-ECG specifies the content and structure of the information to be interchanged. Data-encoding and data-compression methodologies are defined. A minimum set of control and query messages for cart-to-cart and cart-to-host interchange is included. A low-level transport protocol between an ECG cart and a host based on an enhanced X-Modem protocol is specified. The message structure is based on a field tag, length, value format. The ECG data-interchange message includes patient identification, diagnoses, physician data, drugs, machine data, parameter measurements, and ECG data.

6.6 Today's Reality and Tomorrow's Directions

The development of standards is driven by perceived need and is influenced by the user community, vendors, consultants, and government. If a standard is developed as an academic exercise and is before its time, the standard is often unused. If a standard is too late in development, it is difficult to change the patterns of what people do. The pace of standards development is controlled by the rate at which vendors and users are willing to change. New technology often makes the acceptance of standards easier. Clearly, the demand for standards by those who are willing to pay define today's reality. Tomorrow's directions depend on predictions of for what users will be willing to pay.

6.6.1 The Interface: Standards and Workstations

Much of the early work in creating standards for data exchange was in the area of exchanging data between distributed systems, most often in the background and unsolicited. As the online use of information systems by professional users increases, and as the need to bring in data from distributed systems escalates, data-interchange standards requirements will expand to support a request mode, which will allow specific data elements from disparate sources to be integrated at the desktop.

Much of the work to date on data-interchange standards will certainly be useful in connecting health professionals' workstations to the rest of the world. We must recognize, however, that data-messaging standards have thus far focused primarily on exchanging medical data in a way that is largely driven by the desired function—to support an admission, test ordering, or results reporting. Only casual work has been done in developing standards for queries from users to such data sources. Queries will tend to return many more data than the workstations need unless new standards are developed. Should queries for workstations be based on the de facto database query standard, SQL (see Chapter 4)? If so, what modifications will be required to support queries from workstations while building on other ideas of data exchange?

User queries will need to identify the patient and either to request or transmit data elements to other components of the distributed environment. Query methods will be required to support a variety of scenarios: a single test value with date and time, a set of vital signs, a problem list, a list of allergies, a complete data set for an outpatient encounter, a complete data set for a hospitalization, current drugs, or a complete patient record. Invariably, each such exchange of data must control and pass along the patient's rights and wishes regarding access to and use of the data (see Chapter 7).

Standardized access to knowledge systems and bibliographic systems must support scripting and data-entry mechanisms to ensure that a data system can properly and accurately provide a response. Workstations typically permit cut and paste from one module to another; the data representation must thus accommodate a standard linkage to enable user-directed transfer between systems. The global use of decision-support systems will require high-speed query and response for the typically large number of data elements required to execute the decision logic, as well as high computational speeds to process the information and to provide an acceptable real-time response on the workstation.

Patient information will be retrieved not only by patient name or identification number but also by patient characteristics. For example, a physician at a workstation may ask for data on all patients who have coronary-artery disease with more than three-vessel involvement, who have had a myocardial infarction (heart attack), who are diabetic, who were treated surgically, and who have lived more than 5 years. The underlying system must use a variety of standards to translate this query into a manageable task, returning the correct data and preserving access constraints.

How good are the standards that are available today? What do users have to do to incorporate today's operational versions of standards into systems that they are implementing? First, much negotiation is necessary among vendors who are interfacing systems. There are two reasons for this need. Different parts of the various standards have different levels of maturity. For example, in HL7, the ADT version of the standard is defined more completely than is the observation-reporting section when the latter is used to transmit complete clinical data. Most of the standards are not complete, except for their support of some well-defined documents, such as insurance-claim forms. Standards are only now beginning to use an object-oriented model of the data to minimize ambiguity and to ensure completeness.[5] Vendors may interpret the use of a field differently, depending on their perspective or orientation. A billing vendor may understand the meaning of a field entirely differently from a clinical system vendor. The incompleteness of the standards—for example, in managing a complex set of trigger events—may lead one vendor to make assumptions not obvious to another vendor. The issue of optionality creates confusion and requires negotiation among vendors for a well-structured interface. Vocabulary standards also are not adequate for seamless interfaces. The second problem faced by vendors lies in the lower levels of the OSI reference model. Most of the standards bodies are now addressing the lower levels by

[5]See the HL7 website at http://www.hl7.org for more details.

defining strategies and rules for the lower-level protocols, most frequently using TCP/IP rather than pure OSI protocols.

From a user's perspective, the problem lies in how closely the vendor's implementation adheres to the standard. In many cases, the vendor defines standard compliance loosely, and the user purchases a system that cannot be easily interfaced. The only solution to this problem is certification by some agency—an unpopular task at best. Legal concerns and the difficulty of certifying compliance to the standards are obstacles that must be overcome.

Do today's standards reduce costs? The answer depends on the vendor. Some vendors charge little or nothing for standard interfaces; others charge the same as they do for custom interfaces. Over time, however, the cost of the interface will be driven down considerably by the users. In the case of imaging standards, the standards are necessary to develop the market for displaying images in a variety of settings.

6.6.2 Future Directions

The General Accounting Office reported in a study from the early 1990s that several hundred standards would be required by the healthcare industry (United States General Accounting Office, 1993). Other authors have estimated the numbers to be in the thousands. We believe that the most probable need will be 20 to 30 standards. One problem in trying to standardize everything is the conflict between a standard and the opportunity for a vendor to use creativity in a product to enhance sales. Standards should not stifle creativity but rather encourage it. For example, standardization of the screen displays for a computer-based patient-record system is unlikely to occur, because individual vendors have different beliefs about the best designs. On the other hand, it is likely that components of the displays may be standardized. The use of the mouse (e.g., single and double clicks, right and left clicks) needs to be standardized in function. The use of visual objects also needs to be (and can be) standardized. It is likely that icons that represent functions also will be standardized in time.

At the present time, standards do not exist to support fully the requirements of health-professional workstations. A standard is necessary whenever someone other than the originator of the data must understand and use the data received electronically. For seamless electronic interchange of clinical data, standard formats need to be defined to include all types of data representation—images, signals and waveforms, sound and voice, and video, including motion video. Other candidate issues where the definition of standards would be helpful include specifying the location of data (in terms of both physical location and database characteristics) and defining the rules for the retention of data and for tighter coupling of data.

Core data sets for healthcare specialty groups and defined healthcare scenarios are likely candidates for standardization. The Centers for Disease Control and Prevention, for example, has defined a set of standard codes for the emergency department. Forms, such as discharge summaries, operative notes, and so on, can be exchanged meaningfully between organizations if they use a standard format.

Decision-support algorithms and clinical guidelines will be more widely used and accepted if they go through a consensus standardization process.

The future of messaging standards seems bright. The prevailing attitude in all the existing standards groups—in Europe and in the United States—favors developing workable standards so that we can solve new problems. Participants favor working together; proprietary and "not-invented-here" concerns are minimal. The willingness to separate data content from syntax is important. The development of a common, global data model is critical. Definitions of vocabulary, coding, and standard data structures are approaching reality. Clearly, the goals of "plug and play" have not yet been realized, but they may be obtainable within the next few years.

Suggested Readings

Abbey L.M., Zimmerman J. (Eds.) (1991). *Dental Informatics: Integrating Technology into the Dental Environment.* New York: Springer-Verlag.

This text demonstrates that the issues of standards extend throughout the areas of application of medical informatics. The standards issues discussed in this chapter for clinical medicine are shown to be equally pertinent for dentistry.

Chute C.G. (1998). *Electronic Medical Record Infrastructures: An Overview of Critical Standards and Classifications.* New York: Springer-Verlag.

This text provides more in-depth coverage of the structure, content, and issues related to coded terminologies, nomenclatures, and vocabularies in health care.

Stallings W. (1987). *Handbook of Computer-Communications Standards.* New York: Macmillan Publishing Company.

This text provides excellent details on the Open Systems Interconnection mode of the International Standards Organization.

Stallings W. (1997). *Data and Computer Communications.* Englewood Cliffs, NJ: Prentice Hall.

This text provides details on communications architecture and protocols and on local and wide area networks.

Steedman D. (1990). *Abstract Syntax Notation One: The Tutorial and Reference.* Great Britain: Technology Appraisals Ltd.

This text is definitive on the definition and content of Abstract Syntax Notation One (ASN.1) and includes illustrative examples.

Questions for Discussion

1. What are five possible approaches to accelerating the creation of standards?
2. Define five healthcare standards, not mentioned in the chapter, that might also be needed?
3. What role should the government play in the creation of standards?
4. At what level might a standard interfere with a vendor's ability to produce a unique product?
5. Define a hypothetical standard for one of the areas mentioned in the text for which no current standard exists. Include the conceptualization and discussion points. Specifically state the scope of the standard.

7
Ethics and Health Informatics: Users, Standards, and Outcomes

KENNETH W. GOODMAN AND RANDOLPH A. MILLER

After reading this chapter, you should know the answers to these questions:

- Why is ethics important to informatics?
- What are the leading ethical issues that arise in healthcare informatics?
- What are examples of appropriate and inappropriate uses and users for health-related software?
- Why does the establishment of standards touch on ethical issues?
- Why does system evaluation involve ethical issues?
- What challenges does informatics pose for patient and provider confidentiality?
- How can the tension between the obligation to protect confidentiality and that to share data be minimized?
- How might computational health care alter the traditional provider–patient relationship?
- What ethical issues arise at the intersection of informatics and managed care?
- What are the leading issues in the debate over governmental regulation of healthcare computing tools?

7.1 Ethical Issues in Health Informatics

> More and more the tendency is towards the use of mechanical aids to diagnosis; nevertheless, the five senses of the doctor do still, and must always, play the preponderating part in the examination of the sick patient. Careful observation can never be replaced by the tests of the laboratory. The good physician now or in the future will never be a diagnostic robot.
>
> —The surgeon Sir William Arbuthnot Lane, writing in the November 1936 issue of *New Health*

Human values should govern research and practice in the health professions. Healthcare informatics, like other health professions, encompasses issues of appropriate and inappropriate behavior, of honorable and disreputable actions, and of right and wrong. Students and practitioners of the health sciences, including informatics, share an important obligation to explore the moral underpinnings and ethical challenges related to their research and practice.

Although ethical questions in medicine, nursing, human-subjects research, psychology, social work, and affiliated fields continue to evolve, the key issues are generally well known. Major questions in bioethics have been addressed in numerous professional, scholarly, and educational contexts. Ethical matters in health informatics are, in general, less familiar, even though certain of them have received attention for decades (de Dombal, 1987; Miller et al., 1985; Szolovits & Pauker, 1979). Indeed, informatics now constitutes a source of some of the most important and interesting ethical debates in all the health professions.

People often assume that the confidentiality of electronically stored patient information is the primary source of ethical attention in informatics. Although confidentiality and privacy are indeed of vital importance and significant concern, the field is rich with other ethical issues, including the appropriate selection and use of informatics tools in clinical settings; the determination of who should use such tools; the role of system evaluation; the obligations of system developers, maintainers, and vendors; and the use of computers to track clinical outcomes to guide future practice. In addition, informatics engenders many important legal and regulatory questions.

To consider ethical issues in healthcare informatics is to explore a significant intersection among several professions—healthcare delivery and administration, applied computing, and ethics—each of which is a vast field of inquiry. Fortunately, growing interest in bioethics and computer-related ethics has produced a starting point for such exploration. An initial ensemble of guiding principles, or ethical criteria, has emerged to orient decision-making in healthcare informatics. These criteria are of practical utility to health informatics.

7.2 Health-Informatics Applications: Appropriate Use, Users, and Contexts

Application of computer-based technologies in the health professions can build on previous experience in adopting other devices, tools, and methods. Before they perform most health-related interventions (e.g., genetic testing, prescription of medication, surgical and other therapeutic procedures), clinicians generally evaluate appropriate evidence, standards, presuppositions, and values. Indeed, the very evolution of the health professions entails the evolution of evidence, of standards, of presuppositions, and of values.

To answer the clinical question "What should be done in this case?" we must pay attention to a number of subsidiary questions, such as

1. What is the problem?
2. What am I competent to do?
3. What will produce the most desirable results?
4. What will maintain or improve patient care?

5. How strong are my beliefs in the accuracy of my answers to questions 1 through 4?

Similar considerations determine the appropriate use of informatics tools.

7.2.1 The Standard View of Appropriate Use

Excitement often accompanies initial use of computer-based tools in clinical settings. Based on the uncertainties that surround any new technology, however, scientific evidence counsels caution and prudence. As in other clinical areas, evidence and reason determine the appropriate level of caution. For instance, there is considerable evidence that electronic laboratory information systems improve access to clinical data when compared with manual, paper-based test-result distribution methods. To the extent that such systems improve care at an acceptable cost in time and money, there is an obligation to use computers to store and retrieve clinical laboratory results. There is less evidence, however, that existing (circa 2000) **clinical expert systems** can improve patient care in typical practice settings at an acceptable cost in time and money.

Clinical expert systems (see Chapter 16) are intended to provide decision support for diagnosis and therapy more detailed and sophisticated than that provided by simple reminder systems (Duda & Shortliffe, 1983). Creation of expert systems and maintenance of related knowledge bases still involves leading-edge research and development. It is also important to recognize that humans are still superior to electronic systems at understanding patients and their problems, at efficient collection of pertinent data across the spectrum of clinical practice, at the interpretation and representation of data, and at clinical synthesis. Humans may always be superior at these tasks, although such a claim must be subjected to empirical testing from time to time.

What has been called the *standard view* of computer-assisted clinical diagnosis (Miller, 1990) holds in part that human cognitive processes, being more suited to the complex task of diagnosis than machine intelligence, should not be overridden or trumped by computers. The standard view states that, when adequate (and even exemplary) decision-support tools are developed, they should be viewed and used as supplementary and subservient to human clinical judgment. They should take this role because the clinician caring for the patient knows and understands the patient's situation and can make compassionate judgments better than can computer programs; they are also the individuals whom the state licenses, and specialty boards accredit, to practice medicine, surgery, nursing, pharmacy, or other health-related activities. Corollaries of the standard view are that (1) practitioners have an obligation to use any computer-based tool responsibly, through adequate user training and by developing an understanding of the system's abilities and limitations; and (2) practitioners must not abrogate their clinical judgment reflexively when using computer-based decision aids. Because the skills required for diagnosis are in many respects different from those required for the acquisition, storage, and retrieval of laboratory data, there is no contradiction in urging extensive use of electronic laboratory information systems, but cautious or limited use (for the time being) of expert diagnostic decision-support tools.

The standard view addresses one aspect of the question, "How and when should computers be used in clinical practice?" by capturing important moral intuitions about error avoidance and evolving standards. Error avoidance and the benefits that follow from it shape the obligations of practitioners. In computer-software use, as in all other areas of clinical practice, good intentions alone may be insufficient to insulate recklessness from culpability. Thus, the standard view may be seen as a tool for both error avoidance and ethically optimized action.

Ethical software use is evaluated against a broad background of evidence for actions that produce favorable outcomes. Because informatics is a science in extraordinary ferment, system improvements and evidence of such improvements are constantly emerging. Clinicians have an obligation to be familiar with this evidence after attaining minimal acceptable levels of familiarity with informatics in general and with the clinical systems they use in particular.

7.2.2 Appropriate Users and Educational Standards

Efficient and effective use of healthcare informatics systems requires training, experience, and education. Indeed, such requirements resemble those for other tools used in health care and in other domains. Inadequate preparation in the use of tools is an invitation to catastrophe. When the stakes are high and the domain large and complex—as is the case in the health professions—education and training take on moral significance.

Who should use a healthcare-related computer application? Consider expert decision-support systems as an example. An early paper on ethical issues in informatics noted that potential users of such systems include physicians, nurses, physicians' assistants, paramedical personnel, students of the health sciences, patients, and insurance and government evaluators (Miller et al., 1985). Are members of all these groups appropriate users? We cannot answer the question until we are clear about the precise intended use for the system (i.e., the exact clinical questions the system will address). The appropriate level of training must be correlated with the question at hand. At one end of an appropriate-use spectrum, we can posit that medical and nursing students should employ decision-support systems for educational purposes; this assertion is relatively free of controversy once it has been verified that such tools convey accurately a sufficient quantity and quality of educational content. But it is less clear that patients, administrators, or managed-care gatekeepers, for example, should use expert decision-support systems for assistance in making diagnoses, in selecting therapies, or in evaluating the appropriateness of health professionals' actions. To the extent that some systems present general medical advice in hypermedia format, such as might occur with Dr. Spock's print-based child-care primer, use by laypersons may be condoned. There are additional legal concerns related to negligence and product liability, however, when health-related products are sold directly to patients rather than to licensed practitioners and when such products give patient-specific counsel rather than general clinical advice.

Suitable use of a software program that helps a user to suggest diagnoses, to select therapies, or to render prognoses must be plotted against an array of goals and best practices for achieving those goals, including consideration of the characteristics and requirements of individual patients. For example, the multiply interconnected inferential strategies required for arriving at an accurate diagnosis depend on knowledge of facts; experience with procedures; and familiarity with human behavior, motivation, and values. **Diagnosis** is a process, rather than an event (Miller, 1990), so even well-validated diagnostic systems must be used appropriately in the overall context of patient care.

To use a diagnostic decision-support system, the clinician must be able to recognize when the computer program has erred, and, when it is accurate, what the output means and how it should be interpreted. This ability requires knowledge of both the diagnostic sciences and the software applications and their limitations. After assigning a diagnostic label, the clinician must communicate the diagnosis, prognosis, and implications to a patient and must do so in ways both appropriate to the patient's educational background and conducive to future treatment goals. It is not enough to be able to tell patients that they have cancer, human immunodeficiency virus (HIV), diabetes, or heart disease and simply to hand over a number of prescriptions. The care provider must also offer context when available, comfort when needed, and hope as appropriate. The reason many jurisdictions require pretest and post-test HIV counseling, for instance, is not to vex busy health professionals but rather to ensure that comprehensive, high-quality care—rather than just diagnostic labeling—has been delivered.

This discussion points to the following set of ethical principles for appropriate use of decision-support systems:

1. A computer program should be used in clinical practice only after appropriate evaluation of its efficacy and documentation that it performs its intended task at an acceptable cost in time and money.
2. Users of most clinical systems should be health professionals who are qualified to address the question at hand on the basis of their licensure, clinical training, and experience. Software systems should be used to augment or supplement, rather than to replace or supplant, such individuals' decision-making.
3. All uses of informatics tools, especially in patient care, should be preceded by adequate training and instruction, which should include review of all available forms of previous product evaluations.

Such principles and claims should be thought of as analogous to other standards or rules in clinical medicine and nursing.

7.2.3 Obligations and Standards for System Developers and Maintainers

Users of clinical programs must rely on the work of other people who are often far removed from the context of use. Users depend on the developers and maintainers of a system and must trust evaluators who have validated a system for clinical use. Healthcare software applications are among the most complex tools in the technological armamentarium. Although this complexity imposes certain obligations on end users, it also commits a system's developers, designers, and maintainers to adhere to reasonable standards and, indeed, to acknowledge their moral responsibility for doing so.

Ethics, Standards, and Scientific Progress

The very idea of a **standard of care** embodies a number of complex assumptions linking ethics, evidence, outcomes, and professional training. To say that a nurse or physician must adhere to a standard is to say, in part, that she ought not to stray from procedures that have been shown or are generally believed to work better than other procedures. Whether a procedure or device "works better" than another can be difficult to determine. Such determinations in the health sciences constitute progress and indicate that we know more than we used to know. Criteria for evidence and proof are applied. Evidence from randomized controlled trials is preferable to evidence from uncontrolled retrospective studies, and verification by independent investigators is required before the most recent reports are put into common practice.

People who develop, maintain, and sell healthcare computing systems and components have obligations that parallel those of system users. These obligations include holding patient care as the leading value. The Hippocratic injunction *primum non nocere* (first do no harm) applies to developers as well as to practitioners. Although this principle is easy to suggest and, generally, to defend, it invites subtle, and sometimes overt, resistance from people who hold profit or fame as primary motivators. To be sure, quests for fame and fortune often produce good outcomes and improved care, at least eventually. Even so, that approach fails to take into account the role of intention as a moral criterion.

In medicine and nursing, a number of models of the **professional–patient relationship** place trust and advocacy at the apex of a hierarchy of values. Such a stance cannot be maintained if goals and intentions other than patient well-being are (generally) assigned primacy. The same principles apply to people who produce and attend to healthcare information systems. Because these systems are *healthcare* systems—and are not devices for accounting, entertainment, real estate, and so on—and because the domain is shaped by pain, vulnerability, illness, and death, it is essential that the threads of trust run throughout the fabric of clinical system design and maintenance.

System purchasers, users, and patients must trust developers and maintainers to recognize the potentially grave consequences of errors or carelessness, trust them to care about the uses to which the systems will be put, and trust them to value the reduced suffering of other people at least as much as they value their own personal gain. We emphatically do not mean to suggest that system designers and maintainers are blameworthy or unethical if they hope and strive to profit from their diligence, creativity, and effort. Rather, we suggest that no amount of financial benefit for a designer can counterbalance bad outcomes or ill consequences that result from recklessness, avarice, or inattention to the needs of clinicians and their patients.

Quality standards should stimulate scientific progress and innovation while safeguarding against system error and abuse. These goals might seem incompatible, but they are not. Let us postulate a standard that requires timely updating and testing of knowledge bases that are used by decision-support systems. To the extent that database accuracy is needed to maximize the accuracy of inferential engines, it is trivially clear how such a standard will help to prevent decision-support mistakes. Furthermore, the standard should be seen to foster progress and innovation in the same way that any insistence on best possible accuracy helps to protect scientists and clinicians from pursuing false leads or wasting time in testing poorly wrought hypotheses. It will not do for a database maintainer to insist that he is busy doing the more productive or scientifically stimulating work of improving knowledge representation, say, or database design. Although such tasks are important, they do not supplant the tasks of updating and testing tools in their current configuration or structure. Put differently, scientific and technical standards are perfectly able to stimulate progress while taking a cautious or even conservative stance toward permissible risk in patient care.

This approach has been described as "progressive caution": "Medical informatics is, happily, here to stay, but users and society have extensive responsibilities to ensure that we use our tools appropriately. This might cause us to move more deliberately or slowly than some would like. Ethically speaking, that is just too bad" (Goodman, 1998b).

System Evaluation as an Ethical Imperative

Any move toward "best practices" in health informatics is shallow and feckless if it does not include a way to measure whether a system performs as intended. This and related measurements provide the grounding for quality control and, as such, are the obligations of system developers, maintainers, users, administrators, and perhaps other players (see Chapter 8).

> Medical computing is not merely about medicine or computing. It is about the introduction of new tools into environments with established social norms and practices. The effects of computing systems in health care are subject to analysis not only of accuracy and performance but of acceptance by users, of consequences for social and professional interaction, and of the context of use. We suggest that system evaluation can illuminate social and ethical issues in medical computing, and in so doing improve patient care. That being the case, there is an ethical imperative for such evaluation. (Anderson & Aydin, 1998)

To give a flavor of how a comprehensive evaluation program can ethically optimize implementation and use of an informatics system, consider these 10 criteria for system scrutiny (Anderson & Aydin, 1994):

1. Does the system work as designed?
2. Is it used as anticipated?
3. Does it produce the desired results?
4. Does it work better than the procedures it replaced?
5. Is it cost effective?
6. How well have individuals been trained to use it?
7. What are the anticipated long-term effects on how departments interact?
8. What are the long-term effects on the delivery of medical care?
9. Will the system have an impact on control in the organization?
10. To what extent do effects depend on practice setting?

Another way to look at this important point is that *people* use computer systems. Even the finest system might be misused, misunderstood, or mistakenly allowed to alter or erode previously productive human relationships. Evaluation of health-information systems in their contexts of use should be taken as a moral imperative. Such evaluations require consideration of a broader conceptualization of "what works best" and must look toward improving the overall healthcare delivery system rather than only that system's technologically based components. These higher goals entail the creation of a corresponding mechanism for ensuring institutional oversight and responsibility (Miller & Gardner, 1997a,b).

7.3 Privacy, Confidentiality, and Data Sharing

Some of the greatest challenges of the Information Age arise from placing computer applications in healthcare settings while upholding traditional principles. One challenge involves balancing two competing values: free *access* to information and protection of patients' **privacy** and **confidentiality.**

Only computers can manage the vast amount of information generated during clinical encounters and other healthcare transactions; at least in principle, such information should be easily available to health professionals so that they can care for patients effectively. Yet, making this information readily available creates opportunities for access by extraneous individuals. Access may be available to curious healthcare workers who do not need the information to fulfill job-related responsibilities, and, even more worrisome, to other people who might use the information to harm patients physically, emotionally, or financially. Seemingly, clinical system administrators must therefore choose between either improving care through use of computer systems or protecting confidentiality by restricting use of computer systems. Fortunately, it is a mistake to view these objectives as incompatible.

7.3.1 Foundations of Health Privacy and Confidentiality

Privacy and confidentiality are necessary for people to mature as individuals, to form relationships, and to serve as functioning members of society. Imagine what would happen if the local newspaper produced a daily account detailing everyone's actions, meetings, and conversations! It is not that most people have terrible secrets to hide but rather that the concepts of solitude, intimacy, and the desire to be left alone make no sense without the expectation that our actions and words will be kept private and held in confidence.

The terms *privacy* and *confidentiality* are not synonymous. *Privacy* generally applies to people, including their desire not to suffer eavesdropping, whereas *confidentiality* is best applied to information. One way to think of the difference is as follows: If someone follows you and spies on you entering an AIDS clinic, your privacy is violated; if someone sneaks into the clinic and looks at your healthcare record, your record's confidentiality is breached. In discussions of the electronic healthcare record, the term *privacy* may also refer to individuals' desire to restrict the disclosure of personal data (National Research Council, 1997).

There are several important reasons to protect privacy and confidentiality. One is that privacy and confidentiality are widely regarded as *rights* of all people, and such protections help to accord them respect. On this account, people do not need to provide a justification for keeping their health data secret; privacy and confidentiality are entitlements that a person does not need to earn, to argue for, or to defend. Another reason is more practical: Protecting privacy and confidentiality benefits both individuals and society. Patients who know that their healthcare data will not be shared inappropriately are more comfortable disclosing those data to clinicians. This trust is vital for the successful physician–patient or nurse–patient relationship, and it helps practitioners to do their jobs.

Privacy and confidentiality protections also benefit public health. People who fear disclosure of personal information are less likely to seek out professional assistance, increasing the risks that contagion will be spread and maladies will go untreated. In addition, and sadly, people still suffer discrimination, bias, and stigma when certain health data do fall into the wrong hands. Financial harm may occur if insurers are given unlimited access to family members' records, or access to patients' genetic-testing results, because some insurers might be tempted to increase the price of insurance for individuals at higher risk of illness.

The ancient idea that physicians should hold healthcare information in confidence is therefore applicable whether the data are written on paper, etched in stone, or embedded in silicon. The obligations to protect privacy and to keep confidences fall to system designers and maintainers, to administrators, and, ultimately, to the physicians, nurses, and other people who elicit the information in the first place. The upshot for all of them is this: Protection of privacy and confidentiality is not an option, a favor, or a helping hand offered to patients with embarrassing healthcare problems; it is a duty that does not vary with the malady or the data-storage medium.

Some sound clinical practice and public-health traditions run counter to the idea of absolute confidentiality. When a patient is hospitalized, it is expected that all appropriate (and no inappropriate) employees of the institution—primary-care physicians, consultants, nurses, therapists, and technicians—will be given access to the patient's medical records when it is in the interest of patient care to do so. In most communities of the United States, the contacts of patients who have active tuberculosis or certain sexually transmitted diseases are routinely identified so that they may receive proper medical attention; the public interest is protected because the likelihood is decreased that they will transmit an infection unknowingly to other people. In addition, it is essential for healthcare researchers to be able to pool data from patient cases that meet specified conditions to determine the natural history of disease and the effects of various treatments. Examples of benefits from such pooled data analyses range from the ongoing results generated by regional collaborative chemotherapy trials to the discovery, more than two decades ago, of the appropriateness of shorter lengths of stay for patients with myocardial infarction (McNeer et al., 1975).

7.3.2 Electronic Clinical and Research Data

Access to electronic patient records holds extraordinary promise for clinicians and for other people who need timely, accurate patient data. Institutions that are not using computer-based patient records may be falling behind, a position that may eventually become blameworthy. On the other hand, systems that make it easy for clinicians to access data also make it easy for other people to access it. Failure to prevent inappropriate access is at least as wrong as failure to provide adequate and appropriate access. It might therefore seem that the computer-based patient record imposes contradictory burdens on system overseers and users.

In fact, there is no contradiction between the obligation to maintain a certain standard of care (in this case, regarding minimal levels of computer use) and ensuring that such a technical standard does not imperil the rights of patients. Threats to confidentiality and privacy are fairly well known. They include economic abuses, or discrimination by third-party payers, employers, and others who take advantage of the burgeoning market in health data; insider abuse, or record snooping by hospital or clinic workers who are not directly involved in a patient's care but examine a record out of curiosity, for blackmail, and so on; and malevolent hackers, or people who, via networks or other means, copy, delete, or alter confidential information (National Research Council, 1997). Indeed, the National Research Council has noted problems arising from widespread dissemination of information throughout the healthcare system—dissemination that often occurs without explicit patient consent. Healthcare providers, third-party payers, managers of pharmaceutical benefits programs, equipment suppliers, and oversight organizations collect large amounts of patient-identifiable health information for use in managing care, conducting quality and utilization reviews, processing claims, combating fraud, and analyzing markets for health products and services (National Research Council, 1997).

The proper approach to such challenges is one that will ensure both that (1) appropriate clinicians and other people have rapid, easy access to patient records and that (2) other people do not have access. Is that another contradictory burden? No. There are several ways to restrict inappropriate access to electronic records. They are generally divided into technological methods and institutional or policy approaches (Alpert, 1998):

- *Technological methods:* Computers can provide the means for maximizing their own security, including authenticating users, by making sure that users are who they say they are; prohibiting people without a professional need from accessing health information; and using audit trails, or logs, of people who do inspect confidential records so that patients and other people can review the logs.
- *Policy approaches:* The National Research Council has recommended that hospitals and other healthcare organizations create security and confidentiality committees and establish education and training programs. These recommendations parallel an approach that has worked well elsewhere in hospitals for matters ranging from infection control to bioethics.

Such recommendations are all the more important when health data are accessible through networks. The rapid growth of **integrated delivery networks** (IDNs) (see Chapter 10) and **community health information networks** (CHINs), for example, illustrates the need to view health data not as a well into which one drops a bucket but rather as an irrigation system that makes its contents available over a broad—sometimes an *extremely* broad—area. It is not yet clear whether privacy and confidentiality protections that are appropriate in hospitals will be valid in a networked environment. System developers, users, and administrators are obliged to identify appropriate measures. There is no excuse for failing to make ethics a top priority throughout the data-storage and sharing environment.

Electronic Data and Human Subjects Research

The use of patient information for **clinical research** and for quality assessment raises interesting ethical challenges. The presumption of a right to confidentiality seems to include the idea that patient records are inextricably linked to patient names or to other identifying data. In an optimal environment, then, patients can monitor who is looking at *their* records. But if all unique identifiers have been stripped from the records, is there any sense in talking about confidentiality?

The benefits to **public health** loom large in considering record-based research. A valuable benefit of the electronic healthcare record is the ability to access vast numbers of patient records to determine the incidence and prevalence of various maladies, to track the efficacy of clinical interventions, and to plan efficient resource allocation (see Chapter 11). Such research and planning would, however, impose onerous or intractable burdens if informed or valid consent had to be obtained from every patient whose record was represented in the sample. To cite confidentiality as an impediment to all such research is to stand on ceremony that not only fails to protect patients but also forecloses on potentially beneficial scientific investigations.

A more practical course is to establish safeguards that optimize the research ethically. This goal can be reached via a number of paths. The first is to establish mechanisms to anonymize the information in individual records or to decouple the data contained in the records from any unique patient identifiers. This task is not always straightforward: A specific job description ("this 30-year-old starting quarterback of the Wildcats professional football team was admitted with a shattered collarbone"), or a rare disease diagnosis coupled with demographic data, or a nine-digit postal code may act as a surrogate unique identifier; that is, detailed information can serve as a data fingerprint that picks out an individual patient even though the patient's name, Social Security number, or other (official) unique identifier has been removed from the record.

Such challenges point to a second means of optimizing database research ethically: the use of institutional panels, such as **medical-record committees** or institutional review boards. Submission of database research to appropriate institutional scrutiny is one way to make the best use of more or less anonymous electronic patient data. Competent panel members should be educated in the research potential of electronic healthcare records, as well as in ethical issues in epidemiology and public health. Scrutiny by such committees could also ethically optimize internal research for quality control, outcomes monitoring, and so on (Goodman, 1998b; Miller & Gardner, 1997a,b).

Challenges in Bioinformatics

Safeguards are increasingly likely to be challenged as genetic information makes its way into the healthcare record (see Chapter 18). The risks of bias, discrimination, and social stigma increase dramatically as **genetic data** become available to clinicians and investigators. Indeed, genetic information "goes beyond the ordinary varieties of medical information in its predictive value" (Macklin, 1992). Genetic data also may be valuable to people predicting outcomes, allocating resources, and the like (Table 7.1). In addition, genetic data are rarely associated with only a single person; they may provide information about relatives, including relatives who do not want to know about their genetic makeup or maladies, as well as relatives who would love dearly to know more about their kin's genome. There is still much work to be done in sorting out and addressing the ethical issues related to electronic storage, sharing, and retrieval of genetic data (Goodman, 1996).

Bioinformatics offers excellent opportunities to increase our knowledge of genetics, genetic diseases, and public health. These opportunities, however, are accompanied by responsibilities to attend to the ethical issues raised by methods, applications, and consequences.

TABLE 7.1. Correlation of clinical findings with genetic data.[a]

Syndrome	Number of signs	Clinical findings
Atkin-Flaitz	3	Short stature, Obesity, Hypertelorism
Young-Hughes	2	Short stature, Obesity
Vasquez	2	Short stature, Obestity
Stoll	2	Short stature, Obesity
Simpson-Golabi-Behemel	2	Obesity, Hypertelorism
Otopalato-Digital	2	Short stature, Hypertelorism
FG	2	Short stature, Hypertelorism
Chudley	2	Short stature, Obesity
Borjeson	2	Short stature, Obesity
Albright Hereditary Osteodystrophy	2	Short stature, Obesity
Aarskog	2	Short stature, Hypertelorism

[a]Databases with genetic information can be used to help correlate clinical findings with diagnoses of genetic maladies. Here are the results of a "Make Diagnosis" query based on short stature, obesity, and hypertelorism (abnormally large distance between paired organs, especially eyes) performed on the X-Linked Recessive Mental Retardation Database at the University of Miami. (*Source:* Division of Genetics, Department of Pediatrics, University of Miami School of Medicine.)

7.4 Social Challenges and Ethical Obligations

The expansion of **evidence-based medicine** and, in the United States, of managed care places a high premium on the tools of health informatics. The need for data on clinical outcomes is driven by a number of important social and scientific factors. Perhaps the most important among these factors is the increasing unwillingness of governments and insurers to pay for interventions and therapies that do not work or that do not work well enough to justify their cost.

Health informatics helps clinicians, administrators, third-party payers, governments, researchers, and other parties to collect, store, retrieve, analyze, and scrutinize vast amounts of data. Such tasks may be undertaken not for the sake of any individual patient but rather for cost analysis and review, quality assessment, scientific research, and so forth. These functions are important, and, if computers can improve their quality or accuracy, then so much the better. Challenges arise when intelligent machines are mistaken for decision-making surrogates or when institutional or public policy recommends or demands that computer output stand proxy for human cognition.

7.4.1 Informatics and Managed Care

Consider the extraordinary utility of **prognostic scoring systems** or machines that use physiological and mortality data to compare new critical-care patients with thousands of previous patients (Knaus et al., 1991). Such systems allow hospitals to track the performance of their critical-care units by, say, comparing the previous year's outcomes to this year's or by comparing one hospital to another. If, for instance, patients with a particular profile tend to survive longer than their predecessors, then it might be inferred that **critical care** has improved. Such scoring systems can be useful for internal research and for quality management (Fig. 7.1).

Now suppose that most previous patients with a particular physiological profile have died in critical-care units. This information might be used to identify ways to improve care of such patients—or it might be used in support of arguments to contain costs by denying care to subsequent patients fitting the profile.

An argument in support of such a nonresearch application might be that decisions to withdraw or withhold care are often and customarily made on the basis of subjective and fragmented evidence; so it is preferable to make such decisions on the basis of objective data of the sort that otherwise underly sound clinical practice. Such **outcomes data** are precisely what fuels the engines of managed care, wherein health professionals and institutions compete on the basis of cost and outcomes (see Chapter 19). Why, people may argue, should society, or a managed-care organization, or an insurance company pay for critical care when there is objective evidence that such care will not be efficacious? Contrarily, consider the effect of denying care to such patients on the basis of future scientific insights. Scientific progress is often made by noticing that certain patients do

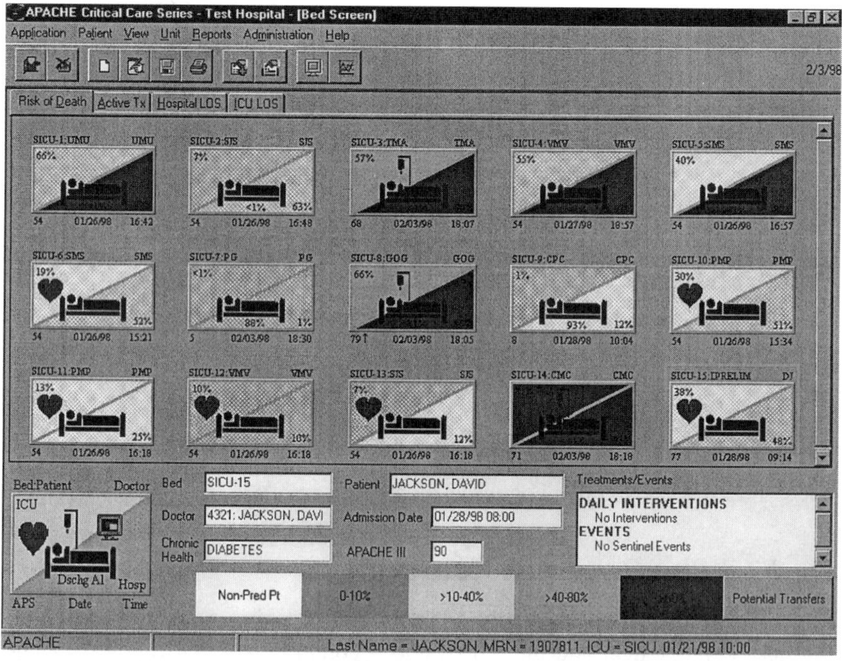

Figure 7.1. "Risk of Death" screen image from the APACHE III Critical Care Series. Using APACHE, clinicians in the intensive-care units are able to monitor critical events and required interventions, and administrators are able to manage the units' staffing based on the acuity of the patients on the units. (*Source:* Courtesy of APACHE Medical Systems, Inc.)

better under certain circumstances, and investigation of such phenomena leads to better treatments. If all patients meeting certain criteria were denied therapy on the basis of a predictive tool, it would become a self-fulfilling prophecy for a much longer time that all such patients would not do well.

Now consider use of a decision-support system to evaluate, review, or challenge decisions by human clinicians; indeed, imagine an insurance company using a diagnostic expert system to determine whether a physician should be reimbursed for a particular procedure. If the expert system has a track record for accuracy and reliability, and if the system "disagrees" with the human's diagnosis or treatment plan, then the insurance company can contend that reimbursement for the procedure would be a mistake. After all, why pay a provider for doing a procedure that is not indicated, at least according to the computer?

In the two examples just offered (a prognostic scoring system is used to justify termination of treatment to conserve resources, and a diagnostic expert system is used to deny a physician reimbursement for procedures deemed inappropriate), there seems to be justification for adhering to the computer output. There are, however, three reasons why it is problematic to use clinical computer programs to guide policy or practice in these ways:

1. As we saw earlier with the standard view of computational diagnosis (and, by easy extension, prognosis), human cognition is still superior to machine intelligence. The act of rendering a diagnosis or prognosis is not merely a statistical operation performed on uninterpreted data. Rather, identifying a malady and predicting its course requires understanding a complex ensemble of causal relations, interactions among a large number of variables, and having a store of salient background knowledge.
2. Decisions about whether to treat a given patient are often value laden and must be made relative to treatment goals. In other words, it might be that a treatment will improve the quality of life but not extend life, or vice versa (Youngner, 1988). Whether such treatment is appropriate cannot be determined scientifically or statistically (Brody, 1989).
3. Applying computational operations on aggregate data to individual patients runs the risk of including individuals in groups they resemble but to which they do not actually belong. Of course, human clinicians run this risk all the time—the challenge of inferring correctly that an individual is a member of a set, group, or class is one of the oldest problems in logic and in the philosophy of science. The point is that computers have not solved this problem, yet, and allowing policy to be guided by simple or unanalyzed correlations constitutes a conceptual error.

The idea is not that diagnostic or prognostic computers are always wrong—we know that they are not—but rather there are numerous instances in which we do not know whether they are right. It is one thing to allow aggregate data to guide policy; doing so is just using scientific evidence to maximize good outcomes. But it is altogether different to require that a policy disallow individual **clinical judgment** and expertise.

Informatics can contribute in many ways to healthcare reform. Indeed, computer-based tools can help to illuminate ways to reduce costs, to optimize clinical outcomes, and to improve care. Scientific research, quality assessment, and the like are, for the most part, no longer possible without computers. But it does not follow that the insights from such research apply in all instances to the myriad variety of actual clinical cases at which competent human clinicians excel.

7.4.2 *Effects of Informatics on Traditional Relationships*

Patients are often sick, scared, and vulnerable. Treating illness, easing fear, and respecting vulnerability are among the core obligations of physicians and nurses. The growth of health informatics should be seen as posing exciting challenges to complement these traditional duties and the relationships that the duties govern. We have pointed out that medical decisions are shaped by nonscientific considerations. This point is important when we assess the effects of informatics on human relationships. Thus:

> The practice of medicine or nursing is not exclusively and clearly scientific, statistical, or procedural, and hence is not, so far, computationally tractable. This is not to make a hoary appeal to the "art and science" of medicine; it is to say that the science is in many contexts inadequate or inapplicable: Many clinical decisions are not exclusively medical—they have social, personal, ethical, psychological, financial, familial, legal, and other components; even art might play a role. (Miller & Goodman, 1998)

Professional–Patient Relationships

If computers, databases, and networks can improve physician–patient or nurse–patient relationships, perhaps by improving communication, then we shall have achieved a happy result. If reliance on computers impedes the abilities of health professionals to establish trust and to communicate compassionately, however, or further contributes to the dehumanization of patients (Shortliffe, 1994), then we may have paid too dearly for our use of these machines.

Suppose that a physician uses a decision-support system to test a diagnostic hypothesis or to generate differential diagnoses, and suppose further that a decision to order a particular test or treatment is based on that system's output. A physician who is not able to articulate the proper role of computational support in his decision to treat or test will risk alienating those patients who, for one reason or another, will be disappointed, angered, or confused by the use of computers in their care. To be sure, he might just withhold this information from patients, but such deception carries its own threats to trust in the relationship.

Patients are not completely ignorant about the processes that constitute human decision-making. What they do understand, however, may be subverted when their doctors and nurses use machines to assist delicate cognitive functions. We must ask whether patients should be told the accuracy rate of decision machines—when they have yet to be given comparable data for humans. Would such knowledge improve the informed-consent process, or would it "constitute another befuddling ratio that inspires doubt more than it informs rationality?" (Miller & Goodman, 1998).

To raise such questions is consistent with promoting the responsible use of computers in clinical practice. The question whether computer use will alienate patients is an empirical one; it is a question we have inadequate data to answer. (Do patients respond well to e-mail messages from their doctors, or do they not?) To address the question now anticipates potential future problems. We must ensure that the exciting potential of health informatics is not subverted by our forgetting that the practice of medicine, nursing, and allied professions is deeply human and fundamentally intimate and personal.

Consumer Health Informatics

The growth of the World Wide Web and the commensurate evolution of clinical and health resources on the Internet also raise issues for professional–patient relationships. **Consumer health informatics**—technologies focused on patients as the primary users—makes vast amounts of information available to patients. There is also, however, misinformation—even outright falsehoods and quackery—posted on some sites (see Chapter 11). If physicians and nurses have not established relationships based on trust, the erosive potential of apparently authoritative Internet resources can be great. Physicians accustomed to newspaper-inspired patient requests for drugs and treatments can expect ever-increasing demands that are informed by web browsing. The following issues will gain in ethical importance over the next decade:

- *Peer review:* How and by whom is the quality of a website to be evaluated? Who is responsible for the accuracy of information communicated to patients?
- *Online consultations:* There is yet no standard of care for online medical consultations. What risks do physicians and nurses run by giving advice to patients whom they have not met or examined? This question is especially important in the context of **telemedicine** or **remote-presence health care,** the use of video teleconferencing, image transmission, and other technologies that allow clinicians to evaluate and treat patients in other than face-to-face situations (see Chapter 20).
- *Support groups:* Internet support groups can provide succor and advice to the sick, but there is a chance that someone who might benefit from seeing a physician will not do so because of comforts and information otherwise attained and that her not doing so will lead to bad consequences. How should this problem be addressed?

That a resource is touted as worthwhile does not mean that it is. We lack evidence to illuminate the utility of consumer health informatics and its effects on professional–patient relationships. Such resources should not be ignored, and they often are useful for improving health. But we insist that here—as with decision support, appropriate use and users, evaluation, and privacy and confidentiality—

there is an ethical imperative to proceed with caution. Informatics, like other health technologies, will thrive if our enthusiasm is open to greater evidence and is wed to deep reflection on human values.

7.5 Legal and Regulatory Matters

The use of clinical computing systems in health care raises a number of legal and regulatory questions.

7.5.1 Difference Between Law and Ethics

As might be anticipated, ethical and legal issues often overlap. Ethical considerations apply in attempts to determine what is good or meritorious and which behaviors are desirable or correct in accordance with higher principles. Legal principles are generally derived from ethical ones but deal with the practical regulation of morality or behaviors and activities. Many legal principles deal with the inadequacies and imperfections in human nature and the less-than-ideal behaviors of individuals or groups. **Ethics** offers conceptual tools to evaluate and guide moral decision-making. Laws directly tell us how to behave (or not to behave) under various specific circumstances and prescribe remedies or punishments for individuals who do not comply with the law. Historical precedent, matters of definition, issues related to detectability and enforceability, and evolution of new circumstances affect legal practices more than they influence ethical requirements.

7.5.2 Legal Issues in Healthcare Informatics

Major **legal issues** related to the use of software applications in clinical practice and in biomedical research include liability under tort law; potential use of computer applications as expert witnesses in the courtroom; legislation governing privacy and confidentiality; and copyrights, patents, and intellectual property issues.

Liability Under Tort Law

In the United States and in many other nations, principles of tort law govern situations in which harm or injuries result from the manufacture and sale of goods and services (Miller et al., 1985). Because there are few, if any, U.S. legal precedents directly involving harm or injury to patients resulting from use of clinical software applications (as opposed to a small number of well-documented instances where software associated with medical devices has caused harm), the following discussion is hypothetical. The principles involved are, however, well established with voluminous legal precedents outside the realm of clinical software.

A key legal distinction is the difference between products and services. **Products** are physical objects, such as stethoscopes, that go through the processes of design, manufacture, distribution, sale, and subsequent use by purchasers. **Ser-**

vices are intangible activities provided to consumers at a price by (presumably) qualified individuals.

The practice of clinical medicine has been deemed a service through well-established legal precedents. On the other hand, clinical software applications can be viewed as either goods (software programs designed, tested, debugged, placed on diskettes or other media, and distributed physically to purchasers) or services (applications that provide advice to practitioners engaged in a service such as delivering health care). There are few legal precedents to determine unequivocally how software will be viewed by the courts, and it is possible that clinical software programs will be treated as goods under some circumstances and as services under others.

Two ideas from tort law potentially apply to the clinical use of software systems. The first is **negligence theory;** the second is **strict product liability.** Providers of goods and services are expected to uphold the standards of the community in producing goods and delivering services. When individuals suffer harm due to substandard goods or services, they may sue the service providers or goods manufacturers to recover damages. **Malpractice** litigation in health care is based on negligence theory.

Because the law views delivery of health care as a service (provided by clinicians), it is clear that negligence theory will provide the minimum legal standard for clinicians who use software during the delivery of care. Patients who are harmed by clinical practices based on imperfect software applications may sue the health-care providers for negligence or malpractice, just as patients may sue attending physicians who rely on the imperfect advice of a human consultant (Miller et al., 1985). Similarly, a patient might sue a practitioner who has *not* used a decision-support system when it can be shown that use of the decision-support system is part of the current *standard of care* and that use of the program might have prevented the clinical error that occurred (Miller, 1989). It is not clear whether the patients in such circumstances can also sue the software manufacturers, as it is the responsibility of the licensed practitioner, and not of the software vendor, to uphold the standard of care in the community through exercising sound clinical judgment. Based on a successful malpractice suit against a clinician who used a clinical software system, it might be possible for the practitioner to sue the manufacturer or vendor for negligence in manufacturing a defective clinical software product, but cases of this sort have not yet been filed. If there were such suits, it might be difficult for a court to discriminate between instances of improper use of a blameless system and proper use of a less than perfect system.

In contrast to negligence, strict product liability applies only to harm caused by defective products and is not applicable to services. The primary purpose of strict product liability is to compensate the injured parties rather than to deter or punish negligent individuals (Miller et al., 1985). For strict product liability to apply, three conditions must be met:

1. The product must be purchased and used by an individual.
2. The purchaser must suffer physical harm as a result of a design or manufacturing defect in the product.

3. The product must be shown in court to be "unreasonably dangerous" in a manner that is the demonstrable cause of the purchaser's injury.

Note that negligence theory allows for adverse outcomes. Even when care is delivered in a competent, caring, and compassionate manner, some patients with some illnesses will not do well. Negligence theory protects providers from being held responsible for all individuals who suffer bad outcomes. As long as the quality of care has met the standards, the practitioner should not be found liable in a malpractice case (Miller et al., 1985). Strict product liability, on the other hand, is not as forgiving or understanding. No matter how good or exemplary are a manufacturer's designs and manufacturing processes, if even 1 in ten million products is defective, and that one product defect is the cause of a purchaser's injury, then the purchaser may collect damages (Miller et al., 1985). The plaintiff needs to show only that the product was unreasonably dangerous and that its defect led to harm. In that sense, the standard of care for strict product liability is 100 percent perfection. To some extent, appropriate product labeling (e.g., "Do not use this metal ladder near electrical wiring") may protect manufacturers in certain strict-product-liability suits in that clear, visible labeling may educate the purchaser to avoid "unreasonably dangerous" circumstances. Appropriate labeling standards may benefit users and manufacturers of clinical expert systems (Geissbuhler & Miller, 1997).

Healthcare programs sold to clinicians who use them as decision-support tools in their practices are likely to be treated under negligence theory as services. When advice-giving clinical programs are sold directly to patients, however, and there is less opportunity for intervention by a licensed practitioner, it is more likely that the courts will treat them as products, using strict product liability, because the purchaser of the program is more likely to be the individual who is injured if the product is defective.

Computer Programs as Potential Expert Witnesses

Individuals may consider using expert clinical decision-support systems as **expert witnesses** in future malpractice trials (Miller, 1989). There are at least two good reasons that this use will not be possible, however, given current technology (Frank, 1988). The first is that witnesses must be able to be sworn to tell the truth. Expert systems cannot be made to do so in any meaningful manner. Second, courts do not admit **hearsay evidence**—external information that cannot be subjected to interactive questioning by opposing lawyers and by judges in the courtroom. At present, expert computer programs are not easily cross-examined and cannot, in general, answer free-form, natural-language questions.

Privacy and Confidentiality

The ethical basis for privacy and confidentiality in health care is discussed in Section 7.3.1. It is unfortunate that the legal state of affairs for privacy and confidentiality of electronic health records is at present chaotic (as it is for written records, to some extent). This state of affairs has not significantly changed in the three decades since it was described in a classic *New England Journal of Medicine* article (Curran et al., 1969).

In the United States, a key federal initiative, the Health Insurance Portability and Accountability Act (HIPAA) of 1996, called for the legislative or executive branch of government to establish the first-ever nationwide protection of electronic patient records. In late 1999, after Congress failed to act under the HIPAA provisions, the Secretary of the Department of Health and Human Services proposed wide-ranging federal privacy regulations, initiating a period of intense public and legislative debate. In the meantime, there are 50 different standards—one for each state—and they vary greatly. An electronic medical record prepared in a clinic near the border between two states may meet the requirements of the state in which it was initially prepared, but transfer of that record, along with the patient, to a hospital in the adjacent state may violate the laws of the adjacent state. In the absence of legal standards, institutions would do well to implement the recommendations (discussed in Section 7.3.2) of the 1997 National Research Council report *For the Record: Protecting Electronic Health Information.*

Copyright, Patents, and Intellectual Property

Another underdeveloped area of the law, with respect to clinical information systems, is the **intellectual-property** protection afforded to developers of software programs, biomedical knowledge bases, and World Wide Web pages. Although there are long traditions of copyright and patent protections for nonelectronic media, their applicability to computer-based resources is not clear. **Copyright law** protects intellectual property from being copied verbatim, and **patents** protect specific methods of implementing or instantiating ideas. The number of lawsuits in which one company claimed that another copied the functionality of its copyrighted program (i.e., its "look and feel") has grown, however, and it is clear that copyright law does not protect the "look and feel" of a program beyond certain limits. Consider, for example, the unsuccessful suit in the 1980s by Apple Computer, Inc., against Microsoft, Inc., over the "look and feel" of Microsoft Windows as compared with the Apple Macintosh interface (which itself resembled the earlier Xerox Alto interface).

It is not straightforward to obtain copyright protection for a list that is a compilation of existing names, data, facts, or objects (e.g., the telephone directory of a city), unless you can argue that the result of compiling the compendium creates a unique object (e.g., a new organizational scheme for the information) (Tysyer, 1997). Even when the compilation is unique and copyrightable, the individual components, such as facts in a database, may not be copyrightable. That they are not has implications for the ability of creators of biomedical databases to protect database content as intellectual property. How many individual, unprotected facts can someone copy from a copyright-protected database before legal protections prevent additional copying?

A related concern is the intellectual-property rights of the developers of materials made available through the World Wide Web. Usually, information made accessible to the public that does not contain copyright annotations is considered to be in the public domain. It is tempting to build from the work of other people in placing material on the Web, but copyright protections must be respected. Similarly, if you develop potentially copyrightable material, the act of placing it on the Web, in the public domain, would allow other people to treat your material as not protected by copyright. Resolution of this and related questions may await workable commercial models for electronic publication on the World Wide Web, whereby authors could be compensated fairly when other people use or access their materials. Electronic commerce should eventually provide copyright protection and revenue similar to the age-old models that now apply to paper-based print media; for instance, to use printed books and journals, you must generally borrow them from a library or purchase them.

7.5.3 Regulation and Monitoring of Computer Applications in Health Care

In 1996, the U.S. **Food and Drug Administration** (FDA) announced that it would hold public meetings to discuss new methods and approaches to regulating clinical software systems as medical devices. In response, a consortium of professional organizations related to healthcare information (the American Medical Informatics Association, the Center for Healthcare Information Management, the Computer-Based Patient Record Institute, the American Health Information Management Association, the Medical Library Association, the Association of Academic Health Science Libraries, and the American Nurses Association) drafted a position paper published in both summary format and as a longer discussion with detailed background and explanation (Miller & Gardner, 1997a,b). The position paper was subsequently endorsed by the boards of directors of all the organizations (except the Center for Healthcare Information Management) and by the American College of Physicians Board of Regents.

The recommendations from the consortium include these:

- Recognition of four categories of clinical system risks and four classes of monitoring and regulatory actions that can be applied based on the level of risk in a given setting
- Local oversight of clinical software systems, whenever possible, through the creation of autonomous **software-oversight committees,** in a manner partially analogous to the institutional review boards that are federally mandated to oversee protection of human subjects in biomedical research. Experience with prototypical software-oversight committees at pilot sites should be gained before any national dissemination
- Adoption by healthcare-information system developers of a code of good business practices

TABLE 7.2. Consortium recommendations for monitoring and regulating clinical software systems*

Variable	Regulatory class			
	A	B	C	D
Supervision by FDA	Exempt from regulation	Excluded from regulation	Simple registration and postmarket surveillance required	Premarket approval and postmarket surveillance required
Local software oversight committee	Optional	Mandatory	Mandatory	Mandatory
Role of software oversight committee	Monitor locally	Monitor locally instead of monitoring by FDA	Monitor locally and report problems to FDA as appropriate	Assure adequate local monitoring without replicating FDA activity
Software risk category				
0: Informational or generic systems†	All software in category	—	—	—
1: Patient-specific systems that provide low-risk assistance with clinical problems‡	—	All software in category	—	—
2: Patient-specific systems that provide intermediate-risk support on clinical problems§	—	Locally developed or locally modified systems	Commercially developed systems that are not modified locally	—
3: High-risk, patient-specific systems‖	—	Locally developed, non-commercial systems	—	Commercial systems

* FDA = Food and Drug Administration.

† Includes systems that provide factual content or simple, generic advice (such as "give flu vaccine to eligible patients in mid-autumn") and generic programs, such as spreadsheets and databases.

‡ Systems that give simple advice (such as suggesting alternative diagnoses or therapies without stating preferences) and give ample opportunity for users to ignore or override suggestions.

§ Systems that have higher clinical risk (such as those that generate diagnoses or therapies ranked by score) but allow users to ignore or override suggestions easily; net risk is therefore intermediate.

‖ Systems that have great clinical risk and give users little or no opportunity to intervene (such as a closed-loop system that automatically regulates ventilator settings).

(*Source:* Miller R.A., Gardner R.M. Summary recommendations for responsible monitoring and regulation of clinical software systems. *Annals of Internal Medicine* [1997], 127(9):842).

- Recognition that budgetary, logistic, and other constraints limit the type and number of systems that the FDA can regulate effectively
- Concentration of FDA regulation on those systems posing highest clinical risk, with limited opportunities for competent human intervention, and FDA exemption of most other clinical software systems

The recommendations for combined local and FDA monitoring are summarized in Table 7.2.

7.6 Summary and Conclusions

Ethical issues are important to health informatics. An initial ensemble of guiding principles, or ethical criteria, has emerged to orient decision-making:

1. Specially trained humans remain, so far, best able to provide health care for other humans. Hence, computer software should not be allowed to overrule a human decision.
2. Practitioners who use informatics tools should be clinically qualified and adequately trained in using the software products.
3. The tools themselves should be carefully evaluated and validated.
4. Health informatics tools and applications should be evaluated not only in terms of performance, including efficacy, but also in terms of their influences on institutions, institutional cultures, and workplace social forces.
5. Ethical obligations should extend to system developers, maintainers, and supervisors as well as to clinician users.
6. Education programs and security measures should be considered essential for protecting confidentiality and privacy while improving appropriate access to personal patient information.
7. Adequate oversight should be maintained to optimize ethical use of electronic patient information for scientific and institutional research.

New sciences and technologies always raise interesting and important ethical issues. Much the same is true for legal issues, although in the absence of precedent or legislation any legal analysis will remain vague. Similarly important challenges confront people who are trying to determine the appropriate role for government in regulating healthcare software. The lack of clear public policy for such software underscores the importance of ethical insight and education as the exciting new tools of health informatics become more common.

Suggested Readings

Goodman K.W. (Ed.) (1998). *Ethics, Computing, and Medicine: Informatics and the Transformation of Health Care.* Cambridge: Cambridge University Press.

This volume—the first devoted to the intersection of ethics and informatics—contains chapters on informatics and human values, responsibility for computer-based decisions, evaluation of medical information systems, confidentiality and privacy, decision support, outcomes research and prognostic scoring systems, and meta-analysis.

Miller R.A. (1990). Why the standard view is standard: People, not machines, understand patients' problems. *Journal of Medicine and Philosophy,* 15:581–591.

This contribution lays out the standard view of health informatics. This view holds, in part, that because only humans have the diverse skills necessary to practice medicine or nursing, machine intelligence should never override human clinicians.

Miller R.A., Schaffner K.F., Meisel, A. (1985). Ethical and legal issues related to the use of computer programs in clinical medicine. *Annals of Internal Medicine* 102:529–536.

This article constitutes a major early effort to identify and address ethical issues in informatics. By emphasizing the questions of appropriate use, confidentiality, and validation, among others, it sets the stage for all subsequent work.

National Research Council. (1997). *For the Record: Protecting Electronic Health Information.* Washington, D.C.: National Academy Press.

A major policy report, this document outlines leading challenges for privacy and confidentiality in medical information systems and makes several important recommendations for institutions and policy-makers.

Questions for Discussion

1. What is meant by the standard view of appropriate use of medical information systems? Identify three key criteria for determining whether a particular use or user is appropriate.
2. Can quality standards for system developers and maintainers simultaneously safeguard against error and abuse *and* stimulate scientific progress? Explain your answers. Why is there an ethical obligation to adhere to a standard of care?
3. Identify (a) two major threats to patient confidentiality and (b) policies or strategies that you propose for protecting confidentiality against these threats.
4. Many prognoses by humans are subjective and are based on faulty memory or incomplete knowledge of previous cases. What are two drawbacks to using objective prognostic scoring systems to determine whether to allocate care to individual patients?
5. People who are educated about their illnesses tend to understand and to follow instructions, to ask insightful questions, and so on. How can the World Wide Web improve patient education? How, on the other hand, might web access hurt traditional physician–patient and nurse–patient relationships?

8 Evaluation and Technology Assessment

CHARLES P. FRIEDMAN, DOUGLAS K. OWENS, AND JEREMY C. WYATT

After reading this chapter, you should know the answers to these questions:

- Why are empirical studies based on the methods of evaluation and technology assessment important to the successful implementation of information resources to improve health care?
- What challenges make studies in informatics difficult to carry out? How are these challenges addressed in practice?
- Why can all evaluations be classified as empirical studies?
- What are the major assumptions underlying objectivist and subjectivist approaches to evaluation? What are the advantages and disadvantages of each?
- What are the factors that distinguish the three stages of technology assessment?
- How does one distinguish measurement and demonstration aspects of objectivist studies, and why are both aspects necessary?
- What steps are typically undertaken in a measurement study? What designs are typically used in demonstration studies?
- What is the difference between cost-effectiveness and cost-benefit analyses? How can investigators address issues of cost effectiveness and cost benefit of medical information resources?
- What steps are followed in a subjectivist study? What techniques are employed by subjectivist investigators to ensure rigor and credibility of their findings?
- Why is communication between investigators and clients central to the success of any evaluation?

8.1 Introduction and Definitions of Terms

This chapter is about the formal study of medical information resources—computer systems that support health care, education, research, and biomedical research—to address questions of importance to developers, users, and other people. We explore the methods of performing such studies, which are essential to the field of informatics but are often challenging to carry out successfully. Fortunately, every study is not designed from a blank tablet. To guide us, there exist two closely related and highly overlapping bodies of methodological knowledge: evaluation and technology assessment. These methodological fields, which have largely developed over the past four decades, are together the subject of this chapter.[1]

8.1.1 Evaluation and Technology Assessment

Most people understand the term *evaluation* to mean a measurement or description of an organized, purposeful activity. Evaluations are usually conducted to answer questions or to help make decisions. Whether we are choosing a holiday destination or a word processor, we evaluate what the options are and how well they fit key objectives or personal preferences. The forms of the evaluation differ widely, according to what is being evaluated and how important the decision is. Thus, in the case of holiday destinations, we may ask our friend which Hawaiian island she prefers and may browse color brochures from the travel agent; for a word processor, we may gather technical details, such as the time to open and spell check a 1,000-word document or the compatibility with our printer. Thus, the term **evaluation** describes a wide range of data-collection activities, designed to answer questions ranging from the casual, "What does my friend think of Maui?" to the more focused, "Is word processor A faster than word processor B on my personal computer?"

In medical informatics, we study the collection, processing, and dissemination of healthcare information and build **information resources**—usually consisting of computer hardware or software—to facilitate these activities. Such information resources include systems to collect, store, and retrieve data about specific patients (e.g., clinical workstations and databases) and systems to assemble, store, and reason about medical knowledge (e.g., medical knowledge-acquisition tools, knowledge bases, decision-support systems, and multimedia educational systems). Thus, there is a wide range of medical information resources to evaluate.

Further complicating the picture, each information resource has many different aspects that can be evaluated. The technically minded might focus on inherent characteristics, asking such questions as, "How many columns of data are there per database table?" or "How many probability calculations per second can this tool sustain?" Clinicians, however, might ask more pragmatic questions, such as, "Is the information in this system completely up to date?" or "How long must we wait until the decision-support system produces its recommendations?" People who have a broader perspective might wish to understand the influence of these resources on users or patients, asking questions such as, "How well does this database support a clinical audit?" or "What effects will this decision-support system have on working relationships and responsibilities?" Thus, evaluation methods in medical informatics must address a wide range of issues, from technical characteristics of specific systems to systems' effects on people and organizations.

---

[1]This chapter is heavily drawn from the textbook on evaluation by co-authors Friedman and Wyatt (1997a); refer to that text for further details.

Technology assessment is a field of study closely aligned with evaluation (Garber & Owens, 1994). The Institute of Medicine (1985, p. 2) defines technology assessment as "any process of examining and reporting properties of a medical technology used in health care, such as safety, efficacy, feasibility, and indication for use, cost, and cost-effectiveness, as well as social, economic, and ethical consequences, whether intended or unintended."

But what is a medical technology? **Medical technology** usually is defined broadly and consists of the "techniques, drugs, equipment, and procedures used by healthcare professionals in delivering medical care to individuals, and the systems within which such care is delivered" (Institute of Medicine, 1985, pp. 1–2). Medical information resources clearly fit within this definition. Technology assessment is relevant to informatics because many of the techniques from this field are applicable to the study of information resources.

We shall not dwell here on the differences between evaluation and technology assessment. Such differences are ones of emphasis and focus. Individuals who do evaluation and technology assessment are interested in much the same issues and use similar methods.

8.1.2 Reasons for Performing Studies

Like all complex and time-consuming activities, evaluation and technology assessment can serve multiple purposes. There are five major reasons why we study clinical information resources (Wyatt & Spiegelhalter, 1990):

- *Promotional:* If we are to encourage the use of information resources in medicine, we must be able to reassure physicians that these systems are safe and that they benefit both patients and institutions through improved cost effectiveness.
- *Scholarly:* One of the main activities in medical informatics is developing clinical information resources using computer-based tools. To obtain a deeper understanding of the links between the structure, function, and effects of these information resources on clinical decisions and actions requires careful evaluation. The knowledge we gain from such studies will help to build the foundations of medical informatics as a discipline (Heathfield & Wyatt, 1995).
- *Pragmatic:* Without evaluating their systems, developers will never know which techniques or methods are more effective or why certain approaches failed. Equally, other developers will not be able to learn from previous mistakes and may reinvent a square wheel.
- *Ethical:* Clinical professionals are under an obligation to practice within an ethical framework. For example, before using an information resource, healthcare providers must ensure that it is safe. Equally, those responsible for commissioning the purchase of a hospital-wide clinical information system costing several million dollars must be able to justify this in preference to other information resources or the many other healthcare innovations that compete for the same budget.

- *Medicolegal:* To reduce the risk of liability, developers of an information resource should obtain accurate information to allow them to assure users that the resource is safe and effective. Users need evaluation results to enable them to exercise their professional judgment before using systems so that the law will regard these users as "learned intermediaries." An information resource that treats users merely as automata, without allowing them to exercise their skills and judgment, risks being judged by the strict laws of product liability instead of by the more lenient principles applied to provision of professional services (Brahams & Wyatt, 1989) (also see Chapter 7).

The motivation for every study is one or more of these factors. Awareness of the major reason for conducting an evaluation will often help the investigators to frame the questions to be addressed and to avoid disappointment.

8.1.3 The Stakeholders in Evaluation Studies and Their Roles

Figure 8.1 shows actors who pay for (solid arrows) and regulate (shaded arrows) the healthcare process. Each of them may be affected by a medical information resource, and each may have a unique view of what constitutes benefit. More

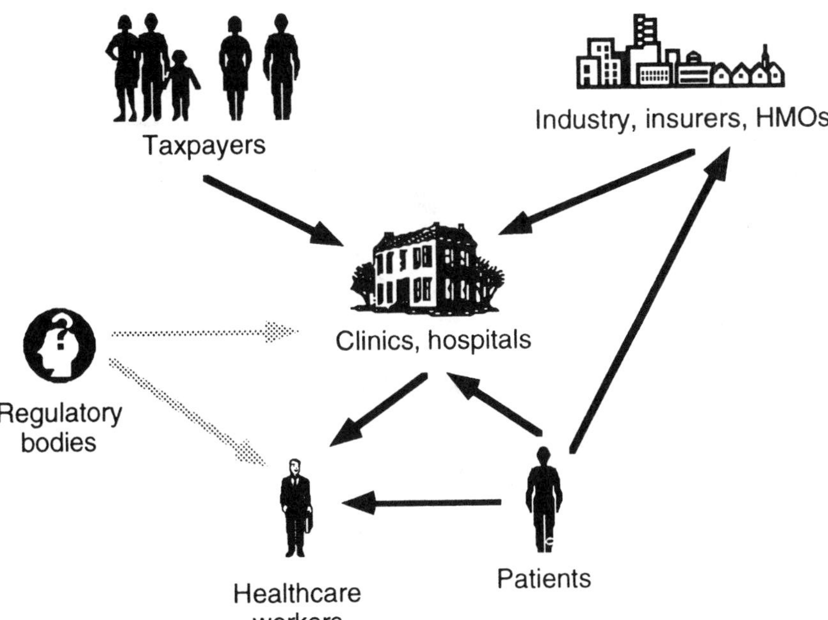

Figure 8.1. Some of the actors involved in healthcare delivery, administration, policy-making, and regulation, each of whom may have a stake in an evaluation study. (*Source:* Friedman & Wyatt, 1997a.)

specifically, in a typical clinical-information resource project, the key stakeholders are the developers, the users, the patients whose management may be affected, and the people responsible for purchasing and maintaining the system. Each may have different questions to be answered (Fig. 8.2).

Whenever we design evaluation or technology-assessment studies, it is important to consider the perspectives of all stakeholders in the information resource. Because studies are often designed to answer specific questions, any one study is unlikely to satisfy all of the questions that concern stakeholders. Sometimes, due to the intricacy of healthcare systems and processes, it can be a challenge for an evaluator to identify all the relevant stakeholders and to distinguish those whose questions must be satisfied from those whose satisfaction is optional.

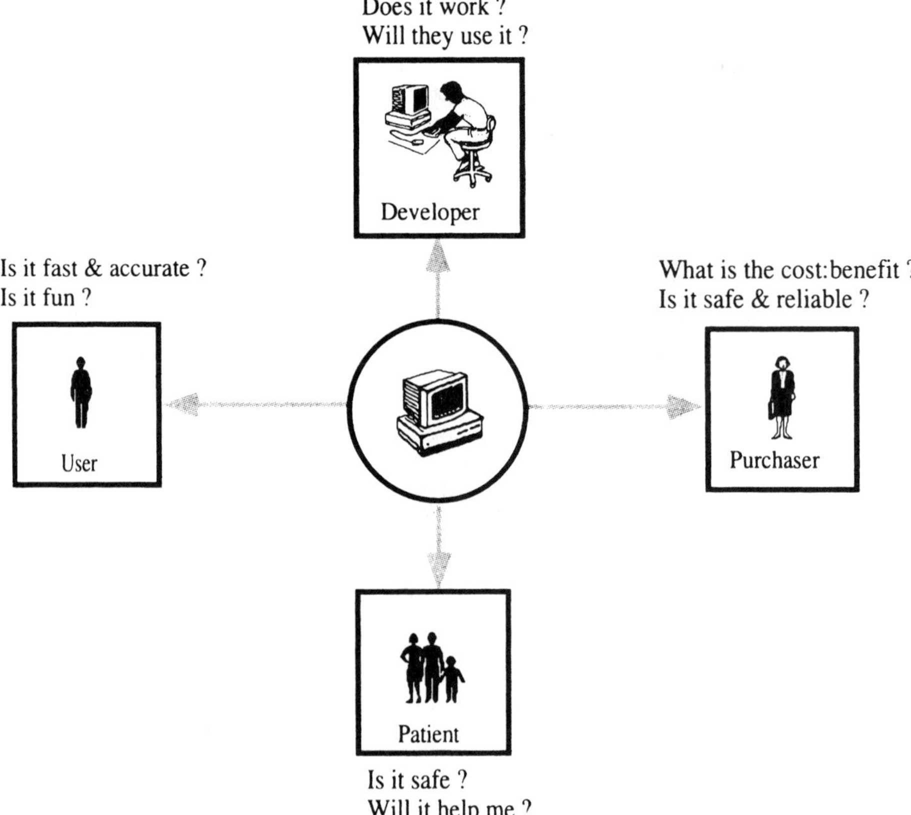

FIGURE 8.2. Different stakeholders may have quite different perspectives on a clinical information resource and questions that they wish to be answered by an evaluation study. (*Source:* Friedman & Wyatt, 1997a.)

8.2 The Challenges of Study Design and Conduct

The work of evaluation and technology assessment in informatics lies at the intersection of three areas, each notorious for its complexity: medicine and healthcare delivery, computer-based information systems, and the general methodology of study conduct itself. Because of the complexity of each area, any work that combines them necessarily poses serious challenges.

8.2.1 The Complexity of Medicine and Healthcare Delivery

Donabedian (1996) informs us that any healthcare innovation may influence three aspects of the healthcare system. The first is the healthcare system's *structure*, including the space it takes up; the equipment available; the financial resources required; and the number, skills, and interrelationships of the staff. The second is the *processes* that take place during healthcare activity, such as the number and appropriateness of diagnoses and the investigations and therapies administered. The third is the healthcare *outcomes* for both individual patients and the community, such as quality of life, complications of procedures, and length of survival. Thus, when we study the influence of an information resource on a healthcare system, we may see effects on any of these three aspects. An information resource may lead to an improvement in one area (e.g., patient outcomes) but to deterioration in another (e.g., the costs of running the service).

Also, it is well known that the roles of nursing and clinical personnel are well defined and hierarchical in comparison to those in many other professions. Thus information resources designed for one specific group of professionals, such as a residents' information system designed for one hospital (Young, 1980), may be of little benefit to other groups.

Because health care is a safety-critical area, with more limited budgets and a less tangible currency than, for example, retail or manufacturing, rigorous proof of safety and effectiveness is required in evaluation studies of clinical information resources. Complex regulations apply to people who develop or market clinical therapies or investigational technology. It is not yet clear whether these regulations apply to all computer-based information resources or to only those that manage patients directly, without a human intermediary (Brannigan, 1991).

Medicine is well known to be a complex domain: Students spend a minimum of seven years gaining qualifications. A single internal-medicine textbook contains approximately 600,000 facts (Wyatt, 1991b); practicing experts have as many as 2 to 5 million facts at their finger tips (Pauker et al., 1976). Also, medical knowledge itself (Wyatt, 1991b), and methods of healthcare delivery, change rapidly, so the goalposts for a medical information resource may move during the course of an evaluation study.

Patients often suffer from multiple diseases, which may evolve over time at differing rates and may be subject to a number of interventions and other influences over the course of the study period, confounding the effects of changes in information management. There is even variation in how doctors interpret patient data (for example, prostate-specific antigen results) across medical centers. Thus, simply because an information resource is safe and effective when used in one center on patients who have a given diagnosis, we are not entitled to prejudge the results of using it in another center or with patients who have a different disease profile.

The causal links between introducing an information resource and achieving improvements in patient outcome are long and complex compared with those for direct patient-care interventions such as medications. In addition, the functioning and influence of an information resource may depend critically on input from healthcare workers or patients. It is thus unrealistic to look for quantifiable changes in patient outcomes after the introduction of many information resources until we have documented changes in the structure or processes of healthcare delivery.

The processes of medical decision-making are complex and have been studied extensively (Elstein et al., 1978; Evans & Patel, 1989). Clinicians make many kinds of decisions—including diagnosis, monitoring, therapy, and prognosis—using incomplete and fuzzy data, some of which are appreciated intuitively and are not recorded in the clinical notes. If an information resource generates more effective management of both patient data and medical knowledge, it may intervene in the process of medical decision-making in a number of ways, making difficult the determination of which component of the resource is responsible for observed changes.

There is a general lack of gold standards in medicine. Thus, for example, diagnoses are rarely known with 100 percent certainty, because it is unethical to do all possible tests on every patient, (to follow-up patients without good cause), because tests and ability to interpret them are imperfect, and because the human body is simply too complex. When a clinician attempts to establish a diagnosis or the cause of death, even if it is possible to perform a postmortem examination, correlating the patients' symptoms or clinical findings before death with the observed changes may prove impossible. Determining the correct management for a patient is even more complicated, because there is wide variation in **consensus opinions** (Leitch, 1989), as reflected in wide variations in clinical practice even in neighboring areas.

Doctors practice under strict legal and ethical obligations to give their patients the best care that is available, to do patients no harm, to keep patients informed about the risks of all procedures and therapies, and to maintain confidentiality. These obligations may well impinge on the design of evaluation studies. For example, because healthcare workers have imperfect memories and patients take holidays and participate in the unpredictable activities of real life, it is impossible to impose strict discipline in data recording, and study data are often incomplete. Similarly, before a randomized controlled trial can be undertaken, healthcare workers and patients are entitled to a full explanation of the possible benefits and disadvantages of being allocated to the control and intervention groups before giving their consent.

8.2.2 The Complexity of Computer-Based Information Resources

From the perspective of a computer scientist, the goal of evaluating a computer-based information resource might be to predict that resource's function and effects from a knowledge of its structure. Although software engineering and formal methods for specifying, coding, and evaluating computer programs have become more sophisticated, even systems of modest complexity challenge these techniques. To formally verify a program rigorously (to obtain proof that it performs all and only those functions specified), we must invest effort that increases exponentially with the program's size—the problem is "**NP hard**." Put simply, to test a program rigorously requires the application of every combination of possible input data in all possible orders. Thus, it entails at least *n* factorial experiments, where *n* is the number of input data items. The size of *n* factorial increases exponentially with small increases in *n*, so the task rapidly becomes unfeasible. In some technology-led projects, the goals of the new information resources are not defined precisely. Developers may be attracted by technology and may produce applications without first demonstrating the existence of a clinical problem that the application is designed to meet (Heathfield & Wyatt, 1993). An example was a conference entitled "Medicine Meets Virtual Reality: *Discovering Applications* for 3D Multimedia" (our italics). The lack of a clear need for an information resource makes it hard to evaluate the ability of the information resource to alleviate a clinical problem. Although one can still evaluate the structure and function of the system in isolation, it will be hard to interpret the results of such an evaluation in clinical terms.

Some computer-based systems are able to adapt themselves to their users or to data already acquired, or they may be deliberately tailored to a given institution; it may then be difficult to compare the results of one evaluation with a study of the same information resource conducted at a different time or in another location. Also, the notoriously rapid evolution of computer hardware and software means that the time course of an evaluation study may be greater than the lifetime of the information resource itself.

Medical information resources often contain several distinct components, including the interface, database, reasoning and maintenance programs, patient data, static medical knowledge, and dynamic inferences about the patient, the user and the current activity of the user. Such information resources may perform a wide range of functions for users. Thus, if evaluators are to answer questions such as, "What part of the information resource is responsible for the observed effect?" or "Why did the information resource fail?," they must be familiar with each component of the information resource, know its functions, and understand potential interactions (Wyatt, 1989, 1991a).

8.2.3 The Complexity of Study Methods

Studies do not focus solely on the structure and function of an information resource; they also address the resource's effects on the care providers who are customarily its users and on patient outcomes. To understand users' actions, investigators must confront the gulfs among peoples' private opinions, public statements, and actual behavior. Humans vary widely in their responses to stimuli, both from minute to minute and from one to another, making the results of measurements subject to random and systematic errors. Thus, studies of medical information resources require analytical tools from the behavioral and social sciences, statistics, and other fields.

Studies require test material, such as clinical cases, and information resource users, such as physicians or nurses. Both are often in shorter supply than the study design requires; the availability of patients also is usually overestimated, sometimes many times over. In addition, it may be unclear what kind of cases or users should be recruited for a study. Often, study designers are faced with a trade-off between selecting cases, users, and study settings with high fidelity to real life and selecting those who will help to achieve adequate experimental control. Finally, one of the more important determinants of the results of an evaluation study is the manner in which case data are abstracted and presented to users. For example, we would expect differing results in a study of an information resource's accuracy depending on whether the test data were abstracted by the developers or by the intended users.

There are many reasons for performing studies, ranging from assessing a student's work to formulating health policy to understanding a specific technical advance. Such reasons will in turn determine the kinds of questions that will be asked about the information resource. To help those who are trying to determine the broad goals of an evaluation study, in Table 8.1 we list some of the many questions that can arise about information resources and about their influence on users, patients, and the healthcare system.

TABLE 8.1. Possible questions that may arise during the study of a medical information resource.

About the resource itself	About the resource's impact
Is there a clinical need for it?	Do people use it?
Does it work?	Do people like it?
Is it reliable?	Does it improve users' efficiency?
Is it accurate?	Does it influence the collection of data?
Is it fast enough?	Does it influence users' decisions?
Is data entry reliable?	For how long do the observed effects last?
Are people likely to use it?	Does it influence users' knowledge or skills?
Which parts cause the effects?	Does it help patients?
How can it be maintained?	Does it change consumption of resources?
How can it be improved?	What might ensue from widespread use?

Source: Friedman and Wyatt (1997a).

8.3 The Full Range of What Can Be Studied

When evaluating a medical information resource, there are five major aspects of interest: the clinical need the resource is intended to address; the process used to develop the resource; the resource's intrinsic structure; the functions that the resource carries out; and the resource's influence on users, patients, and other aspects of the clinical environment. In a theoretically complete evaluation, separate studies of a particular resource might address each aspect. In the real world, however, it is difficult to be comprehensive. Over the course of its development and deployment, a resource may be studied many times, with the studies in their totality touching on many or most of these aspects, but few resources will be studied completely, and many will, inevitably, be studied only minimally.

The evaluation focus changes as we study the different aspects:

1. *The need for the resource:* Evaluators study the clinical status quo absent the resource. They determine the nature of the problems that the resource is intended to address and the frequency with which these problems arise.
2. *The development process:* Evaluators study the skills of the development team and the methodologies employed to understand whether the design is likely to be sound.
3. *The resource's intrinsic structure:* Evaluators study specifications, flowcharts, program codes, and other representations of the resource that they can inspect without running the program.
4. *The resource's functions:* Evaluators study how the resource performs when it is used.
5. *The resource's effects:* Evaluators study not the resource itself but rather its influence on users, patients, and healthcare organizations.

Several factors characterize an evaluation study:

- *The focus of study:* The focus can be the status quo before introduction of the information resource, the design process adopted, the resource's structure or function, the resource users' simulated decisions or real decisions, or the clinical actions and patient outcomes once the resource is made available in the workplace.
- *Study setting:* Studies of the design process, the resource's structure, and the resource's functions can be conducted outside the active clinical environment, in a laboratory setting, which is easier logistically and may allow greater control over the evaluation process. Studies to elucidate the need for a resource and studies of the resource's effects on users both usually take place in clinical settings. The effects of a resource on patients and healthcare organizations can take place in only a true clinical setting where the resource is available for use at the time and place where patient-management decisions are made.
- *Clinical data employed:* For many studies, the resource will actually be run. That will require clinical data, which can be simulated data, data abstracted from real patients' records, or actual patient data. Clearly, the kind of data em-

ployed in a study has serious implications for the study results and the conclusions that can be drawn.

- *User of the resource:* Most information resources function in interaction with one or more users. In any particular study, the users of the resource can be members of the development team or the evaluation team or other individuals not representative of those people who will interact with the resource after it is deployed; or the users in a study could be representative of the end users for whose use the resource is ultimately designed. Again, the selection of resource users can affect study results profoundly.
- *The decisions affected by use of the resource:* Many information resources, by providing information or advice to clinicians, seek to influence the decisions made by these clinicians. As a study moves from the laboratory to the clinical setting, the information provided by the resource potentially has greater implications for the decisions being made. Depending on a study's design and purposes, only simulated decisions may be affected (clinicians are asked what they would do, but no action is taken), or real decisions involved in the care of actual patients may be affected.

Table 8.2 lists eight broad types of studies of clinical information resources that can be conducted, the focus of each type, the setting in which it occurs, the kind

TABLE 8.2. Generic types of evaluation studies of clinical information resources.

Type of study	Focus of study	Study setting	Kind of patient data	User of resource	Clinical decisions affected by use of the resource
Need validation	The status quo	Field	Real data	None	None
Design validation	Resource design process	Laboratory	None	None	None
Structure validation	Resource structure	Laboratory	None	None	None
Laboratory function	Resource function	Laboratory	Simulated or abstracted data	Developer evaluator, or clinician	None
Field function	Resource function	Field	Real data	Developer evaluator, or clinician	None
Laboratory user impact	Simulated decisions	Laboratory	Simulated or abstracted data	Clinician	Clinicians' simulated decisions
Field user impact	Simulated decisions	Field	Real data	Clinician	Clinicians' simulated decisions
Clinical impact	Patient care and outcomes	Field	Real data	Clinician	Clinicians' real decisions

Source: Friedman and Wyatt (1997a).

of clinical data employed as input to the resource, the person who uses the resource during the study, and the kind of clinical decisions affected by the resource during the study. For example, a *laboratory-user* impact study would be conducted outside the active clinical environment based on simulated or abstracted clinical data. Although it would involve individuals representative of the end-user population, the study would yield primary results derived from simulated clinical decisions, so the clinical care of patients would not be affected. Read across each row of the table to obtain a feel for the contrasts among these study types.

8.4 Approaches to Study Design

Having established a large number of reasons why it can be difficult to study medical information resources, we now introduce the methods that have been developed to address these challenges. We begin by describing a generic structure that all studies share. Then we introduce, in turn, more specific methods of evaluation and the closely related methods of technology assessment.

8.4.1 The Anatomy of All Studies

The structural elements that all studies share are illustrated in Figure 8.3. Evaluations are guided by someone's or some group's need to know. No matter who that someone is—the development team, the funding agency, or other individuals and groups—the evaluation must begin with a process of negotiation to identify the questions that will be a starting point for the study. The outcomes of these negotiations are an understanding of how the evaluation is to be conducted, usually stated in a written contract or agreement, and an initial expression of the questions the evaluation seeks to answer. The next element of the study is investigation: the collection of data to address these questions and, depending on the approach selected, possibly other questions that

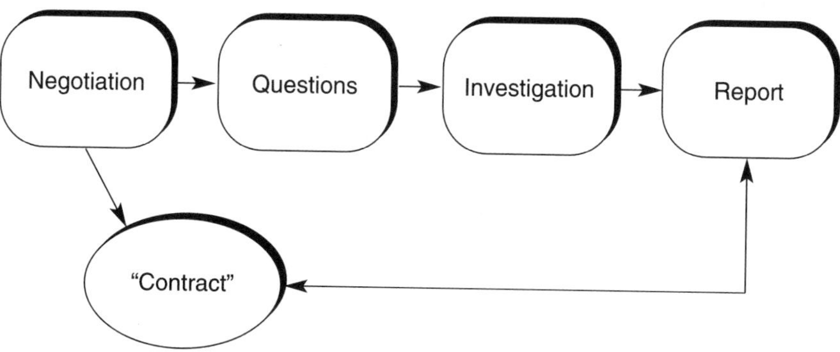

FIGURE 8.3. Anatomy of all evaluation studies. (*Source:* Friedman & Wyatt, 1997a.)

arise during the study. The mechanisms are numerous, ranging from the performance of the resource on a series of benchmark tasks to observations of users working with the resource.

The next element is a mechanism for reporting the information back to the individuals who need to know it. The format of the report must be in line with the stipulations of the contract; the content of the report follows from the questions asked and the data collected. The report is most often a written document, but it does not have to be—the purposes of some evaluations are well served by oral reports or by live demonstrations. We emphasize that it is the evaluator's obligation to establish a process through which the results of her study are communicated, thus creating the potential for the study's findings to be put to constructive use. No investigator can guarantee a constructive outcome for a study, but there is much she can do to increase the likelihood of a salutary result. Also note that a salutary result of a study is not necessarily one that casts the resource under study in a positive light. A salutary result is one where the stakeholders learn important information from the study findings.

8.4.2 *Philosophical Bases of Approaches to Evaluation*

Several authors have developed classifications, or **typologies**, of evaluation methods or approaches. Among the best is that developed in 1980 by Ernest House. A major advantage of House's typology is that each approach is linked elegantly to an underlying philosophical model, as detailed in his book. This classification divides current practice into eight discrete approaches, four of which may be viewed as **objectivist** and four of which may be viewed as **subjectivist.** This distinction is very important. Note that these approaches are *not* entitled *objective* and *subjective*, because those words carry strong and fundamentally misleading connotations: of scientific precision in the former case and of imprecise intellectual voyeurism in the latter.

The objectivist approaches derive from a **logical–positivist** philosophical orientation—the same orientation that underlies the classic experimental sciences. The major premises underlying the objectivist approaches are as follows:

- In general, attributes of interest are properties of the resource under study. More specifically, this position suggests that the merit and worth of an information resource—the attributes of most interest in evaluation—can in principle be measured with all observations yielding the same result. It also assumes that an investigator can measure these attributes without affecting how the resource under study functions or is used.
- Rational persons can and should agree on what attributes of a resource are important to measure and what results of these measurements would be identified as a most desirable, correct, or positive outcome. In medical informatics, making this assertion is tantamount to stating that a gold standard of resource performance can always be identified and that all rational individuals can be brought to consensus on what this gold standard is.

- Because numerical measurement allows precise statistical analysis of performance over time or performance in comparison with some alternative, numerical measurement is *prima facie* superior to a verbal description. Verbal, descriptive data (generally known as qualitative data) are useful in only preliminary studies to identify hypotheses for subsequent, precise analysis using quantitative methods.
- Through these kinds of comparisons, it is possible to prove beyond reasonable doubt that a resource is or is not superior to what it replaced or to a competing resource.

Contrast these assumptions with a set of assumptions that derives from an **intuitionist–pluralist** philosophical position that spawns a set of subjectivist approaches to evaluation:

- What is observed about a resource depends in fundamental ways on the observer. Different observers of the same phenomenon might legitimately come to different conclusions. Both can be objective in their appraisals even if they do not agree; it is not necessary that one is right and the other wrong.
- Merit and worth must be explored in context. The value of a resource emerges through study of the resource as it functions in a particular patient-care or educational environment.
- Individuals and groups can legitimately hold different perspectives on what constitutes the most desirable outcome of introducing a resource into an environment. There is no reason to expect them to agree, and it may be counterproductive to try to lead them to consensus. An important aspect of an evaluation would be to document the ways in which they disagree.
- Verbal description can be highly illuminating. Qualitative data are valuable, in and of themselves, and can lead to conclusions as convincing as those drawn from quantitative data. The value of qualitative data, therefore, goes far beyond that of identifying issues for later "precise" exploration using quantitative methods.
- Evaluation should be viewed as an exercise in argument, rather than as a demonstration, because any study appears equivocal when subjected to serious scrutiny.

The approaches to evaluation that derive from this subjectivist philosophical perspective may seem strange, imprecise, and unscientific when considered for the first time. This perception stems in large part from the widespread acceptance of the objectivist worldview in biomedicine. The importance and utility of subjectivist approaches in evaluation is, however, emerging. Within medical informatics, there is growing support for such approaches (Anderson et al., 1995; Forsythe & Buchanan, 1992; Rothschild et al., 1990). As stated earlier, the evaluation mindset includes methodological eclecticism. It is important for people trained in classic experimental methods at least to understand, and possibly even to embrace, the subjectivist worldview if they are to conduct fully informative evaluation studies.

8.4.3 Multiple Approaches to Evaluation

House (1980) classifies evaluation into eight approaches. Although most evaluation studies conducted in the real world can be unambiguously tied to one of these approaches, some studies exhibit properties of several approaches and are not cleanly classified. The first four approaches derive from the objectivist position; the second four are subjectivist.

Comparison Based

The **comparison-based approach** employs experiments and quasi-experiments. The information resource under study is compared with a control condition, a placebo, or a contrasting resource. The comparison is based on a relatively small number of **outcome variables** that are assessed in all groups; randomization, controls, and statistical inference are used to argue that the information resource was the cause of any differences observed. Examples of comparison-based studies include McDonald's work on physician reminders (McDonald et al., 1984a) and the studies from Stanford on rule-based systems (Hickam et al., 1985a; Yu et al., 1979a). The 28 controlled trials of medical decision-support systems reviewed by Johnson and associates (1994) fall under the comparison-based approach. The Turing test (Turing, 1950) can be seen as a specific model for a comparison-based evaluation.

Objectives Based

The **objectives-based approach** seeks to determine whether a resource meets its designers' objectives. Ideally, such objectives are stated in great detail, so there is little ambiguity in developing procedures to measure their degree of attainment. These studies are comparative only in the sense that the observed performance of the resource is viewed in relation to stated objectives. The concern is whether the resource is performing up to expectations; it is not whether the resource is outperforming what it replaced. The objectives that are the benchmarks for these studies are typically stated at an early stage of resource development. Although clearly suited to laboratory testing of a new resource, this approach can also be applied to testing of an installed resource. Consider the example of a resource to provide advice to emergency-room physicians (Wyatt, 1989). The designers might set as an objective that the system's advice be available within 15 minutes of the time the patient is first seen. An evaluation study that measured the time for this advice to be delivered, and compared that time with this objective, would be objectives based.

Decision Facilitation

In the **decision-facilitation approach**, evaluation seeks to resolve issues important to developers and administrators so that these individuals can make decisions about the future of the resource. The questions that are posed are those that the decision-makers state, although the people conducting the evaluation may help the decision-makers to frame these questions to be amenable to study. The data-collection methods follow from the questions posed. These studies tend to be *formative* in focus. The results of studies conducted at the early stages of resource development are used to chart the course of further development, which in turn generates new questions for further study. A systematic study of alternative formats for computer-generated advisories, conducted while the resource to generate the advisories is still under development, is a good example of this approach (de Bliek et al., 1988).

Goal Free

In the three approaches described, the evaluation is guided by a set of goals for the information resource or by specific questions that the developers either state or play a profound role in shaping. Any such study will be polarized by these manifest goals and may be more sensitive to anticipated than to unanticipated effects. In the **goal-free approach,** the people conducting the evaluation are purposefully blinded to the intended effects of an information resource and pursue whatever evidence they can gather to enable them to identify *all* the effects of the resource, intended or not (Scriven, 1973). This approach is rarely applied in practice, but it is useful to individuals designing evaluations to remind them of the many effects an information resource can engender.

Quasi-Legal

The **quasi-legal approach** establishes a *mock trial*, or other formal adversary proceeding, to judge a resource. Proponents and opponents of the resource offer testimony and may be examined and cross-examined in a manner resembling standard courtroom procedure. A jury that is witness to the proceedings can then, on the basis of this testimony, make a decision about the merit of the resource. As in a debate, the issue can be decided by the persuasive power of rhetoric as well as by the persuasive power of what is portrayed as fact. There are few examples of this technique formally applied to medical informatics, but the technique has been applied to facilitate difficult decisions in other medical areas such as treatment of sickle cell disease (Smith, 1992).

Art Criticism

The **art criticism approach** relies on methods of art criticism and the principle of connoisseurship (Eisner, 1991). Under this approach, an experienced and respected critic, who may or may not be trained in the domain of the resource but who has a great deal of experience with resources of this generic type, works with the resource. She then writes a review highlighting the benefits and shortcomings of the resource. Clearly, the art-criticism approach cannot be definitive if the critic is not expert in the subject domain of a medical informatics resource, because she will be unable to judge the clinical or scientific accuracy of the resource's knowledge base or of the advice that it provides. Nonetheless, the thoughtful and articulate comments of an experienced reviewer can help other people to appreciate important features of a resource. Software reviews are examples of this approach in common practice.

Professional Review

The **professional-review approach** is well known in the form of **site visits**. This approach employs panels of experienced peers who spend several days in the environment where the resource is installed. Site visits are often guided by a set of guidelines specific to the type of project under study but sufficiently generic to accord the reviewers a great deal of control over the conduct of any particular visit. The reviewers are generally free to speak with whomever they wish and to ask these individuals whatever they consider important to know. They may also request documents for review. Over the course of a site visit, unanticipated issues may emerge. The site visitors typically explore both the anticipated issues and questions articulated in the guidelines and those that emerge during the site visit itself. The result is a report usually drafted on site or very soon after the visit is completed.

Responsive–Illuminative

The **responsive–illuminative approach** seeks to represent the viewpoints of both users of the resource and people who are an otherwise significant part of the clinical environment where the resource operates (Hamilton et al., 1977). The goal is understanding or illumination rather than judgment. The methods used derive largely from ethnography. The investigators immerse themselves in the environment where the resource is operational. The designs of these studies are not rigidly predetermined. They develop dynamically as the investigators' experience accumulates. The study team begins with a minimal set of orienting questions; the deeper questions that receive thoroughgoing study evolve over time. Many examples of studies using this approach can be found in the literature of medical informatics (Fafchamps et al., 1991; Forsythe, 1992; Kaplan & Duchon, 1988).

Note that the study types described in Table 8.2 relate to the purposes, foci, settings, and logistics of evaluation studies. The evaluation approaches introduced in this section address a complementary issue: what methods will be used to identify specific questions and to collect data as part of the actual conduct of these studies. Although it is perhaps extreme to state that every evaluation approach can apply to every type of study, there is certainly potential to use both objectivist and subjectivist approaches throughout Table 8.2. At the two extremes, for example, both need-validation studies and clinical-effects studies provide opportunities for application of subjectivist as well as objectivist approaches.

8.4.4 Stages of Technology Assessment

Yet another way to categorize studies is according to the three stages of technology assessment (Fuchs & Garber, 1990; Garber & Owens, 1994). The first stage emphasizes **technical characteristics**, such as the response time of an information system to a query or the degree of resolution of an imaging system. The second stage emphasizes the **efficacy** or effectiveness of a device, information system, or diagnostic or therapeutic strategy (Fuchs & Garber, 1990). Clinical trials of information systems usually fit this category, as do randomized trials of clinical interventions. The trials often use **process measures**, such as the degree of physician compliance with computer-generated reminders or the change in laboratory parameters in response to treatment rather than the endpoints that matter to patients: mortality, morbidity, and cost. Studies that determine the sensitivity and specificity of diagnostic tests are another example of second-stage assessments (see Chapter 3).

Third-stage assessments directly evaluate health and economic **outcomes**; therefore, these evaluations are the most comprehensive technology assessments (Fuchs & Garber, 1990). A third-stage evaluation of a computer-based reminder system for breast-cancer screening would examine changes in mortality or morbidity from breast cancer rather than physician compliance with guidelines. Typically, a third-stage evaluation also would evaluate the costs of such a system. When outcomes are infrequent or occur after a long delay (such as the occurrence of breast cancer), third-stage evaluations may be substantially more difficult to perform than are second-stage evaluations; thus, third-stage assessments are uncommon in medical informatics (Johnston et al., 1994). Third-stage evaluations also may consider the importance of patients' preferences in assessing the outcomes of an intervention (Nease & Owens, 1994; Owens, 1998a).

We examine the types of evaluations that investigators may initiate for each of the stages of technology assessment.

Stage I Assessments: Technical Characteristics

The choice of what to evaluate during a first-stage technology assessment depends on the purpose of the evaluation (Friedman & Wyatt, 1997b). Possibilities include the evaluation of the design and development process of a clinical information resource or of the structure of the resource (the hardware, input and output devices, user interface, internal data, knowledge structures, processor, algorithms, or inference methods). An assessment of the design and development process could evaluate the software engineering of the resource. Such an evaluation might be important to assess how the resource could be integrated with other systems or platforms. The rationale for studying the structure of the resource is the assumption that, if the resource contains appropriately designed components linked together in a suitable architecture, the system is more likely to function correctly.

Stage II Assessments: Clinical Efficacy

Second-stage assessments move beyond evaluation of operating parameters to an evaluation of the function of the information resource. These evaluations are increasingly common: Recent overviews report over 100 clinical trials of information resources (Balas et al., 1996; Johnston et al., 1994; Shea et al., 1996). Examples of second-stage evaluations include studies of computer-assisted drug dosing, preventive care reminder systems, and computer-aided quality assurance programs for active medical problems. The majority of these second-stage evaluations assess the effect of information resources on the process of care. Did the clinician prescribe the right drug dose? Did the patient receive an influenza vaccine? In situations in which a process measure correlates closely with health outcome (e.g., use of thrombolytic therapy for patients who have heart attacks correlates closely with decreased mortality rates), use of the process measure will not adversely affect validity and will increase the feasibility of the study (Mant & Hicks, 1995). The link from many interventions to the intended health and economic outcomes is not, however, well defined; in these circumstances, a second-stage technology assessment may not be sufficient to justify implementation of a system, particularly if the system is costly.

Stage III Assessments: Comprehensive Clinical, Economic, and Social Outcomes

Rising healthcare costs have forced policy-makers, clinicians, and developers to assess whether health interventions provide sufficient value for the required economic investment. Thus, a demonstration of efficacy is often not sufficient: Proponents of a technology must also establish its cost effectiveness (see Section 8.5.5 for a more detailed explanation of cost-effectiveness studies). The third stage of technology assessment encompasses these more sophisticated assessments. The hallmark of these evaluations is a comprehensive assessment of health and economic outcomes. Studies that evaluate comprehensive outcomes will be more useful than studies that evaluates narrowly defined outcomes. Thus, a study that evaluates the cost effectiveness of an information resource in terms of dollars per quality-adjusted life years saved (see Chapter 3) would enable clinicians and policy-makers to compare the cost effectiveness of an information resource to a wide variety of interventions. In contrast, a study that evaluates an information resource in terms of dollars per cases of cancer prevented would provide a useful comparison only for other interventions that prevent cancer.

The choice of outcome measures for a third-stage assessment depends on the purpose of the study and on the cost and feasibility of measuring the outcome. Common choices include the number of lives saved, life-years saved, quality-adjusted life years saved, cancers prevented, and cases of disease averted. For example, a third-stage evaluation of a computer-generated protocol for treatment of hypertension could measure changes in blood pressure of patients whose care was governed by the protocol. The evaluation could also assess the costs of implementing the protocol and subsequently the cost effectiveness of the implementation of the computer-generated protocol. An evaluation of computer-based guidelines for care of people who have human immunodeficiency virus (HIV) evaluated the effect of the guideline on the rate of hospitalization for opportunistic infection (Safran et al., 1995). The study found that, under the guidelines, providers responded more rapidly to changes in patient status (such as abnormal laboratory tests), but this prompt action did not change the rate of hospitalization. This study highlights the difficulty of demonstrating that a beneficial change in the process of care has led to improved health outcomes. In fact, few studies have demonstrated that information resources improve health outcomes (Johnston et al., 1994). The studies may not show benefit because of inadequate sample sizes, use of outcome measures that are difficult to assess, inadequate follow-up, other weaknesses in study design, or interventions that do not work (Rotman et al., 1996).

In summary, the requirements of a technology assessment have expanded to include comprehensive health, economic, and social outcomes. Third-stage technology assessment is a particular challenge in medical informatics. Although the use of process measures will be appropriate in certain circumstances, when feasible economically and logistically, investigators should plan evaluations that incorporate comprehensive health and economic outcomes.

8.5 Conduct of Objectivist Studies

In this section, we focus on the comparison-based approach, which is the most widely used objectivist approach and which also is the basis of most work in technology assessment.

8.5.1 Structure and Terminology of Comparative Studies

In a comparative study, the investigator typically creates a contrasting set of conditions to compare the effects of one with those of another. Usually, the goal is to attribute cause and effect or to answer scientific questions raised by other kinds of studies. After identifying a sample of subjects for his study, the researcher assigns each subject, often randomly, to one or a set of conditions. Some variable of interest is measured for each subject. The aggregated values of this variable are compared across the conditions. To understand the many issues that affect design of comparative studies, we must develop a precise terminology.

The **subjects** in a study are the entities about which data are collected. A specific study will employ one sample of subjects, although this sample might be subdivided if, for example, subjects are assigned to conditions in a comparative design. It is key to emphasize that subjects are often people—either care providers or recipients—but also may be information resources, groups of people, or organizations. In informatics, medical care is conducted in hierarchical settings with naturally occurring groups (a "doctor's patients"; the "care providers in a ward team"), so we often face the challenging question of exactly who the subjects are.

Variables are specific characteristics of subjects that either are measured purposefully by the investigator or are self-evident properties of the subjects that do not require measurement. In the simplest study, there may be only one variable, for example, the time required for an information system to complete a particular task.

Some variables take on a continous range of values. Others have a discrete set of **levels** corresponding to each of the measured values that that variable can have. For example, in a hospital setting, physician members of a ward team can be classified as residents, fellows, or attendings. In this case, the variable "physician's level of qualification" has three levels.

In studies in which computers or people solve problems or work through clinical cases, we use the term **task** to refer generically to those problems or cases. Designing or choosing tasks can be the most challenging aspect of an evaluation.

The **dependent variables** form a subset of the variables in the study that captures the outcomes of interest to the investigator. For this reason, dependent variables are also called **outcome variables**. A study may have one or more dependent variables. In a typical study, the dependent variable will be computed, for each subject, as an average over a number of tasks. For example, clinicians' diagnostic performance may be measured over a set of cases that provide a range of diagnostic challenges.

The **independent variables** are included in a study to explain the measured values of the dependent variables. For example, whether a computer system is available, or not, to support certain clinical tasks could be the major independent variable in a study designed to evaluate that system. A purely descriptive study has no independent variables; comparative studies can have one or many independent variables.

Measurement challenges almost always arise in the assessment of the outcome or dependent variable for a study. Often, for example, the dependent variable is some type of performance measure that invokes concerns about reliability (precision) and validity (accuracy) of measurement. Depending on the study, the independent variables may also raise measurement challenges. When the independent variable is gender, for example, the measurement problems are relatively straightforward. If the independent variable is an attitude, level of experience, or extent of resource use, however, profound measurement challenges can arise.

8.5.2 Issues of Measurement

Measurement is the process of assigning a value corresponding to the presence, absence, or degree of a specific attribute in a specific object, as illustrated in Figure 8.4. Measurement usually results in either (1) the assignment of a numerical score representing the extent to which the attribute of interest is present in the object or (2) the assignment of an object to a specific category. Taking the temperature (attribute) of a patient (object) is an example of the process of measurement.

From the premises underlying objectivist studies (see Section 8.4.2), it follows that proper execution of such studies requires careful and specific attention to

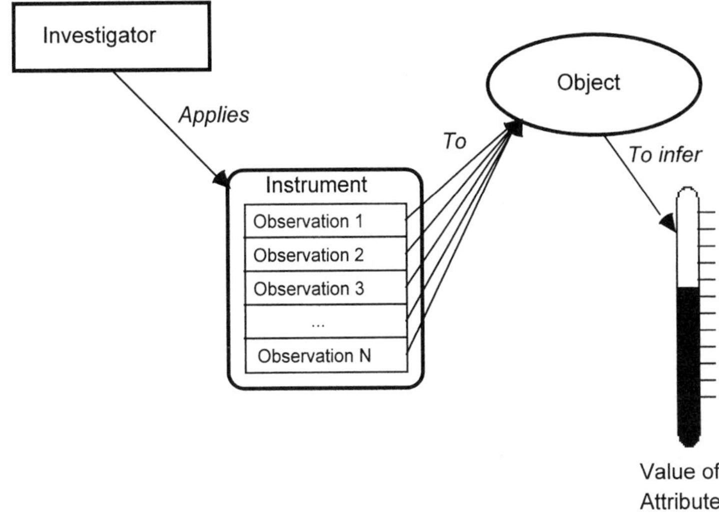

FIGURE 8.4. The process of measurement. (*Source:* Friedman & Wyatt, 1997a.)

methods of measurement. It can never be assumed, particularly in informatics, that attributes of interest are measured without error. Accurate and precise measurement must not be an afterthought. Measurement is of particular importance in medical informatics because, as a relatively young field, informatics does not have a well-established tradition of "variables worth measuring" or proven instruments for measuring them. By and large, people planning studies are faced first with the task of deciding what to measure and then with that of developing their own measurement methods. For most researchers, these tasks prove to be harder and more time consuming than initially anticipated. In some cases, informatics investigators can adapt the measures used by other investigators, but often they need to apply their measures to a different setting where prior experience may not apply.

We can underscore the importance of measurement by establishing a formal distinction between studies undertaken to develop methods for making measurements, which we call *measurement studies,* and the subsequent use of these methods to address questions of direct importance in informatics, which we call *demonstration studies.* **Measurement studies** seek to determine how accurately an attribute of interest can be measured in a population of objects. In an ideal objectivist measurement, all observers will agree on the result of the measurement. Any disagreement is therefore due to error, which should be minimized. The more agreement among observers or across observations, the better the measurement. Measurement procedures developed and validated through measurement studies provide researchers with what they need to conduct **demonstration studies** that directly address questions of substantive and practical concern. Once we know how accurately we can measure an attribute using a particular procedure, we can employ the measured values of this attribute as a variable in a demonstration study to draw inferences about the performance, perceptions, or effects of an information resource. For example, once a measurement study has explored how accurately the speed of an information resource can be measured, a related demonstration study would explore whether a particular resource has sufficient speed—speed being measured using methods developed in the measurement study—to meet the needs of busy clinicians.

A detailed discussion of measurement issues is beyond the scope of this chapter. The bottom line is that investigators should know that their measurement methods will be adequate before they collect data for their studies. It is necessary to perform a measurement study, involving data collection on a small scale, to establish the adequacy of all measurement procedures if the measures to be used do not have an established track record. Even if the measurement procedures of interest do have a track record in a particular healthcare environment and with a specific mix of cases and care providers, they may not perform equally well in a different environment, so measurement studies may still be necessary. Researchers should always ask themselves, "How good are my measures in this particular setting?" whenever they are planning a study, before they proceed to the demonstration phase. The importance of measurement studies for informatics was explained in 1990 by Michaelis and coworkers.

8.5.3 Control Strategies in Comparative Studies

One of the most challenging questions in comparative study design is how to obtain control. We need a way to monitor all the other changes taking place that are not attributable to the information resource. In clinical medicine, it is occasionally possible to predict patient outcomes with good accuracy from a small set of initial clinical findings—for example, the survival of patients in intensive care (Knaus et al., 1991). In these unusual circumstances, where we have a mechanism to tell us what would have happened to patients if we had not intervened, we can compare what actually happens with what is predicted to draw tentative conclusions about the benefit of the information resource. Such accurate **predictive models** are, however, extremely unusual in medicine (Wyatt & Altman, 1995). Instead, we use various types of **controls**: subjects who complete tasks that are not affected by the intervention of interest.

In the following sections we review a series of control strategies. We employ as a running example a reminder system that prompts doctors to order prophylactic antibiotics for orthopedic patients to prevent postoperative infections. In this example, the intervention is the installation and commissioning of the reminder system; the subjects are the physicians; and the tasks are the patients cared for by the physicians. The dependent variables derive from the outcome measurements made and would include physicians' ordering of antibiotics and the rate of postoperative infections averaged across the patients cared for by each physician.

Descriptive (Uncontrolled) Studies

In the simplest possible design, a **descriptive** or uncontrolled **study**, we install the reminder system, allow a suitable period for training, and then make our measurements. There is no independent variable. Suppose that we discover that the overall postoperative infection rate is five percent and that physicians order prophylactic antibiotics in 60 percent of orthopedic cases. Although we have two measured dependent variables, it is hard to interpret these figures without any comparison—it is possible that there has been no change due to the system.

Historically Controlled Experiments

As a first improvement to a descriptive study, let us consider a **historically controlled experiment**, sometimes called a **before–after study**. The investigator makes **baseline** measurements of antibiotic ordering and postoperative infection rates before the information resource is installed and then makes the same measurements after the information resource is in routine use. The independent variable is time and has two levels: before and after resource installation. Let us say that, at baseline, the postoperative infection rates were 10 percent and doctors ordered prophylactic antibiotics in only 40 percent of cases; the postintervention figures are the same as before (see Table 8.3).

The evaluators may claim that the halving of the infection rate can be safely ascribed to the information resource, especially because it was accompanied by a 20 percent improvement in doctors' antibiotic prescribing. Many other factors might, however, have changed in the interim to cause these results, especially if there was a long interval between the baseline and postintervention measurements. New staff could have taken over, the case mix of patients could have altered, new prophylactic antibiotics may have been introduced, or clinical audit meetings may have highlighted the infection problem and thus caused greater clinical awareness. Simply assuming that the reminder system alone caused the reduction in infection rates is naive. Other factors, known or unknown, could have changed meanwhile, making untenable the simple assumption that our intervention is responsible for all of the observed effects.

Simultaneous Nonrandomized Controls

To address some of the problems with historical controls, we might use **simultaneous controls**, which requires us to make our outcome measurements in doc-

TABLE 8.3. Hypothetical results of historically controlled study of an antibiotic reminder system.

	Antibiotic prescribing rate	Postoperative infection rate
Baseline results (before installation)	40%	10%
Postinstallation results	60%	5%

Source: Friedman and Wyatt (1997a).

tors and patients who are not influenced by the prophylactic antibiotic reminder system but who are subject to the other changes taking place in the environment. Taking measurements both before and during the intervention strengthens the design, because it gives an estimate of the changes due to the nonspecific factors taking place during the study period.

This study design would be a parallel group comparative study with simultaneous controls. Table 8.4 gives hypothetical results of such a study, focusing on postoperative-infection rates as a single outcome measure or dependent variable. The independent variables are time and group, both of which have two levels of intervention and control. There is the same improvement in the group where reminders were available, but no improvement—indeed a slight deterioration—where no reminders were available. This design provides suggestive evidence of an improvement that is most likely to be due to the reminder system. This inference is stronger if the same doctors worked in the same wards during the period the system was introduced and if similar kinds of patients, subject to the same nonspecific influences, were being operated on during the whole time period.

Even though the controls in this example are simultaneous, skeptics may still refute our argument by claiming that there is some systematic, unknown difference between the clinicians or patients in the two groups. For example, if the two groups comprised the patients and clinicians in two adjacent wards, the difference in the infection rates could be attributable to systematic or chance differences between the wards. Perhaps hospital staffing levels improved in some wards but not in others or there was cross infection by a multiply resistant organism among only the patients in the control ward. To overcome such criticisms, we could expand the study to include all wards in the hospital—or even other hospitals—but that would clearly take considerable resources. We could try to measure everything that happens to every patient in both wards and to build complete psychological profiles of all staff to rule out systematic differences. We would still, however, be vulnerable to the accusation that some variable that we did not measure—did not even know about—explains the difference between the two wards. A better strategy is to ensure that the controls really are comparable by randomizing them.

Simultaneous Randomized Controls

The crucial problem in the previous example is that, although the controls were simultaneous, there may have been systematic, unmeasured differences between

Table 8.4. Hypothetical results of simultaneous controlled study of antibiotic reminder system.

	Postoperative infection rates	
	Reminder group	Control group
Baseline results	10%	10%
Postintervention results	5%	11%

Source: Friedman and Wyatt (1997a).

Table 8.5. Hypothetical results of a simultaneous randomized controlled study of antibiotic reminder system.

	Postoperative infection rates	
	Reminder physicians	Control physicians
Baseline results	11%	10%
Postinstallation results	6%	8%

Source: Friedman and Wyatt (1997a).

them and the subjects receiving the intervention. A simple and effective way of removing systematic differences, whether due to known or unknown factors, is to randomize the assignment of subjects to control or intervention groups. Thus, we could randomly allocate one-half of the doctors on both wards to receive the antibiotic reminders and the remaining doctors to work normally. We would then measure and compare postoperative infection rates in patients managed by doctors in the reminder and control groups. Provided that the doctors never look after one anothers' patients, any difference that is statistically "significant" (conventionally, for which the p value is less than 0.05) can be attributed reliably to the reminders. The only way other differences could have emerged is by chance.

Table 8.5 shows the hypothethetical results of such a study. The baseline infection rates in the patients managed by the two groups of doctors are similar, as we would expect, because the patients were allocated to the groups by chance. There is a greater reduction in infection rates in patients of reminder physicians compared with those of control physicians. Because random assignment means that there was no systematic difference in patient characteristics between groups, the only systematic difference between the two groups of patients is receipt of reminders by their doctors.

Provided that the sample size is large enough for these results to be statistically significant, we might begin to conclude with some confidence that providing doctors with reminders caused the reduction in infection rates. One lingering question is why there was also a small reduction, from baseline to installation, in infection rates in control cases, even though the control group should have received no reminders.

8.5.4 Threats to Inference and Validity

We all want our studies to be valid. There are two aspects to this: internal and external validity. If a study has **internal validity**, we can be confident in the conclusions drawn from the specific circumstances of the experiment—the population of subjects studied, the measurements made, and the interventions provided. Are we justified in concluding that the differences observed are due to the attributed causes? Even if all threats to internal validity are overcome to our satisfaction, we would also like our study to have **external validity**, such that the conclusions can be generalized from the specific setting, subjects, and intervention studied to the broader range of settings that other people will encounter.

Thus, even if we demonstrate convincingly that our antibiotic reminder system reduces postoperative infection rates in our own hospital, this finding is of little interest to other clinicians unless we can convince them that the results can be generalized safely to other reminder systems or to the same system in other hospitals.

When we conduct a comparative study, there are four possible outcomes. We illustrate them in the context of a study that explores the effectiveness of an information resource and that uses an appropriate comparative design.

1. The information resource was effective, and our study shows that it was.
2. The information resource was ineffective, and our study shows that it was.
3. The information resource was effective, but for some reason our study mistakenly failed to show that it was (a type II error).
4. The information resource was ineffective, but for some reason our study mistakenly suggested that it was effective (a type I error).

Outcomes 1 and 2 are salutary from a methodological viewpoint; the results of the study mirror reality. Outcome 3 is a false-negative result, or **type II error**. In the language of inferential statistics, we mistakenly accept the **null hypothesis**. Type II errors can arise because the size of the information resource's effect on the measure of interest is small and too few subjects have been included for the study to detect it (Freiman et al., 1978). Alternatively, we may have failed to measure the outcome variable on which the example resource is having an effect. In outcome 4, we have concluded that the resource is valuable when it is not: We have a false-positive result or **type I error**. We have mistakenly rejected the null hypothesis. A risk of a type I error is built into every study. When we accept, for example, the conventional value of $p < 0.05$ as a criterion for statistical significance, we are consciously accepting a five percent risk of making a type I error as a consequence of using randomization as a mechanism of experimental control. If we feel uncomfortable with this five percent risk of a type I or false positive error, we can reduce it by reducing the threshold for statistical significance to 0.01, which carries only a 1 percent chance of a type I error.

The more important threats to internal validity of studies are the following:

- **Assessment bias**: It is important to ensure that all persons involved in a study do not allow their own feelings and beliefs about an information resource—positive or negative—to bias the results. Consider a study in which the same clinicians who are users of an antibiotic reminder system also collect the clinical data used for determining whether the advice generated by the system is correct, such as the incidence of significant wound or chest infections. If they had some prejudice against the reminder system and wished to undermine it, they might massage the clinical infection data to prove themselves right and the reminder system wrong in certain patients. Thus, they might record that a patient was suffering from a nonexistent postoperative cough with productive sputum to justify an antibiotic prescription that the reminder system had not advised.

- **Allocation bias**: Early studies of information resources often take place in the environment in which the resources were developed and often arouse strong (positive or negative) feelings among study subjects. In a study where patients are randomized and the subjects have strong beliefs about the information resource, two biases may arise. Investigators may cheat the randomization method and systematically allocate easier (or more difficult) cases to the information-resource group (allocation bias), or they may avoid recruiting a particularly easy (or difficult) case to the study if they know in advance that the next patient will be allocated to the control group (Schulz et al., 1995).
- **The Hawthorne effect**: The Hawthorne effect is the tendency for humans to improve their performance if they know it is being studied. Psychologists measured the effect of ambient lighting on workers' productivity at the Hawthorne factory in Chicago (Roethligsburger & Dickson, 1939). Productivity increased as the room illumination level was raised, but productivity increased again when the illumination level was accidentally reduced. The study itself, rather than changes in illumination, caused the increases. During a study of a medical information resource, the attention of the investigators can lead to an improvement in the performance of all subjects in all study groups, intervention and control, due to the Hawthorne effect.
- **The checklist effect**: The checklist effect is the improvement observed in decision-making due to more complete and better-structured data collection when paper-based or computer-based forms are used to collect patient data. The effect of forms on decision-making can equal that of computer-generated advice (Adams et al., 1986), so it must either be controlled for or quantified. To control for the checklist effect, investigators should collect the same data in the same way in the control and information-resource groups, even though the information resource's output is available in only the latter group (see, e.g., Wyatt, 1989).
- **The placebo effect**: In some drug trials, simply giving patients an inactive tablet or other placebo can cause a measurable improvement in some clinical variables such as well being, sleep pattern, and exercise tolerance, because patients feel good about receiving attention and potentially useful medication. This placebo effect may be more powerful than the drug effect itself and may obscure a complete absence of pharmaceutical benefit. In a study of a medical information resource, if some patients watch their doctors consult an impressive workstation while others have no such experience, this experience could unbalance the groups and overestimate the value of the information resource. Alternatively, some patients might believe that a care provider who needs a computer workstation is less competent than one who can manage without. Several studies have, however, shown that patients show more confidence in clinicians who use technology than in those who get by without it.

These and a number of other biases that may apply in certain kinds of studies are more fully discussed in Chapter 7 of Friedman and Wyatt (1997a).

8.5.5 *Cost-Effectiveness and Cost-Benefit Studies*

The purpose of cost-effectiveness and cost-benefit analyses is to assess quantitatively the benefits obtained from a health intervention relative to the costs of the intervention. In short, cost-effectiveness and cost-benefit analyses provide a mechanism to assess the relative value of different interventions in producing health benefits, such as longer life or greater quality of life. Our description of these analyses is brief; for further details, see Gold (1996), Weinstein and Fineberg (1980), and Sox et al. (1988). In a **cost-effectiveness analysis**, the analyst expresses the health benefits in units of health outcomes (e.g., lives saved) and the costs in dollars. The analyst can choose the health outcomes that she believes are appropriate for the purpose of the analysis, such as life years saved, quality-adjusted life years saved, or cases of disease prevented. Usually she seeks to compare the cost and health effects of one treatment relative to the costs and health effects of another treatment. In such a situation, the appropriate estimate of the relative value of the interventions is the **marginal cost-effectiveness ratio**. To calculate the marginal cost-effectiveness ratio for intervention *b* relative to intervention *a*, we divide the difference in the costs with the two interventions by the difference in health benefits. For example, for interventions whose benefits are measured as increases in life expectancy (LE), we calculate the marginal cost-effectiveness ratio for intervention *b* relative to intervention *a* as

$$\frac{C_b - C_a}{LE_b - LE_a},$$

where C_b is the cost of intervention *b*, C_a is the cost of intervention *a*, LE_b is the life expectancy with intervention *b*, and LE_a is life expectancy with intervention *a*.

In contrast to cost-effectiveness analyses, a **cost-benefit analysis** values all benefits and costs in dollars. Thus, if a health intervention averts a death, the analyst must express the value of that averted death in dollars. The goal of such an analysis is to determine whether the benefit (expressed in dollars) is larger than the cost (expressed in dollars).

To perform a cost-effectiveness analysis, the analyst must perform the following steps (Gold et al., 1996; Office of Technology Assessment, 1980): (1) define the problem, including identification of the objective and perspective of the analysis and the alternative interventions under consideration; (2) identify and analyze the benefits; (3) identify and analyze the costs; (4) perform discounting; (5) analyze uncertainties; (6) address ethical questions; and (7) interpret the results. We shall illustrate these concepts with the example that we used in Section 8.5.3 of a computer-based reminder system that prompts physicians to order prophylactic antibiotics before orthopedic surgery.

The first step of a cost-effectiveness analysis is to define the problem clearly. Failure to define the problem carefully can lead to many difficulties. One approach to defining the problem is to determine the decision context: What decision does the analyst, or the consumer of the analysis, need to make? Is the decision whether to implement a computer-based antibiotic reminder system or a manual system? Or, is the decision which computer-based antibiotic reminder system to implement? Or, do the decision-makers seek to know whether to implement a computer-based system or to hire a nurse practitioner to check the antibiotic orders? Answers to these questions will enable the analyst to frame the analysis appropriately.

To ensure that the cost-effectiveness ratio that she calculates will be helpful for the decision-makers, the analyst also should identify the objective of the study. Is the objective to reduce hospital costs or all costs? A program that reduced hospital costs could do so by shifting certain costs to the outpatient setting. Is that a concern? The analyst also should determine the perspective of the analysis, because the perspective determines whose costs and whose benefits belong in the analysis. For example, if the perspective is that of the hospital, outpatient costs may not matter. If the perspective of the analysis is societal, however, as is typically true, the analyst should include outpatient costs. Finally, the analyst should identify the alternatives that the decision-makers will (or should) consider. Rather than install an expensive hospital information system, perhaps the hospital should sign a contract with another hospital to perform all orthopedic surgeries. If the analyst has evaluated the decision context carefully, the important alternatives should be clear.

The next step in a cost-effectiveness analysis is to identify and analyze the health outcomes and costs of the alternative interventions. How should the analyst evaluate the cost effectiveness of the antibiotic reminder system? First, she should decide how to measure the health benefit of the system. She could quantify the health benefit by assessing the number of postoperative infections before and after implementation of the computer-based system. The units of the cost-effectiveness ratio would therefore be dollars expended per postoperative infection prevented. Such a ratio may be helpful to decision-makers, but the decision-makers could compare the cost effectiveness of the system only to other interventions that prevent postoperative infections; for example, they could not compare the cost effectiveness of the system to that of a computer-based reminder system for breast-cancer screening. To remedy this problem, the analyst could choose a more comprehensive measure of health outcome, such as quality-adjusted life years (see Chapter 3). The analysts would then estimate the number of quality-adjusted life years saved for each postoperative infection prevented. Decision modeling provides one approach to make such estimates (see Chapter 3). Thus, use of quality-adjusted life years would enable policy-makers to evaluate the cost effectiveness of the antibiotic reminder system relative to other interventions, but would impose an additional analytic burden on the analyst.

To evaluate the marginal cost effectiveness of the reminder system, the analysts must also estimate the costs with the old system and the costs with the computer-based system. The literature often refers to *direct costs* and *indirect costs*, but these terms are not used consistently. We shall follow the definitions and conventions of Gold and colleagues (1996) and refer to costs as either *direct costs* or *productivity costs*. With this approach, certain costs that we classify as direct costs formerly were considered as indirect costs. The **direct costs** include the value of all the goods, services, and other resources that are required to produce an intervention, including resources consumed because of future consequences (intended or unintended) of the intervention (Gold et al., 1996). Direct costs include changes in the use of healthcare resources, of nonhealthcare resources, of informal caregiver time, and of patient time. The direct healthcare costs include the costs of drugs, tests, procedures, supplies, healthcare personnel, and facilities. For the antibiotic reminder system, the direct healthcare costs include the costs of installation, maintenance, personnel, supplies, drugs (antibiotics), and the future cost savings that may result from a reduction in postoperative infection, among others. Direct nonhealthcare costs include other services required for the delivery of an intervention, such as patients' transportation costs associated with medical care. If family members provide ancillary care, the value of their time also is a cost of the intervention. The time a patient must spend to receive the intervention also is a cost. Because implementation of an antibiotic reminder system would not change these costs, the analyst does not need to include them in an analysis. **Productivity costs** are those costs that accrue because of changes in productivity due to illness or death; they could be relevant to the analysis of the antibiotic reminder system if prevention of postoperative infection changed substantially the time away from work for patients in whom infection was prevented (for further discussion, see Gold et al., 1996).

To complete the analysis, the analyst should discount health and economic outcomes, address uncertainty and ethical considerations, and interpret the results. **Discounting** enables the analyst to account for time preference in the analysis: Expenditures and health benefits that occur in the future have less value than do those expenditures or benefits that occur immediately. The analyst performs discounting by calculating the net present value of health outcomes and costs; this calculation reduces the influence of future health and economic outcomes relative to those that occur in the present (for further explanations see Gold et al., 1996). Both health and economic outcomes should be discounted (Gold et al., 1996). Sensitivity analyses (described in Chapter 3) provide a mechanism for assessing the importance of uncertainty. Ethical concerns include how to ensure equity in policy alternatives, how to value outcomes, and how to choose a cost-effectiveness threshold (also see Chapter 7). The **cost-effectiveness threshold** (e.g., $50,000 per quality-adjusted life year saved) reflects the value judgment of the decision-makers about the maximum value of a year of life saved. Although currently there is not a consensus on the appropriate threshold, many interventions that are used widely cost less than $50,000 to $60,000 per quality-adjusted life year gained (Owens, 1998b). Interpretation of the results should incorporate statements both about the influence of uncertainty on the estimated cost-effectiveness ratio and about ethical concerns.

Cost-effectiveness and cost-benefit analyses provide tools for helping policy-makers and clinicians to understand the relationship between the health outcomes and costs of alternative health interventions, including information resources. We emphasize that they provide information about one important aspect of an intervention, or information system, but are insufficient alone for decision-making.

Other social, ethical, and political factors will be important for most decisions. Evaluation of comprehensive information systems poses formidable challenges because the benefits of such systems may be diffuse, varied, and difficult to quantify. Nonetheless, like other healthcare interventions and innovations, information resources must provide sufficient benefit to justify their expense.

8.6 Conduct of Subjectivist Studies

The objectivist approaches to evaluation, described in the previous section, are useful for addressing some, but not all, of the interesting and important questions that challenge investigators in medical informatics. The subjectivist approaches described here address the problem of evaluation from a different set of premises. They use different, but equally rigorous methods.

8.6.1 The Rationale for Subjectivist Studies

Subjectivist methods enable us to address the deeper questions that arise in informatics: the detailed "whys" and "according to whoms" in addition to the aggregate "whethers" and "whats." As defined earlier, the responsive–illuminative approach, within the subjectivist family of approaches, seeks to represent the viewpoints of people who are users of the resource or are otherwise significant participants in the clinical environment where the resource operates. The goal is *illumination* rather than judgment. The investigators seek to build an argument that promotes deeper understanding of the information resource or environment of which it is a part. The methods used derive largely from **ethnography**. The investigators immerse themselves physically in the environment where the information resource is or will be operational, and they collect data primarily through observations, interviews, and reviews of documents. The designs—the data-collection plans—of these studies are not rigidly predetermined and do not unfold in a fixed sequence. They develop dynamically and nonlinearly as the investigators' experience accumulates.

Although subjectivist approaches may run counter to common ideas of how we ought to conduct empirical investigations, these methods and their conceptual underpinnings are not altogether foreign to the worlds of information and computer science. The pluralistic, nonlinear thinking that underlies subjectivist investigation shares many features with modern conceptualizations of the information-resource design process. For example, Winograd and Flores (1987, p. 170) argued as follows:

> In designing computer-based devices, we are not in the position of creating a formal "system" that covers the functioning of the organization and the people within it. When this is attempted, the resulting system (and the space of potential action for people within it) is inflexible and unable to cope with new breakdowns or potentials. Instead we design additions and changes to the network of equipment (some of it computer based) within which people work. The computer is like a tool, in that it is

> brought up for use by people engaged in some domain of action. The use of the tool shapes the potential for what those actions are and how they are conducted. Its power does not lie in having a single purpose . . . but in its connection to the larger network of communication (electronic, telephone, paper-based) in which organizations operate.

Another connection is to the methodology of **formal systems analysis**, which is generally accepted as an essential component of information resource development. Systems analysis uses many methods that resemble closely the subjectivist methods for evaluation that we introduce here. People recognize that systems analysis requires a process of information gathering, heavily reliant on interviews with people who use the existing system in various ways. Information gathering for systems analysis is typically portrayed as a cyclic, iterative process rather than as a linear process (Davis, 1994). In the literature of systems analysis, we find admonitions, analogous to those made by proponents of subjectivist evaluation, that an overly structured approach can misportray the capabilities of workers in the system's environment, misportray the role of informal communication in the work accomplished, underestimate the prevalence of exceptions, and fail to account for political forces within every organization that shape much of what actually happens (Bansler & Bødker, 1993). Within the field of systems analysis, then, there has developed an appreciation of some of the shortcomings of objectivist methods and of the potential value of subjectivist methods (Zachary et al., 1984).

8.6.2 A Rigorous, but Different, Methodology

The subjectivist approaches to evaluation, like their objectivist counterparts, are empirical methods. Although it is easy to focus on only their differences, these two broad classes of evaluation approaches share many features. In all empirical studies, for example, evidence is collected with great care; the investigator is always aware of what she is doing and why. The evidence is then compiled, interpreted, and ultimately reported. Investigators keep records of their procedures, and these records are open to audit by the investigators themselves or by individuals outside the study team. The principal investigator or evaluation-team leader is under an almost sacred scientific obligation to report his methods. Failure to do so will invalidate a study. Both classes of approaches also share a dependence on theories that guide investigators to explanations of the observed phenomena, as well as to a dependence on the pertinent empirical literature: published studies that address similar phenomena or similar settings. In both approaches, there are rules of good practice that are generally accepted; it is therefore possible to distinguish a good study from a bad one.

There are, however, fundamental differences between objectivist and subjectivist approaches. First, subjectivist studies are **emergent** in design. Objectivist studies typically begin with a set of hypotheses or specific questions and with a plan for addressing each member of this set. The investigator assumes that, barring major unforeseen developments, the plan will be followed exactly. Deviation, in fact, might introduce bias: The investigator who sees negative results emerging from the exploration of a particular question or use of a particular measurement instrument might change strategies in hope of obtaining more positive findings. In contrast, subjectivist studies typically begin with general **orienting issues** that stimulate the early stages of investigation. Through these initial investigations, the important questions for further study emerge. The subjectivist investigator is willing, at virtually any point, to adjust future aspects of the study in light of the most recent information obtained. Subjectivist investigators tend to be **incrementalists**; they change their plans from day to day and have a high tolerance for ambiguity and uncertainty. In this respect, they are much like good software developers. Also like software developers, subjectivist investigators must develop the ability to recognize when a project is finished: when further benefit can be obtained only at too great a cost in time, money, or work.

A second feature of subjectivist studies is a **naturalistic** orientation: a reluctance to manipulate the setting of the study, which in most cases is the environment into which the information resource is introduced. They do not alter the environment to study it. Control groups, placebos, purposeful altering of information resources to create contrasting interventions, and other techniques that are central to the construction of objectivist studies typically are not used. Subjectivist studies will, however, employ quantitative data for descriptive purposes and may offer quantitative comparisons when the research setting offers a "natural experiment" where such comparisons can be made without deliberate intervention. For example, when physicians and nurses both use a clinical system to enter orders, their experiences with the system offer a natural basis for comparison. Subjectivist researchers are opportunists where pertinent information is concerned; they will use what they see as the best information available to illuminate a question under investigation.

A third important distinguishing feature of subjectivist studies is that their end product is a report written in narrative prose. These reports may be lengthy and may require significant time investment from the reader; no technical understanding of quantitative research methodology or statistics is required to comprehend them. Results of subjectivist studies are therefore accessible—and may even be entertaining—to a broad community in a way that results of objectivist studies are not. Objectivist study reports often can be results of inferential statistical analyses that most readers will not find easy to read and will typically not understand. Reports of subjectivist studies seek to engage their audience.

8.6.3 Natural History of a Subjectivist Study

As a first step in describing the methodology of subjectivist evaluation, Figure 8.5 illustrates the stages or natural history of a study. These stages constitute a general sequence, but, as we mentioned, the subjectivist investigator must always be prepared to revise his thinking and possibly return to earlier stages in light of new evidence. Backtracking is a legitimate step in this model.

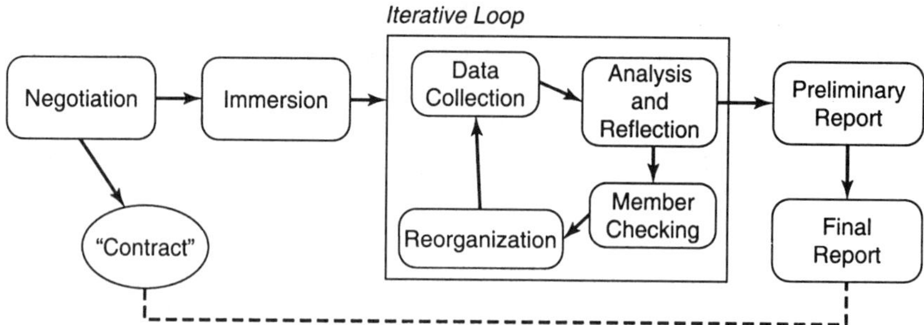

FIGURE 8.5. Natural history of subjectivist studies. (*Source:* Friedman & Wyatt, 1997a.)

1. *Negotiation of the ground rules of the study:* In any empirical research, and particularly in evaluation studies, it is important to negotiate an understanding between the study team and the people commissioning the study. This understanding should embrace the general aims of the study; the kinds of methods to be used; the access to various sources of information, including healthcare providers, patients, and various documents; and the format for interim and final reports. The aims of the study may be formulated in a set of initial **orienting questions**. Ideally, this understanding will be expressed in a **memorandum of understanding**, analogous to a contract.
2. *Immersion into the environment:* At this stage, the investigators begin spending time in the work environment. Their activities range from formal introductions, to informal conversations, to silent presence at meetings and other events. Investigators use the generic term **field** to refer to the setting, which may be multiple physical locations, where the work under study is carried out. Trust and openness between the investigators and the people in the field are essential elements of subjectivist studies to ensure full and candid exchange of information.

   Even as immersion is taking place, the investigator is already collecting data to sharpen the initial questions or issues guiding the study. Early discussions with people in the field, and other activities primarily targeted toward immersion, inevitably begin to shape the investigators' views. Almost from the outset, the investigator is typically addressing several aspects of the study simultaneously.
3. *Iterative loop:* At this point, the procedural structure of the study becomes akin to an iterative loop, as the investigator engages in cycles of data collection, analysis and reflection, member checking, and reorganization. Data collection involves interview, observation, document analysis, and other methods. Data are collected on planned occasions, as well as serendipidously or spontaneously. The data are recorded carefully and are interpreted in the context of what is already known. Analysis and reflection entail the contemplation of the new findings during each cycle of the loop. **Member checking** is the sharing of the investigator's emerging thoughts and beliefs with the par-

ticipants themselves. Reorganization results in a revised agenda for data collection in the next cycle of the loop.

Although each cycle within the iterative loop is depicted as linear, this representation is misleading. Net progress through the loop is clockwise, as shown in Figure 8.5, but backward steps are natural and inevitable. They are not reflective of mistakes or errors. An investigator may, after conducting a series of interviews and studying what participants have said, decide to speak again with one or two participants to clarify their positions on a particular issue.

4. *Preliminary report:* The first draft of the final report should itself be viewed as a research instrument. By sharing this report with a variety of individuals, the investigator obtains a major check on the validity of the findings. Typically, reactions to the preliminary report will generate useful clarifications and a general sharpening of the study findings. Because the report usually is a narrative, it is vitally important that it be well written, in language understandable by all intended audiences. Circulation of the report in draft can ensure that the final document communicates as intended. Use of anonymous quotations from interviews and documents makes a report highly vivid and meaningful to readers.
5. *Final report:* The final report, once completed, should be distributed as negotiated in the original memorandum of understanding. Distribution is often accompanied by "meet the investigator" sessions that allow interested persons to ask the author of the report to expand or explain what has been written.

8.6.4 Data-Collection and Data-Analysis Methods

What data-collection strategies are in the subjectivist researcher's black bag? There are several, and they are typically used in combination. We shall discuss each one, assuming a typical setting for a subjectivist study in medical informatics: the introduction of an information resource into patient-care activities in a hospital.

Observation

The investigator typically immerses himself into the setting under study in one of two ways. The investigator may act purely as a detached observer, becoming a trusted and unobtrusive feature of the environment but not a participant in the day-to-day work and thus reliant on multiple "informants" as sources of information. True to the naturalistic feature of this kind of study, great care is taken to diminish the possibility that the presence of the observer will skew the work activities that occur or that the observer will be rejected outright by the ward team. An alternative approach is participant observation, where the investigator becomes a member of the work team. Participant observation is more difficult to engineer; it may require the investigator to have specialized training in the study domain. It is time consuming but can give the investigator a more vivid impression of life in the work environment. During both kinds of observation, data accrue continuously. These data are qualitative and may be of several varieties: statements by healthcare providers and patients, gestures and other nonverbal expressions of these same individuals, and characteristics of the physical setting that seem to affect the delivery of health care.

Interviews

Subjectivist studies rely heavily on interviews. Formal interviews are occasions where both the investigator and interviewee are aware that the answers to questions are being recorded (on paper or tape) for direct contribution to the evaluation study. Formal interviews vary in their degree of structure. At one extreme is the **unstructured interview**, where there are no predetermined questions. Between the extremes is the **semistructured interview**, where the investigator specifies in advance a set of topics that he would like to address but is flexible as to the order in which these topics are addressed and is open to discussion of topics not on the prespecified list. At the other extreme is the **structured interview**, with a schedule of questions that are always presented in the same words and in the same order. In general, the unstructured and semistructured interviews are preferred in subjectivist research. Informal interviews—spontaneous discussions between the investigators and members of a ward team, as occur during routine observation—are also part of the data-collection process. Informal interviews are invariably considered a source of important data.

Document and Artifact Analysis

Every project produces a trail of papers and other artifacts. These include patient charts, the various versions of a computer program and its documentation, memoranda prepared by the project team, perhaps a cartoon hung on the office door by a ward clerk. Unlike the day-to-day events of patient care, these artifacts do not change once created or introduced. They can be examined retrospectively and referred to repeatedly, as necessary, over the course of a study. Also included under this heading are **unobtrusive measures**, which are records accrued as part of the routine use of the information resource. They include, for example, user trace files of an information resource. Data from these measures are often quantifiable.

Anything Else That Seems Useful

Subjectivist investigators are supreme opportunists. As questions of importance to a study emerge, the investigator will collect any information that he perceives as bearing on these questions. This data collection could include clinical chart reviews, questionnaires, tests, simulated patients, and other methods more commonly associated with the objectivist approaches. There are many procedures for analysis of qualitative data. The important point is that the analysis is conducted systematically. In general terms, the investigator looks for themes or trends emerging from several different sources. He collates individual statements and observations by theme, as well as by source. Some investigators transfer these observations to file cards so they can be sorted and resorted in a variety of ways. Others use software especially designed to facilitate analysis of qualitative data (Fielding & Lee, 1991). At the present level of the technology, the investigator must key in all his handwritten notes, but the flexibility afforded by the software often justifies the effort. Hand-held and pen-based computers may eventually change the way subjectivist research is carried out.

The analysis process is fluid, with analytic goals shifting as the study matures. At an early stage, the goal is primarily to focus the questions that themselves will be the targets of further data elicitation. At the later stages of study, the primary goal is to collate data that address these questions.

8.7 Conclusions: The Mindset of Evaluation and Technology Assessment

The previous sections probably make evaluation and technology assessment look difficult. If scholars of the field disagree in fundamental ways about how these studies should be done, how can relative novices proceed at all, much less with confidence? To address this dilemma, we close this chapter by offering a mindset for evaluation: a general orientation that anyone conducting an evaluation might constructively bring to her work. The components of this mindset apply, to varying degrees, across all study types and approaches.

- *Tailor the study to the problem:* Every study is made to order. Evaluation and technology assessment differ from mainstream views of research in that a study derives importance from the needs of clients rather than from the unanswered questions of an academic discipline. If an evaluation contributes new knowledge of general importance to an academic discipline, that is a serendipitous byproduct.
- *Collect data that will be useful to make decisions:* There is no theoretical limit to the questions that can be asked and, consequently, to the data that can be collected in a study. What is done is determined by the decisions that need ultimately to be made and the information seen as useful to inform these decisions.
- *Look for intended and unintended effects:* Whenever a new information resource is introduced into an environment, there can be many consequences, only some of which relate to the stated purpose of the resource. In a complete evaluation, it is important to look for and document effects that were anticipated as well as those that were not and to continue the study long enough to allow these effects to manifest themselves.
- *Study the resource while it is under development and after it is installed:* In general, the kinds of decisions evaluation can facilitate are of two types. **Formative decisions** are made as a result of studies undertaken while a resource is under development. They affect the resource before it can go on-line. **Summative decisions** are made after a resource is installed in its envisioned envi-

ronment and deal explicitly with how effectively the resource performs in that environment. Often, it will take many years for an installed resource to stabilize within an environment. Before summative studies are conducted, it may be necessary for this amount of time to pass.

- *Study the resource in the laboratory and in the field:* Completely different questions arise when an information resource is still in the laboratory and when it is in the field. In vitro studies, conducted in the developer's laboratory, and in vivo studies, conducted in an ongoing clinical or educational environment, are both important aspects of evaluation.
- *Go beyond the developer's point of view:* The developers of an information resource usually are empathic only up to a point and are often not predisposed to be detached and objective about the resource's performance and utility. People doing evaluation often see it as part of their job to get close to the end user and to portray the resource as the user sees it.
- *Take the environment into account:* Anyone who conducts an evaluation study must be, in part, an ecologist. The function of an information resource must be viewed as an interaction among the resource itself, a set of users of the resource, and the social, organizational, and cultural context that largely determines how work is carried out in that environment. Whether a new resource functions effectively is determined as much by its goodness of fit with its environment as by its compliance with the resource designers' operational specifications as measured in the laboratory.
- *Let the key issues emerge over time:* Evaluation studies are dynamic. The design for a study, as it might be stated in a project proposal, is often just a starting point. Rarely are the important questions known, with total precision or confidence, at the outset of a study. In the real world, evaluation designs, even those employing objectivist approaches, must have some leeway to evolve as the important issues come into focus.
- *Be methodologically Catholic and eclectic:* It is best to derive data-collection methods from the questions to be explored rather than to bring predetermined methods or instruments to a study. Certain questions are better answered with qualitative data collected through open-ended interviews and observation. Others are better answered with quantitative data collected via structured questionnaires, patient chart audits, and logs of user behavior.

Finally, remember that the perfect study has never been performed and probably never will be. This chapter has introduced various approaches to study design and execution that can minimize bias and maximize credibility, but the findings of every study can be questioned. It is sufficient for a study to be guiding, clarifying, or illuminating.

Suggested Readings

Anderson J.G., Aydin C.E., Jay S.J. (Eds.) (1994). *Evaluating Health Care Information Systems: Methods and Applications.* Thousand Oaks, CA: Sage Publications.

This is an excellent edited volume that covers a wide range of methodological and substantive issues in evaluation, including both objectivist and subjectivist approaches. Although not formally constructed as a textbook, it is written at a basic level for individuals more familiar with medical informatics than study methodology.

Cohen P.R. (91995). *Empirical Methods for Artificial Intelligence*. Cambridge, MA: MIT Press.

This is a nicely written, detailed book that is focused on evaluation of artificial intelligence applications, not necessarily those operating in medical domains. It emphasizes objectivist methods and could serve as a basic statistics course for computer science students.

Friedman C.P., Wyatt J.C. (1997). *Evaluation Methods in Medical Informatics*. New York: Springer-Verlag.

This is the book on which the current chapter is based. It offers expanded discussion of almost all issues and concepts raised in the current chapter.

Jain R. (1991). *The Art of Computer Systems Performance Analysis: Techniques for Experimental Design, Measurement, Simulation, and Modeling*. New York: John Wiley & Sons.

This work offers a technical discussion of a range of objectivist methods used to study computer systems. The scope is broader than Cohen's book (1995) described earlier. It contains many case studies and examples and assumes knowledge of basic statistics.

Lincoln Y.S., Guba E.G. (1985). *Naturalistic Inquiry*. Beverly Hills, CA: Sage Publications.

This is a classic book on subjectivist methods. The work is very rigorous but also very easy to read. Because it does not focus on medical domains or information systems, readers must make their own extrapolations.

Rossi P.H., Freeman H.E. (1989). *Evaluation: A Systematic Approach*, Fourth Edition. Newbury Park, CA: Sage Publications.

This is a valuable textbook on evaluation, emphasizing objectivist methods, and is very well written. Like the book of Lincoln and Guba (1985), described earlier, it is generic in scope, and the reader must relate the content to medical informatics. There are several excellent chapters addressing pragmatic issues of evaluation. These nicely complement the chapters on statistics and formal study designs.

Questions for Discussion

1. Choose any alternative area of biomedicine (e.g., drug trials) as a point of comparison, and list at least four factors that make studies in medical informatics more difficult to conduct successfully than in that area. Given these difficulties, discuss whether it is worthwhile to conduct empirical studies in medical informatics or whether we should use intuition or the marketplace as the primary indicators of the value of an information resource.
2. Assume that you run a philanthropic organization that supports medical informatics. In investing the scarce resources of your organization, you have to choose between funding a new system or resource development or funding empirical studies of resources already developed. What would you choose? How would you justify your decision?

3. To what extent is it possible to be certain how effective a medical informatics resource really is? What are the most important criteria of effectiveness?
4. Do you believe that independent, unbiased observers of the same behavior or outcome should agree on the quality of that outcome?
5. Many of the evaluation approaches assert that a single unbiased observer is a legitimate source of information in an evaluation, even if that observer's data or judgments are unsubstantiated by other people. Give examples drawn from our society where we vest important decisions in a single experienced and presumed impartial individual.
6. Do you agree with the statement that all evaluations appear equivocal when subjected to serious scrutiny? Explain your answer.
7. Associate each of the following hypothetical studies with a particular approach to evaluation[2]:
   a. A comparison of different user interfaces for a computer-based medical-record system, conducted while the system is under development
   b. A site visit by the U.S. National Library of Medicine's Biomedical Library Review Committee to the submitters of a competing renewal of a research grant
   c. A noted consultant on user interface design being invited to spend a day at an academic department to offer suggestions regarding the prototype of a new system
   d. Patient-chart reviews conducted before and after the introduction of an information resource, without the reviewer being told anything about the nature of the information resource or even that the intervention is the information resource
   e. Videotapes of attending rounds on a service where a knowledge resource has been implemented and periodic interviews with members of the ward team
   f. Determination of whether a new version of a resource executes a standard set of performance tests at the speed the designers projected
   g. Patients being randomly assigned such that their medical records are maintained either by a new computer system or by standard procedures, and then an investigator seeking to determine whether the new system affects clinical protocol recruitment and compliance
   h. A mock debate at a research-group retreat.
8. For each of the following hypothetical evaluation scenarios, list which of the eight types of studies in Table 8.2 they include. Some scenarios may include more than one type of study.[3]

---

[2]Answers: a, decision facilitation; b, professional review; c, art criticism; d, goal free; e, responsive–illuminative; f, objectives based; g, comparison based; h, quasi-legal.

[3]Answers: a, clinical impact; b, need validation; c, structure validation; d, field function; e, design validation and need validation; f, laboratory function; g, laboratory user impact, laboratory function; h, clinical impact.

a. An order-communication system is implemented in a small hospital. Changes in laboratory workload are assessed.
b. A study team performs a thorough analysis of the information required by psychiatrists to whom patients are referred by community social workers.
c. A medical-informatics expert is asked for her opinion about a doctoral student's project. She requests copies of the student's programming code and documentation for review.
d. A new intensive-care unit system is implemented alongside manual paper charting for one month. Then, the qualities of the computer-based data and of the data recorded on the paper charts are compared. A panel of intensive care physicians is asked to identify episodes of hypotension from each dataset, independently.
e. A medical-informatics professor is invited to join the steering group for a clinical-workstation project in a local hospital. The only documentation available for her to critique at the first meeting is a statement of the project goals, a description of the planned development method, and the advertisements and job descriptions for team members.
f. Developers invite clinicians to test a prototype of a computer-aided-learning system as part of a workshop on user-centered design.
g. A program is built that generates a predicted 24-hour blood-glucose profile using seven clinical parameters. Another program uses this profile and other patient data to advise on insulin dosages. Diabetologists are asked to prescribe insulin for the patient given the 24-hour profile alone and then again after seeing the computer-generated advice. They are also asked their opinion of the advice.
h. A program to generate drug-interaction alerts is installed in a geriatric clinic that already has a computer-based medical-record system. Rates of clinically significant drug interactions are compared before and after installation of the alerting resource.

Unit II
Medical Computing Applications

9
Computer-Based Patient-Record Systems

PAUL C. TANG AND CLEMENT J. MCDONALD

After reading this chapter, you should know the answers to these questions:

- What is the definition of a computer-based patient record (CPR)?
- How does a CPR differ from the paper record?
- What are the functional components of a CPR?
- What are the benefits of a CPR?
- What are the impediments to development and use of a CPR?

9.1 What Is a Computer-Based Patient Record?

The preceding chapters introduced the conceptual basis for the field of medical informatics, including the use of patient data in clinical practice and research. We now focus attention on the **patient record**, commonly referred to as the patient's **chart** or **medical record**. The patient record is an amalgam of all the data acquired and created during a patient's course through the healthcare system. The use of medical data was covered extensively in Chapter 2. We also discussed the limitations of the paper record in serving the many users of patient information. In this chapter, we examine the definition and use of computer-based patient-record systems, discuss their potential benefits and costs, and describe the remaining challenges to address in their dissemination.

9.1.1 Purposes of a Patient Record

Stanley Reiser (1991) wrote that the purpose of a patient record is "to recall observations, to inform others, to instruct students, to gain knowledge, to monitor performance, and to justify interventions." The many uses described in this statement, although diverse, have a single goal—to further the application of health sciences in ways that improve the well-being of patients. Yet, observational studies of physicians' use of the paper-based record find that logistical, organizational, and other practical limitations reduce the effectiveness of traditional records for storing and organizing an ever-increasing number of diverse data. A computer-based patient record is designed to overcome many of these limitations, as well as to provide additional benefits that cannot be attained by a static view of events.

A **computer-based patient record** (CPR) is a repository of electronically maintained information about an individual's lifetime health status and health care, stored such that it can serve the multiple legitimate users of the record. Traditionally, the patient record was a record of care provided when a patient is ill. Managed care (discussed in Chapter 19) encourages healthcare providers to focus on the continuum of health and health care from wellness to illness and recovery. Consequently, the record must integrate elements regarding a patient's health and illness acquired by multiple providers across diverse settings. In addition, the data should be stored such that different views of those data can be presented to serve the many uses described in Chapter 2.

A **computer-based patient-record system** adds information-management tools to provide clinical reminders and alerts, linkages with knowledge sources for health-care decision support, and analysis of aggregate data. To use a paper-based patient record, the reader must manipulate data either mentally or on paper to glean important clinical information. In contrast, a CPR system provides computer-based tools to help the reader organize, interpret, and react to data. Examples of tools provided in current CPR systems are discussed in Section 9.3.

9.1.2 Ways in Which a Computer-Based Patient Record Differs from a Paper-Based Record

In contrast to a traditional patient record, whose functionality is tethered by the static nature of paper—a single copy of the data stored in a single format for data entry and retrieval—a CPR is flexible and adaptable. Data may be entered in a format that simplifies the input process (which includes electronic interfaces to other computers where patient data are stored) and displayed in different formats suitable for their interpretation. Data can be used to guide care for a single patient or in aggregate form to help administrators develop policies for a population. Hence, when considering the functions of a CPR, we do not confine discussion to the uses of a single, serial recording of provider–patient encounters. A CPR system extends the usefulness of patient data by applying information-management tools to the data.

Inaccessibility is a common drawback of paper records. In large organizations, the traditional record may be unavailable to others for days while the clinician finishes documentation of an encounter. For example, paper records are often sequestered in a medical records department until the discharge summary is completed and every document is signed. During this time, special permission and extra effort are required to locate and retrieve the record. Individual physicians often borrow records for their convenience, with the same effect. With computer-stored records, all authorized personnel can access patient data immediately as the need arises. Remote access to CPRs also is possible. When the data are stored on a secure network, authorized clinicians with a need to know can access them from the office, home, or emergency room, to make timely informed decisions.

Documentation in a CPR is usually more legible because it is recorded as printed text rather than as hand writing, and it is better organized because structure is imposed on input. The computer can even improve completeness and quality by automatically applying validity checks on data as they are entered. For example, numerical results can be checked against reference ranges. Typographical errors can be detected if a datum fails a reference range check. Moreover, an interactive system can prompt the user for additional information. In this case, the data repository not only stores data but also enhances their completeness.

Data entered into a computer can be reused. For example, a physician could reuse her clinic visit note in the letter to the referring physician and the admission note. Reusability of data is one way that a CPR increases efficiency of the provider's workflow. Reuse of data also increases the quality of data. The more users and uses that depend on a data element, the more likely that it will be reviewed and be kept up to date.

The degree to which a particular CPR demonstrates these benefits depends on several factors:

1. *Comprehensiveness of information.* Does the CPR contain information about health as well as illness? Does it include information from all clinicians who participated in a patient's care? Does it cover all settings in which care was delivered (e.g., office practice, hospital)? Does it include the full spectrum of clinical data, including clinicians' notes, laboratory test results, medication details, and so on?
2. *Duration of use and retention of data.* A record that has accumulated patient data over 5 years will be more valuable than is one that contains records of only the visits made during 1 month.
3. *Degree of structure of data.* Medical data that are stored simply as narrative text entries will be more legible and accessible than are similar entries in a paper medical record. Uncoded information, however, is not standardized (see Chapter 6), and inconsistent use of medical terminology limits the ability to search for data. Use of a controlled, predefined vocabulary facilitates automated aggregation and summarization of data provided by different physicians or by the same physician at different times. Coded information is also required for computer-supported decision making and clinical research.
4. *Ubiquity of access.* A system that is accessible from a few sites will be less valuable than one accessible from any computer by an authorized user (see Chapter 4).

A computer-stored medical record system has disadvantages. It requires a larger initial investment than its paper counterpart due to hardware, software, training, and support costs. Key personnel may have to spend time away from their practice to learn how to use the system and to redesign their workflow to use the system efficiently. Physicians will also have to spend time learning how to use the system. Their workflow and their interactions with their patients may change. Converting from a paper-based medical-record system to a CPR involves substantial time, resources, determination, and leadership. The human and organizational factors often dominate the technical challenges.

Another risk associated with computer-based systems is the potential for subtle as well as catastrophic failures. If the computer system fails, stored information may be unavailable for an indeterminate time. Paper records fail one chart at a time. On the other hand, if we consider that a given chart may be unavailable up to 30 percent of the time, the paper-based system may be considered to be down 30 percent of the time for any given patient. Organizations can take steps to decrease the risk of CPR outages by providing redundancy for everything from computers and disk drives to networks and personal workstations. As a last resort, temporary paper records can act as a backup system until the computer system becomes available again.

Physicians record large amounts of clinical information in their history, physical examination, and progress notes. Capture of this information directly from the physician format is a major goal of medical informatics because it provides the most timely, accurate, and useful content. However, the goal is elusive. The time cost of physician input can be high, and many physicians initially resist the use of computers to enter data. Although new input devices are introduced or improved each year (e.g., pen-based entry, speech input), problems with convenience, portability, cost, and accuracy have made it difficult for these devices to compete with pen and paper. Dictation remains an option for data entry, but the turnaround time required for the dictation to be transcribed and for someone to review, correct, sign, and file the transcribed document creates delays. The lack of encoding further reduces the benefits of using a CPR.

To avoid the problem of data entry by physicians, some institutions have resorted to scanning physicians' notes into the computer (Teich, 1997). Scanned documents do solve the availability problems of the paper chart because they can be retrieved and viewed from any computer device. A typical scanned document occupies 50,000 bytes, however, so the downloading time can be slow, and there is no option for searching or analyzing the content of a scanned document without an abstraction step.

Although it takes time to learn how to use the system and to change workflows, we expect the long-term benefits of a CPR to compensate for the short-term costs. Thus far, however, there are few empirical data from large-scale evaluations of CPR systems. Hence, a strong belief in the anticipated benefits of CPR systems by senior leadership is required to embark on the process of migrating from paper to electronic records.

9.2 Historical Perspective

The historical development of the medical record parallels the development of science in clinical care. The development of automated systems for dealing with healthcare data parallels the need for data to comply with reimbursement requirements. Early healthcare systems focused on inpatient-charge capture to meet billing requirements in a fee-for-service environment. Contemporary systems need to capture clinical information in a managed-care environment focusing on clinical outcomes in ambulatory care.

9.2.1 Early Hospital Focus

The Flexner report on medical education was the first formal statement made about the function and contents of the medical record (Flexner, 1910). In advocating a scientific approach to medical education, it also encouraged physicians to keep a patient-oriented medical record. The contents of medical records in hospitals became the object of scrutiny in the 1940s, when hospital-accrediting bodies began to insist on the availability of accurate, well-organized medical records as a condition for accreditation. Since then, these organizations also have required that hospitals abstract certain information from the medical record and submit that information to national data centers. Such discharge abstracts contain (1) demographic information, (2) admission and discharge diagnoses, (3) length of stay, and (4) major procedures performed. The national centers produce statistical summaries of these case abstracts; an individual hospital can then compare its own statistical profile with that of similar institutions.

In the late 1960s, computer-based hospital information systems (HISs) began to emerge (see also Chapter 10). These systems were intended primarily for communication. They collected orders from nursing stations, routed the orders to various parts of the hospital, and identified all chargeable services. They also gave clinicians electronic access to results of laboratory tests and other diagnostic procedures. Although they contained some clinical information (e.g., test results, drug orders), their major purpose was to capture charges rather than to assist with clinical care. Many of the early HISs stored and presented much of their information as text, which is difficult to analyze. Moreover, these early systems rarely retained the content for more than a few days after a patient's discharge.

The introduction of the **problem-oriented medical record** (POMR) by Lawrence Weed (1969) influenced medical thinking about both manual and automated medical records. Weed was among the first to recognize the importance of an internal structure of a medical record, whether stored on paper or in a computer. He suggested that the primary organization of the medical record should be by the medical problem; all diagnostic and therapeutic plans should be linked to a specific problem.

Morris Collen (1983) was an early pioneer in the use of hospital-based systems to store and present laboratory-test results as part of preventive care. Use of computers to screen for early warning signs of illness was a basic tenet of health-maintenance organizations (HMOs). Other early university hospital-based systems provided feedback to physicians that affected clinical decisions and ultimately patient outcomes. The HELP system (Pryor, 1988) at LDS Hospital and the CCC system at Beth Israel Deaconess Medical Center (Bleich et al., 1985) continue to add more clinical data and decision-support functionality.

9.2.2 Influence of Managed Care and the Integrated Delivery System

Until recently, the ambulatory-care record has received less attention from the commercial vendors than the hospital record because of differences in financing and regulatory requirements. The status of ambulatory care records was reviewed in a 1982 report (Kuhn et al., 1984). Under the influence of managed care (described in detail in Chapter 19), the reimbursement model has shifted from a **fee-for-service model** (payers pay providers for all services the provider deemed necessary) toward a payment scheme where providers are paid a **fixed fee** for a specific service (payers pay a fixed amount for services approved by the payer). In some regions of the country, health-care–financing models are progressing toward a **capitated system** where providers are given a fixed fee to take care of all the health-care needs of a population of patients. In such managed-care environments, providers are motivated to reduce the cost of care by keeping their population of clients healthy and out of hospitals. Information-management tools that facilitate effective management of patients outside of the hospital setting help providers to achieve these goals. The emphasis on ambulatory care brought new attention to the ambulatory care record.

Thirty years ago, a single family physician provided almost all of an individual's medical care. Today, however, responsibility for ambulatory care is shifting to teams of health-care professionals in outpatient clinics and HMOs (see Chapter 19). Ambulatory care records may contain lengthy notes written by many different health-care providers, large numbers of laboratory-test results, and a diverse set of other data elements, such as X-ray–examination and pathology reports and hospital-discharge summaries. Accordingly, the need for information tools in ambulatory practice has increased. Among the early systems that focused on ambulatory care, COSTAR (Barnett, 1984), the Regenstrief Medical Record System (RMRS) (McDonald et al., 1992), STOR (Whiting-O'Keefe et al., 1985), and TMR (Stead & Hammond, 1988) are still available today.

9.3 Functional Components of a Computer-Based Patient-Record System

As we explain in Section 9.1.2, a CPR is not simply an electronic version of the paper record. When the record is part of a comprehensive CPR system, there are linkages and tools available to facilitate communication and decision-making. In

Sections 9.3.1 to 9.3.5, we summarize components of a comprehensive CPR system and illustrate functionality with examples from systems currently in use. The five functional components are:

- Integrated view of patient data
- Clinical decision support
- Clinician order entry
- Access to knowledge resources
- Integrated communication support

9.3.1 Integrated View of Patient Data

Clearly, providing integrated access to all patient data is a primary purpose of a CPR. Although this task may seem relatively simple, the growing volume of data for a patient from different sources (e.g., clinical laboratories, radiology departments, free-standing magnetic resonance imaging (MRI) centers, pharmacy outlets, home health agencies) make it difficult. For example, at present in the United States, no national patient identifier (similar to a social security number) exists for linking patient data obtained from many sites (patient indexes to link disparate patient identifiers are discussed in Chapter 10). Because different patient-data source systems use different identifiers, data-content terminologies, and data formats, most CPRs use **interface engines** to translate data content and formats from the sending system to ones that are acceptable to the receiving system. Although clinical data can be delivered to CPRs via **Health Level 7** (HL7), a relatively mature message standard (see Chapter 6), differences among implementations of HL7 must be resolved by interface engines. Figure 9.1 shows an example architecture to integrate data from multiple source systems. The database interface depicted not only provides message-handling capability but should also map the terminology of the sending system to a common vocabulary. Each receiving system that needs information about patients registers that interest with the interface engine to be sure that it receives appropriate updates (e.g., patient demographics). The interface engine often provides a technical and translation buffer between systems manufactured by different vendors. In this way, organizations can mix different vendors' products and still achieve the goal of integrated access to patient data for the clinician.

The idiosyncratic, local terminologies used to identify clinical variables and their values in many source systems represent a major barrier to integration of medical-record data by CPRs. Code systems such as LOINC (Forrey et al., 1996) and SNOMED (Rothwell & Côté, 1996), discussed in Chapter 6, help overcome these barriers.

Clinicians need more than just integrated access to patient data; they also need a specific **view** of patient data. Presenting an appropriate view of data for clinicians depends on an understanding of the context of the patient and of the clinician's data-analysis task. An example of a useful summary view of patient data

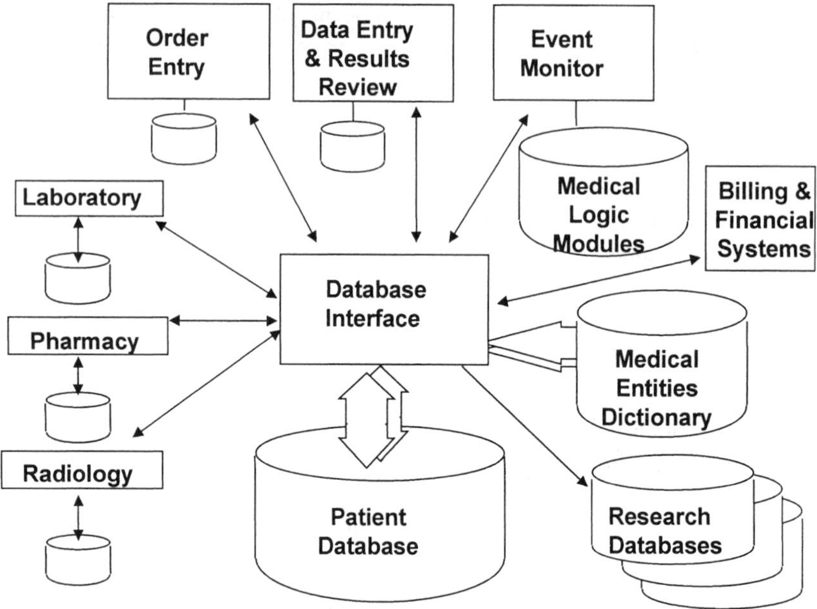

FIGURE 9.1. A block diagram of multiple source-data systems that contribute patient data that ultimately reside in a CPR. The database interface, commonly called an *interface engine*, may perform a number of functions. It may simply be a router of information to the central database. Alternatively, it may provide more intelligent filtering, translating, and alerting functions, as it does at Columbia Presbyterian Medical Center. (*Source*: Courtesy of Columbia Presbyterian Medical Center, New York.)

important for an outpatient clinic visit is shown in Figure 9.2. This summary view of patient data shows the active patient problems, active medications, medication allergies, health-maintenance reminders, and other relevant summary information. Such a view presents a current summary of patient context that is updated automatically at every encounter; such updating is not possible in a paper record.

Cross-platform browsers for finding and viewing information on the Internet (see Chapters 10 and 20) also provide healthcare workers with tools to view patient data from remote systems. Figure 9.3a shows an integrated view of a patient's laboratory-test results from multiple health systems in the city of Indianapolis, which the user sees by using a standard commercial Web browser. Figure 9.3b shows a data-entry screen using a web-browser interface. Advanced security features are required to ensure the confidentiality of patient data transmitted over the public Internet.

9.3.2 Clinical Decision Support

Decision support is most effective when provided at the time that the physician is formulating her assessment of the patient's condition and is making ordering

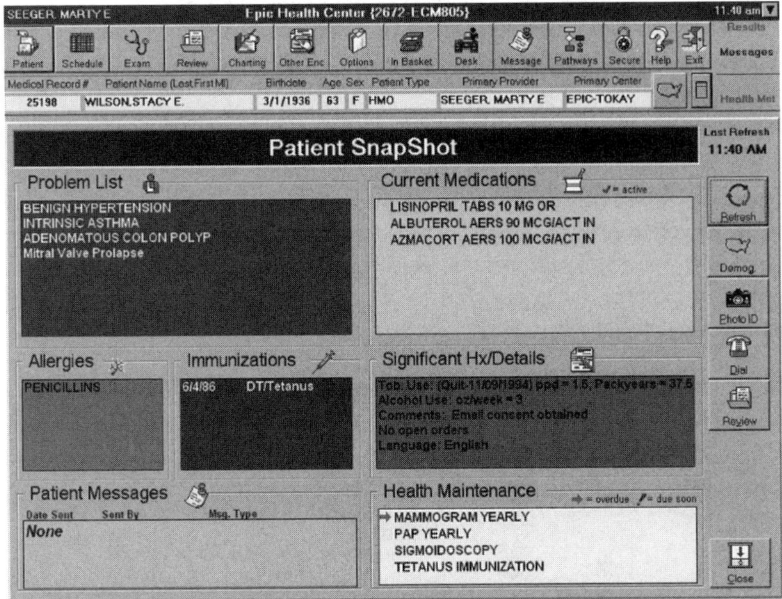

FIGURE 9.2. Quick access to summary information about a patient. The patient's active medical problems, current medications, and drug allergies are among the core data that physicians must keep in mind when making any decision on patient care. An up-to-date snapshot of a patient's context, as depicted in this figure, can save physicians time by providing current information instantly. (*Source*: Courtesy of Epic Systems, Madison, WI.)

decisions. Computer-assisted decision support is only acceptable when it allows the physician to override a system-provided recommendation and choose an alternative action. The most successful decision-support intervention makes complying with the suggested action easy. A brief rationale is generally provided with the recommendation, and complying with the recommendation is as easy as hitting the Enter key or clicking the mouse.

In Figure 9.4, a software module in a large HIS combines information from a variety of data sources regarding a patient's diagnoses and underlying disease and pertinent disease protocols to present recommendations on antibiotic choice, dose, and duration of treatment. Clinicians can view the basis for the recommendations and the logic used. An important part of the program is its solicitation of feedback when the clinician decides not to follow the recommendations. This feedback is used to improve the clinical protocol and the software program. Providing on-line advice on antimicrobial selection has resulted in significantly improved clinical and financial outcomes for patients whose infectious diseases were managed through the use of the program.

Reminders and alerts on a number of matters can be raised during an outpatient encounter as well. Figure 9.5 shows how alerts and reminders are included

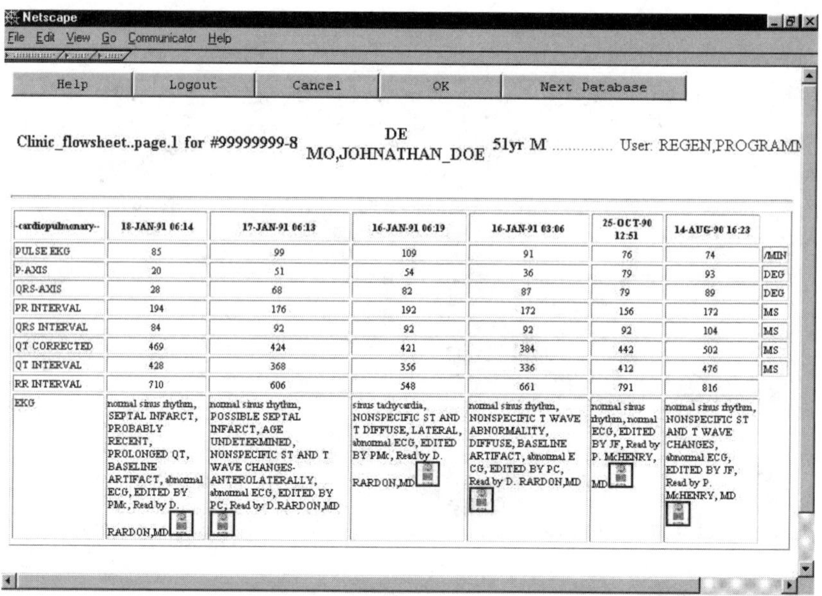

Netscape

File Edit View Go Communicator Help

Help | Logout | Cancel | OK | Next Database

Clinic_flowsheet..page.1 for #99999999-8 DE MO,JOHNATHAN_DOE 51yr M .... User: REGEN,PROGRAMM

-cardiopulmonary--	18-JAN-91 06:14	17-JAN-91 06:13	16-JAN-91 06:19	16-JAN-91 03:06	25-OCT-90 12:51	14-AUG-90 16:23	
PULSE EKG	85	99	109	91	76	74	/MIN
P-AXIS	20	51	54	36	79	93	DEG
QRS-AXIS	28	68	82	87	79	89	DEG
PR INTERVAL	194	176	192	172	156	172	MS
QRS INTERVAL	84	92	92	92	92	104	MS
QT CORRECTED	469	424	421	384	442	502	MS
QT INTERVAL	428	368	356	336	412	476	MS
RR INTERVAL	710	606	548	661	791	816	
EKG	normal sinus rhythm, SEPTAL INFARCT, PROBABLY RECENT, PROLONGED QT, BASELINE ARTIFACT, abnormal ECG, EDITED BY PMc, Read by D. RARDON,MD	normal sinus rhythm, POSSIBLE SEPTAL INFARCT, AGE UNDETERMINED, NONSPECIFIC ST AND T WAVE CHANGES-ANTEROLATERALLY, abnormal ECG, EDITED BY PC, Read by D.RARDON,MD	sinus tachycardia, NONSPECIFIC ST AND T DIFFUSE, LATERAL, abnormal ECG, EDITED BY PMc, Read by D. RARDON,MD	normal sinus rhythm, NONSPECIFIC T WAVE ABNORMALITY, DIFFUSE, BASELINE ARTIFACT, abnormal E CG, EDITED BY PC, Read by D. RARDON,MD	normal sinus rhythm, normal ECG, EDITED BY JF, Read by P. McHENRY, MD	normal sinus rhythm, NONSPECIFIC ST AND T WAVE CHANGES, abnormal ECG, EDITED BY JF, Read by P. McHENRY, MD	

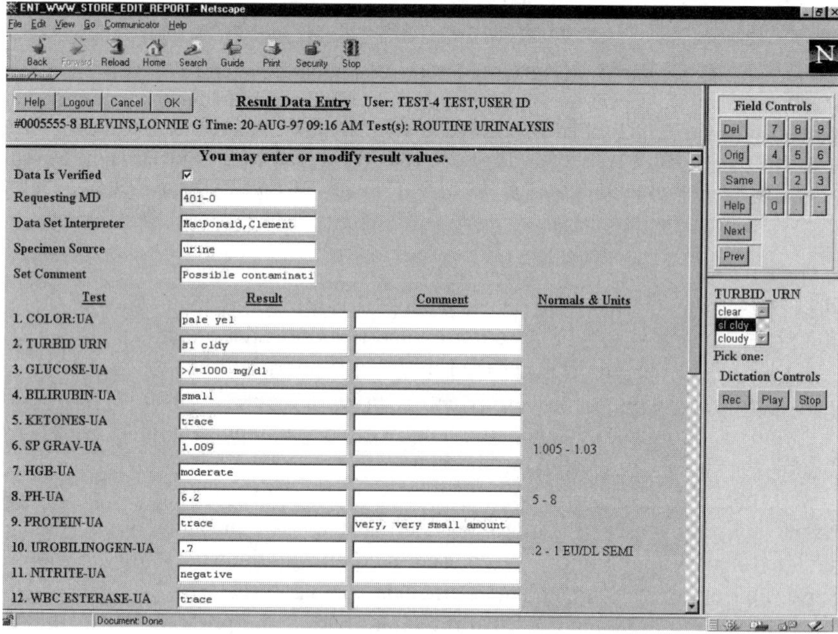

ENT_WWW_STORE_EDIT_REPORT - Netscape

File Edit View Go Communicator Help

Back Forward Reload Home Search Guide Print Security Stop

Help | Logout | Cancel | OK

Result Data Entry User: TEST-4 TEST,USER ID

#0005555-8 BLEVINS,LONNIE G Time: 20-AUG-97 09:16 AM Test(s): ROUTINE URINALYSIS

You may enter or modify result values.

Data Is Verified	☑
Requesting MD	401-0
Data Set Interpreter	MacDonald,Clement
Specimen Source	urine
Set Comment	Possible contaminati

Test	Result	Comment	Normals & Units
1. COLOR:UA	pale yel		
2. TURBID URN	sl cldy		
3. GLUCOSE-UA	>/=1000 mg/dl		
4. BILIRUBIN-UA	small		
5. KETONES-UA	trace		
6. SP GRAV-UA	1.009		1.005 - 1.03
7. HGB-UA	moderate		
8. PH-UA	6.2		5 - 8
9. PROTEIN-UA	trace	very, very small amount	
10. UROBILINOGEN-UA	.7		.2 - 1 EU/DL SEMI
11. NITRITE-UA	negative		
12. WBC ESTERASE-UA	trace		

Field Controls

Del 7 8 9

Orig 4 5 6

Same 1 2 3

Help 0 . -

Next

Prev

TURBID_URN

clear

sl cldy

cloudy

Pick one:

Dictation Controls

Rec Play Stop

Document: Done

FIGURE 9.3. Web resources. *(a)* Web-browser display of ECG results, measurements, and diagnostic impressions. When the user clicks on the icon, the computer displays the full ECG tracing. (*Source*: Courtesy of Regenstrief Institute, Indianapolis, IN). *(b)* A general data-gathering Web page. The form and content are driven by a set term (in this case *urinalysis*). Digital voice input is allowed on any text field (using dictation controls displayed on the right). The system compresses speech to 270 bytes per second using VOXWARE's algorithm. (*Source*: Courtesy of Regenstrief Institute, Indianapolis, IN.)

```
IHC ANTIBIOTIC ASSISTANT & ORDER PROGRAM

  00000000 Doe, John Q.  E999  57yr  M   Dx:PNEUMONIA
  Max 24hr WBC=16.3   (11.1)   Admit:03/27/97.12.15   Max 24hr Temp=38.3 (37.8)
  RENAL FUNCTION: Decreased,  CrCl= 83,    Max 24hr Cr=1.1   (1.7)    IBW: 79kg
  Patient's Diff shows a left shift, Max 24hr Bands = 16   ( 8)
  ANTIBIOTIC ALLERGIES: Penicillin
  CURRENT ANTIBIOTICS:
  1. 03/27/97.17:23  IMIPENEM/CILASTATIN, (PRIMAXIN)  VIAL 500  Q 8 hrs
  IDENTIFIED PATHOGENS                 SITE                  COLLECTED
   Staphylococcus coagulase negative   Subclavian            03/28/97.05:00
   Staphylococcus coagulase negative   Blood                 03/27/97.15:30
   Staphylococcus aureus           Sputum                    03/27/97.15:21
  ABX SUGGESTION        DOSAGE        ROUTE      INTERVAL
   Vancomycin          1000mg          IV          *q24h    (infuse over 1hr)
  Suggested Antibiotic Duration: 14 days
  * Adjusted based on patient's renal function
  <1>Micro, <2>OrganismSuscept, <3>Drug Info, <4>ExplainLogic, <5>Empiric Abx <6>Abx Hx,
<7>ID Rnds, <8>Lab/Abx Levels, <9>Xray, <10>Data Input Screen<Esc>EXIT, <F1>Help,
<0>User Input, <.>OutpatientModels, <+>Change Patient
  ORDERS:<*>Suggested Abx, <Enter>Abx List, </>D/C Abx, <->Modify Abx
```

FIGURE 9.4. Example of the main screen from the Intermountain Health Care Antibiotic Assistant program. The program displays evidence of an infection, relevant patient data (e.g., kidney function, temperature), and recommendations for antibiotics based on the culture results. (*Source*: Courtesy of R. Scott Evans, Stanley L. Pestotnik, David C. Classen, and John P. Burke, LDS Hospital, Salt Lake City, UT.)

on a preprinted encounter form for use during an outpatient visit. The system searches for applicable decision-support rules and prints relevant reminders on the encounter form during batch printing the night before the scheduled visit. Figure 9.6 shows computer-based suggestions regarding health-maintenance topics and potentially efficacious medications to consider. These suggestions were derived from rules that examine the patient's problems and medications and the timing of laboratory-test orders.

9.3.3 Clinician Order Entry

If the ultimate goal of a CPR system is to help clinicians make informed decisions, then the system should present relevant information at the time of order entry. Several systems have the capability of providing decision support during the order-entry process (Steen, 1996; Tierney et al., 1993). For example, a clinical team in the medical intensive-care unit at Vanderbilt University Hospital can use an electronic chart rack to view active orders and enter new orders. The WIZ Order screen integrates information about a patient's active orders, clinical alerts based on current data from the electronic patient record, and abstracts of relevant articles from the literature. Clinical alerts attached to a laboratory-test result can also include suggestions for appropriate actions (Fig. 9.7).

Providing summary information about the patient's status compared with protocols for which the patient is eligible is another way of providing feedback to the clinician when she is considering her orders (Fig. 9.8).

SAMPLE, PATIENT
05-APR-96 317-630-7400
1001 TENTH ST
INDIANAPOLIS 46202

THU AM 2 Dr: MEGREMIS, JIM G
Wishard Memorial Hospital
1001 W Tenth Street
Indianapolis IN 46202

1 CLINIC VISIT, 2 CLINIC CONSULT, 3 CONSULTATION, 4 ASA EVALUATION, 5 LAB ONLY, 6 RX REFILL, 7 NO CHARGE, 8 MC CLINIC VISIT

---- Diagnoses List ----

1 umbilical hernia
2 thrush
3 seborrhea nos /CRADLE CAP
4 cough
5 throat pain
6 well child
7 otitis media
8 SICKLE TRAIT
9
10

--- Observations List ---

1 HEIGHT PEDS ______INCH
2 WEIGHT PEDS ______LBS
3 TEMP ______DEG F
4 TEMP RECTAL ______DEG F
5 TEMP AXILLARY ______DEG F
6 RR ______/MIN
7 PULSE ______/MIN
8 HEAD CIRCUMF ______CM
9 HEAD CIRC %ILE ______%
10 WT %ILE ______%
11 HEIGHT %ILE ______%
12 SYS BP SITTING ______MM HG
13 DIAS BP SITTING ______MM HG
14 TIME COUNSELING ______MIN
15 TOTAL TIME c PAT______MIN
16*IVH GRADE ______

Notes:

Age:
Informant:

Feedings:
Elimination:
Sleep:
Concerns:

PHYSICAL EXAM:
Normal: Significant Findings:
____ Head
____ Skin
____ Eyes/Vision
____ Ears/Hearing
____ Nose/Throat
____ Teeth/Gums
____ Nodes
____ Chest/Lungs
____ Heart
____ Pulses
____ Abdomen
____ Ext Genitalia
____ Hip Abduct
____ Back
____ Extremities
____ Neuro

DEVELOPMENT:
____ Feeds self, crawls
____ Listens and imitates sound
____ Sits without support
____ Gets to sitting position
____ Feeds self crackers
____ Pulls up
____ Vision observed

SOCIAL ASSESSMENT DONE: ____
NUTRITIONAL ASSESSMENT:
WIC: Certified/Letter A
Recert Due: ______
Risk Codes: ___/___/___

NUTRITION/FEEDINGS:
____ Encourage cup
____ Vit/min supp if indicated

SAFETY:
____ Poison control number
____ Syrup of Ipecac
____ Car restraints
____ Safe toys
____ Prevent burns/water heater 125
____ Prevent choking

PARENTING:
____ Temper tantrums/limits
____ Stranger anxiety, separation anxiety
____ Sleep
____ Reading to child
____ Praise/affection
____ Teeth care

IMPRESSIONS:

PLANS:

-------------------- O R D E R S --------------------
* Consider DPT immunization or record previous dates if available.
* Consider OPV immunization or record previous dates if available.
* Consider HEMOPHILUS B VACCINE or record previous dates if available.

Staff: ______________ Signature: ______________

30-JAN-97 Encounter Date	Provider ID	wks months Return	Return Provider	/ / Next Appt Date	PEDIATRICS Service Area

SAMPLE,PATIENT #0999999-6 30-JAN-97 09:15 AM

Printed: 28-Jan-97 Page: 3

ENCOUNTER FORM OPB-8

FIGURE 9.5. Pediatric encounter form. The questions on these forms vary by age. Reminders for routine immunizations appear at the bottom. (*Source*: Courtesy of Regenstrief Institute, Indianapolis, IN.)

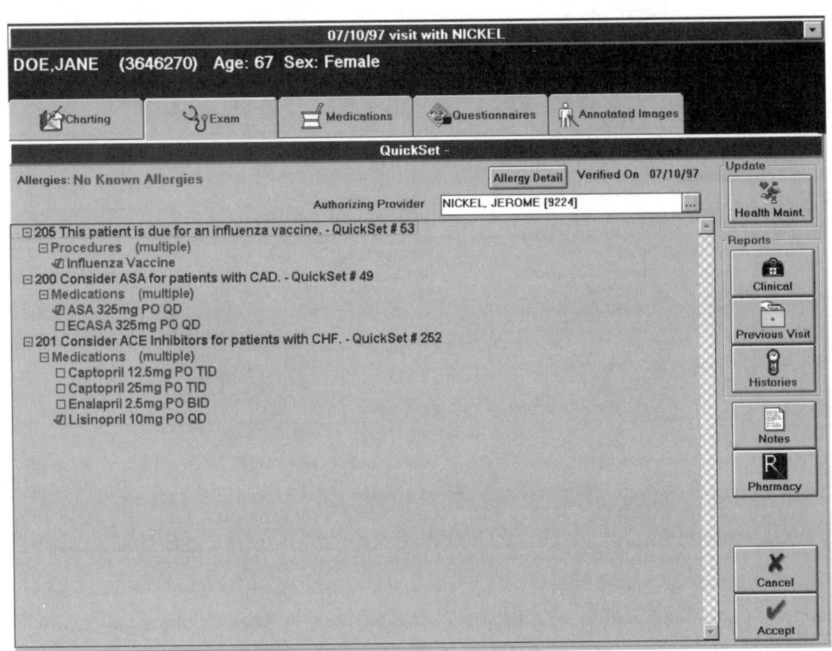

FIGURE 9.6. An example of computer-assisted decision support. The system has examined the patient's problems, medications, age, and health-maintenance record and has determined that she is eligible for certain interventions based on locally approved guidelines. It presents these options for the physician to consider and makes complying with the suggestions as easy as clicking the box (to insert a checkmark). (*Source*: Courtesy of Epic Systems, Madison, WI.)

```
View     PtLookup
Patient: H———,E———        65F  06215446        Adm: 08/17/94 Room: 12B-351
   Time: 10/19/94 05:39 AM    Alert#38269              12B phone: x7865
  Alert: DANGEROUSLY LOW SERUM POTASSIUM
 Reason: <BLOOD> K = 3.2 at 04:22 AM, 10/19/94
         Patient is currently on DIGOXIN.

 Relevant medications:                                   Alert Details
         LASIX 20 MG IV  BID  Starting  on 10/18 (10/17)
         DIGOXIN EVEN days:.125; ODD days:.25 PO        (09/28)

Actions:
      [ ]A   D/C or EDIT relevant medications
      [ ]B   Order POTASSIUM CHLORIDE IV
      [ ]C   Order POTASSIUM CHLORIDE PO
      [ ]D   Order set: STAT EKG
      [ ]E   Order set: STAT K

 Ganesan, Shridar,M.D.,Ph.D.  Bp#2710 was paged on 05:40 AM  Oct 19, 1994
 Covering M.D.: Morrow, David Andrew,M.D. Bp#5336      pAge M.D.
    dOne           <done, Go to OE>        coMments           Logic
Press ALT-O or ALT-G to exit and acknowledge alert.
```

FIGURE 9.7. Clinical alert. Alerts can be attached to a laboratory-test result. Each time that a laboratory test is completed, a set of rules is checked to determine whether the result is sufficiently abnormal to require further action. In this case, the rule checks for a serum potassium level less than 3.3 mEq/L in a patient taking digoxin. The computer pages the patient's doctor directly; when the doctor responds, the above screen shows the relevant information and offers suggested remedial actions, such as ordering administration of more potassium. (*Source*: Courtesy of Brigham and Womens Hospital, Boston, MA.)

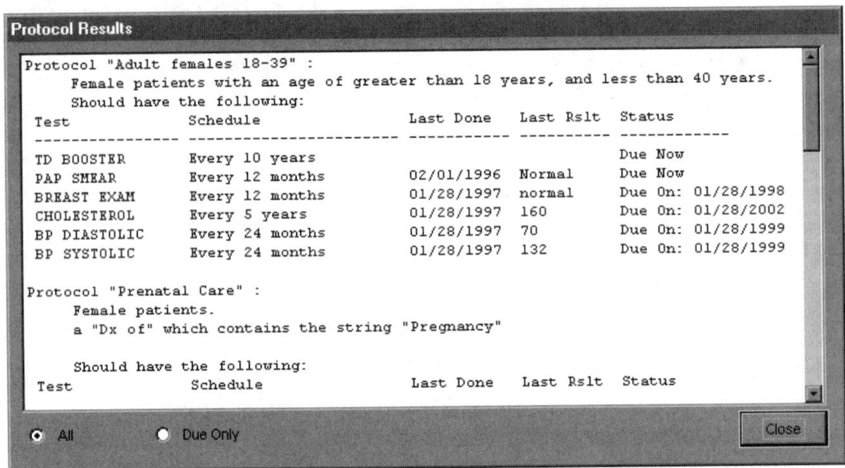

Protocol Results
Protocol "Adult females 18-39" :
Female patients with an age of greater than 18 years, and less than 40 years.
Should have the following:
Test Schedule Last Done Last Rslt Status
TD BOOSTER Every 10 years Due Now
PAP SMEAR Every 12 months 02/01/1996 Normal Due Now
BREAST EXAM Every 12 months 01/28/1997 normal Due On: 01/28/1998
CHOLESTEROL Every 5 years 01/28/1997 160 Due On: 01/28/2002
BP DIASTOLIC Every 24 months 01/28/1997 70 Due On: 01/28/1999
BP SYSTOLIC Every 24 months 01/28/1997 132 Due On: 01/28/1999
Protocol "Prenatal Care" :
Female patients.
a "Dx of" which contains the string "Pregnancy"
Should have the following:
Test Schedule Last Done Last Rslt Status
All
Due Only
Close

FIGURE 9.8. An essential feature of electronic medical records is their ability to use the patient data in combination with protocols or algorithms to provide alerts and reminders to the clinical decision-makers. Here, an advisory shows preventive services due for adult females in the age range 18 to 39 years, as derived from the United States Public Health Service Preventive Services guidelines. (*Source*: Courtesy of MedicaLogic, Inc., Software: Logician Electronic Medical Record, V.4.5, ©1991–1998, Hillsboro, OR.)

Once a physician order-entry system is adopted into the practice culture, simply changing the default drug or dosing based on the latest scientific evidence can significantly change physician ordering behavior. Clinical quality and financial costs can be changed virtually overnight.

9.3.4 Access to Knowledge Resources

Most queries of knowledge resources, whether they are satisfied by consulting another human colleague or by searching through reference materials or the literature, are conducted in the context of a specific patient (Covell et al., 1985). Consequently, the most effective time to provide access to knowledge resources is at the time decisions or orders are being contemplated by the clinician. Furthermore, any method by which the system can provide preformatted queries that anticipate the clinicians' queries will be helpful and will increase the chance that the knowledge will influence clinicians' decisions. Knowledge resources can also help a clinician to decide whether a referral is appropriate and, if one is, which preconsult tests may expedite the consult process (Fig. 9.9).

9.3.5 Integrated Communication Support

As the care function becomes increasingly distributed among multidisciplinary healthcare professionals, the effectiveness and efficiency of communication among the team members affect the overall coordination and timeliness of care

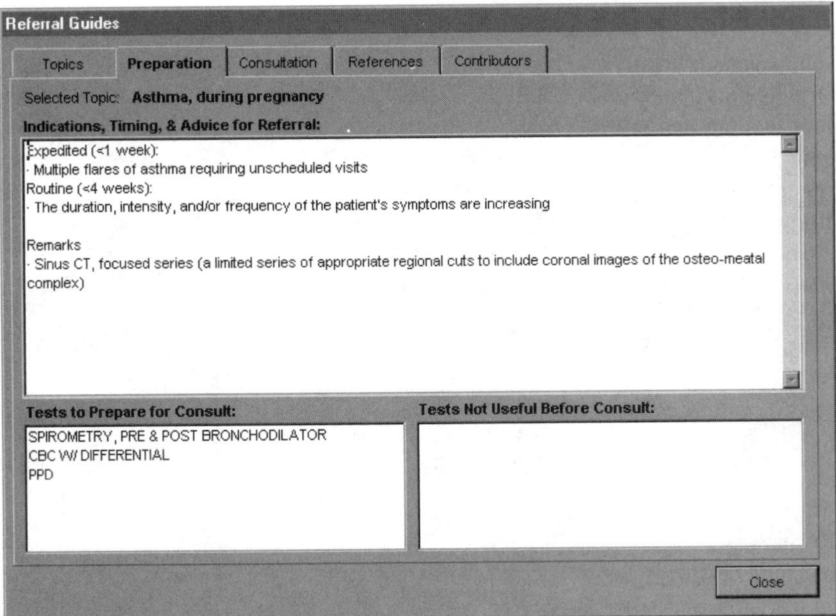

FIGURE 9.9. A CPR linked to knowledge resources so that context-specific information can be displayed at the time of clinical decision-making. For a clinician deciding whether to refer a pregnant patient with asthma to a specialist, a referral guide can provide information that may support decision-making. The guide also may support improved workflow by ensuring that relevant tests and procedures are completed before referral and that unnecessary tests and procedures are avoided. (*Source*: Courtesy of MedicaLogic, Hillsboro, OR.)

provided. Most messages will be associated with a specific patient. Thus, communication tools should be integrated with the CPR system such that messages (including system messages or laboratory-test results) are electronically attached to a patient's record. That is, the patient's record should be available at the touch of a button. Geographic separation of team members creates the demand for networked communication that reaches all sites where providers make decisions on patient care. These sites include the providers' offices, the hospital, the emergency room, and the home. Connectivity to the patient's home will provide an important vehicle for monitoring health (e.g., home blood-glucose monitoring, health-status indicators) and for enabling routine communication.

Figure 9.10 shows an example of a notification message to a primary-care provider that her patient was seen in the emergency room. The patient's complaint and final diagnosis are listed, and the physician can query the system for further information. Notifying the primary-care provider not only provides her with continuity information but also allows her to take proactive steps to follow up on the problem that provoked the unscheduled encounter.

A CPR system can also help with routine patient handoffs, where the responsibility for care is transferred from one clinician to another. Typically, a brief

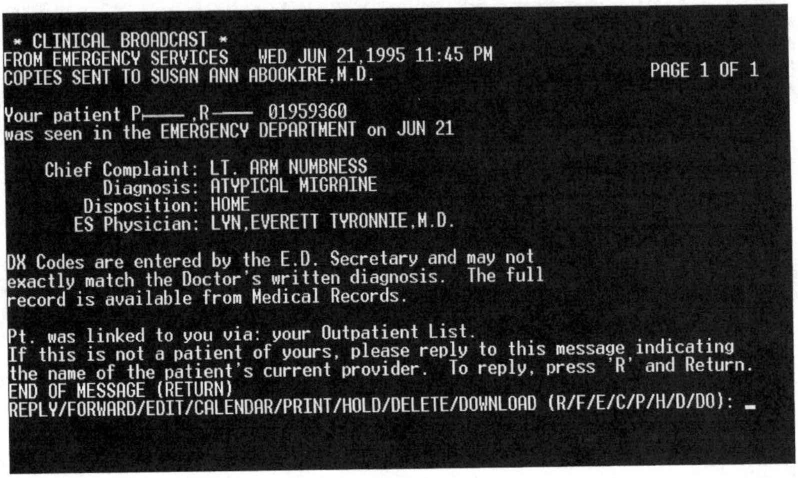

```
* CLINICAL BROADCAST *
FROM EMERGENCY SERVICES    WED JUN 21,1995 11:45 PM
COPIES SENT TO SUSAN ANN ABOOKIRE,M.D.                          PAGE 1 OF 1

Your patient P——,R——   01959360
was seen in the EMERGENCY DEPARTMENT on JUN 21

    Chief Complaint: LT. ARM NUMBNESS
          Diagnosis: ATYPICAL MIGRAINE
        Disposition: HOME
       ES Physician: LYN,EVERETT TYRONNIE,M.D.

DX Codes are entered by the E.D. Secretary and may not
exactly match the Doctor's written diagnosis.  The full
record is available from Medical Records.

Pt. was linked to you via: your Outpatient List.
If this is not a patient of yours, please reply to this message indicating
the name of the patient's current provider.  To reply, press 'R' and Return.
END OF MESSAGE (RETURN)
REPLY/FORWARD/EDIT/CALENDAR/PRINT/HOLD/DELETE/DOWNLOAD (R/F/E/C/P/H/D/DO): _
```

FIGURE 9.10. Communication as part of continuity of care. Whenever a patient completes an emergency-room visit at Brigham and Womens Hospital, an electronic-mail message is sent to the patient's primary provider, outlining the facts of the visit. (*Source*: Courtesy of Brigham and Womens Hospital, Boston, MA.)

verbal or written exchange helps the covering clinician to understand the patient's problems, as is important for making decisions while the primary clinician is unavailable. An example of a screen that contains instructions from the primary physician, as well as system-provided information (e.g., recent laboratory-test results), is shown in Figure 9.11.

Although a patient encounter is usually defined by a face-to-face visit (e.g., outpatient visit, inpatient bedside visit, home health visit), significant information-processing activities occur elsewhere. Responses to patient telephone calls and laboratory-test results are examples of such activities. Ideally, the clinician should be notified of these events and have immediate access to the record to make decisions. Figure 9.12 shows a list of pending information (e.g., new laboratory-test result available, telephone call for a medication refill, telephone call regarding a patient symptom) and buttons linked to information tools that help a clinician to process these new data. The clinician can retrieve the patient's electronic chart, electronically refill a medication, use a template to write a letter informing the patient of normal test results, or dial the patient's telephone number to speak directly with the patient. In addition, when the physician asks the patient to schedule a diagnostic test such as a mammogram, the system can keep track of the time since the order was written and can notify the physician that a test result has not appeared in a specified time. This tracking function prevents diagnostic plans from falling through the cracks. Communication tools that are integrated with a CPR system provide timely notification of patient events in the context of a patient's record and support transmission of appropriate interventions based on that information.

```
POCKET ROUNDS for WARVEL,JEFF            (29 JUL 97 , 04:47PM)      TEST3, PATIENT           - 123123-0
-------------------------------------------------------------------------------------------------------
=======================================================================================================
TEST3, PATIENT                          123123-0
=======================================================================================================
SEX : M     RACE : B      AGE : 61       ADMIT : 17 JAN 1997        WARD : MCU          BED# : D111
ADMITTING INTERN : TEST,INTERN       MED STUDENT : TEST,STUDENT
CODE STATUS : FULL CODE
PROBLEMS     :    1) cor pulmonale /ACTIVE                          4) COPD /ACTIVE
                  2) CHF /ACTIVE                                    5) cigarette smoker /ACTIVE
                  3) ETOH abuse /ACTIVE                             6) coronary artery disease /ACTIVE
ALLERGIES    :    1) PENICILLINS
ACTIVITIES   :  bed rest, With no exceptions
PRECAUTIONS  :  NO SPECIAL PRECAUTIONS
DIET         :  NPO except meds
CALL ORDERS  :  CALL ORDERS DIAS BP, > 110 mm Hg
                CALL ORDERS PULSE, > 120/min < 50/min
                CALL ORDERS RESP RT, > 30/min
                CALL ORDERS SYS BP, > 190 mm Hg < 90 mm Hg
                CALL ORDERS TEMP, > 101.5 F < 96 F
                CALL ORDERS URINE OUT, <240 cc per shift
%%%%%%%%%%%%%%%%%%%%%%%%%%%%%%%%%%%%%%%%%% REMINDERS %%%%%%%%%%%%%%%%%%%%%%%%%%%%%%%%%%%%%%%%%%%%%%%%%%%
 **  Patient on vent: Begin SQ heparin to decrease DVT risk
%%%%%%%%%%%%%%%%%%%%%%%%%%%%%%%%%%%%%%%%%%%%%%%%%%%%%%%%%%%%%%%%%%%%%%%%%%%%%%%%%%%%%%%%%%%%%%%%%%%%%%%
ACTIVE TESTS :
    1) BLD GAS PANEL 1, QAM On 40% oxygen Actv 12 D      5) CXR (PA&LAT), QAM Actv 12 D
    2) BLOOD CELL PROF, QAM Actv 12 D                    6) LYTES, Q AM X indefinitely Actv 12 D
    3) BUN, QAM X indefinitely Actv 5 D                  7) TRIGLYCERIDES Actv 0 D
    4) CREATININE, Draw QAM X indefinitely Actv 5 D
ACTIVE MEDICATIONS :
    1) ALBUTEROL INHL, 4 inhl PO Q4H scheduled. Wait one minute between inhalation, Actv 12 D
    2) ALBUTEROL NEB UNIT DOSE, 1 bottle(3ml) per nebulizer x 1 over 5-15 min per RT -now please, Actv 4 D
    3) ASPIRIN BUFFERED, 325 mg PO QAM -LATE ENTRY, Actv 9 D
    4) CEFTRIAXONE INJ, 1 g IVSP QD -Give first dose now, Actv 5 D
    5) ENTERAL PULMON, Elevate head of bed prior to feeding and hold feeding if residual > 250 ml. Infuse
       50 ml/HOUR of full strength by NG tube.  CHECK RESIDUALS Q4HR. GOAL RATE IS 86 CC/HOUR.  INCREASE BY
       10 CC Q4H IFRESIDUALS ARE OK, Actv 11 D
    6) FE SO4 ELIXIR, 300 mg PO TID AC (iron), Actv 0 D
    7) FOSINOPRIL, 5 mg PO Q day -HOLD FOR SBP < 100, Actv 12 D
    8) HALOPERIDOL INJ, 5 mg iv Q 3 hr -may give an additional 2 mg Q 1 hr prn agitation, Actv 4 D
    9) HEPARIN ARTFLUSH, 1000 units 500 ml LVP inf, Actv 12 D
   10) INHALER SPACER DEVICE, Use with all inhalers, Actv 12 D
   11) IPRATROPIUM INHL, Inhale 4 puffs Q4H, Actv 12 D
   12) IV LOCK (saline flush), WITH ROUTINE FLUSHES, Actv 5 D
   13) LORAZEPAM INJ, 1 mg IV q4h prn agitation., Actv 12 D
   14) NIZATIDINE, 300 mg PO QHS, Actv 12 D
   15) PROPOXYN/ACET 100/650, 1-2 tab PO Q6H PRN pain (maximum of 6 tab/24 hours) -Give first dose now,
       Actv 5 D
ACTIVE OTHER ORDERS :
    1) ANTIEMBOLISM STOCKINGS, to be worn under SCD, Actv 12 D
    2) ARTERIAL LINE, Dressing and heparin flush per routine, Actv 12 D
    3) CARDIAC MONITORING, Continuous monitoring via telemetry or portable monitor, Actv 12 D
    4) CONDOM CATHETER, Apply condom catheter to bedside drainage and measure output Qshift, Actv 5 D
    5) FOLEY CATHETER, Routine nursing care - 07/24/97- May re-anchor foley for decreased urine output
       with condom catheter., Actv 1 D
    6) INTAKE AND OUTPUT, measure all intake and output, Actv 12 D
    7) NEURO CHECKS,  Q2HRS when stable - Q 1HR or more when unstable, Actv 12 D
    8) NG TUBE, Place for medication to gravity, Actv 12 D
    9) OXYGEN THERAPY, Give continuously via Re-breather mask. Use 100% O2 with target oxygen saturation
       of 92% per oxygen titration protocol -- WEAN AS TOLERATED, Actv 4 D
   10) PEAK FLOW, measure and record before and after bronchodilator treatments x7 days then during an
       exacerbation and seek medical care if you cannot reach 80% of your baseline, Actv 4 D
   11) PERCUSSION AND DRAINAGE, Perform to bilateral base q4, Actv 4 D
   12) SEQUENTIAL COMPRESSION DEVICE, Apply to both leg(s) prevent thrombophlebitis, Actv 12 D
   13) VENTILATOR FIO2, 45%, Actv 12 D
   14) VENTILATOR MODE, synchronized IMV, Actv 12 D
   15) VENTILATOR PEEP, 5 cm H2O, Actv 12 D
   16) VENTILATOR PRESSURE SUPPORT, 10 cm H2O, Actv 12 D
   17) VENTILATOR RATE, 6 breaths/min, Actv 12 D
   18) VENTILATOR SETTINGS - (See detailed settings), Actv 12 D
   19) VENTILATOR TIDAL VOL, 800 ML, Actv 12 D
   20) VITALS (TPR&BP), Actv 12 D
   21) WEIGHT KGS, weigh daily, Actv 12 D
STANDARD PARAMETERS :
```

YEAR	1997	1997	1997	1997	1997	1997	1997	1997	1997	1997	1997
DAY-MONTH	29 JUL	29 JUL	28 JUL	27 JUL	27 JUL	27 JUL	26 JUL	26 JUL	26 JUL	25 JUL	25 JUL
HOUR	10:29	04:57	04:28	21:27	17:02	04:30	21:02	20:56	04:14	20:21	20:20
CHEM12											
BUN	-	15	27 h	29 h	-	30 h	30 h	-	21	20	-
GLUCOSE	-	102	81	-	-	109	101	112 h	-	-	128 h
CREATININE	-	0.6	0.7	0.7	-	0.8	1.0	-	0.7	0.7	-
LYTES											
SODIUM	-	140	138	139	-	138	139	-	139	140	-
POTASSIUM	-	4.3	4.8	4.5	-	5.0	4.4	-	4.0	4.5	-
CHLORIDE	-	100	101	102	-	99	102	-	97	97	-

Page 5

FIGURE 9.11 The popular Pocket rounds reports. When folded in half, these reports fit in the pocket of a clinician's white coat. (*Source*: Courtesy of Regenstrief Institute, Indianapolis, IN.)

POCKET ROUNDS for WARVEL,JEFF (29 JUL 97 , 04:47PM) TEST3, PATIENT - 123123-0

YEAR	1997	1997	1997	1997	1997	1997	1997	1997	1997	1997	1997
DAY-MONTH	29 JUL	29 JUL	28 JUL	27 JUL	27 JUL	27 JUL	26 JUL	26 JUL	26 JUL	25 JUL	25 JUL
HOUR	10:29	04:57	04:28	21:27	17:02	04:30	21:02	20:56	04:14	20:21	20:20
LYTES (continued)											
CO2 (TOTAL)	-	32 h	30 h	29 h	-	31 h	31 h	-	33 h	34 h	-
BLOOD CELL PROF											
WBC	-	7.2	6.5	-	-	6.2	-	-	7.2	-	-
RBC	-	4.5	4.7	-	-	4.7	-	-	4.9	-	-
HGB	-	10.9 l	11.1 l	-	-	10.8 l	-	-	11.6 l	-	-
HCT	-	35 l	36 l	-	-	35 l	-	-	37 l	-	-
MCV	-	76 l	76 l	-	-	75 l	-	-	75 l	-	-
MCH	-	24 l	24 l	-	-	23 l	-	-	24 l	-	-
MCHC	-	32	31 l	-	-	31 l	-	-	32	-	-
RDW (CSH)	-	19.1 h	19.1 h	-	-	18.9 h	-	-	18.7 h	-	-
CREATININE URINE	-	-	-	-	194	-	-	-	-	-	-
LYTES RANDOM URINE											
NA+ R-URN	-	-	-	-	21	-	-	-	-	-	-
K+ R-URN	-	-	-	-	69	-	-	-	-	-	-
CL R-URN	-	-	-	-	49	-	-	-	-	-	-
TRIGLYCERIDES	{a}	-	-	-	-	-	-	-	-	-	-
a) 124 Specimen Slightly Hemolyzed											

YEAR	1997	1997	1997	1997	1997	1997	1997	1997	1997	1997	1997
DAY-MONTH	29 JUL	29 JUL	28 JUL	28 JUL	27 JUL	27 JUL	26 JUL	26 JUL	26 JUL	26 JUL	26 JUL
HOUR	11:14	10:53	10:46	04:06	21:20	15:41	23:47	10:57	06:41	05:05	01:10
VITALS											
TEMP AUTO ORAL	-	-	-	-	-	98.6	-	98.4	-	-	-
PULSE AUTO	-	66	72	-	-	78	-	74	-	-	-
RESP RATE AUTO	-	19	8 L	-	-	16	-	16	-	-	-
SYSTOLIC BP AUt	-	116	108	-	-	102	-	123	-	-	-
DIASTOLIC BP At	-	73	68	-	-	62	-	74	-	-	-
WEIGHT VITALNET	-	{a}	{b}	-	-	{c}	-	{d}	-	-	-
a) 281.52 h											
b) 289.02 h											
c) 286.59 h											
d) 278.88 h											
BLD GAS PANEL 1											
PH BLD	7.332 l	-	-	7.360 l	7.381	-	7.373 l	-	7.370 l	7.380	7.398
PCO2	59.5 H	-	-	52.1 h	46.4 h	-	45.7 h	-	61.7 H	48.8 h	53.3 h
PO2	73.0 l	-	-	92.0	65.0 l	-	55.0 l	-	103.0 h	57.0 l	71.0 l
BICAR(HCO3) CAt	31.9 h	-	-	29.7 h	27.8 h	-	26.9 h	-	36.0 h	29.1 h	33.2 h
CO2 TOTAL CALC	33.7 h	-	-	31.3 h	29.2 h	-	28.3 h	-	37.9 h	30.6 h	34.8 h
INSPIRED O2	40	-	-	50	50	-	45	-	50	45	45

YEAR	1997	1997	1997	1997	1997	1997	1997	1997	1997	1997	1997
DAY-MONTH	28 JUL	26 JUL	25 JUL	24 JUL	23 JUL	22 JUL	21 JUL	20 JUL	18 JUL	17 JUL	17 JUL
HOUR										17:02	00:02
ABDOMEN XRAY	-	-	-	-	-	-	-	-	-	{a}	-
a) HOSP NG tube; bibasilar; right pleural effusion											
EXTREMITY ULTRt	-	-	-	-	-	-	-	-	-	-	{a}
a) HOSP no DVT											
CXR FRONTAL	-	{a}	{b}	{c}	{d}	{e}	{f}	{g}	-	-	-
a) 1. Slight interval improvement in pulmonary edema.											
b) Slight increase in amount of opacity in the right lower lobe, could represent alveolar edema.											
c) 1. Bilateral lung infiltrates, which appear slightly improved. 2. Improved right upper lobe atelectasis.											
d) New opacification of the right upper lobe since this morning. This may represent a volume loss vs. a consolidation.											
e) Slight improvement in bilateral lung infiltrates.											
f) Interval improvement in lung aeration bilaterally.											
g) 1. No change in lines and tubes. 2. Slight increase in right effusion and bilateral diffuse infiltrates consistent with pulmonary edema.											
XRAY OTHER	{a}	-	-	-	-	-	-	-	-	-	-
a) Interval increase in lung infiltrates, most consistent with pulmonary edema.											
CXR LAT DECUBIt	-	-	-	-	-	-	-	-	{a}	-	-
a) Large layering right effusion.											
CHEST CT SCAN	-	-	{a}	-	-	-	-	-	-	-	-
a) 1. Bilateral lower lobe partial atelectasis and infiltrate. 2. Small right effusion. 3. Mid atelectasis in the posterior segment of the right upper lobe. There is a few 1 cm to 1.5 cm right peritracheal lymph node.											

FIGURE 9.11 (Continued).

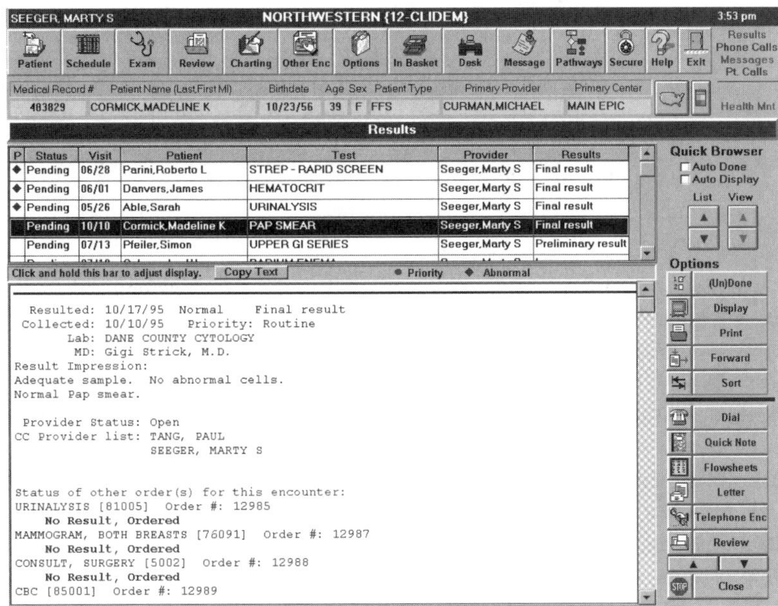

FIGURE 9.12 Prompt notification of laboratory test results. When a messaging system is integrated with the CPR system, test results can be directed to the provider's in-basket as soon as they are available. By clicking on the Review button at the lower right corner, the clinician can retrieve the patient's CPR instantly and with it any relevant information that she reviewed before acting on the most recent result or message. Telephone messages and other patient-related information can be handled in the same manner. (*Source*: Courtesy of Epic Systems, Madison, WI.)

9.4 Fundamental Issues for Computer-Based Patient-Record Systems

The objectives of all medical-record systems are the same, regardless of whether the system is automated or manual. The mechanisms for accomplishing these objectives differ, however. From a user's perspective, the two approaches differ fundamentally in the way data are entered into and information is extracted from the record. In this section, we explore the issues and alternatives related to data entry and then describe the options for displaying and retrieving information from a CPR.

9.4.1 Data Entry

The timely and accurate transfer of patient information into the computer is the most difficult and labor-intensive step in the maintenance of a computer-stored medical record. Yet this step has not received enough attention by developers and potential buyers of such systems, because responsibility for entry of data into the manual record is spread among many different health professionals and because the task is such a habitual part of their daily routines that it is almost invisible.

The transfer of data from its source to the computer requires two separate procedures: data capture and data input.

Data Capture

If the *scope* of the medical record is restricted to the variables under the control of the organization maintaining the record, **data capture** is straightforward, although it requires people's time and resources to interface the data-source systems with the CPR. Capture of comparable information across a patient's hospitalization, visit to the emergency room, and visit to a consulting physician in an independent practice is difficult or impossible. Relevant information may go unnoticed (e.g., the patient fails to mention a recent hospitalization); it may be illegible (e.g., the data recorded on the third carbon of the emergency-room visit form are not legible); or it may be available in insufficient detail (e.g., the consulting physician reports that all the patient's test results were normal but does not specify the tests' actual values). Solutions require personal negotiations with sites that frequently provide care to a practice's patients and place extra work on the part of the practice.

It may be practical to restrict the scope of the medical record to information that is returned to the practice—but such restrictions can limit the computer program's ability to provide intelligent feedback about patient care. A computer system in a medical clinic, for example, cannot make accurate recommendations about the need for cervical Pap testing if most cervical Pap results are requested by, and returned to, a consulting gynecologist from an independent practice group. The clinic would need to develop special procedures to obtain copies of those reports for entry into the medical clinic's computer. Similarly, inpatient CPR systems are constrained in their ability to generate alerts and reminders if data collected in one department are inaccessible to another department. The trend toward larger, more integrated, and more self-contained health-care systems will tend to diminish the problem of data capture. Nevertheless, the standards required to move data faithfully and automatically from source systems to CPRs within a healthcare delivery system remain a significant challenge (see Chapters 6 and 10).

Data Input

The data-input step is burdensome because of the personnel time required. People must interpret or translate the data, as well as enter them into the computer. Data may be entered in **free-text** form, in **coded** form, or in a form that combines both free text and codes. In Chapter 6, we described alternative schemes for classifying diagnoses and medical procedures. The major advantage of coding is that data are classified and standardized, thus facilitating selective retrieval of patient data, clinical research, and information for administrative functions such as billing. Coding lets the computer "understand" the data and thereby process them more intelligently. When there are only a few codes, a selection list can simplify the data input. The major disadvantage of coding is the cost of translating the source text into valid codes. There also is the potential for coding errors—which, in contrast to errors in free-text entry, are difficult to detect, because coded information lacks the internal redundancy of text. For example, a transposition error causing a substitution of code 392 for 329 may not be detected unless the computer displays the associated text and the data-entry operator notices the error.

Trade-offs between the use of codes and narrative text exist. Physicians can record complex information as narrative writing or dictation at the speed of thought. The more detailed the coding system and the more precisely the physician tries to represent a complex description in code, the slower and more costly the coding effort becomes.

Immediate coding by physicians (best through menu selection) yields codes that the CPR can use to guide physicians' decisions. If menus are carefully designed, their use will be more accurate than coding by other personnel. The use of trained coders to abstract physician's notes, however, has the advantages of sparing the physician's time and often of yielding more uniform coding. Various computer sources of coded data, including laboratory systems, pharmacy systems, and electrocardiogram (ECG) carts, exist in health-care settings. Data from these systems can flow automatically to the CPR through message standards such as HL7 (described in Chapter 6). Here, the challenge is the variety of local coding systems. The solution is to use standard coding systems—such as LOINC for identification of laboratory tests and clinical measurements (Forrey et al., 1996) and (in the United States) the National Drug Code for identification of drug products.

Error Prevention

Because of the chance of transcription errors occurring when clinical information is entered into the computer, CPR systems must apply **validity checks** scrupulously. A number of different kinds of checks apply to clinical data (Schwartz et al., 1985). **Range checks** can detect or prevent entry of values that are out of range (e.g., a serum-potassium level of 50.0 mEq/L—the normal range for healthy individuals is 3.5 to 5.0 mEq/L). **Pattern checks** can verify that the entered data have a required pattern (e.g., the three digits, hyphen, and four digits of a local telephone number). **Computed checks** can verify that values have the correct mathematical relationship (e.g., white-blood-cell differential counts [reported as percentages] must sum to 100). **Consistency checks** can detect errors by comparing entered data (e.g., the recording of cancer of the prostate as the diagnosis for a female patient). **Delta checks** warn of large and unlikely differences between the values of a new result and of the previous observations (e.g., a recorded weight that changes by 100 pounds in 2 weeks). **Spelling checks** verify the spelling of individual words. No such syntactic checks can catch all errors.

Physician-Entered Data

Physician-gathered patient information requires special comment because it presents the most difficult challenge to developers and operators of CPR systems. Physicians record four kinds of information:

1. Patient histories
2. Physician's findings from the physical examination
3. Physician's interpretation of the patient's findings
4. Physician's diagnostic and treatment plans

Physicians' notes can be entered via one of three general mechanisms: transcription of dictated or written notes, entry of data recorded on structured encounter forms, or direct data entry by physicians (direct entry may include use of electronic structured encounter forms). Dictation and **transcription** is a common option for data entry of textual information into CPRs because it is widely and comfortably used by physicians. This method is especially attractive when the practice has already invested in dictation services, because then the cost of keying already has been absorbed. If physicians dictate their reports using standard formats (e.g., present illness, past history, physical examinations, and treatment plan), then the transcriptionist maintains this structure in the transcribed document. Furthermore, digital voice dictation itself can also be stored in the CPR and retrieved without transcription, especially with existing and efficient (20:1 real time) data compression algorithms. However, the recorded note must be played back in real time; a clinician cannot skim a recording looking for specific information. In addition, transcription is associated with delays before the notes are available and carries the requirement that the author review, correct, and sign the note. All these steps leave room for errors and delays in completing the record. Interestingly, when CPRs with text-entry capability are introduced into a practice whose members usually dictate their notes, many physicians will choose to type their notes directly into the computer.

The second data-entry method is to have physicians use a **structured encounter form** from which their notes are transcribed (and possibly encoded) by support personnel. This approach has been the most successful to date. The RMRS uses highly tailored turnaround encounter forms (see Figure 9.5) to capture coded information; some forms are tailored to specific patient problems. Encounter forms often contain checklists of common signs, symptoms, and diagnoses, fields where required information may be filled in, and space for free-text comments.

The third alternative is the **direct entry** of data, by a physician, via a computer. Physicians do enter orders directly in some hospitals. Direct order entry can be facilitated by custom menus that contain standing orders for specific problems (e.g., postoperative orders for patients who undergo coronary-artery bypass operations). Menus must be carefully structured; they must not contain lists that are too long, require scrolling, nor impose a rigid hierarchy (Kuhn et al., 1984). Direct entry of the patient's history, physical findings, and progress notes has been challenging because of the extra time it takes the physician to enter such information into the computer compared with scribbling a note. Some physicians who have adopted CPRs into their practice (and consequently do have the complete record available, including progress notes), however, value the benefits of immediate and remote access to their patients' records and consider the initial data-entry time worth the benefits on the retrieval side (Tang & McDonald, unpublished data). **Computer interpretation** of voice input holds promise to eliminate the intermediate step of human transcription because it could permit the computer to understand oral commands and to translate them into the appropriate codes or text. Furthermore, **continuous-speech recognition** has been successful in limited domains (e.g., radiology reports, emergency room visit notes). We expect that speech recognition will eventually alleviate the problem of physician data entry, at least for narrative text, and that early implementations will combine transcription services and speech recognition to speed the transcription process.

9.4.2 Data Display

Once stored in the computer, data can be presented in numerous formats for different purposes without further entry work. In addition, computer-stored records can be produced in novel formats that are unavailable in manual systems. We discuss a few helpful formats.

Flowsheets of Patient Data

A **flowsheet** is similar to a spreadsheet; it organizes patient data according to the time that they were collected, thus emphasizing changes over time. For example, a flowsheet used to monitor patients who have hypertension (high blood pressure) might contain values for weight, blood pressure, heart rate, and doses of medications that control hypertension. Other pertinent information also could be added, such as results of laboratory tests that monitor complications of hypertension itself or of medications used to control hypertension. Flowsheets are designed to be problem specific, patient specific, or specialty specific. The time granularity may change from one setting to another. For example, when a patient is in the intensive-care unit (ICU), minute-to-minute changes in the patient's clinical state may be of interest. On the other hand, an outpatient physician is more likely to want to know how that patient's data have changed over weeks or months. For convenience of human review, the temporal granularity should be appropriate to the intensity of care. Thus, measurement of blood pressures every 20 minutes in an ICU is not of interest to the physician taking care of the same patient later in the clinic after the patient's condition is stabilized.

Summaries and Abstracts

Computer-based patient records can highlight important components (e.g., active allergies, active problems, active treatments, and recent observations) in a clinical summary (Tang et al, 1999). In the future, we can expect more sophisticated summarizing strategies, such as detection of significant changes in observations or aggregation of abnormal observations with a similar meaning (e.g., elevated SGOT, elevated alkaline phosphate, and elevated bilirubin, all of which are indicators of liver dysfunction) into a summary diagnostic statement. We may also see reports that distinguish abnormal changes that have been treated from those that have not and displays that dynamically organize the supporting evidence for existing problems. Ultimately, computers should be able to produce concise and flowing summary reports that are like an experienced physician's hospital discharge summary.

Turnaround Documents

Turnaround documents are computer-tailored reports that both present information to and ask questions of the user. They are the paper equivalent of an input screen on a computer. Visit encounter forms (see Fig. 9.5) can be used as both patient information summary sheets and structured data-input forms. In some settings (Teich, 1997), these forms are entered into the computer when completed. A well-structured turnaround document allows direct capture of clinical information from physicians in many environments. Paper turnaround documents are familiar materials, and people can use them with little training. Obviously, turnaround documents have their greatest application in outpatient care, where there is sufficient time to prepare them before patient visits. They also have been used on inpatient units—for example, to gather drug-administration information and notes from nurses—and as request forms for diagnostic studies. Direct input by clinicians into forms provided on a computer will soon replace most paper intermediaries.

Dynamic Displays

Anyone who has reviewed a patient's chart knows how hard it can be to find a particular piece of information, such as what the interpretation was of the most recent computed tomography scan—or whether one ever was done. From 10 percent (Fries, 1974) to 81 percent (Tang et al., 1994b) of the time, physicians do not find patient information that has been previously recorded and belongs in the medical record. Furthermore, the questions clinicians routinely ask are often the ones that are difficult to answer from perusal of a paper-based record. Common questions include whether a specific test has ever been performed, what kinds of medications have been tried in the past, and how the patient has responded to particular treatments in the past. Physicians constantly ask these questions as they flip back and forth in the chart searching for the facts to support or refute one in a series of evolving hypotheses. Search tools help the physician to locate relevant data, and specialized presentation formats (e.g., flowsheets or graphics) make it easier for them to glean information from the data. Special displays can identify problem-specific parameters to help the physician retrieve relevant information, and a graphical presentation can help the physician to assimilate the information quickly and to draw conclusions (Tang et al., 1994b). Click-and-expand technology, now common on Web pages, will simplify such tasks by using a paradigm that is becoming familiar to everyone.

9.4.3 *Query and Surveillance Systems*

The query and surveillance capabilities of computer-stored records have no counterpart in manual systems. Medical personnel and administrators can use these capabilities to generate alerts about important clinical events, to retrieve a patient's selected medical or administrative characteristics, and to summarize information statistically. **Query** is the retrieval and aggregation of data about groups of similar patients. **Surveillance** across subgroups of patients is the detection and flagging of patient conditions that warrant medical attention.

Although these functions are different, their internal logic is similar. In both, the central procedure is to examine a patient's medical record and, if the record meets prespecified criteria, to generate an appropriate output. Query generally addresses a large subset or all of a patient population; the output is a tabular report of selected raw data on all the patient records retrieved or a statistical summary of the values contained in the records. Surveillance generally addresses only those patients under active care; its output is an **alert** or **reminder message** (McDonald, 1976), such as the message shown in Figure 9.13.

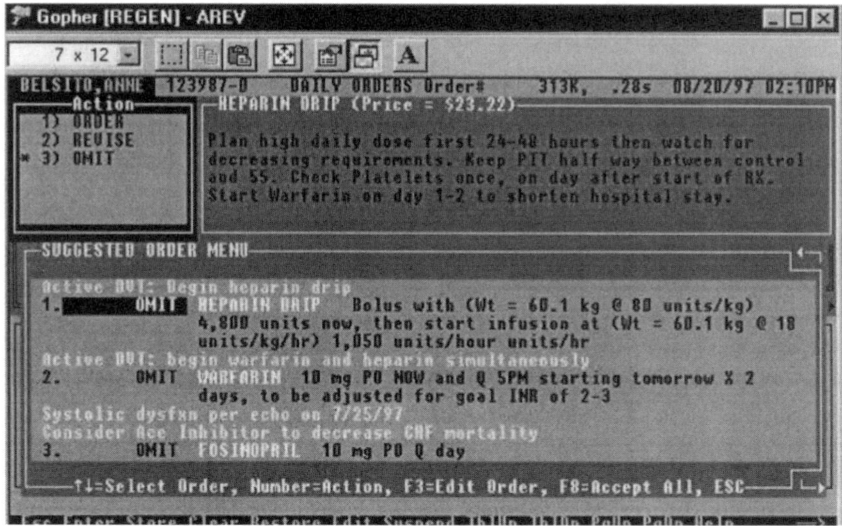

FIGURE 9.13 Display of suggested orders that appears during a physician order-entry session. The suggestions for heparin drip and warfarin arise because the patient has deep venous thrombosis. The suggestion for fosinopril arises because the patient has systolic dysfunction by echocardiography and has no contraindications to angiotensin-converting enzyme inhibitors. (*Source*: Courtesy of Regenstrief Institute, Indianapolis, IN.)

Query and surveillance systems can be used for clinical care, clinical research, retrospective studies, and administration.

Clinical Care

Computer reminders have increased substantially physicians' use of preventive care for eligible patients. Surveillance systems can identify patients who are due for periodic screening examinations such as immunizations, breast examinations, and cervical Pap tests and can remind physicians to perform these procedures during the next visit. For example, physicians given computer reminders quadrupled the use of certain vaccines in eligible patients compared with those who did not receive reminders (McDonald et al., 1984a; McPhee et al., 1991). Query systems are particularly useful for conducting ad hoc searches—for example, to identify and contact patients who have been receiving a drug that is recalled from the market. These systems also can facilitate the completion of quality-management activities, such as accreditation-required care reviews. They can identify candidate patients for concurrent review and can gather many of the data required to complete such audits.

Clinical Research

Query systems can be used to identify patients who meet eligibility requirements for prospective clinical trials. For example, an investigator could identify all patients seen in a medical clinic who were male, were over 50 years of age, and were taking antihypertensive medication. Surveillance facilities can support the execution of a study by tracking patients through their visits and by following the steps of a clinical trial as described in the study protocol to ensure that treatments are given and measurements obtained when required.

Retrospective Studies

Randomized **prospective studies** are the gold standard for clinical investigations, but **retrospective studies** of existing data have contributed much to medical progress. Retrospective studies can obtain answers at a small fraction of the time and cost of comparable prospective studies.

Computer-based patient record systems can provide many of the data required for a retrospective study. They can, for example, identify study cases and comparable control cases, and they can perform the statistical analyses needed to compare the two groups (Bleich et al., 1989; McDonald & Tierney, 1986a).

Computer-stored records do not eliminate all the work required to complete an epidemiologic study; chart reviews and patient interviews may still be necessary if some patient information is recorded as narrative text. The more information that can be retrieved from the record, however, the less frequently and less intensively such time-consuming tasks must be conducted. Computer-stored records are likely to be most complete and accurate with respect to drugs administered, laboratory-test results, and visit diagnoses, especially if the first two types of data are entered directly from automated laboratory and pharmacy systems. Consequently, computer-stored records are most likely to contribute to research on a physician's practice patterns, on the efficacy of tests and treatments, and on the toxicity of drugs.

Administration

As we discuss in Chapter 19, managed care and fixed-cost reimbursement for specific diseases (diagnosis-related groups, or capitation payments) and competitive bidding for healthcare contracts provide incentives for administrators to consider clinical as well as cost information in deciding what services to market, to whom, and at what price. In addition, administrators must be able to monitor physicians' use of resources for various classes of patients and to provide appropriate feedback for physicians whose behavior is significantly different from the norm. Medical query systems can provide information about the relationships among diagnoses, indices of severity of illness, and resource consumption. Thus, query systems are important tools for administrators who wish to make informed decisions in the increasingly cost-sensitive world of health care.

9.5 Challenges Ahead

Although many commercial products are labeled as CPR systems, they do not all satisfy the criteria that we defined at the beginning of this chapter. Even beyond matters of definition, however, it is important to recognize that the concept of a CPR is neither unified nor static. As the capability of technology evolves, the function of the CPR will expand. A review of current products would be obsolete by the time that it was published. We have included examples from various systems in this chapter, both developed by their users and commercially available, to illustrate a portion of the functionality of CPR systems currently in use.

The future of CPR systems depends on both technical and nontechnical considerations (McDonald, 1997a). Hardware technology will continue to advance, with processing power doubling every two years according to Moore's law. Software will improve with more powerful applications, better user interfaces, and more integrated decision support. Perhaps the greater need for leadership and action will be in the social and organizational foundations that must be laid if CPRs are to serve as the information infrastructure for health care. We touch briefly on these challenges in this final section.

9.5.1 Users' Information Needs

We discussed the importance of clinicians directly using the CPR system to achieve maximum benefit from computer-supported decision-making. Consequently, developers of CPR systems must thoroughly understand clinicians' information needs and workflows in the various healthcare settings. The most successful systems have been developed either by clinicians or through close collaborations with practicing clinicians.

Studies of clinicians' information needs reveal that common questions that physicians ask concerning patient information (e.g., Is there evidence to support a specific patient diagnosis? Has a patient ever had a specific test? Has there been any follow up because of a particular laboratory-test result?) are difficult to answer from the perusal of the paper-based chart (Tang et al., 1994a). Regrettably, most clinical systems in use now cannot answer many of the common questions that clinicians ask. Developers of CPR systems must have a thorough grasp of users' needs if they are to produce systems that help healthcare providers to use these tools efficiently to deliver care effectively.

9.5.2 User Interfaces

An intuitive and efficient user interface is an important part of the system. Designers must understand the cognitive aspects of the human and computer interaction if they are to build interfaces that are intuitive and functional. Improving human–computer interfaces will require changes not only in how the system behaves but also in how humans interact with the system. We are learning much from the ubiquity of Web interfaces. What information the provider needs and what tasks the provider performs should influence what and how information is presented. Development of human-interface technology that matches the data-processing power of computers with the cognitive capability of humans to formulate insightful questions and to interpret data is still a rate-limiting step (Tang & Patel, 1993). User interface requirements of clinicians entering patient data are different from the user interfaces developed for clerks entering patient charges. Healthcare applications developers must now focus on specific sets of users (such as clinicians, nurses, and so forth) and must define and address their unique information needs.

9.5.3 Standards

We alluded to the importance of standards earlier in this chapter, when we discussed the architectural requirements of integrating data from multiple sources. Standards were discussed in Chapter 6. Here, we stress the critical importance of national standards in the development, implementation, and use of CPR systems (McDonald et al., 1997). Having standards reduces development costs, increases integration, and facilitates the collection of meaningful aggregate data for quality improvement and health-policy development. Leadership from stakeholders in health care is critical to achieving useful standards. The need for consistent standards throughout the United States, and ideally around the world, requires action and participation of our federal and other countries' governments. Legislation that mandates certain standards has already been enacted (Barrows & Clayton, 1996). Further enabling legislation will be necessary. Those who wish to implement CPRs should promote and adopt clinical information standards.

9.5.4 Legal and Social Issues

In addition to legislation on standards, federal laws and guidelines on other aspects of the use of CPR systems must be established before widespread adoption will occur. Privacy, confidentiality, and security are major areas of concern in CPRs. Federal regulations are needed, because patients and their data pass freely among states, which currently have greatly differing requirements (see Chapter 7). Europe has adopted strict regulations, although their enforcement is spotty. Adequate methods must be defined and legally enforced to protect the private data of our citizens. With appropriate laws and policies, however, computer-stored data can be more secure and confidential than those data maintained in paper-based records (Barrows & Clayton, 1996).

9.5.5 Costs and Benefits

The Institute of Medicine declared the CPR an essential infrastructure for the delivery of health care (Institute of Medicine Committee on Improving the Patient Record, 1997). Like any infrastructure project, the benefits specifically attributable to infrastructure are difficult to establish; an infrastructure plays an enabling role in all projects that take advantage of it. Part of the difficulty in comparing costs and benefits of a CPR is our inability to measure accurately the actual costs and opportunity costs of using paper-based records. Many randomized controlled clinical studies have shown that computer-based decision-support systems that are integrated in a CPR reduce costs and improve quality compared with usual care supported with a paper medical record (Bates et al., 1997; Classen et al., 1997; Tierney et al., 1993). It is difficult, however, to determine the scalability and longevity of such benefits.

Because of the significant resources needed and the significant broad-based potential benefits, the decision to implement a CPR system is a strategic one. Hence, the evaluation of the costs and benefits must consider the effects on the organization's strategic goals, as well as the objectives for individual health care.

9.5.6 Leadership

Leaders from all segments of the healthcare industry must work together to articulate the needs, to define the standards, to fund the development, to implement the social change, and to write the laws to accelerate the development and routine use of CPR systems in health care. Technological change will continue to occur at a rapid pace, driven by consumer demand for entertainment, games, and business tools. Nurturing the use of information technology in health care requires leaders who promote the use of CPR systems and work to overcome the obstacles that impede widespread use of computers for the benefit of health care.

Suggested Readings

Barnett G.O. (1984). The application of computer-based medical-record systems in ambulatory practice. *New England Journal of Medicine*, 310(25):1643–1650.

This seminal article compares the characteristics of manual and automated ambulatory patient record systems, discusses implementation issues, and predicts future developments in technology.

Collen M.F. (1995). *A history of medical informatics in the United States 1950–1990.* Indianapolis: American Medical Informatics Association, Hartman Publishing.

This rich history of medical informatics from the late 1960s to the late 1980s includes an extremely detailed set of references.

Institute of Medicine Committee on Improving the Patient Record. (1997). *The Computer-Based Patient-Record: An Essential Technology for Health Care* (2nd ed). Washington, D.C.: National Academy Press.

This landmark study by the Institute of Medicine defines the CPR, describes the users and uses of the medical record, examines technologies employed in CPRs, and recommends actions to accelerate the development and routine use of CPRs in the United States. The second edition adds commentaries on the status of CPRs in the United States and Europe 5 years after the release of the original report.

McDonald C.J. (Ed.) (1988). Computer-stored medical record systems. *MD Computing,* 5(5):1–62.

This issue of *MD Computing* contains invited papers on the STOR, HELP, RMRS, and TMR systems. The objective of the issue is to describe the design goals, functions, and internal structure of these established, large-scale CPR systems.

McDonald C.J., Tierney W.M. (1986). The medical gopher: A microcomputer system to help find, organize and decide about patient data. *Western Journal of Medicine,* 145(6):823–829.

McDonald and Tierney describe research conducted at the Regenstrief Institute for Health Care in developing a PC-based medical workstation that can help physicians to organize, review, and record medical information.

Osheroff J. (Ed.) (1995). *Computers in Clinical Practices. Managing Patients, Information, and Communication.* Philadelphia: American College of Physicians.

This text looks at the practical use of computers in the office practice with a special emphasis on medical records.

Pryor T.A., Gardner R.M., Clayton P.D., Warner H.R. (1983). The HELP system. *Journal of Medical Systems*, 7(2):87–102.

This article summarizes the HELP system's objectives and describes HELP's use in clinical decision-making.

Van Bemmel J.H., Musen, M.A. (1997). *Handbook of Medical Informatics.* Heidelberg: Bohn Stafleu Van Loghum, Houten.

This book provides a comprehensive survey of work being performed to develop information technology for the clinical workplace.

Weed L.L. (1969): *Medical Records, Medical Evaluation and Patient Care: The Problem-Oriented Record as a Basic Tool.* Chicago: Year Book Medical Publishers.

In this classic book, Weed presents his plan for collecting and structuring patient data to produce a problem-oriented medical record.

Questions for Discussion

1. What is the definition of a CPR? Define a CPR system. What are five advantages of a CPR over a paper-based record? What are three limitations of a CPR?
2. What are the five functional components of a CPR? Think of the information systems used in healthcare institutions in which you work or that you have seen. Which of the components that you named do those systems have? Which are missing? How do the missing elements limit the value to the clinicians or patients?
3. Discuss three ways in which a computer system could facilitate information transfer between hospitals and ambulatory-care facilities, thus enhancing continuity of care for previously hospitalized patients who have been discharged and are now being followed up by their primary physicians.
4. How does the healthcare financing environment affect the use, costs, and benefits of a CPR system? How has the financing environment affected the functionality of information systems? How has it affected the user population?
5. Would a computer scan of a paper-based record be a CPR? What are two advantages and two limitations of this approach?
6. Among the key issues for designing a CPR system are what information should be captured and how it should be entered into the system.
   a. Physicians may enter data directly or may record data on a paper worksheet (encounter form) for later transcription by a data-entry worker. What are two advantages and two disadvantages of each method?
   b. Discuss the relative advantages and disadvantages of entry of free text instead of entry of fully coded information. Describe an intermediate or compromise method.
7. Identify four locations where clinicians need access to the information contained in a CPR. What are the major costs or risks of providing access from each of these locations?
8. What are three important reasons to have physicians enter orders directly into a CPR system? What are three challenges in implementing such a system?
9. Consider the task of creating a summary report for clinical data collected over time and stored in a CPR system. Clinical laboratories traditionally provide summary test results in flowsheet format, thus highlighting clinically important changes over time. A medical-record system that contains information for patients who have chronic diseases must present serial clinical observations, history information, and medications, as well as laboratory-test results. Suggest a suitable format for presenting the information collected during a series of ambulatory-care patient visits.

10. The public demands that the confidentiality of patient data must be maintained in any patient record system. Describe three protections and auditing methods that can be applied to paper-based systems. Describe three technical and three nontechnical measures you would like to see applied to ensure the confidentiality of patient data in a CPR. How do the risks of privacy breaches differ for the two systems?

10 Management of Information in Integrated Delivery Networks

Charles Safran and Leslie E. Perreault

After reading this chapter, you should know the answers to these questions:

- What is an integrated delivery network (IDN)?
- What are an IDN's primary requirements for information?
- What are the clinical and financial factors that drive the need for integrated healthcare information systems?
- How do the information needs of a hospital, an ambulatory clinic, and an IDN differ?
- What are the clinical, financial, and administrative functions provided by an enterprise healthcare information system?
- What are the relative advantages and disadvantages of *central*, *modular*, and *distributed* systems architectures?
- What are the primary considerations in the design and implementation of integrated healthcare information systems to support IDNs?

10.1 Information Management in Healthcare Organizations

Healthcare organizations, like all business entities, are information-intensive enterprises. Health personnel require sufficient data and information management tools to make appropriate decisions, both while caring for patients and while managing and running the enterprise, and to document and communicate plans and activities. Clinicians assess patient status, plan patient care, administer appropriate treatments, and educate patients and families regarding clinical management of various conditions. Primary-care physicians and care managers assess the health status of new members of the health plan. Medical directors evaluate the clinical outcomes, quality, and cost of health services provided. Administrators determine appropriate staffing levels, manage inventories of drugs and supplies, and negotiate payment contracts for services. Governing boards make decisions about investing in new business lines, affiliating with other organizations, and eliminating underutilized services. Collectively, healthcare professionals comprise a heterogeneous group with diverse objectives and information requirements.

The purpose of a **healthcare information system** (HCIS) is to manage the information that health professionals need to perform their jobs effectively and efficiently. Healthcare information systems facilitate communication, integrate information, and coordinate action among multiple healthcare professionals. In addition, they assist in the organization and storage of information, and they perform certain record-keeping functions. Many of the clinical information functions of an HCIS were detailed in our discussion of the computer-based patient record (CPR) in Chapter 9; and systems to support nurses and other care providers are discussed in Chapter 12. An HCIS also supports the financial and administrative functions of a health organization and associated operating units, including the operations of ancillary and other clinical-support departments. The evolving complexities of a healthcare organization's operation place great demands on an HCIS. The HCIS must organize, manage, and integrate a large number of clinical and financial data collected by diverse users in a variety of settings and must provide healthcare workers (and sometimes patients) with timely access to complete, accurate, and up-to-date information presented in a useful format.

10.1.1 Evolution from Hospital Information Systems to Healthcare Information Systems

Chapter 19 details the economic and regulatory factors that have compelled the emergence of managed care and the healthcare reforms that have transformed the delivery-of-care model in the United States. These changes have radically transformed the structure, strategic goals, and operational processes of healthcare organizations by encouraging the consolidation of healthcare providers into **integrated delivery networks** (IDNs) of previously independent organizations—with tremendous implications for information systems.

The evolution of HCISs has paralleled the organizational evolution of the healthcare industry. The earliest HCISs were **hospital information systems** (HISs), developed in the 1960s and early 1970s. These systems were designed to support the information requirements of hospitals and of university-affiliated medical centers—the predominant settings for healthcare delivery. They met the operational needs of the hospitals' units, initially including census management, patient billing, and general accounting. Later, mirroring the facility-centric model of medical care, additional applications were developed to support clinical ancillary departments. By the 1980s, departmental information systems such as laboratory and pharmacy systems were commonly linked into hospital-wide clinical and administrative systems, and the **clinical information system** (CIS) components of HISs offered clinically oriented capabilities, such as order writing and results communications. During the same period, **ambulatory medical record systems** (AMRSs) and **practice management systems** (PMSs) were being developed to support large outpatient clinics and physician offices, respectively. These systems performed functions analogous to those of hospital systems, but were generally less complex, reflecting the lower volume and complexity of patient care delivered in outpatient settings. Typically, these various systems were implemented within organizational boundaries, with no integration between hospital and ambulatory settings.

By the early 1980s, the stage was set for a shift toward corporate medicine, including the growth of for-profit firms providing health services and the reorganization of the healthcare industry as a whole toward greater organizational integration and control (Starr, 1982). The decade of the 1990s was marked by a large number of mergers and affiliations among previously independent and often competitive organizations; there was a major move toward healthcare consolidation to drive excess capacity from the system (e.g., an oversupply of hospital beds) and to secure regional market share. First, hospitals and medical centers began to build satellite ambulatory-care clinics and to reach out to community physician practices in an attempt to feed patient referrals to their specialty services and to fill their increasingly vacant inpatient beds. Later, facing competition with vertically integrated for-profit healthcare chains and with other integrating organizations, hospitals started at first affiliating and then more tightly banding into the regional aggregates of healthcare service providers called IDNs (Fig. 10.1).

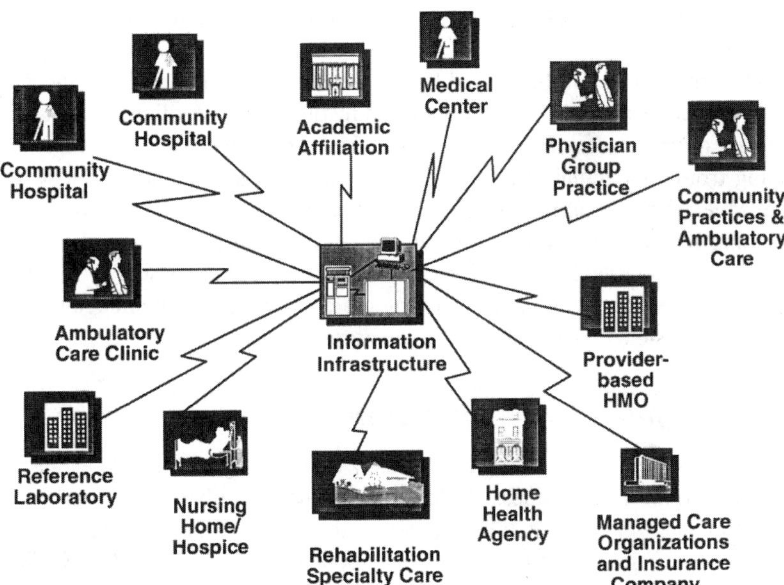

FIGURE 10.1. Major organizational components of an integrated delivery network (IDN). A typical IDN includes multiple acute-care facilities, ambulatory-care clinics, and owned or managed physicians' practices that jointly operate to provide comprehensive health services. In addition, an IDN may own or affiliate with other healthcare facilities, for-profit subcorporations, and managed care or health plan organizations. HMO = Health maintenance organization.

Integrated delivery networks are now prominent in every healthcare market in the United States and may span a large geographic region or multiple states. Each IDN typically consists of multiple acute-care facilities, satellite ambulatory health centers, and owned or managed physicians' practice groups. In addition, the IDNs may have subacute-care facilities, skilled nursing homes, assisted-living facilities, hospices, home-care agencies, and for-profit subcorporations to deliver support services back to the healthcare providers, including regional laboratories, drugs and supplies purchasing and distribution, and remote billing services. Because they control a significant regional market share and are positioned to provide and manage comprehensive health services, IDNs negotiate service contracts with payers or directly with large employers. Some IDNs go further and affiliate with a regional health maintenance organization (HMO) or develop their own health-plan organizations to act as their own insurance carriers. The largest of the IDNs have pooled annual revenues of more than $1 billion, have staffs comprising or contracting with thousands of physicians and nurses, and manage contracts to provide comprehensive care for more than 1 million patients.

These IDNs must coordinate patient care and manage business operations throughout an extensive network of community and regional resources. Although medical centers retain a central role in many emerging IDNs, the focus of attention has shifted to development of the surrounding network of primary-care and ambulatory-care sites, physicians' practice groups, and regional community hospitals.

Today, most IDNs in the United States are *integrating* rather than *integrated,* and most markets are still undergoing rapid institutional consolidation, with multiple new alignments each year. Currently, there are many models of integration, ranging from contractual affiliations to full asset mergers. Although most IDNs have achieved a measure of structural and operational integration, they are only beginning to integrate from a clinical and information perspective (Fig. 10.2). Today's IDN is a melding of diverse organizations, and the associated information systems infrastructure is far from integrated; rather, it is an amalgam of heterogeneous systems, processes, and data stores.

10.1.2 Information Requirements

Clearly, IDNs are complex organizations. From an organizational perspective, they are in flux; their business strategies continue to evolve as the market continues to change. Fundamentally, however, the information requirements of an IDN are no different from those of its component hospitals, ambulatory clinics, physician practices, and other organizations.

From a clinical perspective, the most important function of an HCIS is to provide communication among the many healthcare workers who cooperate in providing health services to patients and to organize and present patient-specific data such that the staff can easily interpret those data and use them in decision-making. From an administrative perspective, the most pressing information needs are those related to the daily operation and management of the organization—bills

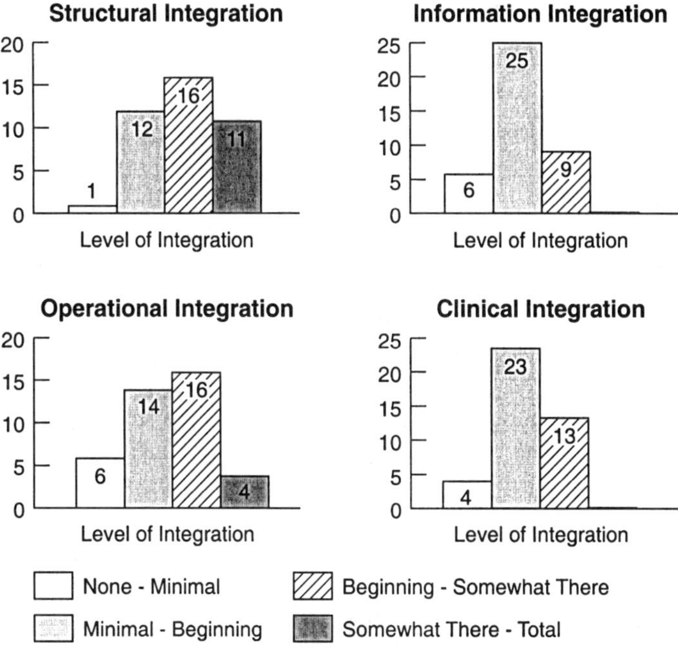

FIGURE 10.2. Relative progress in structural, operational, clinical, and information integration among 40 IDNs from a 1996 survey of organizational members of the Center for Clinical Integration. Clinical integration and information systems typically lag behind structural and operational integration in emerging IDNs. (*Source:* Copyright First Consulting Group. Reprinted with permission.)

must be generated accurately and rapidly, employees and vendors must be paid, supplies must be ordered, and so on. In addition, administrators need information to make short-term and long-term planning decisions. We can classify an IDN's operational information needs into four broad categories of support: daily operations, planning, documentation, and communication.

- *Operational requirements.* Healthcare workers require detailed and up-to-date factual information to perform the daily tasks that keep a hospital, clinic, or physician practice running—the bread-and-butter tasks of the institution. Here are examples of queries for operational information: Where is patient John Smith? What drugs is he receiving? What tests are scheduled for Mr. Smith after his discharge? Who will pay his bill? Is the staffing skill mix sufficient to handle the current volume and special needs of patients in Care Center 3 West? What are the names and telephone numbers of patients who have appointments for tomorrow and need to be called for a reminder? What authorization is needed to perform an ultrasound procedure on Jane Blue under the terms of her health insurance coverage? An HCIS can support these operational requirements for information by organizing data for prompt and easy access.

Because the IDN may have developed product-line specialization within a particular facility (e.g., a diagnostic imaging center or women's health center), however, answering even a simple request may require accessing information held at many different facilities.

- *Planning requirements.* Health professionals also require information to make short-term and long-term decisions about patient care and organizational management. An HCIS should help healthcare personnel to answer queries such as these: What are the organization's clinical guidelines for managing the care of patients with this condition? Have similar patients experienced better clinical outcomes with medical treatment or with surgical intervention? What are the financial and medical implications of closing the maternity service? If we added six nurse practitioners to the outpatient-clinic staff, can we increase visit volume and decrease patient waiting time? Will the proposed contract to provide health services to Medicaid patients be profitable given the current cost structure and current utilization patterns? Often, the data necessary for planning are generated by many sources. An HCIS can help planners by aggregating, analyzing, and summarizing the information relevant to decision-making.
- *Documentation requirements.* The need to maintain records for future reference or analysis makes up the third category of informational requirements. Some requirements are internally imposed. For example, a complete record of each patient's health status and treatment history is necessary to ensure continuity of care across multiple providers and over time. External requirements create a large demand for data collection and record keeping in healthcare organizations. As discussed in Chapter 2, the medical record is a legal document. If necessary, the courts can refer to the record to determine whether a patient received proper care. Insurance companies require itemized billing statements, and medical records substantiate the clinical justification of services provided and charges submitted to them. The Joint Commission for Accreditation of Healthcare Organizations has specific requirements concerning the content and quality of medical records, as well as requirements for organization-wide information-management processes. Furthermore, to qualify for participation in the Medicare and Medicaid programs, hospitals must follow accepted procedures for auditing the medical staff and monitoring the quality of patient care, and they must be able to show that they meet the safety requirements for infectious disease management, buildings, and equipment. Similarly, the National Committee for Quality Assurance has established reporting requirements to allow payers and employers to assess the quality of managed-care plans (see Chapter 11).
- *Communication requirements.* It should be clear that communication and coordination of patient care and operations across multiple personnel, multiple business units, and far-flung geography is not possible without investment in underlying technology infrastructure. For example, the routing of paper medical records, a cumbersome process even within a single hospital, is an impossibility for a regional network of providers trying to act in coordination. Similarly, it is neither timely nor cost effective to copy and distribute hard copy

documents to all participants in a regionally distributed organizational structure. An IDN's technology infrastructure enables information exchange via electronic mail, standard document-management systems, and on-line calendaring systems, as well as providing and controlling HCIS access to authorized users at the place and time that information is required.

The importance of appropriate clinical decision-making is obvious—we devoted all of Chapter 3 to explaining methods to help clinicians select diagnostic tests, interpret test results, and choose treatments for their patients. The decisions made by administrators and managers are no less important in their choices concerning the acquisition and use of healthcare resources. In fact, clinicians and administrators alike must choose wisely in their use of resources to provide high-quality care and excellent service at a competitive price. In the past, waste and inefficiency caused by poor operating procedures and inappropriate choices simply were translated into higher healthcare costs. In an IDN that contracts to care for a member population at a fixed price per member per month, inefficiency translates to loss of revenue, poor member satisfaction, and an inability to remain competitive.

10.1.3 Integration Requirements

In an IDN composed of multiple operating units, the parent corporation can have either a strong centralized governance model that dictates common processes and procedures throughout the organization or a distributed model, whereby the operating units have relatively autonomous decision-making authority. The common objective of all IDNs, however, is the ability to contract jointly to deliver health services—thus implying the need to maintain aggregate management data and to have effective linked voice and data communication throughout the IDN. If an IDN is to manage patient care effectively, to project a unified market identity, and to control its operating costs, it must perform in an integrated manner. For these reasons, information technologies to support data and process integration are recognized as a critical enabler of IDN business strategies. From an IDN perspective, information should be available when and where it is needed; users must have an integrated view, regardless of organizational, system, or geographic boundaries; data must have a consistent interpretation; and adequate security must be in place to ensure access by only authorized personnel for only appropriate uses.

Data Integration

In hospitals, clinical and administrative personnel traditionally held distinct areas of responsibility and performed many of their functions separately. Thus, it is not surprising that administrative and clinical data were often managed separately—administrative data in business offices and clinical data in medical-records departments. When computers were used at all, the hospital's information processing was often performed on separate computers with separate databases, thus minimizing conflicts about priorities in services and investment. Similarly, information systems to support hospital and ambulatory care historically have, with a few notable exceptions (Bleich et al., 1985), developed independently. Many organizations have rich databases for inpatient data but maintain less information for outpatients—often only billing data such as diagnosis and procedure codes and charges for services provided. Even today, relatively few clinical data are available in electronic format for most ambulatory-care clinics and physician offices in the United States, although this disparity is beginning to resolve as IDNs and larger physician group practices make strategic investments in automating their outpatient environments. In contrast, some countries in Western Europe (e.g., the Netherlands, Norway, and Great Britain) have implemented electronic patient records in most primary-care offices.

The lack of integration of data from diverse sources creates a host of problems. If clinical and administrative data are stored on separate systems, then data needed by both must either be entered directly into both systems or be copied from one system to the other. In addition to the expense of redundant data entry and data maintenance incurred by this approach, the consistency of information tends to be poor because data may be updated in one place and not in the other, or information may be copied incorrectly. Within the hospital setting, many of these issues have been addressed through the development of automated interfaces to transfer demographic data, orders, results, and charges between clinical systems and billing systems. Even with interfaces among disparate systems, however, an organization still must solve the thorny issues of synchronization of data and comparability of similar data types.

With the development of IDNs, the sharing of data elements among all operating units becomes more critical and more problematic. Data integration issues are further compounded in IDNs by the acquisition of previously independent organizations that have clinical and administrative information systems incompatible with those of the rest of the IDN. It is still not unusual to encounter minimal automated information exchange among settings in an IDN. Patients register and reregister at the physician's office, diagnostic imaging center, ambulatory surgery facility, and acute-care hospital. Each facility keeps its own clinical records, and *shadow files* include copies of critical information such as operative reports and hospital discharge summaries. Inconsistencies in the databases can result in inappropriate patient management and inappropriate resource allocation. For example, medications that are first given to a patient while she is a hospital inpatient may inadvertently be discontinued when she is transported to an intermediate-care facility such as a nursing home. Also, information about a patient's known allergies and medication history may be unavailable to physicians treating an unconscious patient in an emergency department.

The objectives of coordinated, high-quality, and cost-effective health care cannot be completely satisfied if an IDN's multiple computer systems operate in isolation. Although free-standing systems within IDNs are still common, most such organizations are investing heavily in implementing new common systems in all their facilities or in integrating existing systems to allow data sharing. In Sections 10.3 and 10.4, we discuss architectural components and strategies for data integration.

Process Integration

Healthcare administrators have found the significant task of forging agreements and reorganizing to achieve structural integration the easiest step in developing an IDN. Far more challenging is the implementation of new clinical and administrative processes throughout the organization. The most progressive IDNs have begun to develop new enterprise-wide processes for providing easy and uniform access to health services, for deploying consistent clinical guidelines, and for coordinating and managing patient care across multiple care settings throughout the IDN (Drazen & Metzger, 1999). Integrated information technologies are essential to supporting such enterprise-wide processes.

To be effective, information systems must mesh smoothly with operational workflow and human organizational systems. New IDNs pose significant challenges for process integration from two perspectives. First, the new healthcare-delivery models represent a radical departure from more traditional models of care delivery. They demand, for example, changes in the responsibilities and work patterns of physicians, nurses, and other care providers; the development of entirely new job categories (such as care managers who coordinate a patient's care across facilities and between encounters); and the more active participation of patients in personal health management (Table 10.1). Second, component entities of an IDN typically have evolved substantially different operational policies and procedures, which reflect each component organization's history and

TABLE 10.1. The changing health-care environment and its implications for an IDN's core competencies.

Characteristic	Old care model	New care model
Goal of care	Manage sickness	Manage wellness
Center of delivery system	Hospital	Primary-care providers/ ambulatory settings
Focus of care	Episodic acute and chronic care	Population health, primary, and preventive care
Driver of care decisions	Specialists	Primary-care providers
Metric of system success	Number of admissions	Number of enrollees
Performance optimization	Optimize individual provider performance	Optimize system-wide performance
Utilization controls	Externally controlled	Internally controlled
Quality measures	Defined as inputs to system	Defined as patient outcomes and satisfaction
Physician role	Autonomous and independent	Member of care team; user of system-wide guidelines of care
Patient role	Passive receiver of care	Active partner in care

Source: Copyright First Consulting Group. Reprinted with permission.

leaders. Thus, mechanisms for information management aimed at integrating operations across entities must address not only the migration from legacy systems but also the migration from legacy work processes to new, consistent policies and processes across entities.

The introduction of new information systems almost always changes the workplace. At times, these changes can be fundamental. The implementation of a new system offers an opportunity to rethink and redefine existing work processes to take advantage of the new information-management capabilities, thereby reducing costs, increasing productivity, or improving service levels. For example, providing electronic access to information that was previously accessible only on paper can shorten the overall time required to complete a multistep activity by enabling conversion of serial processes (completed by multiple workers using the same record sequentially) to concurrent processes (completed by the workers accessing an electronic record simultaneously).

Few organizations today have the time or resources to develop entirely new information systems and redesigned processes; therefore, most opt to purchase existing software products or to partner with commercial systems vendors in codevelopment projects. Although these commercial systems allow some degree of custom tailoring, they also reflect an underlying model of work processes that may have evolved through development in other healthcare organizations with different underlying operational policies and procedures. Most clinical sites must adapt their own work processes to those embodied in the systems they are installing. (For example, some commercial systems require care providers to discontinue and then reenter all orders when a patient is admitted to the hospital after being monitored in the emergency department.) Furthermore, once the systems are installed and once workflow has been adapted to them, they become part of the organization's culture—a subsequent change to a new system may be arduous because of these workflow considerations. Thus, decision-makers should take great care when selecting and tailoring a new system to support and enhance desired work processes. Such organizational workflow adaptation represents a significant challenge to the emerging IDN and its systems planners. Some have estimated that less than 50 percent of the potential return on information-technology investments currently flows through the enterprise; inappropriate management practices and suboptimal workflow absorbs the balance.

To meet the requirements of the new healthcare environment, IDNs must change—and they must change quickly. Although an IDN's business plans and information-systems strategies may be reasonable and necessary, changing ingrained organizational behavior can be many times more complex than changing the underlying information systems. Successful process integration requires not only successful deployment of the technology but also sustained commitment of resources; dedicated leadership with the willingness to make difficult, sometimes unpopular decisions; education; and realignment of performance incentives to overcome cultural inertia and politics.

10.1.4 Security and Confidentiality Requirements

As we discussed in Chapter 7, the protection of health information from unwanted or inappropriate use is governed not only by the trust of patients in their health providers but also, in most states, by law. Although federal legislation governing the use of patient information currently does not exist, the public has recognized the need for federal protection, as health information is increasingly shared across traditional institutional and geographic boundaries. A 1997 report of the National Research Council (1997) reviewed current security practices in health-care institutions and recommended 15 measures for such institutions to adopt immediately and five measures to work toward adopting (Table 10.2). Furthermore, in accordance with the Health Insurance Portability and Accountability Act (HIPAA) of 1996, the Secretary of Health and Human Services recommended that "Congress enact national standards that provide fundamental privacy rights for patients and define responsibilities for those who serve them." Such a law would prohibit disclosure of patient-identifiable information except as authorized by the patient or explicitly permitted by legislation. It would provide consumers with significant new rights to be informed about how and by whom their health information has and will be used and would allow for punishment for people who misuse personal health information and redress for people who are harmed by such misuse. The IDN, being a consolidation of many health institutions, will

TABLE 10.2. Fifteen short-term and five longer term security-practice recommendations of the National Research Council.

	Recommended security practices	
	Technical practices and procedures	Organizational practices
Recommended for immediate implementation	• Individual authentication of users • Access controls • Audit trails • Physical security and disaster recovery • Protection of remote access points • Protection of external electronic communications • Software discipline • System assessment	• Security and confidentiality policies • Security and confidentiality committees • Information security officers • Education and training programs • Sanctions • Improved authorization forms • Patient access to audit logs
Recommended for future implementation	• Strong authentication • Enterprise-wide authentication • Access validation • Expanded audit trails • Electronic authentication of records	

Source: National Research Council, 1997.

face numerous challenges in modifying its systems to implement the HIPAA measures, once defined.

Computer systems can be designed to provide security, but only people can promote the trust necessary to protect the confidentiality of patients' clinical information. To achieve the goal of delivering coordinated and cost-effective care, clinicians need access to information on specific patients in many different locations. Unfortunately, it is difficult to predict in advance which clinicians will need access to which patient data. Therefore, an IDN must strike a balance between restricting information access and ensuring the accountability of the users of patient information. To build trust with its patients, an IDN should adopt a three-pronged approach to securing information. First, the IDN needs to develop a uniform security and confidentiality policy, including specification of sanctions, and to enforce this policy rigorously. Second, the IDN needs to adopt a strategy for access control that is consistent and coordinated across operating units. Third, the IDN must use electronic tools such as information audit trails to teach employees and patients that people who access confidential information can be tracked and held accountable.

10.1.5 The Benefits of Healthcare Information Systems

In a 1966 study of three New York hospitals, researchers found that information handling to satisfy requirements such as those discussed in Section 10.1.2 accounted for approximately 25 percent of the hospital's total operating costs (Jydstrup & Gross, 1966). On average, workers in administrative departments spent about three-fourths of their time handling information; workers in nursing units spent about one-fourth of their time on these tasks. Over 30 years later, the basic conclusions of the study still hold true: information management in healthcare organizations is a costly activity. The collection, storage, retrieval, analysis, and dissemination of the clinical and administrative information necessary to support the organization's daily operations, to meet external and internal requirements for documentation, and to support short-term and strategic planning are important and time-consuming aspects of the jobs of healthcare workers.

Today, the justifications for implementing HCISs include cost reduction and quality and service improvement, as well as strategic considerations related to competitive advantage:

- *Cost reduction.* Much of the initial impetus for implementing HCISs was their potential to reduce the costs of information management in hospitals and other facilities. Healthcare organizations continue to make tactical investments in information systems to streamline administrative processes and departmental workflow. Primary benefits that may offset some information-systems costs include reductions in labor requirements, improved productivity of clinicians and other staff, reduced waste (e.g., dated surgical supplies that are ordered but unused or food trays that are delivered to the wrong destination and therefore are wasted), and more efficient management of supplies and other inventories.

Large savings can be gained through efficient scheduling of expensive resources such as operating suites and imaging equipment. In addition, HCISs can help to eliminate inadvertent ordering of duplicate tests and procedures. Once significant patient data are available online, information systems can reduce the costs of storing, retrieving, and transporting charts in the medical-records department.

- *Quality and service improvement.* As HCISs broadened in scope to encompass support for clinical processes, the ability to improve the quality of care became an additional benefit of HCISs. Qualitative benefits of HCISs include improved accuracy and completeness of documentation, reductions in the time clinicians spend documenting (and associated increases in time spent with patients), fewer drug errors, and improved provider-to-provider communication. As described in Chapter 9, the use of clinical decision-support systems in conjunction with an HCIS or CPR can produce impressive benefits, improving the quality of care while reducing costs. (Bates et al., 1997; Classen et al., 1997; Teich et al., 1996; Tierney et al., 1993).
- *Competitive advantage.* Although some organizations still attempt to cost justify all information-systems investments, many IDNs have recognized information technology as a strategic investment that is necessary for survival: Without an enabling technology infrastructure, an IDN cannot meet its needs for integrated operations and coordinated patient care. Information technologies must be deployed appropriately and effectively, but with respect to HCISs, the question is no longer whether to invest, but rather how much and where to invest. As IDNs build their networks of primary-care physician networks and link up with community hospitals, access to clinical information is necessary not only to carry out patient management, but also to attract and retain the loyalty of physicians who care for (and thus control the IDN's access to) the patients. The long-term benefits of clinical systems are the abilities to influence clinical practices by reducing large unnecessary variations in medical practices, to improve patient outcomes, and to reduce costs. Physicians ultimately control the great majority of the resource-utilization decisions in health care through their choices in prescribing drugs, ordering diagnostic tests, and referring patients for specialty care. Thus, providing physicians with access to information on "best practices" based on the latest available clinical evidence, as well as giving them other clinical and financial data to make appropriate decisions, is essential to the success of an IDN.

10.1.6 Managing Information Systems in a Changing Healthcare Environment

Despite the strategic importance of integrated information systems, implementation of HCISs has proved to be a daunting task, requiring a multiyear capital investment of tens to hundreds of millions of dollars and forcing fundamental changes in the types and ways that health professionals perform their jobs. To achieve the potential benefits, health organizations must plan carefully and invest wisely. The grand challenge for an IDN is to design and implement an HCIS that is sufficiently flexible and adaptable to meet the changing needs of the organization. Given the rapidly changing environment and the multiyear effort involved, people must be careful to avoid implementing a system that is obsolete before it becomes operational. Success in implementing an HCIS entails consistent and courageous handling of numerous technical, organizational, and political challenges.

Changing Technologies

As we discussed in Chapter 4, the past decades have seen dramatic changes in computing and networking technologies. These advances are important in that they allow quicker and easier information access, less expensive computational power, greater flexibility, and other performance advantages. A major challenge for IDNs is migration from their patchwork of legacy systems to new integrated systems. Such migration requires integration and selective replacement of diverse systems that are often implemented with closed or nonstandard technologies and medical vocabularies. Furthermore, the end point is not fixed—IDNs must move aggressively to implement new systems, while progress continues in development of standards (see Chapter 6), distributed database architecture, and Internet/Intranet infrastructure. In a sense, it is the information content of the systems that is much more important than the underlying technology—as long as the data are accessible for conversion, the choice of specific technology is less critical. Nonetheless, an understanding of current and emerging technologies enables system developers to avoid choosing closed-ended approaches.

Changing Culture

In the new healthcare environment, physicians are confronted with significant obstacles to the traditional practice of medicine. They face pressure to practice in accordance with institutional standards of care aimed at reducing variation in care, and particularly to avoid use of health resources that do not result in improved outcomes. They are expected to assume responsibility for member wellness, and they often work as members of collaborative patient-care teams. The average patient length of stay in a hospital is decreasing; concomitantly, the complexity of the care provided after discharge is increasing. The time allotted for an individual patient visit in the ambulatory setting has decreased as well, as individual clinicians face economic incentives to increase the number of patients for whom they care per day. To cope with the increasing workload, greater complexity of care, and new skills requirements, both clinicians and health executives must become effective information managers, and the supporting information systems must meet their workflow and information requirements. As the healthcare culture and the roles of clinicians and health executives continue to change, IDNs must constantly reevaluate the role of information technology to ensure that the implemented systems continue to match user requirements.

Changing Process

Developing a new vision of how health care will be delivered and managed, designing processes, and implementing supporting information systems are all critical to the success of the emerging IDN. Changes in process affect the jobs that people do, the skills that people require, and the fundamental ways in which they relate to one another. For example, the new models of cross-continuum care management encourage interdisciplinary care teams that work in symphony to promote health as well as treat illness. Although information systems are not the foremost consideration for people who are redesigning process, a poor information-systems implementation can institutionalize bad processes.

Organizations must and will undertake various process redesign initiatives—and these initiatives can lead to fundamental transformations of the enterprise. Too often, however, the lack of a clear understanding of existing organizational dynamics leads to misalignment of incentives, which is a significant barrier to change. Moreover, organizations, as collections of individuals, have natural fears about and reluctance to change. Even under the best circumstances, there are limits to the amount of change that any organization can absorb. The magnitude of work required to plan and manage organizational change is often underestimated or ignored: It is the handling of people and process issues that has emerged as the most critical success factor for IDNs as they implement new enterprise-wide processes and information systems.

Management and Governance

Figure 10.3 illustrates the information-technology environment of a small IDN composed of two hospitals, an IDN-owned physician practice, affiliated nursing homes and hospice, and several for-profit service organizations. Even this relatively simple environment presents significant challenges for the management and governance of information systems. For example, to what extent will the information management function be controlled centrally versus decentralized to the individual operating units and departments? How should limited resources be allocated between new investment in strategic projects (such as support for regional expansion) and the often critical operational needs of individual entities (e.g., replacement of an obsolete laboratory information system)? Academic medical centers with distinct research and educational needs raise additional issues for managing information across operationally independent and politically powerful constituencies.

Trade-offs between functional and integration requirements, and associated contention between users and information-systems departments, will tend to diminish over time with the development and widespread adoption of technology standards and common clinical-data models and vocabulary. On the other hand, an organization's information-systems "wants" and "needs" will always outstrip its ability to deliver these services. Political battles will persist, as IDNs and their component entities wrestle with the age-old issues of how to distribute scarce resources among competing, similarly worthy projects.

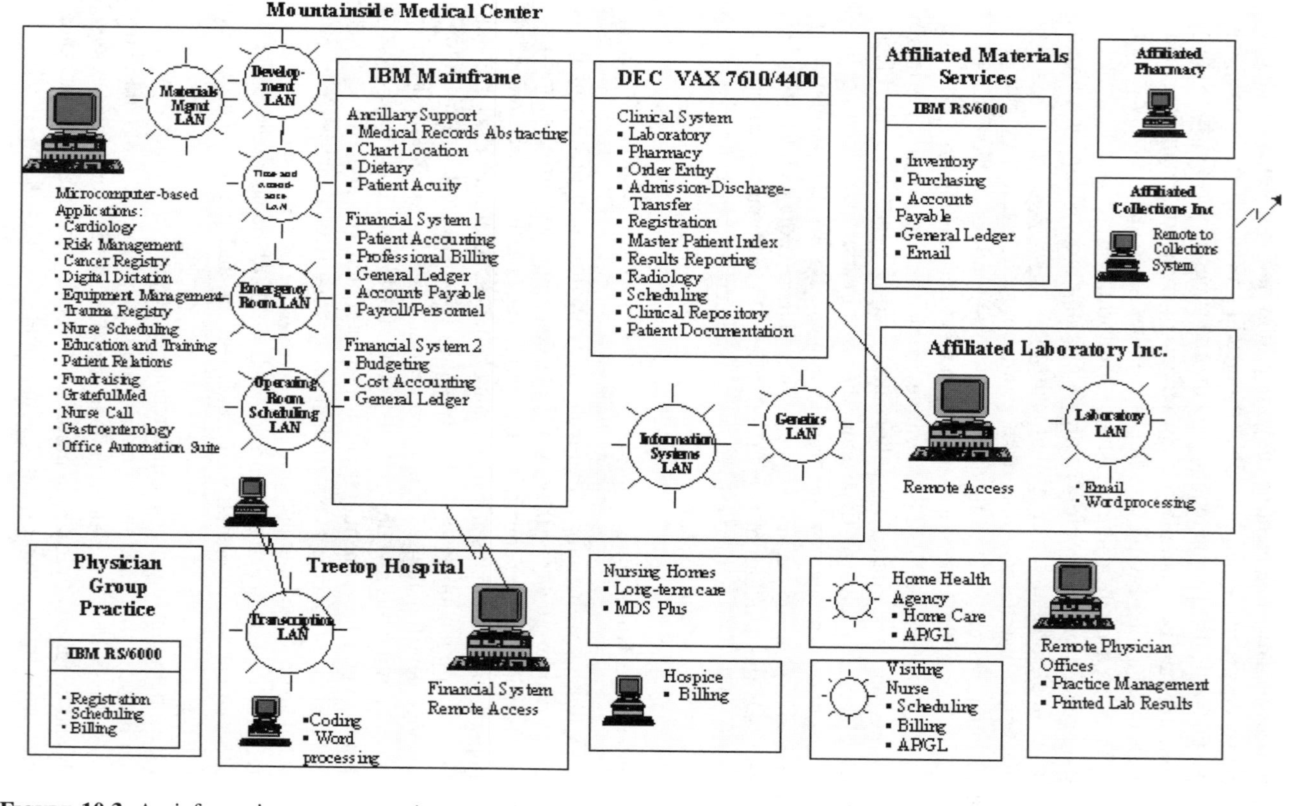

FIGURE 10.3. An information-systems environment for a small IDN. Even this relatively simple IDN has a complex mix of information systems that poses integration and information-management challenges for the organization. MDS = minimum data set; LAN = local area network; AP = accounts payable; GL = general ledger.

A formal governance structure with representation from all major constituents provides a critical forum for direction setting, prioritization, and resource allocation across the IDN (Fig. 10.4). In addition, development of a strategic information-management plan can be a valuable exercise if the process engages the organization's clinical, financial, and administrative leadership and results in their gaining a clear understanding of the highest-priority information technology investments to support the IDN's business priorities. Because of the dynamic nature of both healthcare business strategies and the supporting technologies, a strategic information-management plan should be updated at regular intervals.

10.2 Functions and Components of a Healthcare Information System

A carefully designed computer-based system can increase the effectiveness and productivity of health professionals, improve the quality and reduce the costs of health services, and improve levels of service and of patient satisfaction. As described in Section 10.1, the HCIS supports a variety of functions, including the delivery and management of patient care and the administration of the health organization. From a functional perspective, an HCIS consists of components that support six distinct purposes: (1) patient management, (2) departmental management, (3) care delivery and clinical documentation, (4) clinical decision support, (5) financial and resource management, and (6) managed-care support.

10.2.1 Patient Management

Systems that support patient management perform the basic centralized functions of IDN operations related to patient movement, such as enrollment of new members, identification, registration, scheduling, admission, and discharge. Within hospitals, maintenance of the hospital census was one of the first tasks to be automated. Today, virtually all hospitals and ambulatory centers and many physician offices use a computer-based **master patient index** (MPI) to store patient-identification information; basic demographic data that are acquired during the patient-registration process; and simple encounter-level information such as dates on which and locations where services were provided. The MPI is integrated within the *registration* module of an ambulatory care or physician-practice system. Within the hospital setting, the census is maintained by the **admission–discharge–transfer** (ADT) module, which updates the census whenever a patient is admitted to the hospital, discharged from the hospital, or transferred to a new bed.

Registration and census data serve as a reference base for the financial programs that perform billing functions. When an HCIS is extended to patient-care settings—or to the laboratory, pharmacy, and other ancillary departments—patient-management systems provide a common reference base for use by these systems as well. Without access to the centralized database, these subsystems

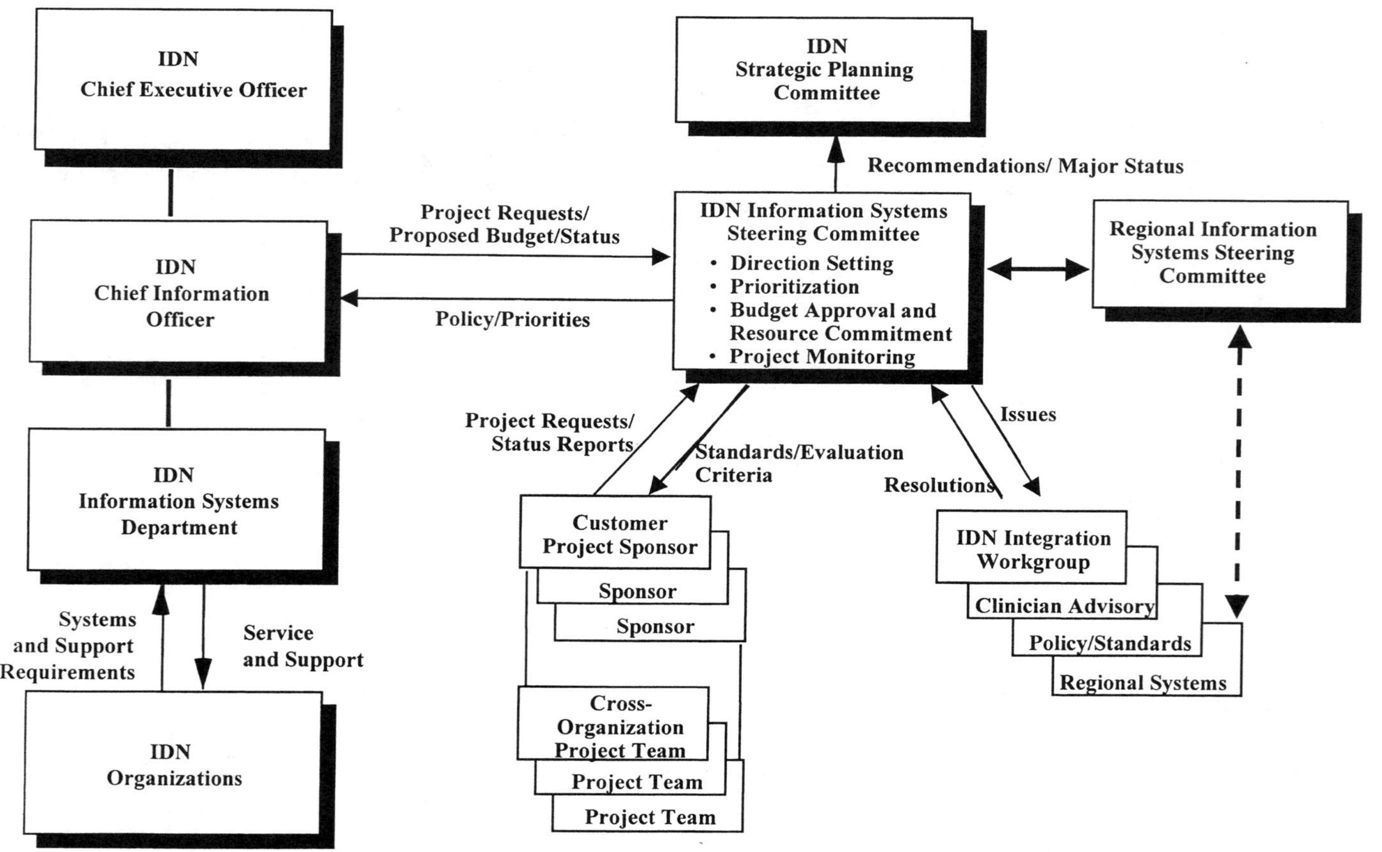

IDN
Chief Executive Officer
IDN
Chief Information
Officer
IDN
Information Systems
Department
IDN
Organizations
Systems
and Support
Requirements
Service
and Support
Project Requests/
Proposed Budget/Status
Policy/Priorities
IDN
Strategic Planning
Committee
Recommendations/ Major Status
IDN Information Systems
Steering Committee
• Direction Setting
• Prioritization
• Budget Approval and
Resource Commitment
• Project Monitoring
Regional Information
Systems Steering
Committee
Project Requests/
Status Reports
Standards/Evaluation
Criteria
Issues
Resolutions
Customer
Project Sponsor
Sponsor
Sponsor
Cross-
Organization
Project Team
Project Team
Project Team
IDN Integration
Workgroup
Clinician Advisory
Policy/Standards
Regional Systems

would have to maintain duplicate patient records. In addition, the transmission of registration data can trigger other activities, such as automatic retrieval of medical records from archival storage for patients scheduled to be seen in the clinic or notification of hospital housekeeping when a bed becomes free.

Scheduling in a healthcare organization is complicated because patient load and resource utilization can vary by season or even through the course of a day simply due to chance. Effective resource management requires that the appropriate resources be on hand to meet ordinary fluctuations in demand. At the same time, resources must not remain unnecessarily idle. The most sophisticated *scheduling* systems have been developed for the operating rooms and radiology departments, where scheduling constraints include matching up the patient not only with the providers but also with special equipment, support staff, and technicians. **Patient-tracking** applications monitor patient movement in multistep processes; for example, they monitor and manage patient wait times in the emergency department.

Within an IDN, the basic tasks of patient management are compounded by the need to manage patient care across multiple settings, many of which are supported by independent information systems. Integrated delivery networks must uniquely identify patients across multiple settings and systems: Is the Patricia C. Brown who was admitted last month to Mountainside Hospital the same Patsy Brown who is registering for her appointment at the Seaview Clinic? Integrated delivery networks ensure unique patient identification either through conversion to common registration systems or, more frequently, through implementation of an enterprise MPI (see Section 10.4) that links patient identifiers and data from multiple registration systems. Similarly, enterprise-wide scheduling systems that manage patient appointments across a network of physician offices and satellite clinics represent a strategic application for most IDNs.

10.2.2 Departmental Management

Ancillary departmental systems support the information needs of individual clinical departments within the IDN. From a systems perspective, those areas most commonly automated are the laboratory, pharmacy, radiology, blood-bank, and medical-records departments. Such systems serve a dual purpose within an IDN. First, ancillary systems perform many circumscribed tasks required for departmental operations. Such tasks include generating specimen-collection lists and capturing results from automated laboratory instruments in the clinical labora-

---

FIGURE 10.4. A simple management and governance structure for a regionally based IDN. The Steering Committee directs information-systems activities for the organization by setting direction, establishing priorities, linking the technology plan to the strategic business plan, and approving budget requests. The information systems department is responsible for implementing and maintaining the IDN's technology and applications environment. IDN = integrated delivery network.

tory, printing medication labels and managing inventory in the pharmacy, and scheduling examinations and transcribing image interpretations in the radiology department. Second, the ancillary systems contribute major data components to on-line patient records, including laboratory-test results and pathology reports, medication profiles, digital images (see Chapter 14), records of blood orders and usage, and various transcribed reports including history and physical examination, operative, and radiology reports. As IDNs consolidate ancillary functions outside hospitals to gain economies of scale—for example, creating outpatient pharmacy centers and regional outreach and reference laboratories—they add complexity to integrated patient management, financial, and billing processes.

10.2.3 Care Delivery and Clinical Documentation

Computer-based patient record systems that support care delivery and clinical documentation are discussed at length in Chapter 9. Although comprehensive CPRs are the ultimate goal of some IDNs, most organizations today are still building more basic clinical-management capabilities. Automated **order entry** and **results reporting** are two important functions provided by the clinical components of an HCIS. Health professionals can use the HCIS to communicate with ancillary departments electronically, eliminating the easily misplaced paper slips and thus minimizing delays in conveying orders. The information then is available on-line, where it is accessible to health professionals who wish to review a patient's medication profile or previous laboratory-test results. Ancillary departmental data represent an important subset of a patient's clinical record. A comprehensive clinical record, however, also includes various data that clinicians have collected by questioning and observing the patient. In the hospital, an HCIS can help health personnel to perform an initial assessment when a patient is admitted to a unit, to maintain patient-specific care plans, to chart vital signs, to maintain medication-administration records, to record diagnostic and therapeutic information, to document patient and family teaching, and to plan for discharge (also see Chapter 12). Many organizations have developed diagnosis-specific **clinical pathways** that identify clinical goals, interventions, and expected outcomes by time period; using the clinical pathway, case managers or care providers can document actual versus expected outcomes and are alerted to intervene when a significant unexpected event occurs.

With the shift toward delivering more care in outpatient settings, clinical systems are becoming more common in ambulatory clinics and physician practices. Such systems allow clinicians to record problems and diagnoses, symptoms and physical examinations, medical and social history, review of systems, functional status, and active and past prescriptions. The most successful of such systems provide additional support for physician workflow and typical clinic functions, such as by documenting telephone follow-up calls or printing prescriptions. Similarly, specialized systems have been developed to meet the specific requirements of intensive-care units (see Chapter 13), long-term care facilities, home-health organizations, and specialized departments such as cardiology and oncology.

10.2.4 Clinical Decision Support

Clinical decision-support systems directly assist clinical personnel in data interpretation and decision-making. Once the basic clinical components of an HCIS are well developed, clinical decision-support systems can use the information stored there to monitor patients and issue alerts, to make diagnostic suggestions, and to provide limited therapy advice. These capabilities are particularly useful when they are integrated with other information-management functions. For example, a useful adjunct to an order-entry system is a decision-support program that alerts physicians to patient drug allergies; helps physicians to calculate patient-specific drug-dosing regimens; performs advanced order logic, such as recommending an order for prophylactic antibiotics before certain surgical procedures; automatically discontinues drugs when appropriate or prompts the physician to reorder them; suggests more cost-effective drugs with the same therapeutic effect; or activates and displays applicable clinical-practice guidelines (see Chapter 9). Clinical-event monitors integrated with results-reporting applications can alert clinicians to abnormal results and drug interactions by electronic mail or page. In the outpatient setting, these event monitors may produce reminders to provide preventive services such as screening mammograms and routine immunizations. The same event monitors might trigger access to the IDN's approved formulary, displaying information that includes costs, indications, contraindications, approved clinical guidelines, and relevant on-line medical literature (Perreault & Metzger, 1999; Teich et al., 1997).

The wish to provide decision support was a major motivation for the developers of the HELP system (see Section 10.5.1). The direct assistance that this system provides in monitoring and interpreting patient information encourages complete and timely recording of the data. We describe other decision-support systems in Chapter 16. Although such capabilities are still at the leading edge of HCIS features, they are developing rapidly.

10.2.5 Financial and Resource Management

Financial and administrative systems are typically among the first functions to be centralized in an IDN. These systems assist with the traditional business functions of the organization and are consolidated across all the integrating entities. Such functions include financial requirements such as managing the payroll, human resources, general ledger, accounts payable, and materials purchasing and inventory. Most of these data-processing tasks are well structured, labor intensive, and repetitious—ideal applications for computers. Furthermore, with the exception of patient-billing functions, the basic financial tasks of an IDN do not differ substantially from those of organizations in other industries.

Conceptually, the tasks of creating a patient bill and tracking payments are straightforward, and financial transactions such as claims submission and electronic funds transfer have been standardized to allow **electronic data interchange** (EDI) among providers and payers. In operation, however, patient accounting requirements are complicated by myriad reimbursement requirements of government and third-party payers. Billing and reimbursement requirements vary substantially by payer, by insurance plan, and by type of facility where service was provided. With the growth of managed care (see Chapter 19), these requirements have become more complex, necessitating processes and information systems to check a patient's health-plan enrollment and eligibility for services, to manage referrals and preauthorization for care, to price claims based on negotiated contracts, and to create documentation required to substantiate the services provided.

10.2.6 Managed Care Support

As IDNs go "at risk" for delivery of health services by negotiating capitated payments (see Chapter 19) to provide comprehensive care for a specified patient population at a preset cost, their incentives shift from reducing the cost per unit service to maintaining the health of members while using health resources effectively and efficiently. Similarly, the IDN's scope of concern shifts from the small population of sick patients to a much larger population of members, most of whom are still well.

Provider-profiling systems support utilization management by tracking each provider's resource utilization (costs of drugs prescribed, diagnostic tests and procedures ordered, and so on) compared with severity-adjusted outcomes of that provider's patients such as their rate of hospital readmission and mortality by diagnosis. **Contract-management systems** have capabilities for estimating the costs and payments associated with potential managed care contracts and comparing actual with expected payments based on the contracts' terms. More advanced managed-care information systems handle **patient triage** and **medical management** functions, helping the IDNs to direct patients to appropriate health services and to proactively manage the care of chronically ill and high-risk patients. Integrated delivery networks that incorporate a health plan also must support payer and insurance functions such as claims administration, premium billing, marketing, and member services.

10.3 Alternative Architectures for Healthcare Information Systems

In this section, we describe three alternative models for an integrated HCIS: the central, modular, and distributed models. In theory, each of these architectures provides the same range of functions; from a user's point of view, the differences among the systems may not be obvious. From the perspective of the computing personnel who design, develop, and maintain the systems, however, the differences are striking. The choice of architecture affects the choice of hardware and the design of software for storing, accessing, and transmitting data. Each architecture has advantages and disadvantages. During the 1960s and 1970s, the relative merits of the central and modular approaches were the subject of much controversy. To a large extent, this debate predated the availability of powerful microcomputers and the development of network technologies. In general, we have seen an evolutionary trend in the development of HCISs from central, to modular, to distributed systems.

10.3.1 Central Systems

The earliest HCISs (typically hospital systems) were designed according to the philosophy that a single comprehensive or **central system** could best meet a healthcare organization's information needs. Advocates of the centralized approach emphasized the importance of first identifying all the hospital's information needs and then designing a single, unified framework to meet these needs. As we discussed in Chapter 5, an information system ideally should be designed to meet a specified set of requirements rather than evolve through a patchwork of solutions to problems in individual application areas. One natural product of this design goal is the development of a system in which a single, large computer performs all information processing and manages all the data files using application-independent file-management programs (Fig. 10.5). Users obtain information via general-purpose video-display terminals (VDTs).

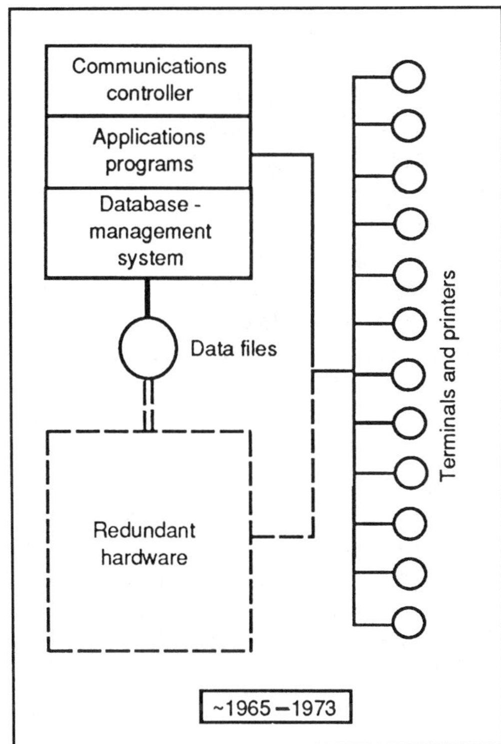

FIGURE 10.5. The earliest HCISs were central systems. In this model a large, central computer serves the information needs of the entire hospital. Users access the computer from video-display terminals via general interface programs.

Central systems integrate and communicate information well because they provide users with a single data store and a general method to access information simply and rapidly. On the other hand, large systems are expensive to implement and operate. Large initial investments are necessary, first by the vendor to develop and test a sufficiently complete product and then by the healthcare organization to bring the entire system into operation. Central systems are difficult to install because many areas of an organization are affected simultaneously, and backup is particularly costly because of the expense of purchasing redundant hardware to be used when the primary computer is unavailable. An insidious problem is that, by the time a vendor has developed a comprehensive system that supports all the functions a healthcare organization might want, technological obsolescence will have crept in. It is not easy to modify a central system to accommodate previously unrecognized or changing needs. Furthermore, central systems often serve poorly those individual users who compete with all other users for the computer's resources.

The biggest limitation of central systems is their inability to accommodate the diverse needs of individual application areas. There is a tradeoff between the uniformity (and relative simplicity) of a general system and the nonuniformity and greater power of custom-designed systems that solve specific problems. Generality—a characteristic that enhances communication and data integration in a homogeneous environment—can be a drawback in an enterprise-wide system because of the complexity and heterogeneity of the information-management tasks.

Of the early medically oriented HCISs, the Technicon Medical Information System (TMIS; the precursor of Eclipsys Corporation's TDS 7000) was the most successful and the most widely distributed. System development began in 1965 as a collaborative project between Lockheed and El Camino Hospital, a community hospital in Mountain View, California. By 1987, TMIS had been installed in more than 85 institutions by TDS Healthcare Systems Corporation, which purchased the system from Lockheed in 1971.

The Technicon Medical Information System was one of the strongest examples of what we should expect from a large, centrally operated HCIS. It ran on a duplex installation of IBM-compatible mainframes. One computer was used for tasks that involved direct interaction with users; the other was used for batch-oriented tasks, such as billing and report generation. The system could also provide backup when the primary computer required maintenance or failed unexpectedly. Depending on the size of the central machine, the TMIS center could support from several to a few thousand hospital beds. Because of this high capacity, one computer installation could serve multiple hospitals in an area. The hospitals were connected via high-speed dedicated telephone lines to the central computer. Within a hospital, a switching station connected the telephone lines to an onsite network that led to stations on all the patient-care units. Each unit had at least one VDT and one printer with which users could access and display information.

10.3.2 Modular Systems

By the 1970s, modular HCISs began to emerge. Decreases in the price of powerful hardware and improvements in software made it feasible for individual departments within a hospital to own and operate their own computers. In a **modular system,** one or a few machines are dedicated to processing within the organization. Distinct software application modules carry out specific tasks (Fig. 10.6), and a common framework, which is specified initially, defines the interfaces that will allow data to be shared among the modules. Major tasks may be performed by free-standing systems. Thus, a healthcare organization can tailor the HCIS to meet its information needs and financial constraints by "plugging in" appropriate modules as desired.

The modular approach solves many of the problems of central systems. Although individual modules are constrained to function with predefined interfaces, they do not have to conform to the general standards of the overall system, so

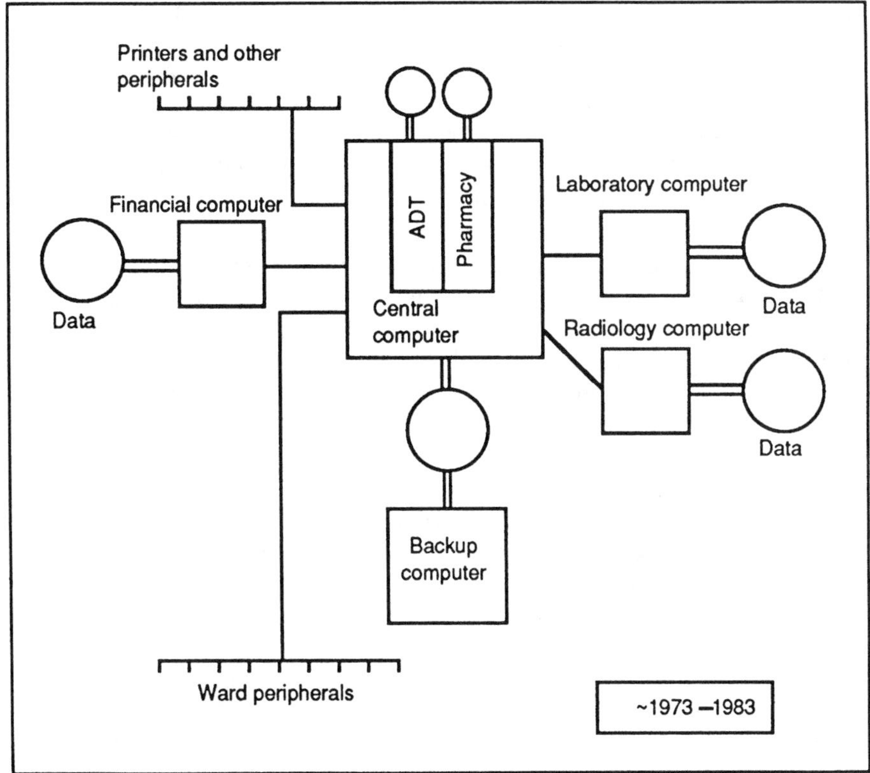

FIGURE 10.6. In modular systems, much information processing is performed locally on dedicated machines that communicate with a central machine via direct interfaces. ADT = admission–discharge–transfer.

they can be designed to accommodate the special needs of specific areas. For example, the processing capabilities and file structures suitable for managing the data acquired from a patient-monitoring system in the intensive-care unit (analog and digital signals acquired in real time) differ from the features that are appropriate for a system that reports radiology results (text storage and text processing). Furthermore, modification of modules, although laborious with any approach, is simpler because of the smaller scope of the system. As long as the interfaces are undisturbed, subsystems can be modified or replaced without the remainder of the HCIS being disrupted.

Modular systems also are more responsive to local users because much processing can be performed locally on the departmental machines. The central machine with shared data files can be smaller, because it does not handle all processing. The price for this greater flexibility is increased difficulty in integrating data and allowing communication among modules. In reality, installing a subsystem never is as easy as simply plugging in the connections.

The most ambitious project based on the modular approach was the Distributed Hospital Computer Program (DHCP) for the Veterans Administration (VA) hospitals. The system had a common database and a database system (Fileman), which was written to be both hardware- and operating-system-independent. A small number of support centers in the VA developed the software modules in cooperation with user groups. The CORE—the first set of applications to be developed and installed—consisted of modules for patient registration, ADT, outpatient scheduling, laboratory, outpatient pharmacy, and inpatient pharmacy. Modules to support other clinical departments (such as radiology, dietetics, surgery, nursing, and mental health) and administrative functions (such as financial and procurement applications) were developed subsequently. By 1985, the VA had installed DHCP in more than one-half of its approximately 300 hospitals and clinics. The software is in the public domain and is also used in private hospitals and other government facilities (Munnecke & Kuhn, 1989).

10.3.3 Distributed Systems

By the 1980s, HCISs based on the new network-communications technology were being developed. As a **distributed system,** an HCIS consists of a federation of independent computers that have been tailored for specific application areas. The computers operate autonomously and share data (and sometimes programs and other resources, such as printers) by exchanging information over a local area network (LAN; see Chapter 4) using a standard protocol for communication (Fig. 10.7).

The advantage of a distributed system is that individual departments have a great deal of flexibility in choosing hardware and software that optimally suits their needs. Smaller ancillary departments that previously could not justify a major computer acquisition because of insufficient workload now can purchase microcomputers and participate in the computer-based information system. Healthcare providers in nursing units (or even at the bedside), physicians in their offices,

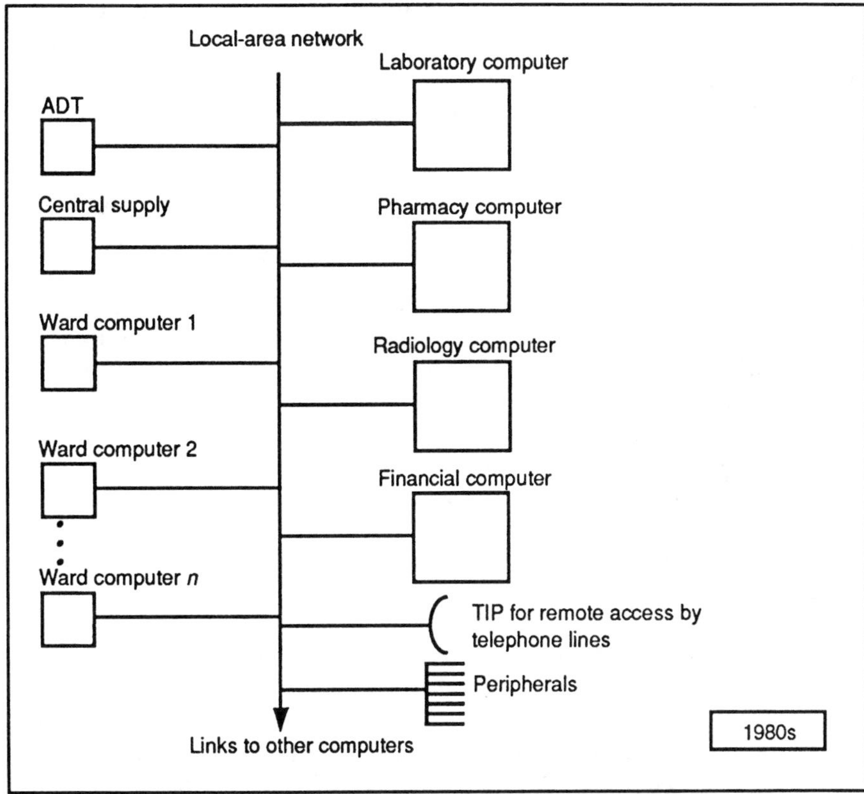

FIGURE 10.7. Network technology that enables users to perform all information processing locally. Independent machines share data over the network by passing messages according to a communication protocol. A terminal-interface processor (TIP) is a utility communications computer that is used to attach video-display terminals and other communications devices to the local-area network. ADT = admission–discharge–transfer.

and managers in the administrative offices can access and analyze data locally using microcomputers. Some computers may handle resources that are shared by all users—for example, the ADT information, the active medical records, the index to archived medical records, and the mail exchanged electronically between individual users. Several LANs can be linked together by gateway computers (see Chapter 4). Thus, networks can provide for communication throughout an IDN—for example, by linking one hospital's systems with the information systems serving affiliated outpatient facilities, nursing homes, and outside laboratories.

The distribution of information processing and the responsibility for data among diverse systems makes the tasks of data integration and communication difficult. The development of industry-wide standard network protocols has eased the technical problems of electronic communication. Still, there are many problems to overcome in managing and controlling access to a patient database that is fragmented over multiple computers, each with its own file structure and method of file management. Furthermore, when no global structure is imposed on an HCIS, individual departments and entities may encode data values in ways that are incompatible with the definitions chosen by other areas of the organization. The promise of sharing among independent departments, entities, and even independent institutions increases the importance of defining clinical data standards (see Chapter 6).

In the early 1980s, researchers at the University of California, San Francisco (UCSF) Hospital successfully implemented one of the first LANs to support communication among several of the hospital's standalone systems. Using technology developed at the Johns Hopkins University, they connected minicomputers serving patient registration, medical records, radiology, the clinical laboratory, and the outpatient pharmacy. In the historical sense, each of the four computers was incompatible with the other three: The computers were made by different manufacturers and ran different operating systems (McDonald et al., 1984a).

The University of Michigan Hospital in Ann Arbor later adopted a hybrid strategy to meet its information needs. The hospital emphasized the central model of architecture and operated a mainframe computer to perform core HCIS functions. In 1986, however, it installed a LAN to allow communication among all its internal clinical laboratories and to allow physicians to obtain laboratory-test results directly from the laboratory information system. At the time of installation, more than 95 percent of all the peripheral devices in the laboratories were connected to the network rather than hardwired to the laboratory computer. One month later, a second clinical host computer, which supported the radiology information system, was added to the LAN, allowing physicians to access radiology reports directly. Although the mainframe HCIS initially was not connected to the LAN, the hospital later adopted the strategy of installing **universal workstations** that could access both the mainframe computer and the clinical hosts via the LAN (Friedman & Dieterle, 1987).

Today, the distributed architecture for information systems is the norm, and all viable commercial systems support a distributed model. Universal workstations are widespread; however, separate access to independent ancillary systems has been largely eliminated by interfaces that join such systems to a core clinical system. For example, whereas staff working in the laboratory would access the laboratory system directly, clinicians would view consolidated clinical results (laboratory, radiology, and so on) stored in the HCIS database by accessing the HCIS clinical applications.

10.4 Architecture for a Changing Environment

The IDN presents new challenges to information systems planners. As we described in Section 10.1, most IDNs have developed through the merger or acquisition of independent organizations. Thus, the information systems environment of a new or evolving IDN usually is a jumble of disparate **legacy systems,** technologies, and architectures. How, in such an environment, can an IDN's information systems planners design systems and processes to support new business strategies (such as a diabetes management program or a central call center) and provide integrated information access throughout the IDN, while maintaining uninterrupted operational support for the IDN's existing business units?

Sometimes, an IDN will selectively replace specific systems to fit its new organizational structure and strategies (e.g., consolidation of the finance and human resources departments and migration to common corporate general ledger, accounts payable, payroll, and human resources systems for all business entities). As always, resources (both money and staff) are limited; and it is simply not feasible for an IDN to replace all legacy systems with new common systems. Therefore, more creativity is required to develop an architecture that can support the emerging IDN and flexibly grow with it as business conditions (and associated information requirements) change.

An IDN's particular legacy systems environment and business strategy present unique information requirements; therefore a single architecture is unlikely to suffice for all. Nonetheless, a few lessons can be learned from past implementations. First, an IDN must develop a strategy for data preservation by providing open access to data and implementing an approach for standardizing the meaning of those data. Second, to the extent possible, an IDN should separate three conceptual layers—data management, applications and business logic, and user interface—to allow greater flexibility (Fig. 10.8).

The first layer of architecture is the **data layer.** Data—the facts of process that are collected as part of the health enterprise—are of central strategic importance. One fundamental mistake that a healthcare organization can make is to fail to provide open access to its data. Organizations that choose information systems based on the functionality available to meet short-term needs may find that these needs are no longer as strategically important when the IDN starts to evolve. For this reason, each organization needs a long-term data strategy that is a separate component of its information-management plan. This plan must include open access to data for applications and a method to ensure that demographic, clinical, and financial data collected across business units are consistent and comparable. Security and confidentiality safeguards (see Section 10.1.4) should also be part of the data strategy.

With respect to clinical data, healthcare organizations need data for both real-time operations and retrospective data analysis. These needs generate different requirements for data management. In the first case, detailed data need to be stored and optimized for retrieval for the individual patient. In the second case, the data need to be optimized for aggregation across a population of patients. Although the terms are sometimes used interchangeably, the distinction should be made between a **clinical data repository** (CDR), which serves the needs of patient care and day-to-day operations, and a **data warehouse,** which serves longer term business and clinical needs such as contract management and outcomes evaluation. Both the CDR and data warehouse should be purchased or developed for

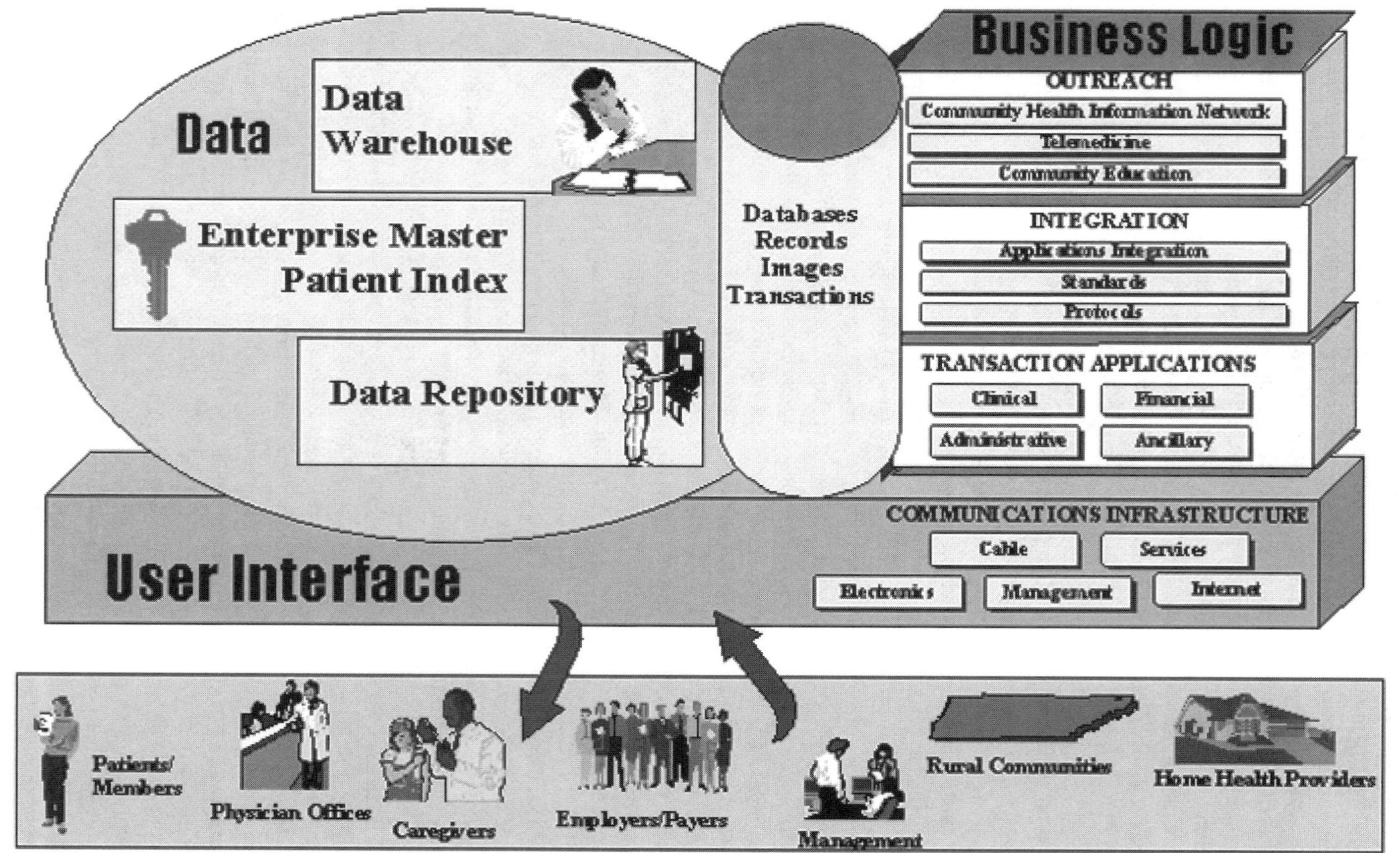

FIGURE 10.8. Three conceptual layers of an IDN's architectural model. Separation of data, business logic, and user interface allows system developers to modify applications and interfaces over time to meet changing needs while preserving the IDN's long-term data asset.

their ability to model, store, and retrieve efficiently the organization's data. Quite often, vendors of a CDR or warehouse also include programs to view and manipulate these data. Conceptually, this packaging makes sense. Why would anyone put data in a repository for which she did not have a browser to view them? A tight interdependency between data, user interface, and business logic layers, however, restricts an IDN's ability to preserve its data independent of the applications that use it.

The second component of a clinical data strategy is an ability to keep patient information comparable. At the simplest level one needs to identify the patient. When a health organization consisted of only one hospital and one major information system, the authority over patient identification was relatively simple and usually resided in the HCIS's admitting or registration module (see Section 10.2.1). As the IDN evolves, there is no one authority that can identify the patient or resolve a conflicting identification. Thus, a new architectural component, the **enterprise master patient index** (EMPI), has arisen as the **name authority.** In its simplest form, the EMPI is an index of patient names and identification numbers used by all information systems in the IDN that store a patient registry. Using this type of EMPI requires considerable manual intervention to ensure data synchrony, but it does enable an IDN to uniquely identify its patients and link their data. Alternatively, an EMPI can be configured as the name authority for all systems that hold the key patient information. Then all systems must interact with the EMPI in order to get a patient-identification number assigned. This type of EMPI requires that all other systems disable their ability to assign identification numbers and use the external—and unique—EMPI-generated identification numbers.

Uniquely identifying patients within the IDN is just a necessary first step in ensuring data comparability and consistency. Healthcare providers also may want to know which of their patients are allergic to penicillin, which patients should be targeted for new cardiac-disease prevention services, or which patients are likely to need home services when they are discharged from the hospital or emergency room. To store and evaluate the data that could be used to make such determinations, an IDN must develop a consistent approach for naming data elements and defining their values. Some institutions, such as Columbia Presbyterian Medical Center in New York City, have developed their own internal vocabulary standards, or **terminology authority.** Columbia Presbyterian Medical Center separates the storage and retrieval of data from the meaning of the terms in the database using a medical entities dictionary (MED) that defines valid database terms and synonyms for use by its clinical applications. An alternative approach is to develop a set of **terminology services** for the IDN. These services fall into three categories: (1) linking or normalizing the data contained within the IDN's legacy databases before these data are copied to a CDR; (2) reregistering all terms used by new applications and linking them to external authoritative vocabulary terms, such as those contained within the Unified Medical Language System's Metathesaurus (see Chapter 6); and (3) providing real-time help in (reproducibly) selecting the appropriate term to describe a clinical situation.

The second layer of architecture is the **business-logic layer.** As we discussed in Section 10.1.6, once a system has been installed, its users will usually resist change. The reason for this inertia is not just that there is a steep learning curve for a new system but also that the old system embodied institutional workflow. Separating the workflow from the database and also from the interface will enable more natural migrations of systems as the IDN evolves. Organizations should not, however, assume that old workflow is correct or should be embodied in new information systems. The point here is that a modern architecture that separates the workflow from the data allows prior data to be carried forward as the systems migrate.

The third layer, the **user-interface layer,** is the one most likely to change within several years. The cost of desktop devices and support represents a significant portion of an IDN's information systems budget—often as much as one-third of the total budget. For example, an IDN that supports 10,000 workstations will incur ongoing costs for hardware and software alone of $10 million per year, assuming a $3,000 unit cost and a 3-year life span per workstation. Network computing, which minimizes processing at the workstation level, could substantially reduce this cost by allowing simpler maintenance and support as well as decreased cost per device.

Although we might be safe in assuming that the future network and computer-system architecture will resemble that of the World Wide Web, these systems are currently better suited for one-way retrieval and presentation of information and cannot adequately support clinicians' input of data. Moreover, the forms of input devices are still changing. For example, new classes of lightweight **personal digital assistants** (PDAs), small handheld devices with electronic schedule, contact list, (modified) handwriting recognition capabilities, and other productivity tools, have become popular. Voice-entry devices have found some utility where noncontinuous speech is supported by good screen design (see Chapter 4). Even computer tablets with handwriting and gesture recognition have been used in specialized clinical applications. Most probably, clinician end users will require a variety of devices—some that are application specific and some that vary with personal preference. The important design consideration is that, if possible, the design of the display and the nature of the input devices should not be so tied to the application that change and modification are difficult.

10.5 A Comparison of Three Healthcare Information Systems

We saw in Section 10.3 how changes in technology have played a role in shaping the evolution of HCISs. The nature of a computer system also is highly dependent on the functional goals of that system's developers. Requirements analysis (problem definition) is the first step of the system-development process (see Chapter 5). Decisions at this earliest phase set the stage for the design and implementation choices that follow. Thus the final form of the system depends greatly on which problems the developers aim to solve. Within an IDN, the form of the enterprise HCIS is highly dependent on the organization's history, including its origins (as either an academic medical center or as a looser affiliation of midsized community hospitals), its rate of growth, and the mix of legacy information systems that it has inherited. We illustrate the importance of the original design goals and the influence of business priorities by describing the evolution of three systems in the United States and Europe.

10.5.1 The HELP System at Intermountain Health Care

The University of Utah's HELP system (also see Chapters 9, 13, and 16) was designed to meet the clinical, teaching, and research needs of hospital personnel; administrative functions were added later. Developed by Warner and colleagues at the Latter Day Saints (LDS) Hospital—a tertiary-care and teaching hospital in Salt Lake City, Utah—HELP was later implemented in many of the other acute-care facilities within the Intermountain Health Care IDN.

The HELP system is notable in that it was among the first to incorporate decision-support logic. Within HELP, modules of specialized decision logic permit the system to react to data as they are entered into patients' files and to generate patient-specific warnings, alerts, diagnostic suggestions, and limited management advice. HELP protocols also can be written that evaluate the patient database at set periodic intervals—for example, to check whether a patient who is receiving a potassium-wasting diuretic has had his serum-potassium level measured during prespecified intervals (Pryor et al., 1983).

Expert collaborators define the search criteria of the HELP frames using a HELP Frame Language that was designed to be easily understood by clinicians (see Chapters 9 and 16). Researchers can analyze the clinical and administrative database by writing HELP protocols to identify study populations that have particular characteristics and to retrieve variables of interest. HELP's research subsystem is interfaced with statistical programs that can analyze the differences among study populations; the results then can be used in clinical research, in administrative audits, or as the basis for the creation of additional HELP frames to assist in patient management

10.5.2 The Center for Clinical Computing System at Beth Israel Deaconess Medical Center

The Center for Clinical Computing (CCC) system, developed by Howard Bleich and Warner Slack as a centralized clinical computing system, was first deployed in 1978 at the Beth Israel Medical Center in Boston (now part of the Beth Israel Deaconess Medical Center and the CareGroup IDN). This system is designed around a single common registry of patients, with tight integration of all its departmental systems. It is remarkable in the intensity of its use by clinicians and in the breadth of its functionality to support physicians. For example, the system records over 70,000 lookups of patient data per week by clinicians. It was the first system to offer hospital-wide electronic mail, as well as end-user access to Medline via PaperChase. In addition, CCC was the first to employ many mechanisms for confidentiality, such as an audit trail of patient lookups, that are now common in most advanced clinical systems. In ambulatory clinics, an electronic patient record including support for problem lists, clinic notes, prescription writing, and other functions is used by over 1,000 clinicians in more than 30 primary-care and specialty areas (Safran et al., 1991). In contrast to HELP, the CCC system provides only limited support for order entry, alerts, and reminders.

The CCC has a MUMPS database that functions as a clinical-data repository and an on-line data warehouse, called ClinQuery (Safran et al., 1989). With records from more than 300,000 consecutive hospitalizations since 1983, the database contains complete data on all test results and medications, as well as ICD-9 and SNOMED diagnosis codes. The CCC was transferred to the Brigham and Women's Hospital in 1983 and has since developed separately as the Brigham Integrated Computer System (BICS), a distributed client–server system.

10.5.3 The DIOGENE System at Geneva Canton University Hospital

Healthcare information systems in Europe started to evolve at about the same time as similar systems in the United States. One example is the DIOGENE System developed by Jean-Raoul Scherrer and his colleagues at the Canton Hospital at the University of Geneva beginning in 1971. Built originally with a centralized architecture, it has migrated successfully to a distributed platform. In contrast to HELP and CCC, DIOGENE was originally designed to perform administrative functions—its earliest applications were personnel management, invoicing, patient admitting, and general accounting, later followed by ancillary departmental and clinical information modules. Today, DIOGENE supports almost all administrative and clinical functions, including a full physician order entry that has been operational for more than a decade. A unique feature of the system is its user interface: DIOGENE primarily prints its reports instead of making them available on clinical workstations. Physicians write orders by telephoning a special operator who types the order while the physician dictates. The physician then views the typing on the computer screen and gives verbal consent (Scherrer et al., 1990, 1995).

10.6 Forces That Will Shape the Future of Healthcare Information Systems

As we have discussed throughout this chapter, the changing landscape of the healthcare industry and the strategic and operational requirements of IDNs have accelerated the acquisition and implementation of HCISs. Although there are many obstacles to implementation and acceptance of smoothly functioning, fully integrated HCISs, few people today would debate the critical role of information technologies in an IDN's achievement of clinical and operational integration.

We have emphasized the dynamic nature of today's healthcare environment and the associated implications for HCISs. The information architecture described in Section 10.4 can help to carry IDNs through this dynamic time, but a host of new requirements loom that will challenge today's available solutions. We anticipate additional requirements associated with the changing organizational landscape, technological advances, and broader societal changes.

10.6.1 Changing Organizational Landscape

Although the concept of an IDN is no longer new, the underlying organizational form and business strategies of these complex organizations continue to evolve. In fact, to date, IDNs have largely failed to achieve the operational improvements and cost reductions they were designed to deliver. It is possible that we will witness the emergence of entirely new forms of IDNs or even a reversal of the trend toward consolidation. Key to understanding the magnitude of the information systems challenge for IDNs is recognizing the pace of change—IDNs reorganize services, merge, uncouple, acquire, sell off, and strategically align in a matter of weeks or months. On the other hand, today's state-of-the-art systems (computer systems and people processes) may require months or years to build and refine.

All too frequently, the business deals are cut with insufficient regard to the cost and time required to create the supporting information infrastructure. Even in the best of circumstances, the cultural and organizational challenges of linking diverse users and care-delivery settings will tax an IDN's ability to change its information systems environment quickly enough. These issues will increase in acuity as operational budgets continue to shrink—today's IDNs are spending 25 to 75 percent of their capital budgets on information-systems investments. In turn, these new investments translate into increased annual operating costs (costs of regular system upgrades, maintenance, user support, and staffing). Still only 3 to 6 percent of total revenues for most healthcare organizations, information systems operating budgets typically run 10 to 15 percent of revenues in other information-intensive industries.

10.6.2 Technological Changes Affecting Healthcare Organizations

Although future changes in technology are hard to predict (e.g., we have heard for over a decade that voice-entry systems are 5 years from practical use!), the best clues to the future may be found in our recent past. First, the emergence of the powerful microprocessor and the cost performance of storage media will continue to be a dominant factor in future health-systems design. These technologies ensure that sufficient processing and storage will be available for almost any healthcare application that currently can be imagined. Second, trends in the communications industry to integrate voice, video, and data will ensure that the IDN will have broadband capacity not only within its traditional domain but also to an extended enterprise that may include even patients' homes, schools, and workplaces. Third, the design of modern software based on modular components with an emphasis on communication and information standards should evolve to more flexible information-technology systems. These three technological trends all contribute to the emergence of the World Wide Web as the single technological event most likely to affect IDNs.

If security and confidentiality concerns can be resolved, the emergence of a networked society will profoundly change our thinking about the nature of healthcare delivery. Health services are still primarily delivered locally—we seldom leave our local communities to receive health care except under the most dire of circumstances. In the future, providers and even patients will have access to healthcare experts that are dispersed over state, national, and even international boundaries (we see the beginnings of these capabilities in the growth of consumer-health resources on the Internet [see Chapter 11]). Distributed healthcare capabilities will enable the implementation of collaborative models that could include virtual house calls and routine remote monitoring via telemedical linkages (see Chapter 20).

10.6.3 Societal Change

At the beginning of the twenty-first century, clinicians find themselves spending less time with each patient and spending more time with administrative and regulatory concerns. This decrease in clinician–patient contact has contributed to declining patient and provider satisfaction with care-delivery systems. At the same time, empowered health consumers interested in self-help and unconventional approaches have access to more health information than ever before. These factors are changing the interplay among care teams, patients, and external (regulatory and financial) forces. The changing model of care, coupled with changing economic incentives, places a greater focus on wellness and preventative and lifelong care. Although we might agree that aligning economic incentives with wellness is a good thing, this realignment also implies a shift in responsibility. For instance, basic nursing care after an abbreviated hospital stay is now often provided by a family member in the home.

Like the healthcare environment, the technical context of our lives is changing. The Web has already dramatically changed our approaches to information access and system design in the workplace. Concurrent with development of these new standards of information display and exchange is a push led by the entertainment industry (and others) to deliver broadband multimedia into our homes. Such community connectivity will catalyze changing care models more than any other factor we can imagine by bringing fast, interactive, and multimedia capabilities to the household level. Finally, vast amounts of information can now be stored efficiently on movable media. If past performance predicts future availability, we can assume almost unlimited and inexpensive storage of consumer-oriented health information, including, for example, video segments that show the appearance and sounds of normal and abnormal conditions or demonstrate common procedures for home care and health maintenance.

With societal factors pushing our IDNs to change, and the likely availability of extensive computing and communication capacity in the homes, in the work place, and in the schools, health organizations and health providers are free to rethink the basic operating assumptions about how to deliver care. The traditional approach has been facility and physician centric—patients usually come to the physician at a time convenient for the physician. The IDN of the twenty-first century may be truly a healthcare delivery system without walls, where routine health management is conducted in nontraditional settings, such as homes and workplaces, using the power of telemedicine and consumer informatics.

Suggested Readings

Drazen E., Metzger J. (1999). *Strategies for Integrated Health Care.* San Francisco: Jossey-Bass Publishers.

This book reviews descriptive research covering the organizational and information systems aspects of new healthcare delivery strategies being pursued by pioneering IDNs. Prominent in the book are discussions of new models for providing access to health services, for delivering coordinated services across distributed care settings, and for integrating physician and IDN patient care activities.

Gross M.S., Lohman P. (1997). The technology and tactics of physician integration. *Journal of the Healthcare Information and Management Systems Society,* 11(2):23–41.

This article discusses physician integration, which is the process of aligning the activities and incentives of individual and groups of physicians with the other components of an IDN. The article examines alternative IDN models, common problems associated with physicians' changing roles, and the influence of physician culture on these problems. The article recommends integration tactics and discusses how management style and information technology can address the goals of the IDN and the interests of its physicians.

Lorenzi N. M., Riley R.T., Blyth A.J., Southon G., Dixon, B.J. (1997). Antecedents of the people and organizational aspects of medical informatics: review of the literature. *Journal of the American Medical Informatics Association,* 4(2):79–93.

This article reviews the contributions of behavioral science and organizational management disciplines and their implications for processes for creating future direction, managing complex change processes, involving individuals and groups in implementation projects, and managing the altered organization.

Overhage J. M. (1998). *Proceedings of the Fourth Annual Nicholas E. Davies CPR Recognition Symposium.* July 9–10. Renaissance Mayflower Hotel, Washington, D.C. Computer-based Patient Record Institute, Schaumburg, IL

This conference proceedings includes detailed and organized summaries of the management, function, technology, and effects of provider information systems for the 1998 Davies award-winning organizations. These organizations have demonstrated an ability to integrate data from multiple sources, provide decision support, and be used by caregivers as the primary source of information in patient care. The 1998 winners were Northwestern Memorial Hospital (Chicago) and Kaiser-Permanente Northwest (Portland, OR). Prior years' proceedings summarize the systems of Intermountain Health Care, Columbia Presbyterian Medical Center (New York City), Department of Veterans Affairs (1995); Brigham and Women's Hospital (1996); Kaiser-Permanente of Ohio, North Mississippi Health Services, and the Regenstrief Institute for Health Care (1997). The winning HCISs represent both inhouse-developed and commercial systems.

Proceedings of the 1996 IAIMS Symposium: Building Infrastructure for Integrated Health Systems. (1997). September 27, 1996. Dedicated to Richard T. West. *Journal of the American Medical Informatics Association,* 4(2 Suppl):S1–76.

This special issue—the third in a series of IAIMS symposia—reviews the evolution of the integrated advanced information management systems (IAIMSs) concept; foundation issues of planning, architecture, and organization; areas of ongoing interest; evaluation of effects on cost and quality of care; support for regional affiliate networks; and requirements for basic informatics research.

Questions for Discussion

1. Briefly explain the differences among an IDN's operational, planning, and documentary requirements for information. Give two examples in each category. Choose one of these categories, and discuss similarities and differences in the environments of a tertiary-care medical center, a community-based ambulatory-care clinic, and a specialty-care physician's office. Describe the implied differences in these units' information requirements.
2. Describe three situations in which the separation of clinical and administrative information could lead to inadequate patient care, loss of revenue, or inappropriate administrative decisions. Identify and discuss the challenges and limitations of two methods for improving data integration.
3. Describe three situations in which lack of integration of information systems with clinicians' workflow can lead to inadequate patient care, reduced physician productivity, or poor patient satisfaction with an IDN's services. Identify and discuss the challenges and limitations of two methods for improving process integration.
4. Describe the key philosophies underlying the design of central, modular, and distributed HCISs. What are at least two advantages and two disadvantages of each architecture?
5. Assume that you are the chief information officer of a newly formed IDN. You have just been charged with planning a new HCIS to support a large tertiary care medical center, two smaller community hospitals, a nursing home, and a 40-physician group practice. Each organization currently operates its own set of integrated and standalone technologies and applications. What technical and organizational factors must you consider? What are the three largest challenges you will face over the next 24 months?
6. How do you think the implementation of HCISs will affect the quality of relationships between patients and providers? Discuss at least three potential positive and three potential negative effects. What steps would you take to maximize the positive value of these systems?

11
Public Health and Consumer Uses of Health Information: Education, Research, Policy, Prevention, and Quality Assurance

PATRICIA FLATLEY BRENNAN AND ANDREW FRIEDE

After reading this chapter you should know the answers to these questions:

- What role can informatics play in managing the health of populations?
- How does direct access to health information technologies assist patients in participating in their own health care?
- What are the interdependencies between clinical informatics and public-health informatics in monitoring, surveillance, and policy-making for disease and health states?
- How does public-health informatics support and inform the clinical encounter?

11.1 Public Health and the Emergence of Healthcare Consumerism

Health care in the twenty-first century requires the merging of public and private health concerns. Information technology provides tools that facilitate linking of information about the health of the public with data specific to the care of an individual patient as well as provides clinicians and patients with access to the knowledge that they need to ensure optimum health outcomes. This chapter introduces public health concepts such as "notifiable disease" and "consumer health" and illustrates how maturing computer networks, such as the Internet, make possible a link among public health, medical care, and self-help.

Throughout this chapter, we follow a simple case to explore the role of public-health informatics in the prevention and treatment of disease and disability:

> Baby Sarah K. was delivered at 34 weeks' gestation; her birth weight was 2,000 grams. Her neonatal course was complicated by vertically transmitted Chlamydial Pneumonia, treated successfully with antibiotics. Her parents, Karen and Tony, both age 22 years, were subsequently diagnosed with Chlamydia Trachomatis and were treated similarly.

Until recently, the concept of health was often artificially divided into *private health* (the health of the individual, called simply "medicine" or "medical care") and *public health* (the health of populations, especially poorer ones). This chapter has two basic themes:

1. The implications that the new integration of medicine and public health has for information systems
2. A major consequence of this new integration: the increasingly important role that individuals will have the opportunity—and obligation—to take in their own health care

We do not attempt to catalog the many public-health and consumer-oriented systems, because such a compilation would be outdated at publication; however, a list of the most important information resources from the Centers for Disease Control and Prevention (CDC) is available (Friede & O'Carroll, 1996),[1] and there is a relatively recent bibliography for the field (Selden et al., 1996). Many systems were described in an earlier review (Friede et al., 1995). Rather than discussing systems that are used for public health per se, we emphasize how properly focused information systems can bring population-based thinking into daily medical practice.

11.1.1 Public Health: The Study of Populations

Public health has often been seen as a secondary concern for medical professionals or as the special concern of public administrators or of people interested in tropical infectious diseases. Recent changes in the ecology and epidemiology of disease and, perhaps more important, the financing of health care have prompted a change in this thinking.

With respect to ecology and epidemiology, the global human immunodeficiency virus (HIV) and acquired immune deficiency syndrome (AIDS) pandemic, the reemergence of tuberculosis, and the epidemic of salmonellosis in the United States have forced many people to realize that the better-off population will not be spared from epidemic infectious diseases. Moreover, people now generally recognize that the major controllable causes of morbidity are such traditional public-health topics as smoking, alcohol and drug abuse, injuries, and poor diet (including a diet too high in fat and calories) (Public Health Service, 1991). There is a worldwide concern about what the threats to the environment are and how they affect health through factors such as air pollution (causing asthma), exposure to chemical toxins in our food (perhaps causing cancers and birth defects), and, secondarily, effects from damage to the environment (holes in the ozone layer predisposing to skin cancer). In brief, there is a growing sense of biological interdependence and a perception that we will all sink together or swim together.

Another factor driving an increased appreciation of population-based thinking is the revolution in the financing of health care in the United States (and the be-

---

[1]The full text may be found at http://www.cdc.gov/elecinfo.htm.

ginnings of changes in Europe, perhaps to be followed in other parts of the world). Although there are proposed schemes to try to hold down burgeoning healthcare costs, it appears that some form of managed care (see Chapter 19) will rule in the United States for this generation. Ironically, it is the very triumph of managed care and capitation that has made payers (and hence providers) more cognizant of the *populations* that they contract to protect. The whole equation of medicine has changed. Formerly, medical-services providers made more money when their clients were sick and needed services; now, they make more money when their clients are well. Suddenly, prevention is attractive because it is usually less expensive than treatment and because it can be attractive to potential customers (payers and clients). Now, all medical professionals will have to practice public health.

Hence, it will be incumbent on all healthcare professionals to be knowledgeable about public health and the related special informatics requirements that devolve from public health's roots in surveillance and epidemiology (including modeling) and the analysis of large data sets that describe complex, often mobile, populations.

11.1.2 The Consumer's New Opportunities and Obligations

The patient of the late twentieth century experiences greater demand to participate in his own care than have patients at any time since the development of contemporary health care. Patient participation takes many forms: shared decision-making, self-care, and collaborative practices. In essence, it reflects a shift from the patient as the silent recipient of ministrations from a wise, beneficent clinician to an active collaborator whose values, preferences, and lifestyle not only alter predisposition to certain illnesses but also shape the characteristics of desirable treatments.

The role of the consumer as a full partner in health promotion and disease management has never been more necessary than now. In the distributed-managed-care models of the late twentieth century, consumers serve as their own case managers, brokering care from generalists, specialists, and ancillary groups. Rarely do consumers receive all of their needed clinical services from a single provider. Informatics tools, such as the electronic patient record, provide an integrated record and communication service. Consumers require access to this record so that they can contribute timely observations, monitor their own progress toward health, and comprehend the plethora of clinical interventions available to them.

The development of inexpensive, reliable, telecommunications technology enables healthcare providers, payers, patients, and the general public to access health information and healthcare resources directly from their homes and from public gathering places, such as libraries, schools, and workplaces. Through computer networks, telephone messaging services, and other initiatives, clinicians have a unique opportunity to reach patients and clients with health-promotion, disease-prevention, and illness-management clinical interventions. Telecommunications-based health services also pose unique challenges to modify existing clinical interventions and to devise new ones to take appropriate advantage of the electronic environment.

11.2 Historical Perspective

The end of the twentieth century witnessed a transition in health care and health informatics from a focus on the individual to a focus on populations. In public health, this change is evident in the increased focus on the health of groups. In health informatics, it is evident in the emphasis on networked data and information systems.

11.2.1 Public-Health Informatics: The Special Needs of Public Health

The fundamental science of public health is **epidemiology**, which is the study of the prevalence and determinants of disability and disease in populations. Hence, most public-health information systems have focused on information about aggregate populations. For example, the CDC's HIV/AIDS reporting system, which collects millions of observations concerning people infected with HIV or diagnosed with AIDS and is used to conduct dozens of studies, does not even collect personal identifiers (individuals are tracked by pseudo-identifiers). Similarly, the National Noticeable Diseases Surveillance System, which state epidemiologists use to report the occurrences of some 50 diseases every week to the CDC (and which is the source for statistics reported in the *Morbidity and Mortality Weekly Report*), makes no attempt to track or follow individuals. The CDC's WONDER system (Friede et al., 1994b,1996), which contains tens of millions of observations drawn from some 30 databases, blanks out cells with fewer than three to five (depending on the data set) observations. A wide variety of data and information systems have evolved to serve the needs of public-health agencies in four basic areas: policy development, program management, purchasing (the federal government is the world's largest buyer of health services), and regulation (Harris et al., 1998). They share one unifying feature: They are all about populations—sometimes large populations.

In contrast, most clinical information systems focus almost exclusively on identifying information about *individuals*. For example, almost any clinical laboratory system can quickly find Billy Cross's culture results; however, few such systems can easily track the time trend of antibiotic resistance for the population of all the clinic's patients. Almost no system can track such a trend for the population that the clinic actually serves (the people in the clinic's surrounding area, whether or not they visit the facility). What is needed are systems that can tell us about both individuals *and* the world in which those individuals live.

How did this dichotomy come about? Computer systems developed for traditional medical-informatics applications or businesses often lack features required for public health; therefore, public health specialists have had to develop their systems de novo. For example, standard statistical packages cannot be used easily to perform standardization, to fit mathematical models to disease patterns, or to calculate sample sizes for case-control studies. Commonly available data-entry programs cannot handle the long or complex questionnaires common in public health. General-purpose graphing programs make bar and pie charts but cannot generate histograms or county maps. EpiInfo, specialized computer software developed for public health, can carry out most of these functions (Dean et al., 1991).[2] The CDC is developing the first mapping system that contains the boundaries of public-health jurisdictions in the United States.

Furthermore, public-health data files often contain many millions of records, and accessing these large files quickly requires special database designs. There is also an increasing need to search the full contents of massive text databases, such as publications, reports, and recommendations; tables of summary data; and information about the national population health goals, such as those established in Healthy People 2000 (Public Health Service, 1991). Typically, these documents have no keywords, and their diversity, their dynamic nature, and the unavailability of appropriate keywords in the Medical Subject Headings (MeSH) thesaurus often preclude their being assigned keywords. One of the challenges for public-health informatics is to develop streamlined ways to access complex textual data.

As we mentioned, public-health informaticians have often developed specialized solutions for their specific needs; however, now that the lines between medicine and public health are blurring, these systems will, of necessity, coalesce.

11.2.2 Progress in the Federal Sector

The CDC and other government health agencies increasingly consider information processing and dissemination to be central to their mission. In recognition of this emphasis, in 1992, the CDC initiated the Information Network for Public Health Officials (INPHO), a 14-state consortium of state-based public-health information systems (Baker et al., 1995). The principal thrust of INPHO is to help state and local health departments make use of information technology. INPHO started with the development of a statewide information network in Georgia, funded by a $5 million grant from the Woodruff Foundation (Chapman & Moulton, 1995). By 1997, 12 states had received specific CDC or Foundation funding for this work, and two others had used other monies.

Much of the money has gone to building statewide immunization registries and to tying together formerly standalone systems. More broadly, states have

[2]Software and information can be found through EpiInfo at http://www.cdc.gov.

used the funds to integrate existing standalone systems, a task that can be difficult or impossible to do with categorical (disease-specific) funding, which typically specifies that computer X can be used for only disease Y. Why is this integration important for medical informatics? Once the state health-department systems are integrated, they can be linked to ambulatory-care and hospital clinical systems. Suddenly, the key missing link for monitoring populations—namely, **denominators**—becomes available, and the stage is set for using integrated public health and clinical data to monitor the health of populations.

11.2.3 Community and Regional Health-Information Networks

Many factors are driving the need to integrate healthcare data, including

- Decentralization of care due to increased utilization of outpatient services (e.g., urgent-care centers, primary-care centers, hospices, and home care)
- An increasingly mobile population (the family doctor who knows you over your lifetime is now a rarity)
- Managed care and capitated reimbursement
- The increased emphasis on controlling costs, improving quality, and assessing cost–benefit ratios and cost effectiveness
- Emerging government regulations for healthcare data management and reporting

During the late 1980s and early 1990s, it was widely believed that **community** or **regional health-information networks** (CHINs or RHINs) would develop in population centers throughout the United States. These networks were to be formed as public–private alliances among healthcare providers, pharmacies, public-health departments and, possibly, payers. The goal of such networks was to share health information among all health participants, thereby improving community health and heath care.

There were important experiments in cities such as New Orleans and Indianapolis; however, several factors conspired to block the widespread implementation of CHINs and RHINs. First, the technical difficulties of networking different institutions often proved insurmountable, especially in the absence of compelling financial or political justifications. Second, there were worrisome unresolved concerns about data ownership, especially as they affected confidentiality and marketing strategies of competing organizations. Third, as the healthcare landscape continued to shift daily, it was difficult for many institutions to make long-term commitments to public–private partnerships that often had vague (although noble) long-term objectives.

As healthcare dollars are scrutinized more closely, administrators are under intense pressure to justify each investment financially. The challenge for people interested in community-based network schemes will be to prove that the latter can save money and promote health. For now, CHIN and RHIN alliances are generally on hold. These networks are, however, to be distinguished from new market-based business alliances and mergers among hospitals, group practices, home-healthcare agencies, and other providers (integrated delivery networks; see Chapter 10) and from privatization of nonprofit institutions, such as Blue Cross and Blue Shield—both of which continue apace.

11.3 Informatics as a Tool for Managing the Health of Populations

As we discussed in Chapter 9, a computer-based record of patients' lifetime medical histories can support patient care and provider communication while providing a basis for research. Traditionally, such a record has focused on an individual's personal health and encounters with the health system—however, it also can place the patient in the context of her home and community. What risks are people exposed to through their home situations (e.g., lead dust clinging to a roommate's clothing or the absence of a parent who is caring for his own aging, fragile parent)? What is the pattern of antibiotic-resistant strains of gonorrhea in the community? Is the house at risk of flooding or full of obstacles or structural defects that predispose its occupants to falls (the largest cause of childhood trauma) or the risk of fire?

In the past, these kinds of concerns were generally relegated to public-health departments; managed care has changed all that. Medical informatics must adapt to the new realities by fully embracing public-health information systems. Similarly, public-health information systems will have to serve the needs of health plans. These goals will need to be met in two domains: data content and information systems.

11.3.1 Data Requirements

> Although Baby Sarah K. has chlamydia, the specific etiology exempts this particular case from the CDC notification requirements. Karen's insurance company and her employer, however, both of which participate in a quality-review program, request that any illness matching the primary diagnosis of a notifiable illness be reported and a quality-monitor screen initiated.

As medical practice shifts in emphasis from treatment of illness to promotion of health, the effective medical record will also serve as a public-health document—one that places the individual in the context of her community. Until recently, the primary candidate for a national data set that reflects prevention activities has been the Healthy People 2000 Objectives (Friede, Freedman et al., 1994a; Public Health Service, 1991), which contains 332 measurable objectives and 284 related subobjectives that target minorities and other at-risk populations.

The Healthy People 2000 Objectives have been used widely for program planning and evaluation at the state and national levels; however, many of the indices were designed to make use of available data, and to look at the national picture, rather than to study smaller populations (Harris et al., 1998). The objectives thus have important limitations. For example, consider infant deaths, which are relatively rare in a given covered population. Infant-mortality data are readily available at the state level, but what is of greater interest is to know what is being done to *prevent* infant mortality—for example, the consistency with which low-birth-weight deliveries take place at facilities for high-risk deliveries and neonates. It is an example of the need to collect data intermediate between the presumed cause (expert perinatal care) and the outcome (infant death). The outcome infant death is, at best, a proxy for perinatal care (Harris et al., 1998). This indicator is not available at the national level, but the data can be collected locally.

In fact, it *is* a measure that has been included in the Health Plan Employer Data and Information Set (HEDIS), developed by the National Committee for Quality Assurance (NCQA) (National Committee for Quality Assurance, 1997).[3] The NCQA is a private, not-for-profit organization dedicated to assessing and reporting on the quality of managed-care plans. Its board is made up of employers (including many of the largest firms in the United States), consumer and labor representatives, health-plan representatives, quality experts, regulators, and representatives from medicine.

HEDIS was originally designed to let payers and consumers shop for the best managed-care plan. It was developed by a broad-based constituency that reflects NCQA's governance, with important scientific input from the CDC, the Agency for Healthcare Research and Quality (AHRQ), and the Health Care Financing Administration (which oversees Medicare and Medicaid). There is a special version of HEDIS, called Medicaid HEDIS, that focuses on the special needs of that population.

HEDIS has evolved to be a powerful tool for monitoring prevention activities (Tables 11.1 to 11.3). This emphasis is probably attributable to the heavy input from public-health agencies, especially the CDC. HEDIS did not start out being about prevention, per se, but it has evolved to be a de facto tool for measuring the quality of prevention services provided by a healthcare organization. In 1997, 60 percent of health maintenance organizations (HMOs) used HEDIS to assess performance (Harris et al., 1998). (In addition to these prevention-oriented data, there are also measures of client satisfaction, health-plan stability, costs, and health plan descriptive information.) HEDIS is the current leading candidate data set to serve as a national reference standard for evaluating the ability of health plans to monitor—and to manage proactively—the health of the populations that they cover.

Another important data set is the Indicator Measurement System being promulgated by the Joint Commission on Accreditation of Healthcare Organizations (JCAHO) as part of the ORYX accreditation process. Idiosyncratically named, ORYX was initially designed to apply to only hospitals and long-term care or-

---

[3]Available online at http://www.ncqa.org.

Table 11.1. HEDIS 1999 reporting set measures: effectiveness of care.

Use of services domain
Childhood Immunization Status[a]
Adolescent Immunization Status[a]
Advising Smokers to Quit[a]
Flu Shots for Older Adults[a]
Breast Cancer Screening[a]
Cervical Cancer Screening[a]
Prenatal Care in the First Trimester[a]
Low Birth-Weight Babies
Check-Ups After Delivery[a]
Beta Blocker Treatment After a Heart Attack[a]
Cholesterol Management After Acute Cardiovascular Events
Eye Exams for People with Diabetes[a]
Comprehensive Diabetes Care
Follow-Up After Hospitalization for Mental Illness[a]
Antidepressant Medication Management
The Health of Seniors

[a]These measures and survey instruments are required for reporting. Where measures are not relevant for a given population, plans are not required to report that measure.
Source: National Committee for Quality Assurance.

ganizations; similar requirements are being set for healthcare networks (e.g., health plans and provider-sponsored organizations). ORYX is used to examine the performance of hospitals; it contains measures such as the risks and rates for surgical procedures and associated complications and the appropriateness of drug treatments. It will be valuable for monitoring the quality of care and the performance of an organization but may have less utility for studying population-based prevention strategies. For example, to continue the infant-mortality example, the ORYX gathers data on Apgar scores (quantitative appraisal of neonate functional

Table 11.2. HEDIS 1999 reporting set measures: access/availability of care.

Access/availability of care domain
Adults' Access to Preventive/Ambulatory Health Services
Children's Access to Primary Care Practitioners
Availability of Primary Care Providers
Availability of Behavioral Health Care Providers
Availability of Obstetrical and Prenatal Care Providers
Initiation of Prenatal Care
Low Birth-Weight Deliveries at Facilities for High-Risk Deliveries and Neonates
Annual Dental Visit
Availability of Dentists
Availability of Language Interpretation Services

Source: National Committee for Quality Assurance.

TABLE 11.3. HEDIS 1999 Reporting set measures: use of services.

Use of services domain
Frequency of Ongoing Prenatal Care
Well-Child Visits in the First 15 Months of Life
Well-Child Visits in the Third, Fourth, Fifth and Sixth Year of Life
Adolescent Well-Care Visits
Frequency of Selected Procedures
Inpatient Utilization—General Hospital/Acute Care
Ambulatory Care
Inpatient Utilization—Non-Acute Care
Discharge and Average Length of Stay—Maternity Care
Cesarean Section Rate
Vaginal Birth After Cesarean Rate (VBAC-Rate)
Births and Average Length of Stay, Newborns
Mental Health Utilization—Inpatient Discharges and Average Length of Stay
Mental Health Utilization—Percentage of Members Receiving Inpatient, Day/Night Care and Ambulatory Services
Readmission For Specified Mental Health Disorders
Chemical Dependency Utilization—Inpatient Discharges and Average Length of Stay
Chemical Dependency Utilization—Percentage of Members Receiving Inpatient, Day/Night Care and Ambulatory Services
Readmission for Chemical Dependency
Outpatient Drug Utilization

Source: National Committee for Quality Assurance.

status) of less than 4 at 5 minutes; a requirement for admission to the neonatal intensive care unit within 1 day of delivery for greater than 1 day; and a clinically apparent seizure or significant birth trauma. These outcomes are possibly attributable to obstetrical practice rather than to prevention-oriented interventions.[4]

If we are to make HEDIS, ORYX, and similar programs effective, we will need information systems that are an integral part of medical practice. Various information-systems vendors are vying to be ORYX certified, and JCAHO has put in place an elaborate process for their evaluation, selection, and certification.[5] Many vendors are working on HEDIS-related applications; however, there is much work to be completed on the underlying information feeds to these sys-

[4]See http://www.jcaho.org/perfmeas/ims/imsfrm.htm for a summary of the infant mortality measures.
[5]See http://www.jcaho.org/perfmeas/oryx/oryx_frm.htm.

tems before we will be able to assess prevention activities routinely in known populations.

11.3.2 Surveillance Systems and National Reporting

Most healthcare professionals are surprised to learn that there is no uniform national routine reporting—let alone information system—for most diseases, disabilities, risk factors, or prevention activities in the United States. In contrast, France, Britain, Denmark, Norway, and Sweden have comprehensive systems for selected areas such as occupational injuries, infectious diseases, and cancer. No country, however, has complete reporting for every problem. In fact, it is only births, deaths, and to a lesser extent fetal deaths that are uniformly and relatively completely reported in the United States. If you have an angioplasty and survive, nobody at the state or federal level necessarily knows.

How then do we obtain estimates of, for example, the trends in teenage smoking or in the incidence of breast cancer? How do epidemics come to our attention? Data from periodic surveys and special studies, surveillance systems, and disease registries are handled by numerous standalone information systems. These systems—usually managed by state health departments and federal health agencies (largely the CDC) or their agents—provide periodic estimates of the incidences and prevalences of diseases and of certain risk factors (e.g., smoking and obesity); however, because the data are from population samples, it is usually impossible to obtain estimates at a level of geographic detail finer than that of a region or state. On the level of an individual patient case, the CDC data systems are rarely useful. Moreover, many of the behavioral indices are self-reported by survey respondents (although extensive validation studies have shown that they are good for trending and sometimes are more reliable than are data obtained from clinical systems). In the case of special surveys, such as the National Health and Nutrition Examination Survey (NHANES), there is primary data collection and entry into a CDC system. The data are complete, but the survey costs many millions of dollars and is conducted only every few years; it then takes years for the data to be made available.

There are also disease registries that track—often completely—the incidence of certain diseases, especially cancers. Such registries usually focus on one topic or cover certain diseases for specific time periods. The CDC maintains dozens of surveillance systems that attempt to track completely the incidence of many conditions, including lead poisoning, injuries and deaths in the workplace, and birth defects. (Some of these systems use samples or cover only certain states or cities.) There is also a list of more than 50 **notifiable diseases** (Table 11.4) that the state epidemiologists and the CDC have determined are of national significance and warrant routine, complete reporting. It is up to providers to report the data, however, and reporting is still often done by telephone or mail, resulting in incomplete data capture. Finally, some states do collect complete summaries of all hospital discharges. As more care is delivered in the ambulatory setting, however, these data capture a decreasing fraction of the data of interest.

TABLE 11.4. Infectious diseases notifiable at the national level.

Acquired immunodeficiency syndrome (AIDS)	Anthrax
Botulism	Brucellosis
Chancroid	*Chlamydia trachomatis,* genital infections
Cholera	Coccidioidomycosis
Cryptosporidiosis	Diphtheria
Encephalitis, California serogroup	Encephalitis, eastern equine
Encephalitis, St. Louis	Encephalitis, western equine
Escherichia coli O157:H7	Gonorrhea
Haemophilus influenzae, invasive disease	Hansen disease (leprosy)
Hantavirus pulmonary syndrome	Hemolytic uremic syndrome, post-diarrheal
Hepatitis A	Hepatitis B
Hepatitis, C/non A, non B	HIV infection, pediatric
Legionellosis	Lyme disease
Malaria	Measles
Meningcoccal disease	Mumps
Pertussis	Plague
Poliomyelitis, paralytic	Psittacosis
Rabies, animal	Rabies, human
Rocky Mountain spotted fever	Rubella
Rubella, congenital syndrome	Salmonellosis
Shigellosis	Streptococcal disease, invasive, Group A
Streptococcus pneumoniae, drug-resistant invasive disease	Streptococcal toxic-shock syndrome
Syphilis	Syphilis, congenital
Tetanus	Toxic-shock syndrome
Trichinosis	Tuberculosis
Typhoid fever	Yellow fever

Source: CDC (1998): *Morbidity and Mortality Weekly Report,* November 20, 46(S4):1–87, Table A.

11.3.3 Linking Public-and Private-Health Information

What all these systems have in common is that they rely on special data collection. It is rare that they are interfaced to and fed by clinical information systems used to document patient care. Even such data as hospital infection data are reentered. Why? We discussed the special requirements of public-health systems in Section 11.2.1. These systems were developed in parallel to the systems that were being implemented in hospitals and clinics. Incompatibilites in systems and vocabularies necessitate duplicate data entry, which can result in the data being shallow, delayed, and subject to input error and recall bias. Furthermore, the systems themselves are often unpopular with state agencies and healthcare providers precisely because they require duplicative data entry (e.g., for a child with lead poisoning and salmonella, data must be entered in two different CDC systems).

How can information from public-health and clinical information systems—once they are integrated—be used to practice prevention? Data from surveillance systems and disease registries might be used by a county health officer to estimate the number of doses of measles vaccine needed for an outbreak. A regional planning commission might use census, surveillance, and hospitalization data to project the occupancy of AIDS hospice beds and demand for home hospice services for a city and to prepare related funding requests for the state legislature. An epidemiologist might use surveillance data on lead poisoning to develop hypotheses for an in-depth case-control study. Significant progress is being made on a national system for tracking childhood immunizations. Even before completion, this project has been used to provide valuable planning data to administrators, but making these practices routine and manageable at the local level will require a full integration of clinical systems with one another.

Over time, it is possible that the distinction between medicine and public health will fade and, with it, the boundaries between the associated information systems. For example, Columbia Presbyterian Medical Center and the New York City Department of Health have collaborated on the development of a tuberculosis registry for northern Manhattan, and the Emory University System of Health Care and the Georgia Department of Public Health have built a similar system for tuberculosis monitoring and treatment in Atlanta. It is not by chance that these two cities each developed tuberculosis systems; rather, tuberculosis is a perfect example of what was once a public-health problem (one that affects the poor and underserved) coming into the mainstream population as a result of an emerging infectious disease (AIDS), immigration, increased international travel, multidrug resistance, and the growing prison population. Hence, the changing ecology of disease, coupled with revolutionary changes in how health care is managed and paid for, will necessitate information systems that serve both individual medical and public-health needs.

Better public-health information systems will enhance the identification and investigation of disease outbreaks, promote rapid dissemination of new information to public-health professionals and to the public, and help people provide services, such as clinic appointments for childhood immunizations. Most important, good public-health systems will help to bridge the gap between public health and private health and will help to bring epidemiology, industrial medicine, and ecology—exemplified by patient education and the involvement of patients, their families, and their communities in their own preventive and therapeutic care—into the mainstream of medicine (Greenlick, 1992).

11.4 Consumerism, Self-Help, and Consumer Health Informatics

The legacy of the self-help movement of the 1970s and the consumerism of the 1980s is growth in the importance of the patient as a full participant in health care. Patients participate by self-monitoring, by evaluating and choosing therapeutic strategies from a set of acceptable alternatives, by implementing the therapies, and by evaluating the effects. Recent social and clinical changes in the manner in which care is provided shift clinical-practice activities that were once the purview of licensed professionals to patients and their family caregivers. The failure of 50 years of bioscience research to produce definitive clinical remedies for more than a handful of disease states requires that medical science be tempered with patient preferences (e.g., between surgical and radiation therapies). Furthermore, there is growing belief that behavioral interventions and alternative therapies hold great promise as adjuncts, or even replacements, for traditional medical therapies. These trends contribute to a contemporary healthcare environment that is more diffuse and involves more people than ever before. The home and the community are fast becoming the most common sites where health care is provided. Information technologies necessary to support patients and their family caregivers must not only migrate from the inpatient institution to the community but also be populated with information resources that help to guide patients in complex healthcare decision-making, to communicate with the care providers, and to comprehend their illnesses and appropriate treatments.

These social trends, coupled with the introduction of managed care and the rapid growth of computer tools, networks, and multimedia, led to both an explosion of need for healthcare information by the lay public and a dramatic rise in the use of information technology to meet that need. Lay persons need information about health promotion, illness prevention, and disease management. Special computer programs, health-focused CD-ROMs, and health-related, Internet-based World Wide Web sites all provide information likely to be useful to the lay public in participating in health care. Labeled **consumer-health informatics** (CHI), this application of medical informatics technologies to health care focuses on the patient as the primary user.

11.4.1 Direct Access to Health Information Resources by Consumers

> "Chlamydia?!" thought Karen. "I've never even heard of that. How did I get it? Did Tom give it to me? Did I give it to him? Will it kill the baby? I'm so embarrassed—I don't want to tell the nurse I don't know what it means; I'm so embarrassed I could die!"

Patients like Karen need quick, private access to accurate information that can calm their fears and ensure that they obtain and follow the currently accepted treatment for their illness. Existing healthcare delivery systems are woefully inadequate in providing such information to their patients. At best, a busy clinician may be able to take a few minutes to explain terms and likely consequences and perhaps to provide the patient with additional brochures and printed information. Computer technology can supplement clinicians' teaching with more detailed information that can be referenced repeatedly by a patient in the privacy of her home.

Consumer health informatics resources provide substantive and procedural knowledge about health problems and promising interventions (Table 11.5). Information resources developed for consumers range in content and sophistication. Some of these resources are little more than digitized brochures, presenting in an electronic form exactly what can be found in available printed materials.

TABLE 11.5. Selected consumer health websites on the Internet.

The CDC Prevention Guidelines Database http://aepo-xdv-www.epo.cdc.gov/wonder/prevguid/prevguid.htm
American Heart Association http://www.amhrt.org/index.html
The Natural Resource Directory http://www.nrd.com/
New York Online Access to Health (NOAH) http://noah.cuny.edu/
Patient Resources and Cancer Information site of the Fred Hutchinson Cancer Research Center http://www.fhcrc.org/cipr/
Healthfinder: the Federal Government's Gateway to Consumer Health http://www.healthfinder.gov/
Medicinal Herbs Online http://www.egregore.com
Mayo Clinic Health Oasis http://www.mayohealth.org/

Others include interactive or multimedia presentations of information about specific conditions and appropriate actions to prevent, cure, or ameliorate the problem. Multimedia presentations capitalize on the features of computer systems to enrich the presentation of health-related materials with pictures, short movies, and drawings.

Consumer health informatics resources provide patients with condition-specific and disease-specific information about the problems they face. Some resources explain the etiology and natural histories of disease in terms comprehensible to lay people. Other resources provide procedural information, explain diagnostic procedures or services, detail expected treatment activities, and provide any relevant warnings and precautions. The presentation of CHI is heavily influenced by the perspective of the system developer. Medically oriented clinical resources demonstrate an emphasis on locally accepted medical practice. Community health-oriented resources are more likely to include information relevant to living in the community with a specific disease or condition.

Consumer health informatics resources originate from two major perspectives: professional and self-help. **Professional-developed CHI resources** are those developed by healthcare clinicians and their organizations. Healthcare organizations—such as HMOs, managed-care companies, and group practices—develop information resources as a service to the patient populations that they treat. These resources tend to complement and extend the clinical services offered by the professional group and may be based on a desire to ensure adherence with accepted therapies or to triage and manage access to care for common health problems. Examples include the Kaiser Permanente Health Facts, a program designed to help Kaiser members answer questions about common health problems, and the Mayo *Health Advisor,* a commercially available CD-ROM that any interested person can purchase and use to help manage his health at home. Examples of other commercially available programs that have a professional orientation include *Health Wise* and *Health Desk.* Figures 11.1 and 11.2 show examples of professional-developed CHI resources accessible via the Internet.

Consumer health informatics resources developed from a self-help perspective complement and augment those provided by the formal healthcare delivery system. A self-help perspective is generally more inclusive than a professional perspective. The information may address daily living concerns and lifestyle issues along with, or in place of, content deemed credible by established medical authorities. Figure 11.3 illustrates this perspective.

Many CHI resources represent a combination of professional and self-help perspectives. Web-based resources, such as the Fred Hutchinson Cancer Research Center, provide pointers to other websites that represent professional or self-help perspectives. Commercial vendors, such as HealthGate Data Corporation, provide access via a website to professional-developed and self-help–oriented CHI resources for a subscription or transaction-based fee.

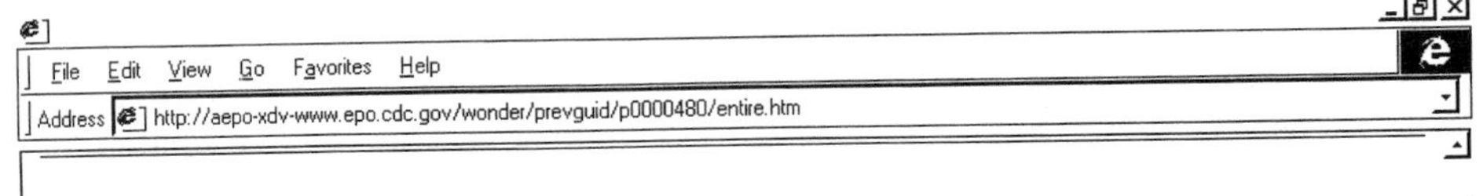

CLINICAL PREVENTION GUIDELINES

The prevention and control of STDs is based on five major concepts: first, education of those at risk on ways to reduce the risk for STDs; second, detection of asymptomatically infected persons and of symptomatic persons unlikely to seek diagnostic and treatment services; third, effective diagnosis and treatment of infected persons; fourth, evaluation, treatment, and counseling of sex partners of persons who are infected with an STD; and fifth, preexposure vaccination of persons at risk for vaccine-preventable STDs. Although this report focuses primarily on the clinical aspects of STD control, prevention of STDs is based on changing the sexual behaviors that place persons at risk for infection. Moreover, because STD control activities reduce the likelihood of transmission to sex partners, prevention for individuals constitutes prevention for the community.

Clinicians have the opportunity to provide client education and counseling and to participate in identifying and treating infected sex partners in addition to interrupting transmission by treating persons who have the curable bacterial and parasitic STDs. The ability of the health-care provider to obtain an accurate sexual history is crucial in prevention and control efforts. Guidance in obtaining a sexual history is available in the chapter "Sexuality and Reproductive Health" in Contraceptive Technology, 16th edition (4). The accurate diagnosis and timely reporting of STDs by the clinician is the basis for effective public health surveillance.

Prevention Messages

Preventing the spread of STDs requires that persons at risk for transmitting or acquiring infections change their behaviors. The essential first step is for the health-care provider to proactively include questions regarding the patient's sexual history as part of the clinical interview. When risk factors have been identified, the provider has an opportunity to deliver prevention messages. Counseling skills (i.e., respect, compassion, and a nonjudgmental attitude) are essential to the effective delivery of prevention messages. Techniques that can be effective in facilitating a rapport with the patient include using open-ended questions, using

Start | 3 webpag... | Inbox - Mi... | Win95b (C: | Collwin | 1998 Gui... | 3:13 PM

FIGURE 11.1. Patient information on chlamydia from CDC Wonder. The CDC's information focuses on the surveillance of this sexually transmitted disease.

Iowa

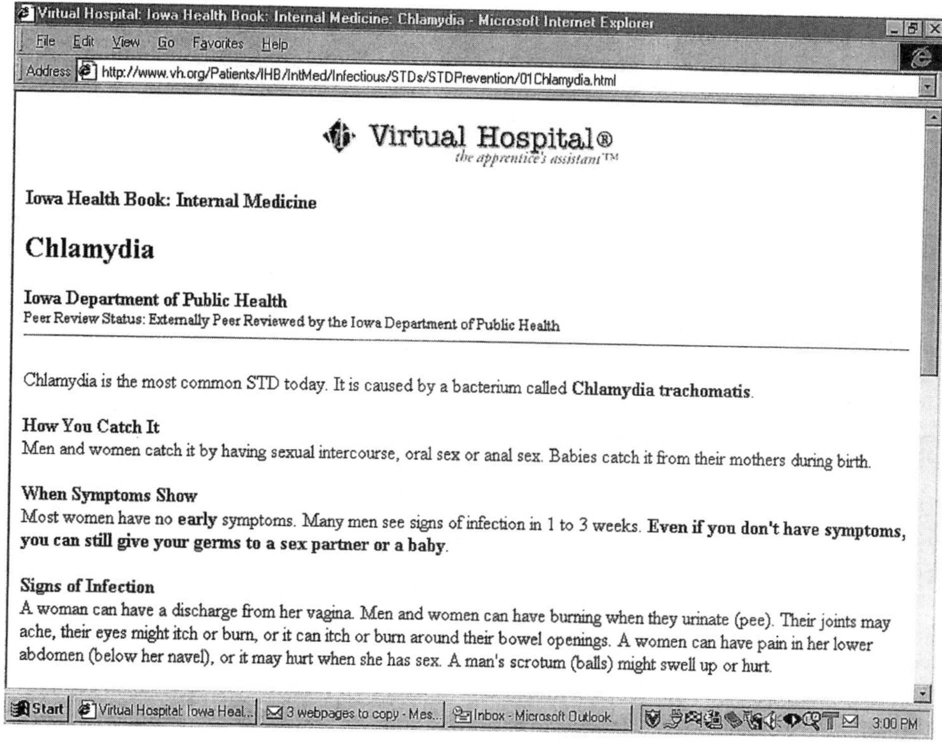

FIGURE 11.2. Patient information on chlamydia from the University of Iowa Virtual Hospital. The information presented is nontechnical and geared to the general public.

11.4.2 Consumer Health Networks

Karen walks her newborn to the public library, where she can use a computer terminal to access the Internet. She types the word "chlamydia" into the network search service and locates several websites addressing the diagnosis and treatment of chlamydia. She first looks at the information provided by the CDC. It appears to be technical and doesn't answer her questions about what chlamydia is and how she got it. Next, she reviews the website of the Women's Health Service of the Major City Academic Medical Center. Here she learns that over 20 percent of all young adults have chlamydia, that it is treatable with antibiotics, and that it is never fatal to either partner or to the baby. Finally, she locates the Women's Wellness Initiative, sponsored by the Regional Women's Collective. This site provides short articles that discuss the possible marital aftereffects of discovering a sexually transmitted disease and give advice and hints about talking with your partner. It also includes a chat room, where other women who have had similar experiences can post and read messages. Karen reviews several messages on the theme of "Talking with Your Partner."

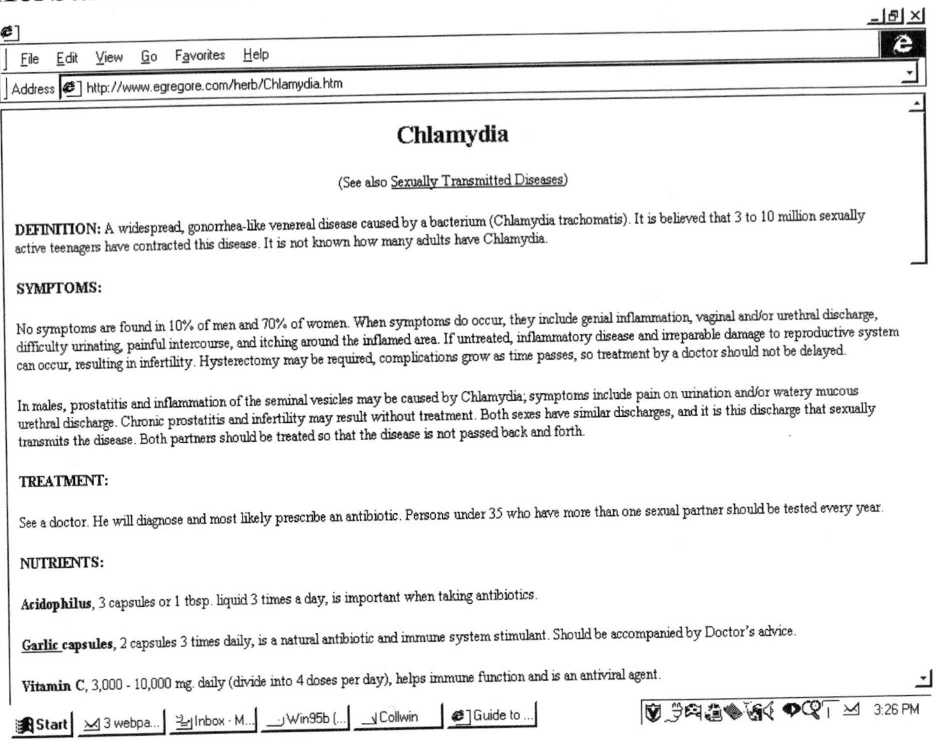
Herbal Remedies

File Edit View Go Favorites Help
Address http://www.egregore.com/herb/Chlamydia.htm

Chlamydia

(See also Sexually Transmitted Diseases)

DEFINITION: A widespread, gonorrhea-like venereal disease caused by a bacterium (Chlamydia trachomatis). It is believed that 3 to 10 million sexually active teenagers have contracted this disease. It is not known how many adults have Chlamydia.

SYMPTOMS:

No symptoms are found in 10% of men and 70% of women. When symptoms do occur, they include genial inflammation, vaginal and/or urethral discharge, difficulty urinating, painful intercourse, and itching around the inflamed area. If untreated, inflammatory disease and irreparable damage to reproductive system can occur, resulting in infertility. Hysterectomy may be required, complications grow as time passes, so treatment by a doctor should not be delayed.

In males, prostatitis and inflammation of the seminal vesicles may be caused by Chlamydia; symptoms include pain on urination and/or watery mucous urethral discharge. Chronic prostatitis and infertility may result without treatment. Both sexes have similar discharges, and it is this discharge that sexually transmits the disease. Both partners should be treated so that the disease is not passed back and forth.

TREATMENT:

See a doctor. He will diagnose and most likely prescribe an antibiotic. Persons under 35 who have more than one sexual partner should be tested every year.

NUTRIENTS:

Acidophilus, 3 capsules or 1 tbsp. liquid 3 times a day, is important when taking antibiotics.

Garlic capsules, 2 capsules 3 times daily, is a natural antibiotic and immune system stimulant. Should be accompanied by Doctor's advice.

Vitamin C, 3,000 - 10,000 mg. daily (divide into 4 doses per day), helps immune function and is an antiviral agent.

Start 3 webpa... Inbox - M... Win95b (... Collwin Guide to ... 3:26 PM

FIGURE 11.3. Self-help perspective on consumer health sexually transmitted disease concerns.

Computer networks not only provide patients with access to information; they provide the additional opportunity for individuals to connect with other people who share similar concerns and with their healthcare providers. Network-based consumer-health services include both specialty and public access networks. Examples of two specialty systems that have been heavily researched are the ComputerLink (Brennan et al., 1995), a specialized computer network service for homebound patients and their caregivers, and the Comprehensive Health Evaluation and Social Support System (CHESS), which targets the needs of people living with AIDS and women diagnosed with breast cancer (Gustafson et al., 1993). Public access systems include the health-related Usenet discussion groups and the health forums available on CompuServe and America Online.

Network-based CHI resources generally provide both static information about health problems and management and specialized health-communications utilities. Some professional-developed CHI resources not only provide information to members of a health plan but also facilitate communication between the patient and the health plan. The Kaiser model allows patients who determine that the health problem they face requires a visit to a clinician to cease the information-resource portion and to activate a communication module that links them to the scheduling desk of their local health clinic, where they can request an appointment to see a clinician. Information resources that reside on the Web generally provide a question-answering service—a utility where interested persons can leave a question to be answered by a professional. Still others support direct electronic mail between patients and clinicians. Some offer discussion groups and chat rooms, where people interested in a specific disease or condition can post and read messages. These discussion areas function as electronic support groups and demonstrate many of the same features found in face-to-face support groups. Professionals participate in these discussions, providing advice or counsel.

Patient-to-patient communication services are generally the most actively used aspects, with a ratio of 10 contacts with a communication service for each access to an information service. These communication services offer great opportunity for health professionals to clarify information, to guide people in wellness behavior, and to recommend specific activities for managing existing health conditions.

Access to informational services may have the greatest positive health benefit (Bass et al., 1998). For some users, even infrequent access to information resources has led to improved health outcomes. Because of their convenience and accessibility, it is possible that the network-based services offer timely, private access to information when needed by the individual. It is also possible that the network access, supporting both communication and information access, permits lay people to obtain factual knowledge in the context of peer support.

11.4.3 Quality of Information and Content Credentialing

The amount of information available to consumers is growing rapidly. This volume of information can be overwhelming. Therefore, consumers may need help in sifting through the mass of available resources. Furthermore, the quality of such information varies widely not only in terms of the extent to which it is accepted by the formal medical industry but also in its basic clinical or scientific accuracy. Therefore, a key issue in CHI lies in determining the quality and relevance of health information found on CD-ROMs or websites. **Credentialing** or certification by recognized bodies, such as respected healthcare providers or clinical professional associations, represents one approach to ensuring the quality of health information available to consumers. This approach bases its quality ratings on reviews and evaluations conducted by established knowledgeable sources. It has the advantage of delivering an imprimatur to a CD-ROM or website, which informs the user that the information presented met a standard of quality. Credentialing is most useful when the credential itself is accompanied by a statement indicating the perspectives and biases of those granting it. Information presented by alternative therapies and other nonclinical groups is no less susceptible to bias than is information presented by professional sources.

Inherent in the credentialing approach are three disadvantages. First, the challenge to ensure that every information element—every link in a decision program or pathway in a website—is tested and evaluated fully exceeds the resources available to do so (see Chapter 8). In many cases, the credentialing approach rests on certification of the group or individuals providing the information rather than approval of the content itself. Second, the credentialing approach leaves control of the authority for healthcare information in the hands of traditional care providers, reflecting both the expertise and the biases of established medical sources. Third, credentialing alone is inherently contradictory to healthcare consumerism, which empowers the consumer to make choices consistent with her own world view. A source's credential is just an additional piece of information that may be considered in making personal health decisions.

An approach to evaluating the quality and relevance of CHI resources that is consistent with a philosophy of patient participation is based on teaching patients and lay people how to evaluate CHI resources. Consumers with sufficient literacy and evaluation skills can locate CHI resources and determine these resources' relevance to their individual health concerns. Consumers can use six criteria to evaluate the quality and relevance of CHI resources to their situations (Table 11.6). Applying the criteria listed in Table 11.6 to the samples presented in Figures 11.1, 11.2, and 11.3 illustrates the strengths and weaknesses of the various presentations.

11.4.4 Challenges to Using the Internet for Public Health and Consumer Health

Because of the public, shared nature of the Internet, its resources are widely accessible by citizens and healthcare organizations. This public nature also presents challenges to the security of data transmitted along the Internet. The openness of the Internet leaves the transmitted data vulnerable to interception and inappropriate access. In its present form, the Internet offers little protection for sensitive health-related data. Without special security features, only aggregate community-level data or general health information can safely be transmitted along the Internet.

Ensuring every citizen access to the Internet represents a second important challenge to the ability to use it for public health and consumer health purposes. Access to the Internet presently requires computer equipment that may be out of reach for persons with marginal income levels. Majority-language literacy and the physical capability to type and read present additional requirements for effective use of the Internet. Preventing unequal access to healthcare resources delivered via the Internet will require that healthcare agencies work with other social service and educational groups to make available the technology necessary to capitalize on this electronic environment for health care.

11.4.5 Roles of Health Professionals in Consumer-Health Informatics

Healthcare professionals play three key roles in CHI. First, professionals serve as sources for content. Working in conjunction with software designers, clini-

TABLE 11.6. Sample criteria for evaluating consumer health information resources on the World Wide Web.

Credibility
Source
Context
Currency
Relevance/utility
Editorial review process
Content
Accuracy
Hierarchy of evidence
Original source stated
Disclaimer
Omissions noted
Disclosure
Purpose of the site
Profiling
Links
Selection
Architecture
Content
Back linkages and description
Design
Accessibility
Logical organization navigability
Internal search engine
Interactivity
Mechanism for feedback
Chat rooms
Tailoring

Source: Criteria for Assessing the Quality of Health Information on the Internet, working draft white paper, October 14, 1997 http://hitiweb.mitretek.org/docs/criteria.html [January 1999].

cians provide relevant information on the nature and course of illnesses and expected treatment. To be most effective as content experts, clinicians should consider not only the physiological causes of disease but also the social and environmental causes and consequences of illnesses. Second, professionals provide important guidance in moderating public electronic discussion groups and responding to patients' electronic messages. This responsibility challenges clinicians to modify existing interventions to ensure proper interpretation and clear communication when interacting with patients electronically. Third, clinicians become information brokers and interpreters for patients, directing patients to relevant resources and using time in the clinical encounter to discuss observations, to help interpret the meaning and relevance of particular information, and to aid patients to translate information into behavioral changes in their lives.

11.5 Future Directions

The shifting focus from treating illness to managing health and wellness requires that clinicians know not only the history of the individuals they treat but also information about the social and environmental context within which those individuals reside. In the chlamydia example, knowledge of the rates of sexually transmitted diseases in an area and the appropriate diagnostic and interventional protocols aid the clinical staff in providing timely and appropriate treatment.

> Encouraged by Karen, Tom goes to see Derek Smith, his family physician. "Karen and the baby have something and they said I have it too." Smith runs a test and confirms the diagnosis of chlamydia. He knows that he should provide Tom with treatment, but he is not sure whether he should instruct Tom about contact tracing for patients with chlamydia. In addition, he recalls from a lecture in school that some diseases are "reportable"—but he is not sure whether chlamydia infection is one of these.

To carry this example further, access to additional information on community issues and characteristics could further help in care planning.

> One year later, Baby Sarah's pediatrician is conducting a well-baby checkup. She confirms that the baby's lung capacity and function are within normal limits. She has learned this week of a warning of potential lead epidemic among toddlers in her town. She consults a Geographic Information System (GIS) map survey of the community. On this map, she sees which neighborhoods have older homes. Children living in older homes have greater risk of exposure to lead in paint dust and from water that has passed through lead pipes. She determines that Baby Sarah's house is not in a designated risk area, so she does not screen for lead, but she does counsel Karen and Tom about paint, use of clay pots, and so on.

Through the Internet and private intranets, a wealth of public health information and provider-oriented information resources is available to clinicians in practice. Workstations connected to secure or public networks facilitate access to public-health information that can help clinicians to diagnose disease and to plan treatment. Using CDC Wonder or the CDC's website, clinicians can verify the reportability of illness or confirm an unusual clinical presentation of an infectious disease. An interface between the clinical information system and the infectious disease reporting system would allow for concurrent recording of the patient's status in the clinical record and automatic reporting of notifiable diseases to public-health authorities.

From the provider perspective, clinicians now encounter patients who come to the appointment prepared with citations from Medline or comments pulled down from an electronic chat group. Working with enlightened patients demands new skills for clinicians and changes the nature of the clinical encounter. Time must be allotted to discuss information patients have read, to help patients interpret the relevance of the information to themselves, and to refer patients to appropriate resources. Clinicians are challenged to become information brokers and to devise new ways to ensure that patients are prepared to participate in the clinical interaction.

Technology alone will not determine the extent to which these changes occur. A major social change is needed on the part of both clinicians and patients if they are to become full partners in health care. Patients have been socialized to assume a passive, dependent role in health care, presenting themselves for diagnosis and treatment with little planning. At the same time, clinicians have enjoyed the privilege of control, holding fast to the possession of expert knowledge and therefore direction to patients. In addition, not all clinicians and patients now or ever will have computers. Furthermore, there will always be many situations where use of technology is not feasible or is inappropriate due to the patient's physical or mental health status, level of literacy, comfort with technology, or access to information resources.

Contemporary pressures to share decision-making with patients and to assume a longitudinal perspective to health problems necessitate that we involve patients early and continuously in their own care. Further development of consumer-health technologies will allow patients access to the knowledge that they need for care and the analytical tools necessary to ensure that they know their own minds. Technology also will increasingly support the clinician in integrating patient preferences, scientific knowledge, and practical realities of care into efficient treatment plans. The availability of new and integrated public-health technologies will ensure the expansion of reference from the individual in the clinic, to her home, community, and life.

Perhaps the greatest long-term effect of the information/communications revolution will be the breaking down of role, geographic, and social barriers. Medicine is already greatly benefiting from this effect. Traditional "doctors and nurses" are collaborating with public health professionals; the sick and the well can easily access information that only 5 years ago was unavailable to the lay public (or did not exist at all); everyone with computer access can potentially communicate with experts around the world. We now have the tools to develop new healthcare models, wherein clinicians, community leaders, families, and friends collaborate to prevent illness, promote health, care for the sick, and develop and administer new therapies. This vision is no longer a pipe dream: We can do it today. The challenge will be to facilitate productive collaborations between patients, their caregivers, biomedical scientists, and information technology experts.

Suggested Readings

Brennan P.F. (1996). The future of clinical communication in an electronic environment. *Holistic Nursing Practice,* 11(1):97–104.

Dyadic interaction forms the core of the clinician–patient relationship. Modifications in familiar skills are needed to form those relationships in a healthcare environment that increasingly relies on technology to maintain contact with patients.

Brennan P.F., Ripich S. (1994). Use of a home-care computer network by persons with AIDS. *International Journal of Technology Assessment in Health Care,* 10(2):258–272.
Thirty people living with AIDS used a computer network to form a small community. The stories of four participants illustrate the various ways that electronic communication fosters, and occasionally inhibits, social support and peer interaction.

Friede A., O'Carroll P.W. (1998). Public health informatics. In Last J.M. (Ed.), *Maxcey-Rosenau-Last Public Health and Preventive Medicine*, 14th ed. Norwalk, CT: Appleton & Lange, pp. 59–65.
This book provides a thorough discussion of public health informatics, including the development and use of public health information systems.

Widman L., Tong D.A. (1997). Requests for medical advice from patients and families to health care providers who publish on the World Wide Web. *Archives of Internal Medicine,* 15(2):209–212.
Provision of advice over the Internet is emerging as a respectable, and important, practice component for some physicians. This article summarizes the kinds of questions posed and the answers provided.

Questions for Discussion

1. Your city wants to build a new community health facility. What public health informatics data and information system resources might inform the political process?
2. Some people involved in CHI advocate that any publicly accessible health information be credentialed (reviewed and certified as accurate) by a professional body. Other people argue that credentialing is antithetical to the consumerist perspective. Assume and defend one of these perspectives.
3. To be optimally useful, public-health interventions require full disclosure of events within the clinical encounter. Identify three key issues of privacy and confidentiality. Prepare a dialogue between a physician and a consumer advocate that enables patients to understand and to choose mindfully how to preserve confidentiality while not disrupting the clinical and public health processes.

12
Patient Care Systems

JUDY G. OZBOLT AND SUZANNE BAKKEN

After reading this chapter, you should know the answers to these questions:

- What are the four major information-management issues in patient care?
- How have patient-care systems evolved during the last three decades?
- How have patient-care systems influenced the process and outcomes of patient care?
- Why are patient-care systems essential to the computer-based patient record?
- How can they be differentiated from the computer-based patient record itself?

12.1 Information Management in Patient Care

Patient care is the focus of many clinical disciplines—medicine, nursing, pharmacy, nutrition, therapies such as respiratory, physical, and occupational, and others. Although the work of the various disciplines sometimes overlaps, each has its own primary focus, emphasis, and methods of care delivery. Each discipline's work is complex in itself, and collaboration among disciplines adds another level of complexity. In all disciplines, the quality of clinical decisions depends in part on the quality of information available to the decision-maker. The systems that manage information for patient care are therefore a critical tool. Their fitness for the job varies, and the systems enhance or detract from patient care accordingly. This chapter describes information-management issues in patient care, the evolution of patient care systems in relation to these issues, and current research. It will also show how patient care systems provide the infrastructure that determines the quality and functions of the computer-based patient record.

12.1.1 Concepts of Patient Care

Patient care is a multidisciplinary process centered on the care recipient in the context of the family, significant others, and community. Typically, patient care includes the services of physicians, nurses, and members of other health disciplines according to patient needs: physical, occupational, and respiratory therapists; nutritionists; psychologists; social workers; and many others. Each of these disciplines brings specialized perspectives and expertise. Specific cognitive processes and therapeutic techniques vary by discipline, but all disciplines share certain commonalities in the provision of care.

In its simplest terms, the process of care begins with collecting data and assessing the patient's current status in comparison to criteria or expectations of normality. Through cognitive processes specific to the discipline, diagnostic labels are applied, therapeutic goals are identified with timelines for evaluation, and therapeutic interventions are selected and implemented. At specified intervals, the patient is reassessed, the effectiveness of care is evaluated, and therapeutic goals and interventions are continued or adjusted as needed. If the reassessment shows that the patient no longer needs care, services are terminated. This process was illustrated for nursing in 1975 (Goodwin & Edwards, 1975) and was updated and made more general in 1984 (Ozbolt et al., 1985). The flowchart reproduced in Figure 12.1 could apply equally well to other patient-care disciplines.

Although this linear flowchart helps to explain some aspects of the process of care, it is, like the solar-system model of the atom, a gross simplification. Frequently, for example, in the process of collecting data for an initial patient assessment, the nurse may recognize (diagnose) that the patient is anxious about her health condition. Simultaneously with continuing the data collection, the nurse sets a therapeutic goal that the patient's anxiety will be reduced to a level that increases the patient's comfort and ability to participate in care. The nurse selects and implements therapeutic actions of modulating the tone of voice, limiting environmental stimuli, maintaining eye contact, using gentle touch, asking about the patient's concerns, and providing information. All the while, the nurse observes the effects on the patient's anxiety and adjusts his behavior accordingly. Thus, the complete care process can occur in a microcosm while one step of the care process—data collection—is underway. This simultaneous, nonlinear quality of patient care poses challenges to informatics in the support of patient care and the capture of clinical data.

Each caregiver's simultaneous attention to multiple aspects of the patient is not the only complicating factor. Just as atoms become molecules by sharing electrons, the care provided by each discipline becomes part of a complex molecule of **multidisciplinary care.** Caregivers and developers of informatics applications to support care must recognize that true multidisciplinary care is as different from the separate contributions of the various disciplines as an organic molecule is from the elements that go into it. The contributions of the various disciplines are not merely additive; as a force acting on the patient, the work of each discipline is transformed by its interaction with the other disciplines in the larger unity of patient care.

For example, a 75-year-old woman with rheumatoid arthritis, high blood pressure, and urinary incontinence might receive care from a physician, a home-care nurse, a nutritionist, a physical therapist, and an occupational therapist. From a

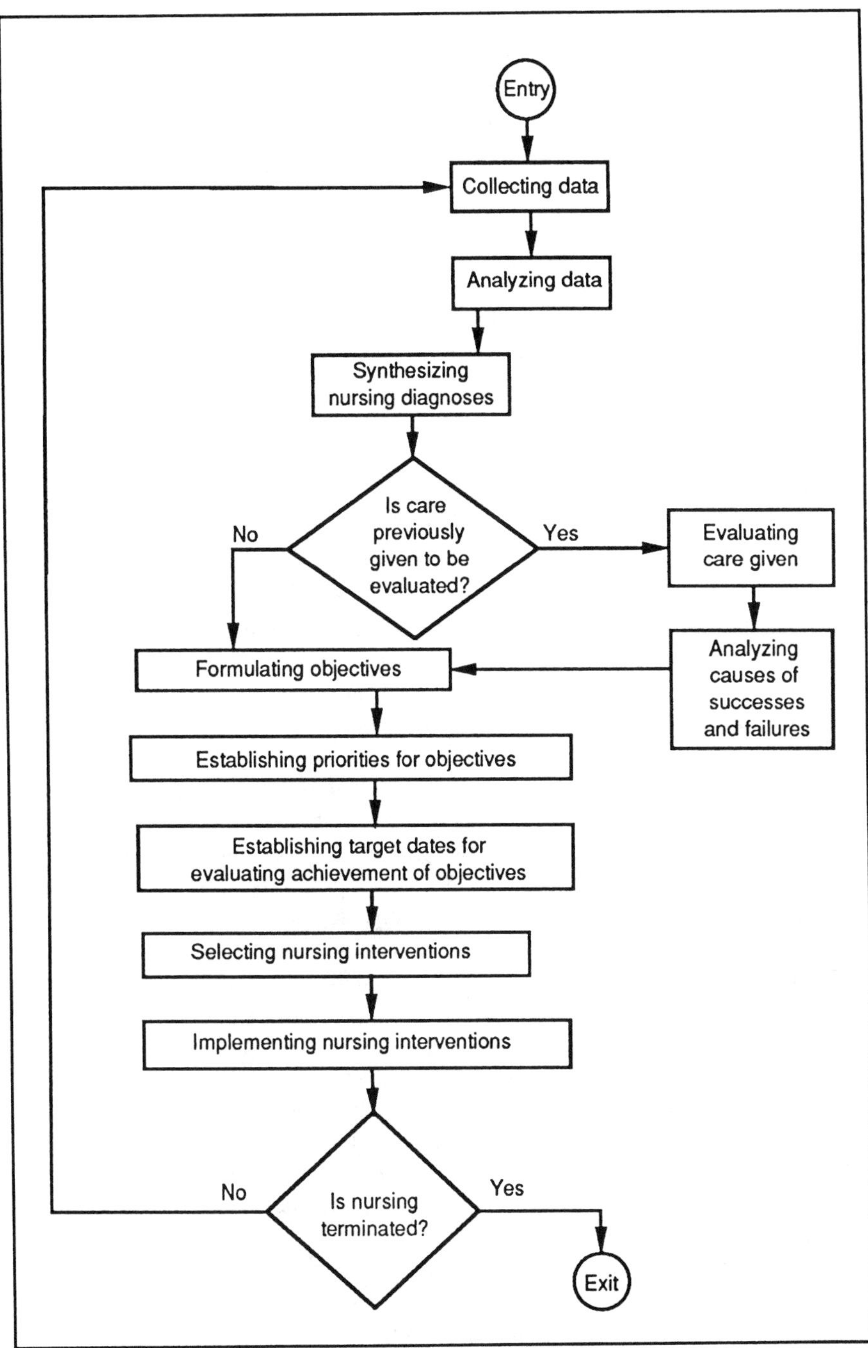

FIGURE 12.1. The provision of nursing care is an iterative process that consists of steps to collect and analyze data, to plan and implement interventions, and to evaluate the results of interventions. (*Source:* Adapted with permission from Ozbolt J.G., et al. [1985]. A proposed expert system for nursing practice. *Journal of Medical Systems,* 9:57–68.

simplistic, additive perspective, each discipline could be said to perform the following functions:

1. Physician: diagnose diseases, prescribe appropriate medications, authorize other care services
2. Nurse: assess patient's understanding of her condition and treatment and her self-care abilities and practices; teach and counsel as needed; help patient to perform exercises at home; report findings to physician and other caregivers
3. Nutritionist: assess patient's nutritional status and eating patterns; prescribe and teach appropriate diet to control blood pressure and build physical strength
4. Physical therapist: prescribe and teach appropriate exercises to improve strength and flexibility and to enhance cardiovascular health, within limitations of arthritis
5. Occupational therapist: assess abilities and limitations for performing activities of daily living; prescribe exercises to improve strength and flexibility of hands and arms; teach adaptive techniques and provide assistive devices as needed

In a collaborative, multidisciplinary practice, the nurse might discover that the patient was not taking walks each day as prescribed because her urinary incontinence was exacerbated by the diuretic prescribed to treat hypertension, and the patient was embarrassed to go out. The nurse would report this to the physician and the other caregivers so that they can understand why the patient was not carrying out the prescribed regime. The physician might then change the strategy for treating hypertension while initiating treatment for urinary incontinence. The nurse would help the patient to understand the interaction of the various treatment regimes, would provide practical advice and assistance in dealing with incontinence, and would help the patient to find personally acceptable ways to follow the prescribed treatments. The nutritionist might work with the patient on the timing of meals and fluid intake so that the patient could exercise and sleep with less risk of urinary incontinence. The physical and the occupational therapists would adjust their recommendations to accommodate the patient's personal needs and preferences while moving toward the therapeutic goals. Finally, the patient, rather than being assailed with sometimes conflicting demands of multiple caregivers, would be supported by an ensemble of services. Such collaboration, however, requires exquisite communication and feedback. The potential for information systems to support or sabotage this kind of care is obvious.

Although the care of individual patients is thus complex, it is far from being the totality of patient care. Because patients receive services from multiple caregivers, someone must coordinate those services. Coordination includes seeing that patients receive all the services they need in logical sequence without scheduling conflicts and ensuring that each caregiver communicates as needed with the others. Sometimes, a **case manager** is designated to do this coordination. In other situations, a physician or a nurse assumes the role by default. Sometimes, coordination is left to chance, and both the processes and the outcomes of care are put at risk.

Delivering and managing the multidisciplinary care of each patient would seem to be sufficiently challenging, but patient care has yet another level of complexity. Each caregiver is usually responsible for the care of multiple patients. In planning and executing the work of caregiving, each professional must consider the competing demands of all the patients for whom she is responsible, as well as the exigencies of all the other professionals involved in each patient's care. Thus, the nurse on a post-operative unit must plan for scheduled treatments for each of her patients to occur near the optimal time for that patient. She must take into account that several patients may require treatments at nearly the same time and that some of them may be receiving other services, such as X-ray or physician's visits, at the time when it might be most convenient for the nurse to administer the treatment. When unexpected needs arise, as they often do—an emergency, an unscheduled patient, observations that could signal an incipient complication—the nurse must set priorities, organize, and delegate to be sure that at least the critical needs are met. Decision-support systems have the potential to provide important assistance for both clinical and organizational decisions.

Finally, caregivers not only deliver services to patients, with all the planning, documenting, collaborating, referring, and consulting attendant on direct care; they are also responsible for **indirect-care** activities, such as teaching and supervising students, attending staff meetings, participating in continuing education, and serving on committees. Each caregiver's plan of work must allow for both the direct-care and the indirect-care activities. Because the caregivers work in concert, these plans must be coordinated.

In summary, patient care is an extremely complex undertaking with multiple levels. Each caregiver's contributions to the care of every patient must take into account the ensemble of contributions of all caregivers and the interactions among them, all coordinated to optimize effectiveness and efficiency. Moreover, these considerations are multiplied by the number of patients for whom each caregiver is responsible. Patient care is further complicated by the indirect-care activities that caregivers must intersperse among the direct-care responsibilities and coordinate with other caregivers. It is little wonder that managing, processing, and communicating data, information, and knowledge are integral and critical to every aspect of patient care.

12.1.2 Information to Support Patient Care

As complex as patient care is, the essential information for direct patient care is defined in the answers to the following questions:

- Who is involved in the care of the patient?
- What information does each professional require to make decisions?
- From where, when, and in what form does the information come?
- What information does each professional generate? Where, when, and in what form is it needed?

The framework described by Zielstorff and others (1993) provides a useful heuristic for understanding the varied types of information required to answer each of these questions. As listed in Table 12.1, this framework delineates three information categories: (1) patient-specific data, which are those data about a particular patient acquired from a variety of data sources; (2) agency-specific data, which are those data relevant to the specific organization under whose auspices the health-care is provided; and (3) domain information and knowledge, which is specific to the health-care disciplines.

The framework further identifies four types of information processes that information systems may apply to each of the three information categories. **Data acquisition** entails the methods by which data become available to the information system. It may include data entry by the care provider or acquisition from a medical device or from another computer-based system. **Data storage** includes the methods, programs, and structures used to organize data for subsequent use. Examples of standardized coding and classification systems useful in representing patient care concepts are listed in Table 12.2. This topic is discussed in greater detail in Chapters 2, 6, and 9. **Data transformation** or **processing** comprises the methods by which stored data or information are acted on according to the needs of the end user—for example, calculation of a decubitus risk-assessment score at admission or calculation of critically ill patients' acute physiology and chronic health evaluation (APACHE) scores. Figure 12.2 illustrates the transformation (abstraction, summarization, aggregation) of patient-specific data for multiple uses. **Presentation** encompasses the forms in which information is delivered to the end user after processing.

Transformed patient-specific data can be presented in a variety of ways. Numeric data may be best presented in chart or graph form to allow the user to examine trends, whereas the compilation of potential diagnoses generated from patient-assessment data lends itself to an alphanumeric-list format. Different types of agency-specific data lend themselves to a variety of presentation formats. Common among all, however, is the need for presentation at the point of patient care; for example, the integration of up-to-the-minute patient-specific data with agency-specific guidelines or parameters can produce alerts, reminders, or other types of notifications for immediate action. See Chapter 13, on patient-monitoring systems, for an overview of this topic. Presentation of domain information and knowledge related to patient care is most frequently accomplished through interaction with databases and knowledge bases, such as Medline or DXplain (see Chapter 15). Another example is the Pressure Ulcer Prevention and Management System that captures coded data about assessment, diagnosis, and intervention and provides guideline-based decision support (Zielstorff et al., 1996).

To support patient care, information systems must be geared to the needs of all the professionals involved in care. The systems should acquire, store, process, and present each type of information (patient, agency, and domain specific) where, when, and how each function is needed by each professional. These systems not only support each professional's care of individual patients but also, through appropriate use of patient-specific information (care requirements),

Table 12.1. Framework for design characteristics of a patient-care information system with examples of patient-specific data, agency-specific data, and domain information and knowledge for patient care.

Types of data	System processes			
	Acquiring	Storing	Transforming	Presenting
Domain-specific	Downloading relevant scientific or clinical literature or practice guidelines	Maintaining information in electronic journals or files, searchable by key words	Linking related literature or published findings; updating guidelines based on research	Displaying relevant literature or guidelines in response to queries
Agency-specific	Scanning, downloading, or keying in agency policies and procedures; keying in personnel, financial, and administrative records	Maintaining information in electronic directories, files, and databases	Editing and updating information; linking related information in response to queries; analyzing information	Displaying on request continuously current policies and procedures shoring relevant policies and procedures in response to queries; generating management reports
Patient-specific	Point-of-care entry of data about patient assessment, diagnoses, treatments planned and delivered, therapeutic goals patient outcomes	Moving patient data into a current electronic record or an aggregate data repository	Combining relevant data on a single patient into a cue for action in a decision-support system; performing statistical analyses on data from many patients	Displaying reminders, alerts probable diagnoses, or suggested treatments; displaying vital signs graphically; displaying statistical results

Source: Framework adapted with permission from *Next Generation Nursing Information Systems*, 1993, American Nurses Association, Washington, DC.

TABLE 12.2. Examples of standardized coding and classification systems with utility for patient care.

System	Problems	Interventions	Outcomes
International Classification of Diseases	x		
NANDA Taxonomy 1	x		
Current Procedural Terminology		x	
Nursing Interventions Classification		x	
Nursing Outcomes Classification			x
Omaha System	x	x	x
Home Health Care Classification	x	x	x
SNOMED International	x	x	x
Patient Care Data Set	x	x	x

agency-specific information (caregivers and their responsibilities and agency policies and procedures), and domain information (guidelines), such systems can greatly aid the coordination of multidisciplinary services for individual patients and the planning and scheduling of each caregiver's work activities. Such integrated systems—still an ideal today—would enhance our understanding of each patient's situation and needs, improve decision-making, facilitate communications, aid coordination, and use clinical data to provide feedback for improving clinical processes.

Clearly, when patient-care information systems fulfill their potential, they will not merely replace oral and paper-based methods of recording and communicat-

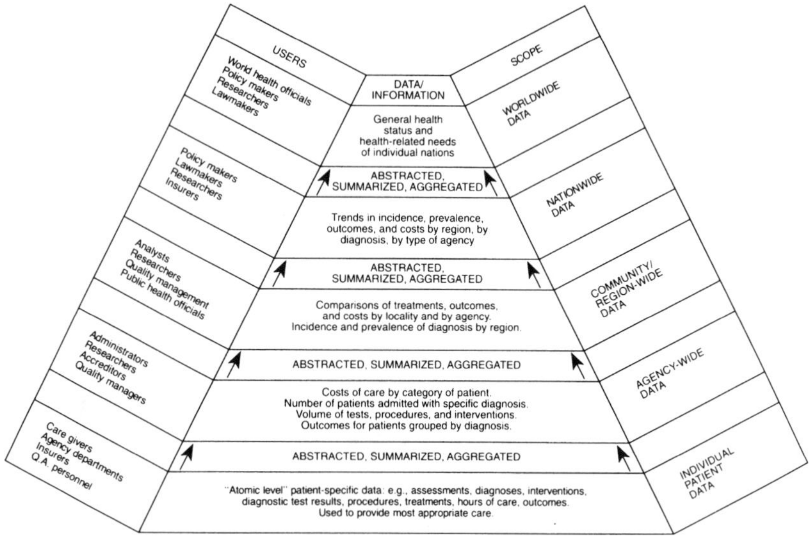

FIGURE 12.2. Examples of uses for atomic-level patient data collected once but used many times. (*Source:* Reprinted with permission from R. D. Zielstorff, C. I. Hudgings, S. J. Grobe, and The National Commission on Nursing Implementation Project Task Force on Nursing Information Systems. *Next-Generation Nursing Information Systems,* © 1993 American Nurses Publishing, American Nurses Foundation/American Nurses Association, Washington, DC.)

ing. They will not only support but also transform patient care. How far have we come toward the ideal? What must we do to continue our progress?

12.2 Historical Evolution of Patient-Care Systems

The genesis of patient care systems occurred in the mid-1960s. One of the first and most successful systems was the Technicon Medical Information System (TMIS), begun in 1965 as a collaborative project between Lockheed and El Camino Hospital in Mountain View, California (see Chapter 10). Designed to simplify documentation through the use of standard order sets and care plans, TMIS defined the state of the art when it was developed. More than three decades later, versions of TMIS are still widely used, but the technology has moved on. The hierarchical, menu-driven arrangement of information in TMIS required users to page through many screens to enter or retrieve data and precluded aggregation of data across patients for statistical analysis. Today's users have a different view of what can be done with data, and they demand systems that support those uses.

Part of what changed users' expectations for patient care systems was the development and evolution of the HELP system (see Chapters 9, 10, and 13) at LDS Hospital in Salt Lake City, Utah. Initially providing decision support to physicians during the process of care (in addition to managing and storing data), HELP has subsequently become able to support nursing care decisions and to aggregate data for research leading to improved patient care. Today, both vendors of information systems and researchers in health-care enterprises are working to incorporate decision support and data aggregation features in systems that use the latest technologies for navigating and linking information.

12.2.1 Societal Influences

The historical evolution of information systems that support patient care is not solely a reflection of the available technologies. Societal forces—including delivery-system structure, practice model, payer model, and quality focus—have influenced the design and implementation of patient-care systems (Table 12.3).

Delivery-System Structure

Authors have noted the significant influence of the organization and its people on the success or failure of informatics innovations (Ash, 1997; Kaplan, 1997; Lorenzi et al., 1997; Southon et al., 1997). As delivery systems have shifted from the predominant single-institution structure of the 1970s to the integrated delivery systems of the 1990s, the information needs have changed, and the challenges of meeting those information needs have increased in complexity. See Chapter 10 for a discussion of managing clinical information in integrated delivery systems.

Table 12.3. Societal forces that have influenced the design and implementation of patient care systems.

	1970s	1980s	1990s
Delivery-system structure	Single institution	Single organization	Integrated delivery systems
Professional-practice model	Team nursing Single or small group physician practice	Primary nursing Group models for physicians	Patient-focused care Multidisciplinary care Case management Variety of constellations of physician group practice models
Payer model	Fee for service	Fee for service Prospective payment, diagnosis-related groups (DRGs)	Capitation Managed Care
Quality focus	Professional Standards Review Organizations (PSROs) Retrospective chart review Joint Commission on Accreditation of Hospitals' Peer Evaluation Program Quality of Patient Care System (QUALPACS)	Continuous quality improvement Joint Commission on Accreditation of Health Care Organization (JCAHO)'s Agenda for Change	Risk-adjusted outcomes Benchmarking Practice guidelines Critical paths/care maps Health Employer Data and Information set (HEDIS)

Professional Practice Models

Professional practice models have also evolved for nurses and physicians. In the 1970s, team nursing was the typical practice model for the hospital, and the nursing care plan—a document for communicating the plan of care among nursing team members—was most frequently the initial application designed for use by nurses. The 1990s have been characterized by a shift to multidisciplinary-care approaches necessitating computer-based applications such as critical paths to support case management of aggregates of patients, usually with a common medical diagnosis, across the **continuum of care**.

Physician practice models have shifted from single physician or small group offices to complex constellations of provider organizations. The structure of the model (e.g., staff model health-maintenance organization, captive-group model health-maintenance organization, or independent-practice association; see Chapter 19) determines the types of relationships among the physicians and the organizations. These include issues—such as location of medical records, control of practice patterns of the physicians, and data-reporting requirements—that have significant implications for the design and implementation of patient-care systems. In addition, the multidisciplinary-care approaches of the 1990s have given impetus to system-design strategies, such as the creation of a single-patient problem list, around which the patient-care record is organized, in place of a separate list for each provider group (e.g., nurses, physicians, respiratory therapists).

Payer Models

Changes in payer models have been a significant driving force for information-system implementation in many organizations. With the shift from fee for service to prospective payment in the 1980s, and then toward capitation in the 1990s, information about costs and quality of care has become an essential commodity for rational decision-making in the increasingly competitive healthcare marketplace. See Chapter 19 for a thorough discussion of the effects of healthcare financing on health-care information systems.

Quality Focus

Demands for information about quality of care have also influenced the design and implementation of patient-care systems. The quality-assurance techniques of the 1970s were primarily based on retrospective chart audit. In the 1980s, continuous-quality-improvement techniques became the *modus operandi* of most healthcare organizations. The quality-management techniques of the 1990s were much more focused on concurrently influencing the care delivered than on retrospectively evaluating its quality. Patient-care systems-based approaches—such as critical paths, practice guidelines, alerts, and reminders—are an essential component of **quality management**. In addition, institutions must have the capacity to capture data for benchmarking purposes and to report process and outcomes data to regulatory and accreditation bodies, as well as to any voluntary reporting programs (e.g., Maryland Hospital Indicator Program) to which they belong.

12.2.2 Patient-Care Systems

The design and implementation of **patient-care systems**, for the most part, occurred separately for hospital and ambulatory-care settings. The components of several hospital information systems (HISs) and ambulatory-care systems are listed in Table 12.4. The systems were selected to provide a snapshot of the period. For a comprehensive review, see Collen (1995).

According to Collen (1995), the most commonly used patient-care systems in hospitals of the 1980s were those that supported nursing care planning and documentation. Systems to support capture of physicians' orders, communications with the pharmacy, and reporting of laboratory results were also widely used. Some systems merged physician orders with the nursing care plan to provide a more comprehensive view of care to be given. This merging, such as allowing physicians and nurses to view information in the part of the record designated for each other's discipline, was a step toward integration of information. It was still, however, a long way from support for truly collaborative multidisciplinary practice.

TABLE 12.4. Patient care components in selected information systems

Patient-care component	Examples: hospital	Examples: ambulatory care
Problem lists	Problem-Oriented Medical Information System (PROMIS), Medical Center Hospital of Vermont, Burlington, VT (Weed, 1975) Tri-Service Medical Information System (TRIMIS), Department of Defense (Bickel, 1979)	Computer-Stored Ambulatory Record (COSTAR), Massachusetts General Hospital, Boston, MA (Barnett, 1976) Summary Time-Oriented Record (STOR), University of California, San Francisco, CA (Whiting-O'Keefe et al., 1980)
Summary reports	Technicon Medical Information System (TMIS), Clinical Center at National Institutes of Health, Bethesda, MD (Hodge, 1990) Distributed Hospital Computer Program (DHCP), Department of Veteran's Affairs (Ivers & Timson, 1985)	Regenstrief, Regenstrief Institute, Indianapolis, IN (McDonald, 1976) Computer-Stored Ambulatory Record (COSTAR), Massachusetts General Hospital, Boston, MA (Barnett, 1976)
Order entry	Health Evaluation Logical Processing (HELP), Latter Day Saints Hospital, Salt Lake City, UT (Kuperman et al., 1991) Technicon Medical Information System (TMIS), Clinical Center at National Institutes of Health, Bethesda, MD (Hodge, 1990)	The Medical Record (TMR), Duke University Medical Center, Durham, NC (Hammond et al., 1980)
Results review	University of Missouri—Columbia System, Columbia, MO (Lindberg, 1965) Decentralized Hospital Computer Program (DHCP), Department of Veteran's Affairs (Ivers & Timson, 1985)	Computer-Stored Ambulatory Record (COSTAR), Massachusetts General Hospital, Boston, MA (Barnett, 1976) Summary Time-Oriented Record (STOR), University of California, San Francisco, CA (Whiting-O'Keefe et al., 1980)
Nursing protocols and care plans	Health Evaluation Logical Processing (HELP), Latter Day Saints Hospital, Salt Lake City, UT (Kuperman et al., 1991) Technicon Medical Information System (TMIS) El Camino Hospital, Mountain View, CA (Watson, 1977)	
Alerts and reminders	Health Evaluation Logical Processing (HELP), Latter Day Saints Hospital, Salt Lake City, UT (Kuperman et al., 1991) Beth Israel Hospital System, Boston, MA (Safran et al., 1989)	Regenstrief, Regenstrief Institute, Indianapolis, IN (McDonald, 1976) The Medical Record (TMR), Duke University Medical Center, Durham, NC (Hammond et al., 1980)

Early ambulatory-care systems most often included paper-based, patient encounter forms that were either computer-scannable mark-sense format or were subsequently entered into the computer by clerical personnel. Current desktop, laptop, or hand-held systems use keyboard, mouse, or pen-based entry of structured information, with free text kept to a minimum. These systems also provide for retrieval of reports and past records. Some systems provide decision support or alerts to remind clinicians about needed care, such as immunizations or screening examinations, and to avoid contraindicated orders for medications or unnecessary laboratory analyses. Depending on network capabilities, systems may facilitate communications among the professionals and settings involved in the patient's care. Voice-recognition technology is advancing and is beginning to permit direct dictation into the record. Although this mode of data entry has the advantages of ease and familiarity to clinicians, free text in the record inhibits search, retrieval, and analysis of data. Before dictated notes can become as useful as structured data, the entry systems will have to become able to recognize the meanings of words and their context and to store the data in databases. Although this level of intelligent processing of natural language remains in the future, systems to support ambulatory care have clearly made great strides. The best provide good support for traditional medical care. Support for comprehensive, collaborative care that gives as much attention to health promotion as to treatment of disease presents a challenge not only to the developers of information systems but also to practitioners and healthcare administrators who must explicate the nature of this practice and the conditions under which agencies will provide it.

Patient-care information systems in use today represent a broad range in the evolution of the field. Versions of some of the earliest systems are still in use. These systems were generally designed to speed documentation and to increase legibility and availability of the records of patients currently receiving care. Most lack the capacity to aggregate data across patients, to query the data about subsets of patients, or to use data collected for clinical purposes to meet informational needs of administrators or researchers. These shortcomings seem glaring today, but they were not apparent when the very idea of using computers to store and communicate patient information required a leap of the imagination.

More recently developed systems attempt with varying success to respond to the edict "collect once, use many times." Selected items of data from patient records are abstracted manually or electronically to aggregate databases where they can be analyzed for administrative reports or for clinical or health-services research. Moreover, these recent systems may offer some degree of coordination of the information and services of the various clinical disciplines into integrated records and plans. Data collected by one caregiver can appear, possibly in a modified representation, in the "view" of the patient record designed for another discipline. When care-planning information has been entered by multiple caregivers, it can be viewed as the care plan to be executed by a discipline, by an individual, or by the multidisciplinary team. Some patient-care systems offer the option to organize care temporally into **clinical pathways** and to have variances from the anticipated activities, sequence, or timing reported automatically.

Many healthcare agencies have substantial investment in legacy systems and cannot simply switch to more modern technology. Finding ways to phase the transition from older systems to newer and more functional ones is a major challenge to health informatics. To make the transition from a patchwork of systems with self-contained functions to truly integrated systems with the capacity to meet emerging information needs is even more challenging (see Chapter 10). Approaches to making this transition are described in the Proceedings of the 1996 IAIMS Symposium (IAIMS, 1996) and in the *Journal of the American Medical Informatics Association* (Stead et al., 1996).

12.2.3 Nursing Informatics

Like every other healthcare discipline, nursing contributes its specialized knowledge and skills to patient care. Unlike other disciplines, however, nursing has historically provided continuous presence with the patient and a domain of professional responsibility that embraces all aspects of the patient's health, illness, and treatment. Thus, physicians diagnose diseases, identify risks of disease, and prescribe preventive or therapeutic interventions. Other caregivers assess patients in their domains of expertise and implement prescribed therapies. Nurses assess patients' responses to illness, health risks, development through the lifespan, and treatments and they also identify ways to enhance coping, to promote health, to facilitate recovery, to reduce suffering, or to find peace and dignity in dying. The broad scope of nursing's responsibilities and the nurse's continuing presence with the patient place nursing at the heart of patient care and at the hub of patient information. This disciplinary experience has given rise to developments in **nursing informatics** that can inform the development of integrated multidisciplinary applications for patient care.

The centrality of patient care to nursing informatics is captured in the National Center for Nursing Research priority panel report entitled "Nursing Informatics: Enhancing Patient Care" and in the research priorities delineated in the report (National Priority Expert Panel on Nursing Informatics, 1993). Because nurses are the primary provider of patient-care in most settings, nursing informatics has influenced the design and implementation of patient-care systems in the hospital, in the home, and in other community-based settings. Indeed, the predominant definition of nursing informatics could, with minor changes in wording, be applied generally to **clinical informatics**: "a combination of computer science, information science, and nursing science designed to assist in the management and processing of nursing data, information and knowledge to support the practice of nursing and the delivery of nursing care" (Graves & Corcoran, 1989). How then can the knowledge and experience developed in nursing informatics foster more general developments in patient-care information systems?

Nursing Vocabularies

The cornerstone of good patient-care systems is the ability to capture clinical data in the process of care, to store the data, to aggregate them, to analyze them, and to produce reports that not only describe care but also yield knowledge of quality, effectiveness, and costs that can be the basis of improved clinical processes. The key to performing these operations is **data standards** (see Chapters 6 and 9). Traditionally, however, nurses' data about patients were recorded in narrative notes, with both content and phrasing as varied and individual as the nurses. This tradition is similar to those in other health disciplines.

The earliest efforts to define a standard vocabulary for nursing arose from the need to name the clinical nursing problems that would be entered into a computer-based record-keeping system. In response to this need, the First National Conference on Classification of Nursing Diagnoses was held at St. Louis University in 1973 (Gordon, 1982). It led to subsequent conferences and eventually to the formation of the North American Nursing Diagnosis Association (NANDA). NANDA's methods of adopting terms into the standard vocabulary have evolved over the years but generally have involved review of nominated terms by a designated group and classification of the terms into categories of diagnoses. Early inductive methods of naming diagnostic categories through recollection of many clinical examples were later augmented by deductive efforts to generate diagnostic categories from a conceptual model of nursing.

By the 1980s, efforts to develop nursing language were gathering momentum. The Omaha Visiting Nurses Association needed a way to simplify clinical record keeping and to generate reports of activities and costs. The nurses developed their own version of standard terms for patient problems, clinical actions, and patient outcomes to facilitate computer-based records and reports (Simmons, 1980). The Omaha System of vocabulary and documentation was subsequently adopted by a number of community-based nursing agencies (Martin & Scheet, 1995). In 1985, Werley and Lang convened an invitational conference on the Nursing Minimum Data Set (NMDS) to identify data elements that should be collected on all patients and abstracted from the records for studies of costs and effectiveness (Werley & Lang, 1988). In 1987, a group at the University of Iowa began a carefully designed research project involving consensus development and validation to name and classify nursing interventions (McCloskey & Bulecheck, 1996). In 1992, we saw creation of the Home Health Care Classification, a set of terms for nursing diagnoses and interventions derived and classified by statistical methods from a national sample of homehealth care patient records (Saba, 1992, 1994). Shortly thereafter, the Patient Care Data Set was developed to identify standard terms for patient problems, patient care actions, and expected patient outcomes used in nine acute-care hospitals across the United States (McDaniel, 1997; Ozbolt, 1996; Ozbolt et al., 1994, 1995).

The sets of terms developed through these projects have provided the basis for nursing-data dictionaries in patient-care systems. More recently, the American

Nurses Association has fostered the inclusion of these nursing-data elements in patient-care systems through a "recognition" program of classification systems that comprise a Unified Nursing Language System (McCormick et al., 1994) and through the creation of an evaluation center, the Nursing Information and Data Systems Evaluation Center (NIDSEC), to accredit that a particular patient-care system meets specific requirements to support the practice of nursing and the delivery of nursing care (American Nurses Association, 1997).

The processes whereby terms have been derived and proposed for standard use in nursing information systems can demonstrate to other health disciplines both productive strategies and pitfalls in creating controlled vocabularies to replace natural-language text. The methods used to generate standard terms range from nomination and consensus to empirical identification in patient records. Each approach has its strengths and limitations. The resulting sets of terms, like many medical vocabularies, have been found to fulfill their intended functions well but to be less suited to other purposes (Henry et al., 1994). The variety of terms provides richness and vigor for capturing clinical events, but no one ideal set of terms predominates as *the* standard. A unified, as opposed to a uniform, language may be the best feasible approach to standard terminology.

Nursing Informatics Education

In addition to vocabulary development, nursing informatics offers examples of ways to prepare clinicians to work in roles related to patient-care systems. The National League for Nursing published guidelines for basic computer education in nursing in 1987. The preparation of advanced-practice nurse informaticists at the Master's level was facilitated through federally funded programs at the University of Maryland, Baltimore, and at the University of Utah, as well as through subspecialization in nursing administration programs (e.g., University of Texas at Austin; University of California, San Francisco). In 1995, a scope of practice for nursing informatics was published by the American Nurses Association, and a certification examination based on the standards was initiated in 1995 (American Nurses Association, 1995). The number of nurses choosing to complete multidisciplinary training in informatics in National Library of Medicine training programs has also increased in recent years. These efforts have produced a cadre of informaticists well prepared for key roles in patient-care-systems design, implementation, and evaluation.

To what degree do other patient-care disciplines need to prepare their practitioners for informatics roles? To the degree that members of the discipline use information in ways unique to the discipline, the field needs members prepared to translate the needs of clinicians to those who develop, implement, and make decisions about information systems. If the information needs are different from those of other disciplines, some practitioners should be prepared as system developers.

This section has only briefly described the influence of nursing informatics on patient-care systems. For an in-depth historical perspective on nursing and computers, see Saba and McCormick (1996).

12.3 Current Research

Friedman (1995) proposed a typology of the science in medical informatics. The four categories build from fundamental conceptualization to evaluation as follows:

- Formulating models for acquisition, representation, processing, display, or transmission of biomedical information or knowledge
- Developing innovative computer-based systems, using these models, that deliver information or knowledge to healthcare providers
- Installing such systems and then making them work reliably in functioning healthcare environments
- Studying the effects of these systems on the reasoning and behavior of healthcare providers, as well as on the organization and delivery of health care

Following are examples of recent research on patient-care systems in each category.

12.3.1 Formulation of Models

Standardized coding and classification (SCC) systems are a prerequisite for patient-care information systems, including databases, knowledge bases, patient records, and expert systems. SCC systems vary in purpose, in scope, in structure, and in the level of granularity (abstract versus atomic) of the data elements. As discussed in Chapter 6 and noted earlier in this chapter (see Table 12.2), extensive work is underway to develop and refine SCC systems for patient care (Forrey et al., 1996; Maas et al., 1996; Martin & Scheet, 1992; McCloskey & Bulecheck, 1996; McFarland & McFarlane, 1993; Rothwell et al., 1993; Saba, 1992). To date, the American Nurses Association's Steering Committee on Databases to Support Nursing Practice (renamed the Clinical Practice Information Infrastructure Committee in 1998) has recognized six systems as part of a Unified Nursing Language System (McCormick et al., 1994). These include the nursing diagnoses identified by NANDA (Warren & Hoskins, 1995); the Home Health Care Classification of nursing diagnoses and interventions (Saba, 1995); the Omaha System of Nursing Diagnoses, Interventions, and Client Outcomes (Martin & Scheet, 1995); the Nursing Interventions Classification (NIC) (Bulecheck et al., 1995); the Nursing Outcomes Classification (NOC) (Maas et al., 1996); and Ozbolt's Patient Care Data Set, encompassing patient problems, therapeutic goals, and patient care orders (Ozbolt, 1996; Ozbolt et al., 1994). Grobe and associates are utilizing natural-language processing techniques to examine both the content and structure of nursing documentation as an extension of the work on the Nursing Intervention Lexicon and Taxonomy (Grobe, 1996). At the international level, the International Council of Nursing, is working on the creation of an International Classification of Nursing Practice to accompany the existing World Health Organization classifications (Clark & Lang, 1992; Mortensen & Nielsen, 1996; Nielsen & Mortensen, 1996).

The evaluation of the adequacy of existing standardized classification schemes to represent clinical data has also been the focus of recent investigations (Campbell et al., 1997; Griffith & Robinson, 1992; Henry et al., 1997; Lange, 1996). One of the broadest studies was conducted by Chute and others for the Computer-Based Patient Record Institute's Work Group on Codes and Structures. They reported on a comparative study of seven SCC systems in coding 3,061 distinct concepts from four medical centers (Chute et al., 1996). The concepts were grouped into Diagnoses, Modifiers, Findings, Treatments and Procedures, and Other. The concept matches were scored as no match, fair match, and complete match. SNOMED (see Chapter 6) had the highest score in each category. Not surprisingly, SCC systems developed to represent a specific domain, Current Procedural Terminology codes for physicians and NANDA diagnoses for nurses, scored lowest. A series of studies by Henry and associates (1994, 1997) provided evidence that disciplines overlap in the terms used for description of patient problems but that discipline-specific intervention schema were required. The evaluation studies have been unanimous in their conclusions that, although each vocabulary served the purpose for which it was designed, no one existing vocabulary or unifying scheme was adequate to represent the broad array of patient-care data.

12.3.2 Development of Innovative Systems

New systems to support patient care often are designed to take advantage of information entered in one context for use in other contexts. For example, the Brigham Integrated Computing System (BICS), a PC-based client–server HIS supporting Brigham and Women's Hospital in Boston, uses information from the order entry, scheduling, and other systems to prepare drafts of the physician's discharge orders and the nurse's discharge abstract, thus minimizing the information to be entered manually. The professionals review the drafts and edit as needed (O'Connell et al., 1996). Similarly, information entered once is used many times in the low-cost bedside workstations for intensive-care units developed at the University Hospital of Giessen, Germany (Michel et al., 1996). The client–server architecture combines local data-processing capabilities with a central relational patient database, permitting, for example, clinical nursing data to be used in calculating workload. These workstations also combine data from many sources, including medical devices, to support the integrated care of physicians, nurses, and other caregivers. Still another system is under development to support case management by prospectively comparing clinical data with defined critical pathways and alerting the responsible professional to variances during the process of care (Bliss-Holtz, 1995).

Even as systems such as these begin to fulfill some of the promises of informatics to support patient care, research and development continue to address the demands that the complexities of patient care place on information systems. Hoy and Hyslop (1995) reported a series of projects directed toward the development of a person-based health record. They found problems with traditional approaches to automating paper-based care-planning systems that resulted in loss of data detail, inability to use data for multiple purposes, and limitations in the capacity to aggregate and query patient data. Hoy and Hyslop (1995) recommended:

- Making the structure of the clinical record (including the care plan) more flexible and extensible to allow summarized higher-level data, with lower-level details where appropriate
- Simplifying the elements of that structure to make data entry and retrieval easier and more effective

Hoy and Hyslop (1995) built a prototype system to demonstrate their recommendations. Like other investigators, they concluded that "the issues of language and structures must be dealt with before the integration of person-based systems can be realized."

12.3.3 Implementation of Systems

Higgins and associates (see Rotman et al., 1996) described the lessons learned from a failed implementation of a computer-based physician workstation that had been designed to facilitate and improve ordering of medications. Those lessons are not identical to, but are consistent with, the recommendations of Leiner and Haux (1996) in their protocol for systematic planning and execution of projects to develop and implement patient-care systems. As these experiences demonstrate, the implementation of patient-care systems is far more complex than the replacement of one technology with another. Such systems transform work and organizational relationships. If the implementation is to succeed, attention must be given to these transformations and to the disruptions that they entail. Southon and colleagues (1997) provided an excellent case study of the role of organizational factors in the failed implementation of a patient-care system that had been successful in another site. To realize the promise of informatics for health and clinical management, people who develop and promote the use of applications must anticipate, evaluate, and accommodate the full range of consequences.

12.3.4 Study of the Effects of Systems

A frequent expectation of systems to support nursing care planning and documentation is that they will decrease the time required for documentation, improve the quality and relevance of data in the record, and increase the proportion of nursing time spent in direct patient care. Pabst and colleagues (1996) found that an automated system designed to replace just 40 percent of manual documentation decreased the time required for documentation by one third, or by 20 minutes per shift. Nurses using the system spent more time in direct patient care and were more likely than were nurses using only manual documentation to complete documentation during their shifts rather than staying over into the next shift. Quality of documentation was not affected. Adderley and associates (1997) described the benefits of a phased implementation of a paperless record as related to accessibility of the record. Verbal orders were eliminated, and progress notes were more likely to be entered. Communications among caregivers were enhanced. Prospective, rather than retrospective, reviews of clinical data provided concurrent assessment of patient progress, care planning, medication use, and ancillary services. Annual cost avoidance from using the electronic patient record was estimated at more than $300,000.

Seeking a more representative assessment of the influence of clinical information systems on nursing practice, Axford and Carter (1996) used qualitative methods to design a survey instrument and then surveyed a random sample of nurses who used and who did not use computers in providing care. The qualitative phase identified the following six categories of impacts of clinical information systems on nursing practice: time, cost, satisfaction with nursing, nursing work itself, professional status, and patient outcomes. The survey showed that users of systems generally had more favorable opinions than nonusers about the influence of the systems on practice. As health informatics evolves, we can anticipate more direct investigations of the effects of information technology on the process of care.

Improving the methods of evaluating information resources was the driving force behind the Institute of Medicine's 1996 report on telemedicine (Field, 1996). Finding assessments of technical performance insufficient, the report recommended that evaluations focus on effects on patient welfare and on the processes and costs of care in comparison to those of reasonable alternatives. Members of the committee who developed the report noted that telemedicine may be considered a subset of medical informatics and that the methods of research and evaluation applicable to telemedicine are like those applicable to other patient-care systems (also see Chapter 8).

12.4 Outlook for the Future

Patient-care systems are changing in two ways. First, legacy systems designed primarily for charge capture and other administrative functions are being replaced by systems designed to support and improve clinical practice, as well as to send clinical data to the various locations where these data are needed for practice, management, and research. Second, systems designed to support each discipline separately are yielding to those based on integrated, multidisciplinary concepts of care. Research is continuing to develop structured clinical languages, standards, and data models; to develop innovative systems; to determine more effective and efficient ways to implement systems; and to investigate the effects of changing information resources on the processes of care and the functioning of the organization.

This environment is a fertile one for the development and growth of patient-care systems. The first decade of the twenty-first century will see the fruits of today's trends, as more and more clinicians gain access to systems that offer intelligent support for clinical decisions; better organization and communication; feedback on clinical effectiveness; linked databases for research; and administrative analyses based on pertinent clinical data. Such tools will make available to clinicians, managers, and policy-makers the data, information, and knowledge required for sound decisions and effective action. By complementing and extending cognitive processes, patient-care systems become an integral and essential technology for patient care.

Suggested Readings

Ball M. (Ed.) (1995). *Introduction to Nursing Informatics*. New York: Springer.

This second edition comprises six units: (1) integration, (2) roles for informatics nurse specialists, (3) clinical applications and nursing informatics, (4) administration and nursing informatics, (5) research and nursing informatics, and (6) education and nursing informatics. The appendices include useful tools such as a site-visit checklist, sample request for proposal, index to computer-assisted instructional software, and list of electronic resources of interest to nurses.

Henry S.B., Holzemer W.L., Tallberg M., Grobe, S. (1996). Informatics: Infrastructure for quality assessment and improvement in nursing. *Proceedings of the Fifth International Nursing Informatics Symposium (NI94) Post-Conference*, Austin, TX.

This proceedings of the Fifth International Nursing Informatics Symposium (NI94) Post-Conference includes papers in four areas: (1) informatics as infrastructure for quality assessment and improvement, (2) national and international perspectives on clinical nursing vocabulary projects, (3) controlling variations in practice, and (4) role of informatics in measuring the outcome of care. Also included are action agendas for clinical practice, education, administration, and research focused on significant questions related to the four areas addressed in the papers.

McCloskey J.C., Bulechek G.M. (1996). *Nursing Interventions Classification* (2nd ed.). St. Louis: C.V. Mosby.

This text provides a comprehensive overview of the development and testing of the Nursing Interventions Classification (NIC). The taxonomic structure of NIC is described. Numeric codes and linkages with NANDA diagnoses are included.

Saba V.K., McCormick K. (1996). *Essentials of Computers for Nurses*. New York: McGraw-Hill.

The second edition of this classic text on computers in nursing provides a comprehensive historical overview of nursing informatics. Also of note in this edition is a new chapter on outcomes and guidelines applications.

Zielstorff R.D., Hudgings C.I., Grobe, S.J. (1993). *Next-Generation Nursing Information Systems: Essential Characteristics for Nursing Practice*. Washington, DC: American Nurses Publishing.

This book describes the principles and guidelines for the nursing component of a system supporting patient care. Included are a framework for organizing patient-care concepts; system benefits; and an action plan, describing the activities of nurses and systems developers, that will hasten the development and implementation of nursing information systems.

Questions for Discussion

1. What is the utility of a linear model of patient care as the basis for a decision-support system? What are two primary limitations? Discuss two challenges that a nonlinear model poses for representing and supporting the care process in an information system?
2. Compare and contrast "segregated" versus "integrated" models of multidisciplinary patient care. What are the advantages and disadvantages of each model as a mode of care delivery? As the basis for developing information systems to plan, document, and support patient care?
3. Imagine a patient-care information system that assists in planning the care of each patient independently of all the other patients in a service center or patient-care unit. What are three advantages to the developer in choosing such an information architecture? What would be the likely result in the real world of practice? Does it make a difference whether the practice setting is hospital, ambulatory care, or home care? What would be the simplest information architecture that would be sufficiently complex to handle real-world demands? Explain.
4. Zielstorff et al. (1993) proposed that data routinely recorded during the process of patient care could be abstracted, aggregated, and analyzed for management reports, policy decisions, and knowledge development. What are three advantages of using patient care data in this way? What are three significant limitations?
5. A number of patient-care information systems designed in the 1970s are still in use. How do the practice models, payer models, and quality focus of today differ from those of the past? What differences do these changes require in information systems? What are two advantages and two disadvantages of "retrofitting" these changes on older systems versus designing new systems "from scratch"?
6. What are three advantages and three disadvantages of free text (including oral narrative entered by dictation) versus structured data for recording observations, assessments, goals, and plans? What is the impact of using free text on the ability to retrieve and aggregate data? Should developmental efforts focus on interpreting natural language or on creating data standards? Explain your position.
7. What are four major purposes of patient care information systems? What criteria should be used to evaluate them? What methods of evaluation could be used to assess the system with respect to these criteria?

13
Patient-Monitoring Systems

REED M. GARDNER AND M. MICHAEL SHABOT

After reading this chapter,[1] you should know the answers to these questions:

- What is patient monitoring, and why is it done?
- What are the primary applications of patient-monitoring systems in the intensive-care unit?
- How do computer-based patient monitors aid health professionals in collecting, analyzing, and displaying data?
- What are the advantages of using microprocessors in bedside monitors?
- What are the important issues for collecting high-quality data either automatically or manually in the intensive-care unit?
- Why is integration of data from many sources in the hospital necessary if a computer is to assist in most critical-care-management decisions?

13.1 What Is Patient Monitoring?

Continuous measurement of patient parameters such as heart rate and rhythm, respiratory rate, blood pressure, blood-oxygen saturation, and many other parameters have become a common feature of the care of critically ill patients. When accurate and immediate decision-making are crucial for effective patient care, electronic monitors frequently are used to collect and display physiological data. Increasingly, such data are collected using non-invasive sensors from less seriously ill patients in a hospital's medical-surgical units, nursing homes, or patients' own homes to detect unexpected life-threatening conditions or to record routine but required data efficiently.

We usually think of a **patient monitor** as something that watches for—and warns against—serious or life-threatening events in patients, critically ill or oth-

[1] Portions of this chapter are based on Shabot M.M., Gardner R.M. (Eds.) (1994). *Decision Support Systems in Critical Care,* Boston, Springer-Verlag; and Gardner R.M., Sittig D.F., Clemmer T.P. (1995). Computers in the ICU: A Match Meant to Be! In Ayers S.M., et al. (Eds.), *Textbook of Critical Care* (3rd ed., p. 1757). Philadelphia, W.B. Saunders.

erwise. **Patient monitoring** can be rigorously defined as "repeated or continuous observations or measurements of the patient, his or her physiological function, and the function of life support equipment, for the purpose of guiding management decisions, including when to make therapeutic interventions, and assessment of those interventions" (Hudson, 1985, p. 630). A patient monitor may not only alert caregivers to potentially life-threatening events; many also provide physiologic input data used to control directly connected life-support devices.

In this chapter, we discuss the use of computers to assist caregivers in the collection, display, storage, and interpretation of physiological data. In the past most physiologic data were in the form of heart and respiratory rates, blood pressures, and flows, but now they include bedside measurements of blood gases, chemistry, and hematology. Although we deal primarily with patients who are in intensive-care units (ICUs), the general principles and techniques are also applicable to other hospitalized patients. For example, patient monitoring may be performed for diagnostic purposes in the emergency room or for therapeutic purposes in the operating room. Techniques that just a few years ago were used only in the ICU are now routinely used on general hospital units and in some cases by patients at home.

13.1.1 A Case Report

A case report provides a perspective on the problems faced by the healthcare team caring for a critically ill patient: A young man is injured in an automobile accident. He has multiple chest and head injuries. His condition is stabilized at the accident scene by skilled paramedics using a microcomputer-based electrocardiogram (ECG) monitor, and he is quickly transported to a trauma center. Once in the trauma center, the young man is connected via sensors to computer-based monitors that determine his heart rate and rhythm and his blood pressure. Because of the head injury, the patient has difficulty breathing, so he is connected to a microprocessor-controlled ventilator. Later, he is transferred to the ICU. A fiberoptic pressure-monitoring sensor is inserted through a bolt drilled through the skull to continuously measure intracranial pressure with another computer-controlled monitor. Clinical chemistry and blood-gas tests are performed in two minutes at the bedside with a microcartridge inserted into the physiologic monitor, and the results are transmitted to the laboratory computer system and the ICU system using a Health Level 7 (HL7) interface over a standard Ethernet network. With intensive treatment, the patient survives the early threats to his life and now begins the long recovery process.

Unfortunately, a few days later, he is beset with a problem common to multiple trauma victims—he has a major nosocomial (hospital-acquired) infection and develops sepsis, adult respiratory distress syndrome (ARDS), and multiple organ failure. As a result, even more monitoring sensors are needed to acquire data and to assist with the patient's treatment; the quantity of information required to care for the patient has increased dramatically.

The ICU computer system provides suggestions about how to care for the specific problems, provides visual alerts for life-threatening situations, and organizes and reports the mass of data so that caregivers can make prompt and reliable treatment decisions. The patient's physicians are automatically alerted to critical laboratory and blood gas results as well as to complex physiological conditions by detailed alphanumeric pager messages. His ARDS is managed with the assistance of a computer-monitored and controlled protocol. Figure 13.1 shows an example of a computer-generated ICU report produced by the HELP system (HELP is discussed in Chapter 10). This report summarizes 24 hours of patient data and is used by physicians to review a patient's status during daily rounds (daily visits by physicians to their hospitalized patients).

13.1.2 Patient Monitoring in Intensive-Care Units

There are at least four categories of patients who need physiological monitoring:

1. Patients with unstable physiological regulatory systems; for example, a patient whose respiratory system is suppressed by a drug overdose or anesthesia
2. Patients with a suspected life-threatening condition; for example, a patient who has findings indicating an acute myocardial infarction (heart attack)
3. Patients at high risk of developing a life-threatening condition; for example, patients immediately after open-heart surgery or a premature infant whose heart and lungs are not fully developed
4. Patients in a critical physiological state; for example, patients with multiple trauma or septic shock.

Care of the critically ill patient requires prompt and accurate decisions so that life-protecting and life-saving therapy can be appropriately applied. Because of these requirements, ICUs have become widely established in hospitals. Such units use computers almost universally for the following purposes:

- To acquire physiological data frequently or continuously, such as blood pressure readings
- To communicate information from data-producing systems to remote locations (e.g., laboratory and radiology departments)
- To store, organize, and report data
- To integrate and correlate data from multiple sources
- To provide clinical alerts and advisories based on multiple sources of data
- To function as a decision-making tool that health professionals may use in planning the care of critically ill patients
- To measure the severity of illness for patient classification purposes
- To analyze the outcomes of ICU care in terms of clinical effectiveness and cost effectiveness

L D S   H O S P I T A L   I C U   R O U N D S   R E P O R T
DATA WITHIN LAST 24 HOURS

NAME: , STEVEN   NO. 10072   ROOM: E609   DATE: JAN 29 14:17
DR. STINSON, JAMES B.   SEX: M   AGE: 43   HEIGHT: 178   WEIGHT: 75.40   BSA: 1.93   BEE: 1697   MOF: 0
ADMT DIAGNOSIS: FEVER UNK ORIGN, S/P KIDNEY TR   ADMIT DATE: 14 DEC 88

CARDIOVASCULAR: 0   EXAM: ________
-- NO CARDIAC OUTPUT DATA AVAILABLE

	SP	DP	MP	HR	LACT	CPK	CPK-MB	LDH-1	LDH-2
LAST VALUES	121	68	89	113					
MAXIMUM	194	97	126	124	( )	( )	( )	( )	( )
MINIMUM	101	58	72	83					

RESPIRATORY: 0

	pH	PCO2	HCO3	BE	HB	CO/MT	PO2	SO2	O2CT	%O2	AVO2	VO2	C.O.	A-a	QS/QT	PK/ PL/PP	MR/SR
29 06:21 A	7.43	27.3	18.0	-4.5	10.0	2/ 1	80	94	13.2	30				66		0/ 0/ 5	17/ 0

SAMPLE # 74, TEMP 38.4, BREATHING STATUS : ASSIST/CONTROL
NORMAL ARTERIAL ACID-BASE CHEMISTRY
SEVERELY REDUCED O2 CONTENT (13.2) DUE TO ANEMIA (LOW HB)

------- machine settings ------- | ---------------------------- patient values ----------------------------

	VENT	MODE	VR	Vt	O2%	PF	IP	MAP	PK	PL	PP	m-Vt	c-Vt	s-Vt	MR	SR	TR	m-VE	s-VE	t-VE	Cth	Pc
29 14:15	B-I	A/C	16	700	30	50			32	26	5	866	731		29			21.2			34.8	
29 06:05	B-I	A/C	16	700	30	50			22	20	5	830	745		19			14.2			49.7	

29 14:15 5/14:16 INTERFACE: TRACH TUBE; ALARMS CHECKED; POSITION: SUPINE; THERAPIST: DAVIS, TERIANNE, CRTT
29 06:05 10/06:08 INTERFACE: TRACH TUBE; ALARMS CHECKED; POSITION: SEMI-FOWLER; PATIENT CONDITION: CALM; SUCTIONED, 3 CC, HEMOPTIC; THERAPIST: TARR, TED, RRT

DATE	TIME	HR	VR	VT	VC	VE	MIP	MEP	MVV	PK FLOW	THERAPIST
01/29/89	07:15	109	20	600		12.0	-60				DAVIS, TERIANNE

EXAM: ________

NEURO AND PSYCH: 0
GLASCOW 6 (08:00) VERBAL ________ EYELIDS ________ MOTOR ________ PUPILS ________ SENSORY ________
DTR ________ BABIN. ________ ICP ________ PSYCH ________

COAGULATION: 0
PT: 14.2 (05:15) PTT: 50 (05:15) PLATELETS: 89 (05:15) FIBRINOGEN: 0(00:00) EXAM: ________
FSP-CON: 0 (00:00) FSP-PT: 0 (00:00) 3P: (00:00)

RENAL, FLUIDS, LYTES: 0
IN 3430 CRYST 1025 COLLOID 1035 BLOOD NG/PO 1340 | NA ( ) K ( ) CL ( )
OUT 2689 URINE 800 NGOUT 500 DRAINS 25 OTHER 1364 | CO2 21.0 (05:15) BUN 51 (05:15) CRE 4.2 (05:15)
NET 741 WT 75.40 WT-CHG S.G. 1.015 | AGAP 16.7 UOSM UNA CRCL

METABOLIC --- NUTRITION: 0
KCAL 2630 GLU 138 (05:15) ALB 2.9 (05:15) | CA 7.7 (05:15) FE .0 (00:00) TIBC 0 (00:00)
KCAL/N2 891 UUN .0 (00:00) N-BAL .0 | PO4 1.9 (05:15) MG 1.9 (05:15) CHOL 228 (05:15)

GI, LIVER, AND PANCREAS: 0   EXAM:
HCT 29.4 (05:15) TOTAL BILI 23.1 (05:15) SGOT 73 (05:15) ALKPO4 957 (05:15) GGT 768 (05:15) ________
GUAIAC ( ) DIRECT BILI 17.4 (05:15) SGPT 99 (05:15) LDH 237 (05:15) AMYLASE 0 (00:00) ________

INFECTION: 0
WBC 5.2(05:15) TEMP 40.3 (28/06:00) DIFF 26 B, 70P, 3L, 1M, E (05:15) GRAM STAIN: SPUTUM ________ OTHER ________

SKIN AND EXTREMITIES:
PULSES ________ RASH ________ DECUBITI ________

TUBES:
VEN ________ ART ________ SG ________ NG ________ FOLEY ________ ET ________ TRACH ________ DRAIN ________
CHEST ________ RECTAL ________ JEJUNAL ________ DIALYSIS ________ OTHER ________

MEDICATIONS:

MORPHINE, INJ	MGM	IV	20
MEPERIDINE (DEMEROL), INJ	MGM	IV	150
PHENYTOIN (DILANTIN), SUSPENSION	MGM	NG	300
MIDAZOLAM (VERSED), INJ	MGM	IV	5
AMPHOTERICIN B, INJ	MGM	IV	40
CEFTAZIDIME (FORTAZ), INJ	MGM	IV	1000
SUCRALFATE (CARAFATE), TAB	MGM	NG	4000
FAMOTIDINE (PEPCID), INJ	MGM	IV	40
AMPHOJEL, LIQUID	ML	NG	30
DIPHENHYDRAMINE (BENADRYL), INJ	MGM	IV	100
HYDROCORTISONE NA SUCCINATE (SOLU-CORTEF)	MGM,	IV	200
AMIN-AID FULL STRENGTH, LIQUID	ML	NG D	1380
TAP WATER, LIQUID	ML	NG	60
MAGNESIUM SULFATE 50%, INJ	GM	IV	2
POTASSIUM CHLORIDE, INJ	MEQ	IV	20
NOVOLIN REGULAR, INJ	UNITS	IV	58

#087 - pg1

FIGURE 13.1. Rounds report used at LDS Hospital in Salt Lake City for evaluation of patients each day during teaching and decision-making rounds. The report abstracts data from diverse locations and sources and organizes them to reflect the physiological systems of interest. Listed at the top of the report is patient-identification and patient-characterization information. Next is information about the cardiovascular system; data for other systems follow. (*Source:* Courtesy of LDS Hospital.)

13.2 Historical Perspective

The earliest foundations for acquiring physiological data date to the end of the Renaissance period.[2] In 1625, Santorio, who lived in Venice at the time, published his methods for measuring body temperature with the spirit thermometer and for timing the pulse (heart) rate with a pendulum. The principles for both devices had been established by Galileo, a close friend. Galileo worked out the uniform periodicity of the pendulum by timing the period of the swinging chandelier in the Cathedral of Pisa, using his own pulse rate as a timer. The results of this early biomedical-engineering collaboration, however, were ignored. The first scientific report of the pulse rate did not appear until Sir John Floyer published "Pulse-Watch" in 1707. The first published course of fever for a patient was plotted by Ludwig Taube in 1852. With subsequent improvements in the clock and the thermometer, the temperature, pulse rate, and respiratory rate became the standard **vital signs.**

In 1896, Scipione Riva-Rocci introduced the sphygmomanometer (blood-pressure cuff), which permitted the fourth vital sign, arterial blood pressure, to be measured. A Russian physician, Nikolai Korotkoff, applied Riva-Rocci's cuff with a stethoscope developed by the French physician Rene Laennec to allow the auscultatory measurement[3] of both systolic and diastolic arterial pressure. Harvey Cushing, a preeminent U.S. neurosurgeon of the early 1900s, predicted the need for and later insisted on routine arterial blood pressure monitoring in the operating room. Cushing also raised two questions familiar even at the turn of the century: (1) Are we collecting too much data? (2) Are the instruments used in clinical medicine too accurate? Would not approximated values be just as good? Cushing answered his own questions by stating that vital-sign measurements should be made routinely and that accuracy was important (Cushing, 1903).

Since the 1920s, the four vital signs—temperature, respiratory rate, heart rate, and arterial blood pressures—have been recorded in all patient charts. In 1903, Willem Einthoven devised the string galvanometer for measuring the ECG, for which he was awarded the 1924 Nobel Prize in physiology. The ECG has become an important adjunct to the clinician's inventory of tests for both acutely and chronically ill patients. Continuous measurement of physiological variables has become a routine part of the monitoring of critically ill patients.

At the same time that advances in monitoring were made, major changes in the therapy of life-threatening disorders were also occurring. Prompt quantitative evaluation of measured physiological and biochemical variables became essential in the decision-making process as physicians applied new therapeutic interventions. For example, it is now possible—and in many cases essen-

---

[2] This section has been adapted, with permission, from Glaeser D.H., Thomas L.J. Jr. (1975). Computer monitoring in patient care. *Annual Review of Biophysics and Bioengineering,* 4:449–476, copyright Annual Reviews, Inc.

[3] In medicine, auscultation is the process of listening to the sounds made by structures within the body, such as by the heart or by the blood moving within the vessels.

tial—to use ventilators when a patient cannot breathe independently, cardiopulmonary bypass equipment when a patient undergoes open-heart surgery, hemodialysis when a patient's kidneys fail, and intravenous (IV) nutritional and electrolyte (e.g., potassium and sodium) support when a patient is unable to eat or drink.

13.2.1 Development of Intensive-Care Units

To meet the increasing demands for more acute and intensive care required by patients with complex disorders, new organizational units—the ICUs—were established in hospitals beginning in the 1950s. The earliest units were simply post-operative recovery rooms used for prolonged stays after open-heart surgery. Intensive-care units proliferated rapidly during the late 1960s and 1970s. The types of units include burn, coronary, general surgery, open-heart surgery, pediatric, neonatal, respiratory, and multipurpose medical-surgical units. Today there are an estimated 75,000 adult, pediatric, and neonatal intensive care beds in the United States.

The development of **transducers** and electronic instrumentation during World War II dramatically increased the number of physiological variables that could be monitored. Analog-computer technology was widely available, as were oscilloscopes, electronic devices used to picture changes in electrical potential on a cathode-ray tube (CRT) screen. These devices were soon used in specialized cardiac-catheterization[4] laboratories, and they rapidly found their way to the bedside.

Treatment for serious cardiac arrhythmias (rhythm disturbances) and cardiac arrest (abrupt cessation of heartbeat)—major causes of death after myocardial infarctions—became possible. As a result, there was a need to monitor the ECGs of patients who had suffered heart attacks so that these episodes could be noticed and treated immediately. In 1963, Day reported that treatment of postmyocardial-infarction patients in a coronary-care unit reduced mortality by 60 percent. As a consequence, coronary-care units—with ECG monitors—proliferated. The addition of online blood-pressure monitoring quickly followed. **Pressure transducers,** already used in the cardiac-catheterization laboratory, were easily adapted to the monitors in the ICU.

With the advent of more automated instruments, the ICU nurse could spend less time manually measuring the traditional vital signs and more time observing and caring for the critically ill patient. Simultaneously, a new trend emerged; some nurses moved away from the bedside to a central console where they could monitor the ECG and other vital-sign reports from many patients. Maloney (1968) pointed out that this was an inappropriate use of technology when it deprived the

[4] A procedure whereby a tube (catheter) is passed into the heart through an artery or vein, allowing the cardiologist to measure pressure within the heart's chambers, to obtain blood samples, to inject contrast dye for radiological procedures, and so on.

patient of adequate personal attention at the bedside. He also suggested that having the nurse record vital signs every few hours was "only to assure regular nurse–patient contact" (Maloney, 1968, p. 606).

As monitoring capabilities expanded, physicians and nurses soon were confronted with a bewildering number of instruments; they were threatened by **data overload.** Several investigators suggested that the digital computer might be helpful in solving the problems associated with data collection, review, and reporting.

13.2.2 Development of Computer-Based Monitoring

Teams from several cities in the United States introduced computers for physiological monitoring into the ICU, beginning with Shubin and Weil (1966) in Los Angeles and then Warner and colleagues (1968) in Salt Lake City. These investigators had several motives: (1) to increase the availability and accuracy of data, (2) to compute derived variables that could not be measured directly, (3) to increase patient-care efficacy, (4) to allow display of the time trend of patient data, and (5) to assist in computer-aided decision-making. Each of these teams developed its application on a mainframe computer system, which required a large computer room and special staff to keep the system operational 24 hours per day. The computers used by these developers cost over $200,000 each in 1965 dollars! Other researchers were attacking more specific challenges in patient monitoring. For example, Cox and associates (1972) in St. Louis developed algorithms to analyze the ECG for rhythm disturbances in real-time. The arrhythmia-monitoring system, which was installed in the coronary-care unit of Barnes Hospital in 1969, ran on an inexpensive microcomputer.

As we described in Chapter 4, the advent of integrated circuits and other advances allowed computing power per dollar to increase dramatically. As hardware became smaller, more reliable, and less expensive, and as better software tools were developed, simple analog processing gave way to digital signal processing. Monitoring applications developed by the pioneers using large central computers now became possible using dedicated microprocessor-based machines at the bedside.

The early bedside monitors were built around "bouncing-ball" or conventional oscilloscopes and analog-computer technology (Fig. 13.2). As computer technology has advanced, the definition of **computer-based monitoring** has changed. The early developers spent a major part of their time deriving data from analog physiological signals. Soon the data-storage and decision-making capabilities of the computer monitoring systems came under the investigator's scrutiny. Therefore, what was considered computer-based patient monitoring in the late 1960s and early 1970s (Fig. 13.3) is now built into bedside monitors and is considered simply "patient monitoring." Systems with database functions, report-generation systems, and some decision-making capabilities are usually called **computer-based patient monitors.**

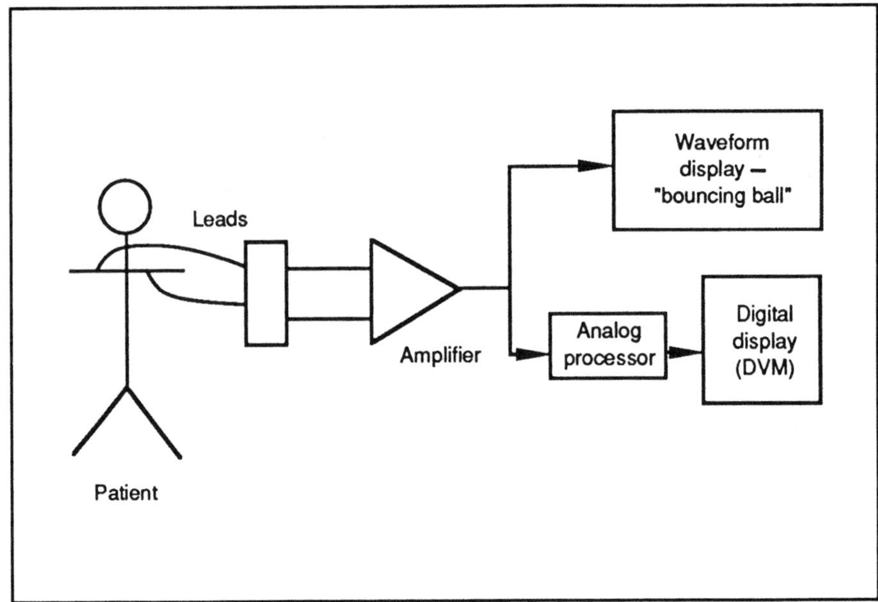

FIGURE 13.2. Block diagram of a typical analog monitor. These systems were developed in the early 1970s and are still in widespread use in hospitals today. DVM = digital volt meter.

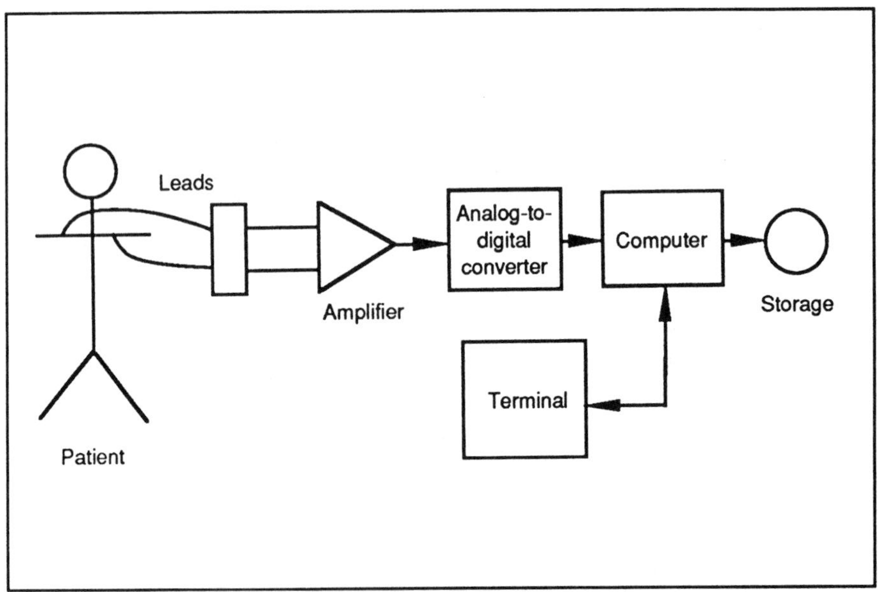

FIGURE 13.3. Analog monitor (see Fig. 13.2) with a minicomputer attached. The system configuration is much like that used more than two decades ago by the developers of early computer-based monitoring systems.

13.3 Data Acquisition and Signal Processing

The use of microcomputers in bedside monitors has revolutionized the acquisition, display, and processing of physiological data. There are virtually no bedside monitors or ventilators marketed today that do not use at least one microcomputer. Figure 13.4 shows a block diagram of a patient connected to sensors and bedside monitors. Sensors convert biological signals (such as pressure, flow, or mechanical movement) into electrical signals.

Some biological signals are already in electrical form, such as the currents that traverse the heart and are recorded as the ECG. Figure 13.5 shows a patient connected to ECG electrodes and an accompanying amplifier. The ECG signal derived from the electrodes at the body surface is small—only a few millivolts in amplitude. The patient is isolated from the electrical current of the monitor, and the analog ECG signal is amplified to a level sufficient for conversion to digital data using an analog-to-digital converter (ADC). Digital data then can be processed and the results displayed (Weinfurt, 1990, p. 130) (Fig. 13.6).

As discussed in Chapter 4, the sampling rate is an important factor that affects the correspondence between an analog signal and that signal's digital representation. Figure 13.7 shows an ECG that has been sampled at four different rates. At a rate of 500 measurements per second (Fig. 13.7a), the digitized representation of the ECG looks like an analog recording of the ECG. All the features of the ECG, including the shape of the P wave (atrial depolarization), the amplitude of the QRS complex (ventricular depolarization), and the shape of the T

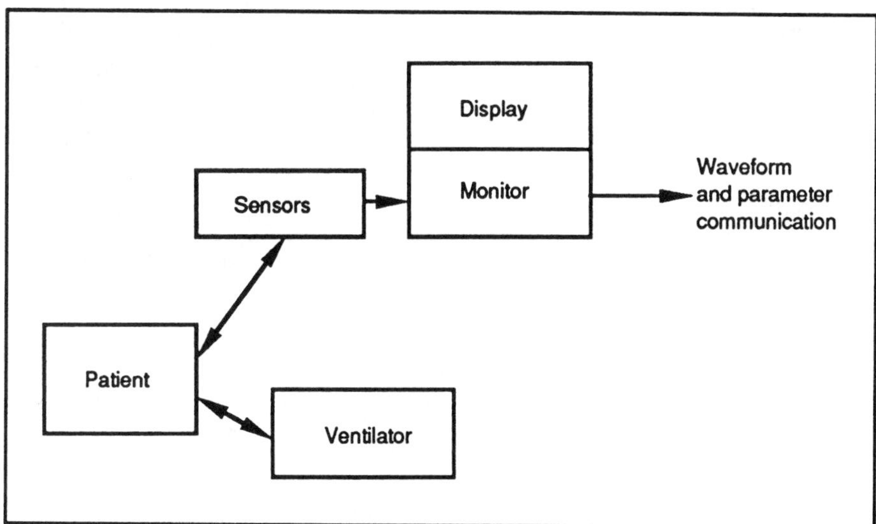

FIGURE 13.4. Block diagram of a simple bedside monitor with sensors attached to the patient. Signals are derived from the patient's physiological states and are communicated as waveforms and derived parameters to a central station display system.

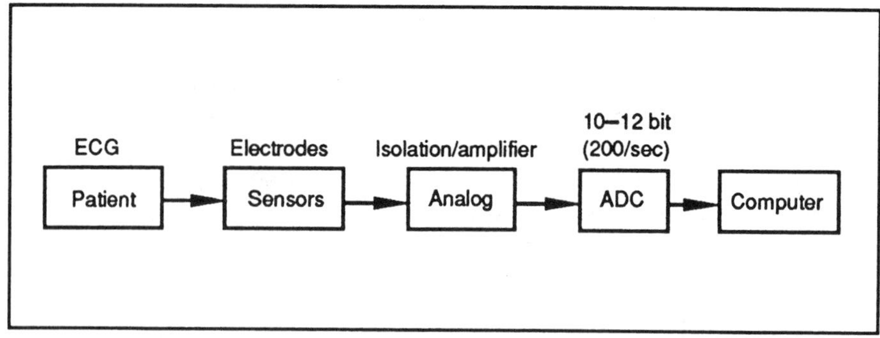

FIGURE 13.5. Front-end signal acquisition for a bedside monitor. The ECG signal is used as an example. The sensors (ECG electrodes) are attached to the patient. The resulting ECG signal is amplified by an electrically isolated analog amplifier and is presented to an analog-to-digital converter (ADC). The signal is sampled at a rate of 200 measurements per second with a 10-bit to 12-bit ADC; then it is presented to the computer for pattern analysis.

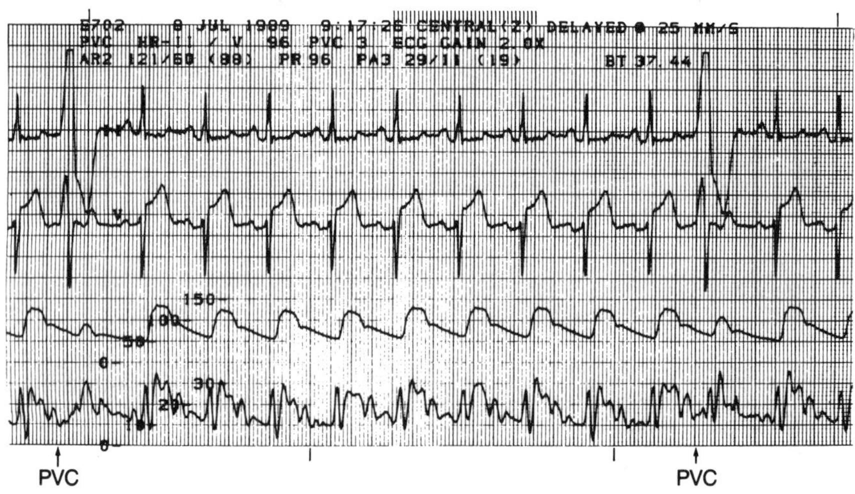

FIGURE 13.6. Electrocardiogram (first and second traces), arterial pressure (third trace), and pulmonary-artery pressure (fourth trace) recorded from a patient's bedside. Annotated on the recording are the bed number (E702), date (8 Jul 1989), and time (9:17:25). Also noted are a regular rhythm, a heart rate from the ECG (V) of 96 beats per minute, a systolic arterial pressure of 121, a diastolic pressure of 60, a mean pressure of 88 mm Hg, and a heart rate from pressure (PR) of 96. The patient is having premature ventricular contractions (PVCs) at a rate of three per minute; two PVCs can be seen in this tracing (at the beginning and near the end). The pulmonary-artery pressure is 29/11, with a mean of 19 mm Hg, and the blood temperature is 37.44°C. The self-contained monitoring system has determined the values and generated the calibrated graphical plot.

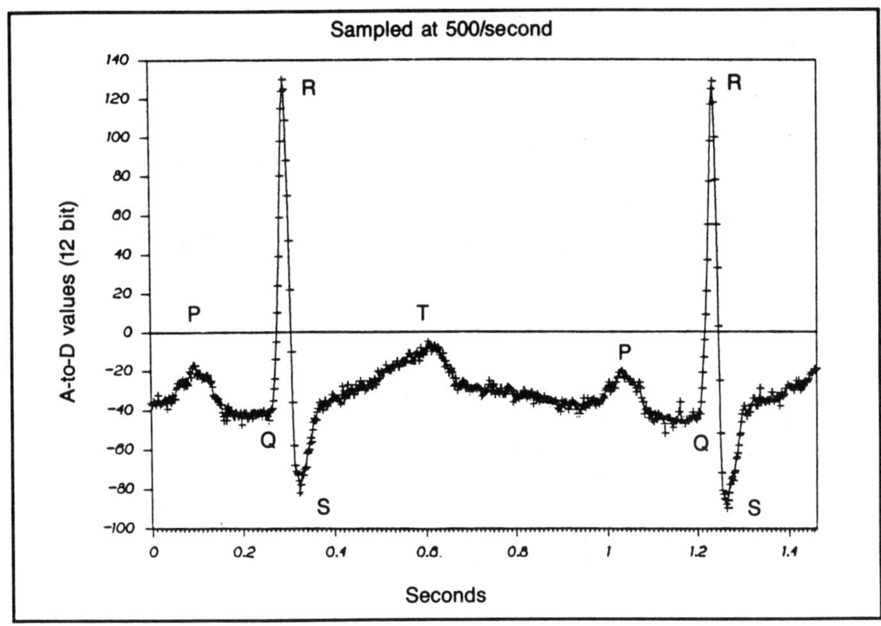

(a)

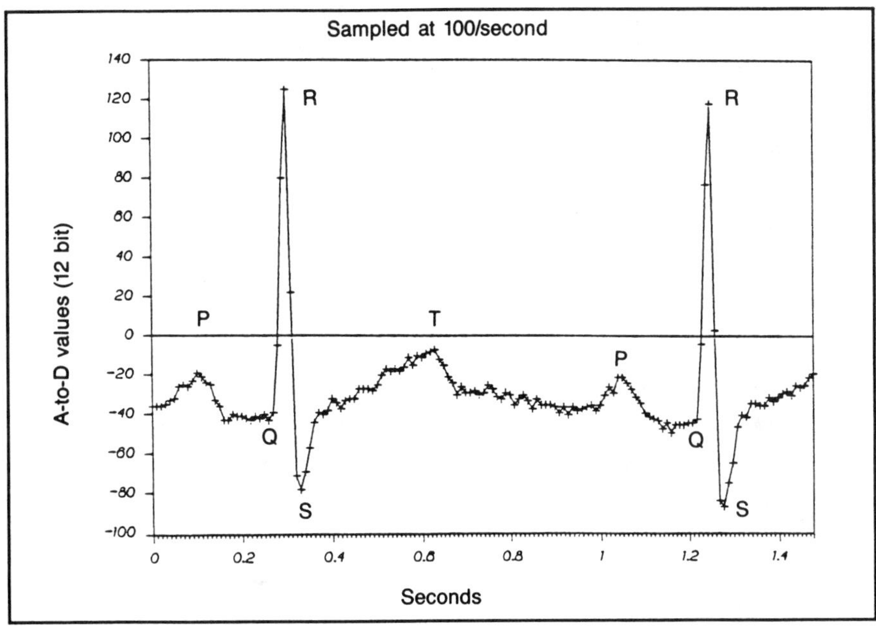

(b)

FIGURE 13.7. The sampling rate of the analog-to-digital converter determines the quality of the ECG. All four panels show the same ECG, sampled at different rates. Note the degradation of the quality of the signal as one proceeds from *a* to *d*. The ECG is sampled at 500 *(a)*, 100 *(b)*, 50 *(c)*, and 25 *(d)* measurements per second.

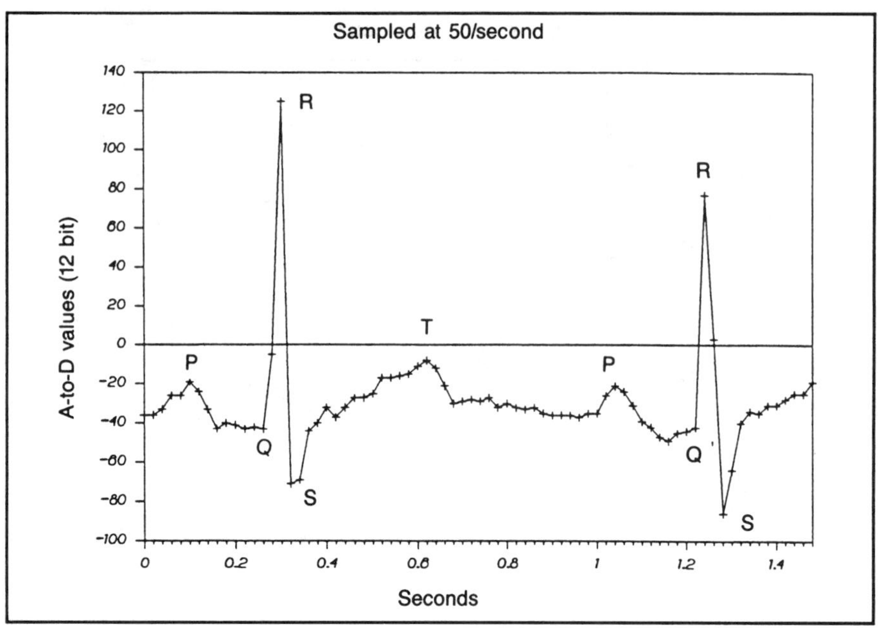

(c)

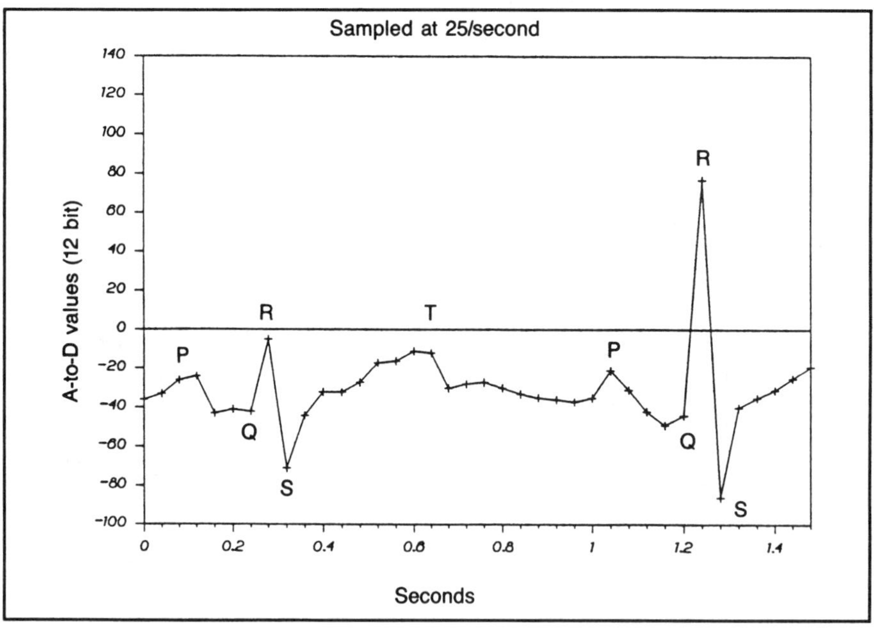

(d)

FIGURE 13.7. (Continued)

wave (ventricular recovery), are reproduced faithfully. When the sampling rate is decreased to 100 measurements per second, however, the amplitude and shape of the QRS complex begin to be distorted. When only 50 observations per second are recorded, the QRS complex is grossly distorted, and the other features also begin to distort. At a recording rate of only 25 measurements per second, gross signal distortion occurs, and even estimating heart rate by measuring intervals from R to R is problematic.

13.3.1 Advantages of Built-In Microcomputers

Today, the newest bedside monitors contain multiple microcomputers, with much more computing power and memory than was available in the systems used by the computer monitoring pioneers (Fig. 13.8). Bedside monitors with built-in mi-

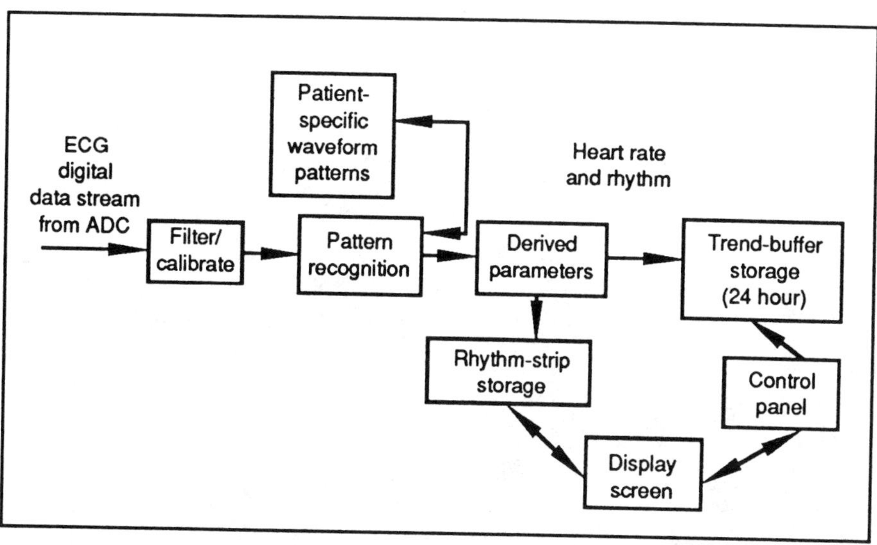

FIGURE 13.8. Block diagram of a microcomputer-based bedside monitor showing how a digital data stream is derived from an analog-to-digital converter (ADC) and how parameters are derived from the signal. First, the signal is calibrated, and unwanted signals are removed (such as the 60-Hz signal from the power line). Next, software pattern-recognition algorithms are applied. For ECG rhythm analysis, patient-specific waveform templates that the microcomputer-based system has learned are compared with each patient waveform. Once the signal characteristics are determined, derived parameters are generated and are stored in time-trend buffers. When special arrhythmia events are detected by the pattern-recognition algorithm, the digitized signals also are transferred to a storage area for ECG recordings. Figure 13.10 shows an example of an ECG recording, or strip. The operator—usually a nurse or a physician—interacts with the monitor via a control panel and display screen.

crocomputers have the following advantages over their analog predecessors (Weinfurt, 1990):

- The digital computer's ability to store patient waveform information such as the ECG permits sophisticated **pattern recognition** and **feature extraction.** Modern microcomputer-based bedside monitors use multiple ECG channels and pattern recognition schemes to identify abnormal waveform patterns and then to classify ECG arrhythmias.
- Signal quality from multiple ECG leads can now be monitored and interference noise minimized. For example, the computer can watch for degradation of ECG skin–electrode contact resistance. If the contact is poor, the monitor can alert the nurse to change the specified problematic electrode.
- Physiological signals can be acquired more efficiently by converting them to digital form early in the processing cycle. The waveform processing (e.g., calibration and filtering, as described in Chapter 4) then can be done in the microcomputer. The same process simplifies the nurse's task of setting up and operating the bedside monitor by eliminating the manual calibration step.

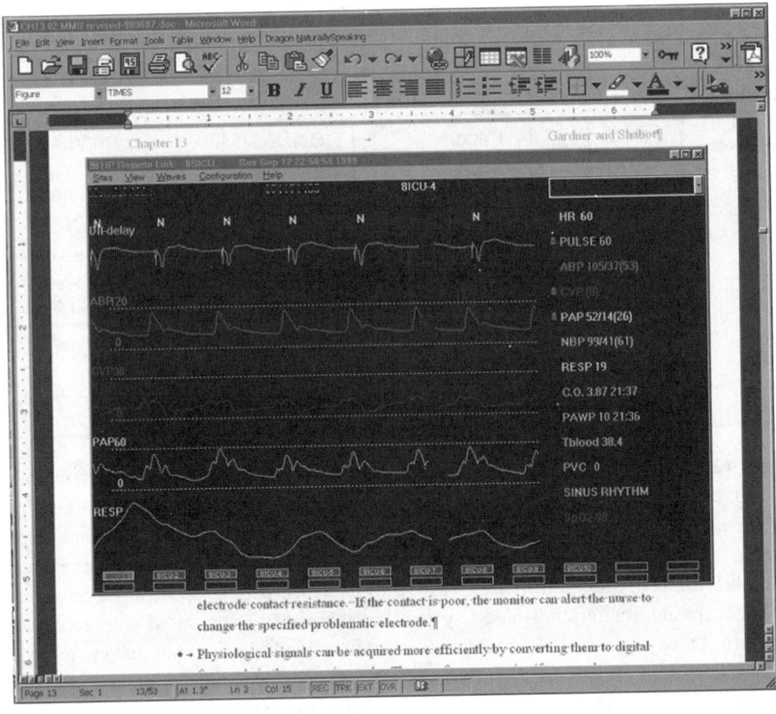

FIGURE 13.9. Screen of a personal computer (PC) showing a remote bedside physiological monitoring window in front of a word processor display. Bedside physiological data are digitized and converted to an HL7 data stream and displayed on a remote PC as a bedside monitor or a central station overview screen.

- Transmission of digitized physiological waveform signals is easier and more reliable. Digital transmission of data is inherently noise-free. As a result, newer monitoring systems allow health-care professionals to review a patient's waveform displays and derived parameters, such as heart rate and blood pressure, at the bedside, at a central station in the ICU, or at home via modem on a laptop computer. For example, the computer screen shown in Figure 13.9 was obtained by Dr. Shabot at his home via an intranet connection to his hospital.
- Selected data can be retained easily if they are digitized. For example, ECG strips of interesting physiological sequences, such as periods of arrhythmias (Fig. 13.10), can be stored in the bedside monitor for later review. Today's monitors typically store all of the waveform data from multiple leads of ECG and blood pressure transducers for at least 24 hours and sometimes for even longer.
- Measured variables, such as heart rate and blood pressure, can be graphed over prolonged periods to aid with detection of life-threatening trends (Fig. 13.11).

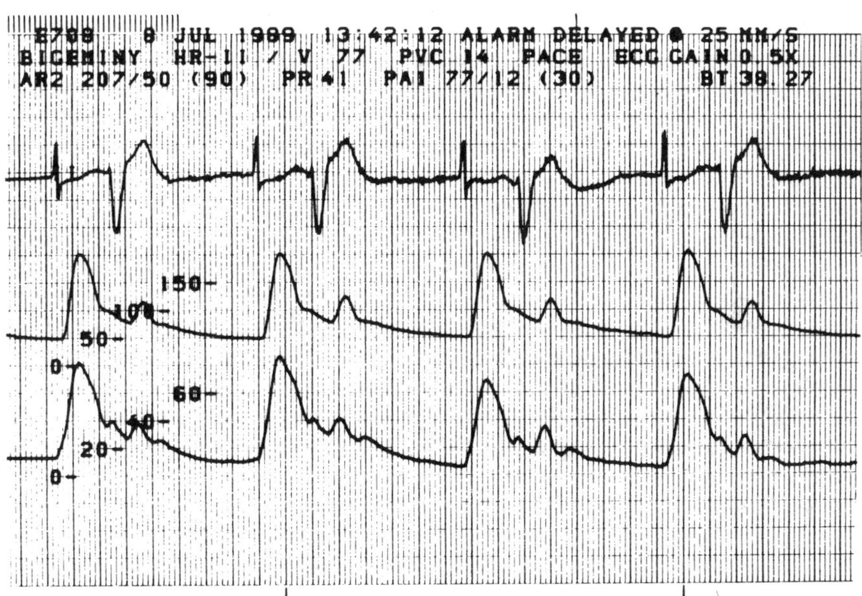

FIGURE 13.10. A strip showing a patient's ECG (upper trace) and arterial (middle trace) and pulmonary-artery (lower trace) pressure waveforms. The patient has a potentially life-threatening arrhythmia in which heart beats occur in pairs—a pattern called *bigeminy*. Note that, for two extra beats on the ECG pattern, the resulting pressure waveform pulsation is unusually small, indicating that the heart has not pumped much blood for that extra beat. The patient's heart rate, as determined from the ECG, is 77 beats per minute, whereas that determined from blood pressure is only 41 beats per minute. The heart is effectively beating at a very slow rate of 41 beats per minute.

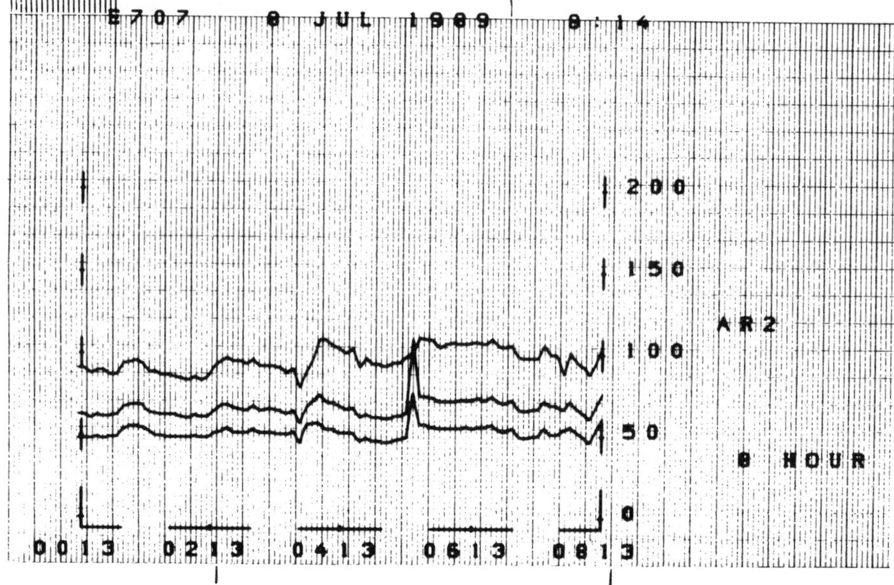

(a)

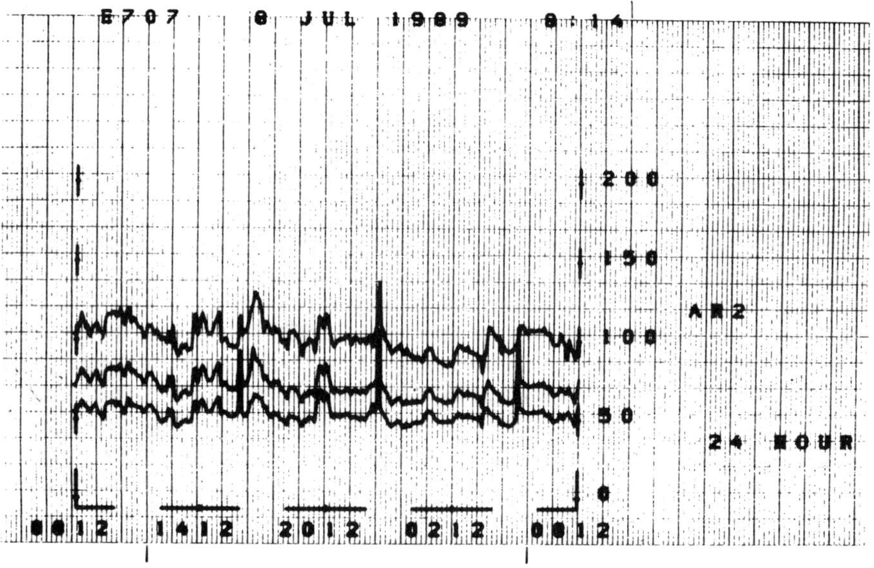

(b)

FIGURE 13.11. Two time-trend plots of systolic, mean, and diastolic pressure: *a,* 8 hours; *b,* 24 hours. Indicated across the bottom are the time of day at each of the tick marks. These plots show relatively stable blood-pressure trends over the 24-hour period.

- Alarms from bedside monitors are now much "smarter"and raise fewer false alarms. In the past, analog alarm systems used only high–low threshold limits and were susceptible to **signal artifacts** (Gardner, 1997). Now, computer-based bedside monitors often can distinguish between artifacts and real alarm situations by using the information derived from one signal to verify that from another and can confidently alert physicians and nurses to real alarms. For example, heart rate can be derived from either the ECG or the arterial blood pressure. If both signals indicate dangerous tachycardia (fast heart rate), the system sounds an alarm. If the two signals do not agree, the monitor can notify the health-care professional about a potential instrumentation or medical problem. The procedure is not unlike that performed by a human verifying possible problems by using redundant information from simpler bedside monitor alarms. Despite these advancements in bedside monitors, however, false alarms are still very prevalent (Tsien & Fackler, 1997).
- Systems can be upgraded easily. Only the software programs in read-only memory (ROM) need to be changed; older analog systems required hardware replacement.

13.3.2 Arrhythmia Monitoring—Signal Acquisition and Processing

Although general-purpose computer-based physiological monitoring systems have not yet been adopted widely, computer-based ECG arrhythmia-monitoring systems were accepted quickly (Weinfurt, 1990). Electrocardiographic arrhythmia analysis is one of the most sophisticated and difficult of the bedside monitoring tasks. Conventional arrhythmia monitoring, which depends on people observing displayed signals, is expensive, unreliable, tedious, and stressful to the observers. One early approach to overcoming these limitations was to purchase an arrhythmia-monitoring system operating on a time-shared central computer. Such minicomputer-based systems usually monitored 8 to 16 patients and cost at least $50,000.

The newest bedside monitors, in contrast, have built-in arrhythmia-monitoring systems. These computers generally use a 16-bit or 32-bit architecture, waveform templates, and real-time feature extraction in which the computer measures such features as the R-R interval and QRS complex width; and template correlation, in which incoming waveforms are compared point by point with already classified waveforms (Weinfurt, 1990). Figure 13.12 shows the output from a commercial bedside monitor. There are four ECG leads attached to the patient, and the computer has correctly classified a rhythm abnormality—in this case, a premature ventricular contraction. The bedside monitor also retains an ECG tracing record in its memory so that at a later time a health professional can review the information.

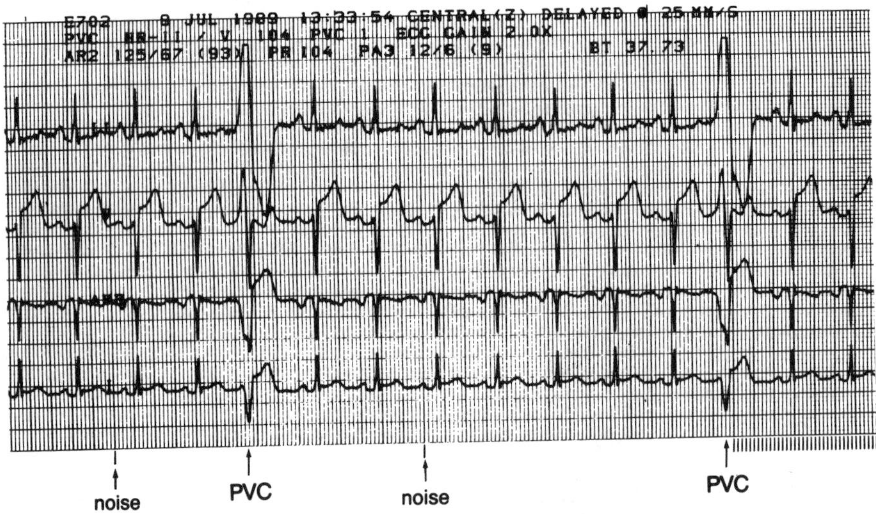

FIGURE 13.12. Four simultaneous lead tracings of ECG for a patient with a premature ventricular contraction (PVC) rate of 1 per minute. (Two PVCs occur—one at the middle left and one at the right of the tracing.) The PVC is most apparent in lead II (top trace); it is much less apparent in lead V (second trace). Multiple-lead recording and computer access permit detection of a much wider variety of arrhythmias and also minimize the effect of artifact (noise), which may occur in only one lead (as shown here in the bottom lead).

Wave Form Classification

Computer algorithms for processing ECG rhythms take sampled data, such as those shown in Figure 13.7, and extract features, such as the amplitude and duration of the QRS complex (Weinfurt, 1990). In most schemes, each time the QRS detector is tripped, it signals a beat classification subprogram, which receives four channels of ECG data at the same time. Such a beat-classification scheme compares the waveform of each incoming beat with that of one or more clinically relevant waveform classes already established for the patient. If the new waveform matches any of those already classified, the "template" of that waveform class is updated to reflect any minor evolutionary changes in the shape. Most beat-classification schemes have the capacity to store up to 30 templates. The performance of these newer multilead monitors has been dramatic; however, such arrhythmia monitors are still not perfect.

Detecting and identifying pacemaker signals poses special problems for digital computer-based monitoring systems. Pacemaker signals do not reliably traverse the analog acquisition circuitry, and the pacemaker "spikes" are very narrow such that they can occur between data samples and be missed entirely. As a result, special analog "injection" methods are used to enhance the pacemaker "spike" so that it can be more easily detected (Weinfurt, 1990).

Full-Disclosure and Multilead ECG Monitoring

Contemporary **central monitors** combine the advantages of digital waveform analysis as described above with high-capacity disk drives to store one or more days worth of continuous waveform data, including ECG. Some of these monitors can support recording **full disclosure** or synthesis of the entire 12-lead ECG on a second by second basis. Figure 13.13 shows a run of ventricular tachycardia in a portion of a 24-hour full disclosure ECG display. Figure 13.14 shows the synthesized 12-lead ECG at the point the arrhythmia began.

ST segment analysis of the ECG has also become very important because ST segment displacement is indicative of ischemic episodes of the heart muscle. Changes in open-heart procedure and administration of thrombolytic therapy is predicated on ST segment analysis. Newer multilead monitors now offer the opportunity to monitor ST segment changes.

ST segment monitoring can be performed on a single ECG lead, multiple leads, or across all leads. Figure 13.15 shows the rapid recovery of the summed ST segments (ST-VM) and QRS vector differences (QRS-VD) in a patient receiving reperfusion therapy for an acute myocardial infarction.

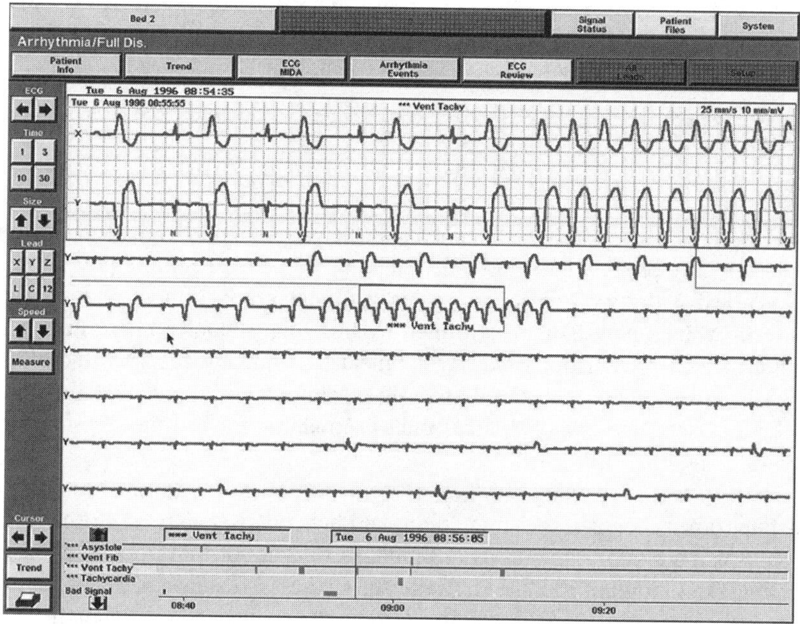

FIGURE 13.13. Full disclosure ECG display showing onset of ventricular tachycardia. This system stores continuous waveforms for 48 hours along with arrhythmia information. Waveforms may be displayed in a highly compressed format similar to Holter displays. (*Source:* Courtesy of Hewlett Packard Company.)

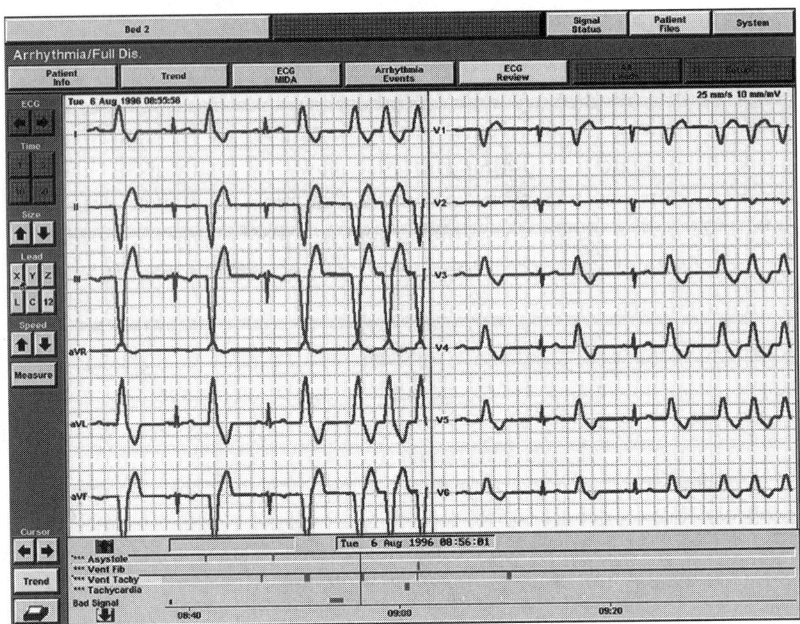

FIGURE 13.14. Synthesized 12-lead ECG display at the onset of ventricular tachycardia. A 12-lead ECG can be reconstructed and displayed for any point in time in the 48-hour ECG database. This function is useful for determining the onset and course of ischemic and arrhythmic events. (*Source:* Courtesy of Hewlett Packard Company.)

13.3.3 Bedside Point of Care Laboratory Testing

Over the past decade, laboratory chemical, hematologic, and blood gas testing processes have progressed from "wet" methods in which specific liquid reagents were mixed with blood or serum to perform analyses to a more or less "dry" phase in which analyses are performed by bringing a blood sample in contact with a reagent pack. Additional development has miniaturized both the blood-analysis cartridge and the blood-analysis machine to the point that the entire analysis system consists of a small plug-in module to a bedside physiological monitor (Fig. 13.16).

Up to 20 tests, including pH, Po_2, Pco_2, Hco_3, electrolytes, glucose, ionized calcium, other chemistries, hemoglobin, and hematocrit, can be performed in 2 minutes using two or three drops of blood. Results are displayed on the bedside physiological monitor and are stored in the monitor's database for comparison with previous results (Fig. 13.17). In addition, the results and corresponding calibration data are automatically transmitted through the monitoring network and hospital's backbone network to the laboratory computer system, and other systems as required, so that the results can be integrated into the patient's long-term records.

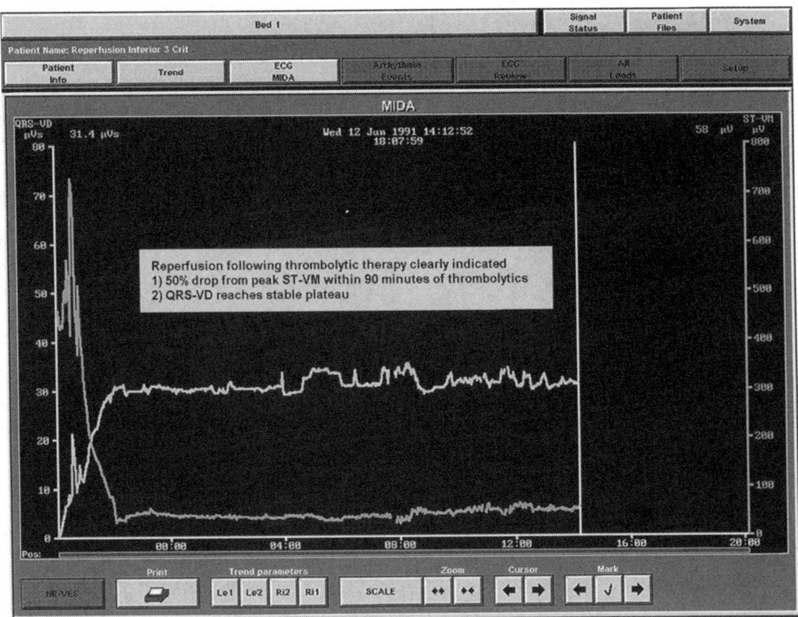

FIGURE 13.15. Computerized display of summed QRS and ST vectors in an acute myocardial infarction with reperfusion. The rapid fall in the summed ST vector display is a powerful indicator of the efficacy of the thrombolytic agent in this case. (*Source:* Courtesy of Hewlett Packard Company.)

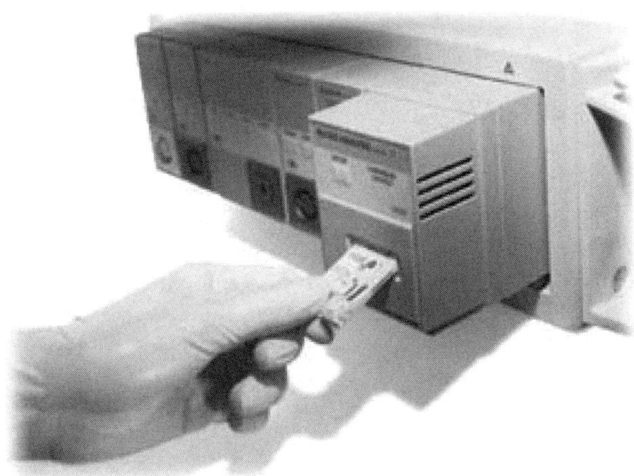

FIGURE 13.16. Blood analysis module and sample cartridge in a bedside physiological monitor. The module rack is for a Hewlett-Packard Component Monitoring System, and the Blood Analysis Module is a joint development of the i-STAT Corporation and Hewlett-Packard. (*Source:* Courtesy of Hewlett Packard Company.)

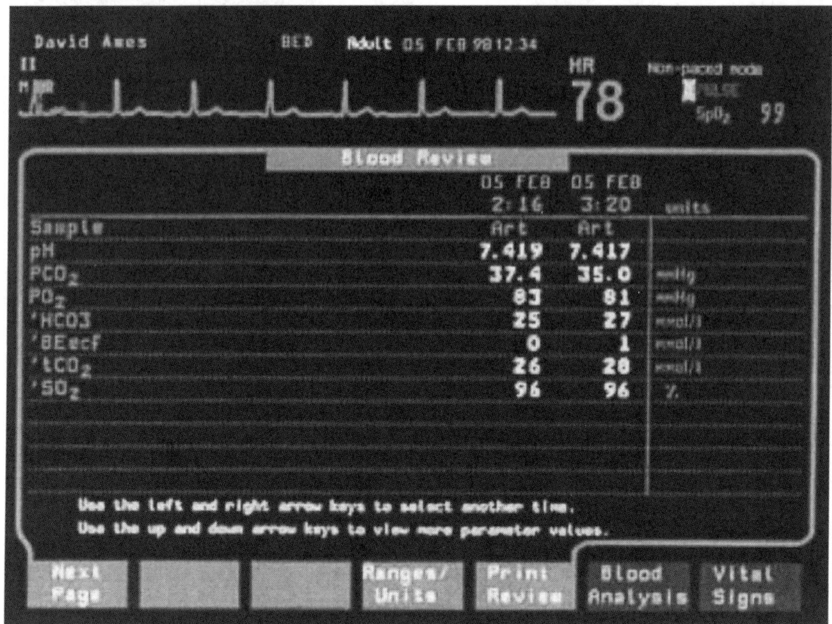

FIGURE 13.17. Hewlett-Packard Component Monitoring System physiological monitor display of bedside blood gas test results. Previous measurements are stored in the monitor and displayed with the current results. (*Source:* Courtesy of Hewlett Packard Company.)

13.3.4 Commercial Development of Computer-Based Monitoring and Intensive-Care-Unit Information Systems

The development of central stations and integrated arrhythmia systems based on standard microcomputer-based server hardware and software platforms has led to wide-scale distribution in the clinical environment. These systems possess database and analysis functions previously reserved for larger systems, and well over 2000 such systems are in use in ICUs worldwide.

In recent years, the bedside monitor has become a focal point for data entry and presentation. In fact, most bedside monitoring systems sold today can also acquire and display data from clinical laboratories, bedside laboratory devices such as blood chemistry machines, and a host of other devices such as ventilators. Unfortunately each of these monitors has its own proprietary communications protocol and data acquisition scheme. As a result, the user community is faced with bedside monitors that function like "mini" patient-data-management systems. Furthermore, the desire to capture and manage all clinical data for patients in a critical care setting (not just patient monitoring data) has resulted in development of specialized ICU information systems (see Section 13.4). It is common for hospitals to acquire computer-based bedside monitors, which must be interfaced to an ICU information system, which in turn may be interfaced with a hospital's clinical information system. Several large, capable, and reputable manufacturers have supplied over 350 computer-based ICU information systems worldwide. Two of the major companies involved in the development of such computer-based charting and monitoring systems are Hewlett-Packard with its CareVue system (Shabot, 1997b) and Eclipsys (formerly EMTEK) with its Continuum 2000 computerized charting application (Brimm, 1987; Cooke & Barie, 1998).

13.4 Information Management in the Intensive-care Unit

The goal of bedside patient monitoring is to detect life-threatening events promptly so that they can be treated before they cause irreversible organ damage or death. Care of the critically ill patient requires considerable skill and necessitates prompt, accurate treatment decisions. Healthcare professionals collect numerous data through frequent observations and testing, and more data are recorded by continuous-monitoring equipment. Physicians generally prescribe complicated therapy for such patients. As a result, enormous numbers of clinical data accumulate (Buchman, 1995; Kahn, 1994; Sailors & East, 1997; Shabot, 1995). Professionals can miss important events and trends if the accumulated data are not presented in a compact, well-organized form. In addition, the problems of managing these patients have been made even more challenging by economic pressures to reduce the cost of diagnostic and therapeutic interventions.

Continuity of care is especially important for critically ill patients. Such patients are generally served by teams of physicians, nurses, and therapists. Data often are transferred from one individual to another (e.g., the laboratory technician calls a unit clerk who reports the information to a nurse who in turn passes it on to the physician who makes a decision). Each step in this transmission process is subject to delay and error. The medical record is the principal instrument for ensuring the continuity of care for patients.

13.4.1 Computer-Based Charting

As discussed in Chapters 2 and 9, the traditional medical record has several limitations. The problems of poor or inflexible organization, illegibility, and lack of physical availability are especially pertinent to the medical records of critically ill patients due to the large number of data collected and the short time allowed for many treatment decisions.

The importance of having a unified medical record was demonstrated by a study conducted at LDS Hospital in the mid-1980s (Bradshaw et al., 1984). Investigators kept detailed records of the data used by physicians to make treatment decisions in a shock–trauma ICU (Fig. 13.18). The investigators were surprised to find that laboratory and blood-gas data were used most frequently (42

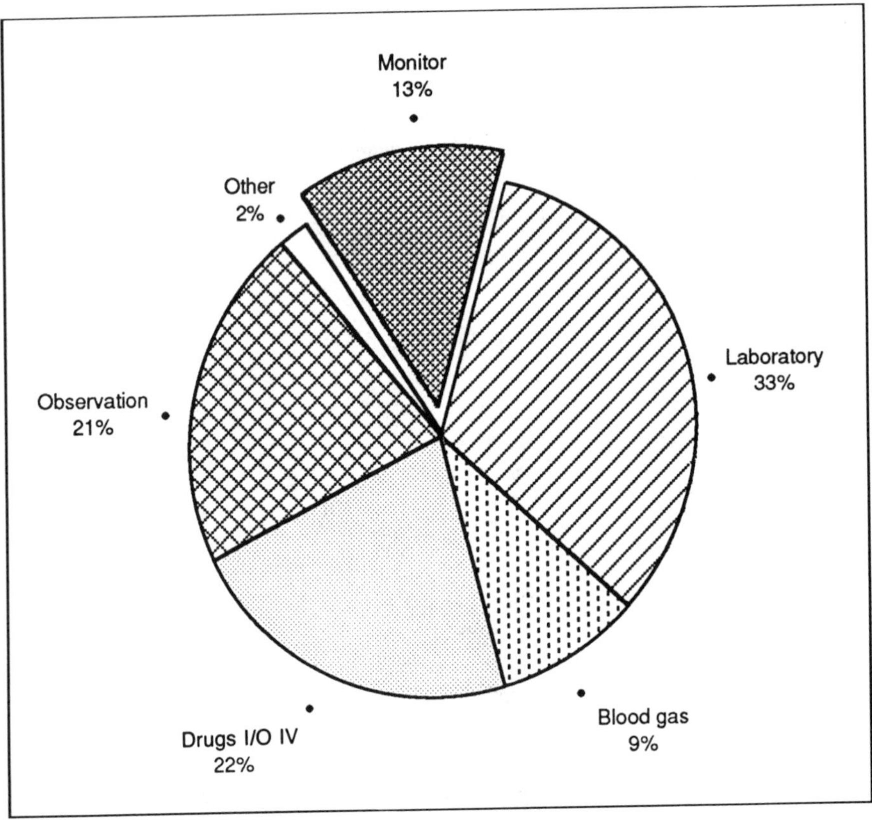

FIGURE 13.18. Pie chart indicating the variety of data physicians use when making treatment decisions in a shock–trauma intensive care unit. I/O = input–output; IV = intravenous.

percent total), given that physiological bedside monitors are always present in the ICU. Clinicians' observations (21 percent) and drug and fluid-balance data (22 percent) also were used frequently. The bedside physiological monitor accounted for only 13 percent of the data used in making therapeutic decisions. These findings clearly indicate that data from several sources, not just from the traditional physiological monitoring devices, must be communicated to and integrated into a unified medical record to permit effective decision-making and treatment in the ICU. More recent studies by investigators at Stanford University further support the need for integrated records and methods to assist in the "communal reasoning" required by the ICU team.

To be effective, computer charting in the ICU must support multiple types of data collection. As Figure 13.18 shows, a large percentage of the data collected comes from what are typically manual tasks, such as administering a medication or auscultating breath or heart sounds. Furthermore, many instruments that present data in electronic form require their data to be taken by a person and entered into the patient chart. Thus, computer charting systems must be able to collect a wide variety of data from automated and remote sites, as well as from health-care providers at the bedside. Dictated and transcribed reports (e.g., history, physical, and X-ray reports) still represent a large and important source of computer readable but uncoded information for the clinical staff in an ICU. Unfortunately, most computer-charting systems have dealt with a limited set of the data that need to be charted (usually only the bedside monitoring data).

Figure 13.19 illustrates the complexity of ICU charting. Modern computerized ICU flowsheet and medication administration record (MAR) displays are shown in Figures 13.20 and 13.21. The chart must document the actions taken by the medical staff to meet both medical and legal requirements (items 1 and 2 in Fig. 13.19).

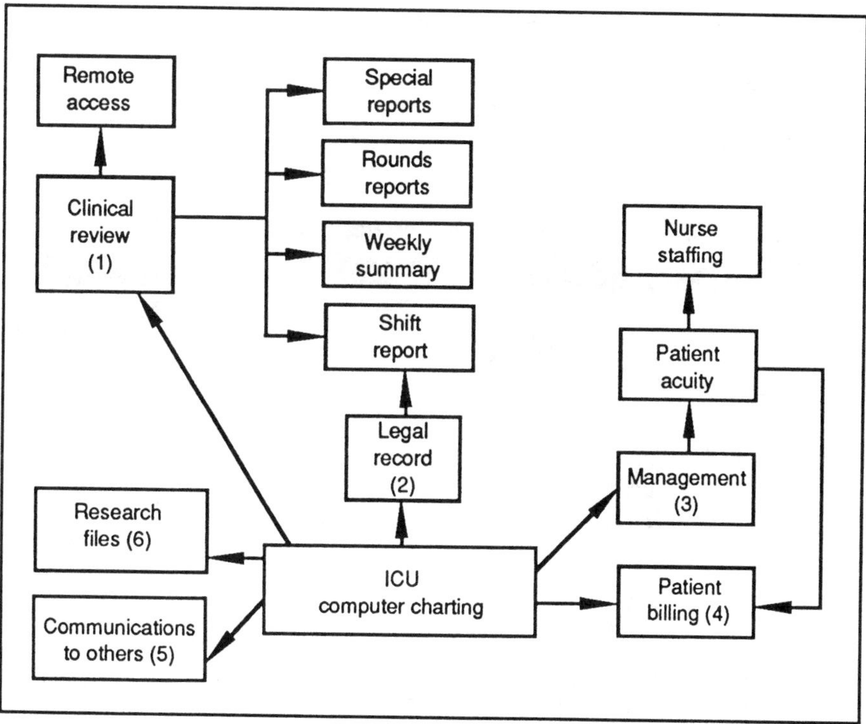

Figure 13.19. Block diagram showing the six major areas in which healthcare professionals interact with computer-based ICU charting to make patient care more effective and efficient. See text for explanations of functions. (*Source:* Reprinted with permission from Gardner R.M., Sittig D.F, Budd, M.C. [1989]. Computers in the intensive care unit: match or mismatch? In Shoemaker W.C., et al. (Eds.), *Textbook of Critical Care* (2nd ed, (p. 249). Philadelphia: W.B. Saunders.

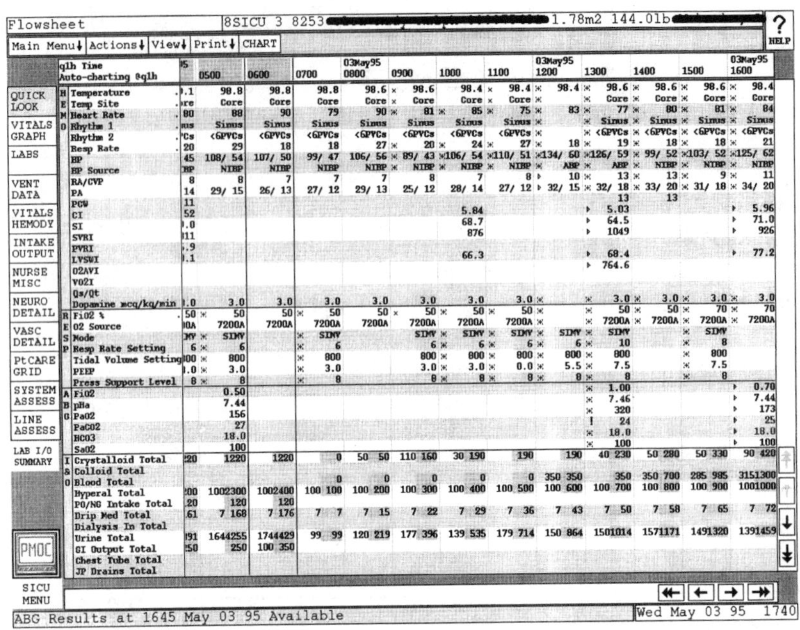

FIGURE 13.20. CareVue QuickLook Summary Display. The Quicklook display contains a summary of important data from different parts of the flowsheet. The content and appearance of the QuickLook display can be configured for each clinical area. (*Source:* M. Michael Shabot.)

Medication Administration: 8SICU 0 8276 1.95m2

Main Menu | Actions | View | Print | CHART

Scheduled | PRN | One-Time STAT | ALL

Allergies: NKA

Date	Medication	Schedule	May 04 98	May 05 98
Scheduled				
May 02 98	Accucheck 1U Diag q6h verified Jeannie Chen PharmD jgchen May 02 98 2320 covered with regular insulin sliding scale Jeannie Chen PharmD jgchen May 02 98 2320	0200 0800 1400 2000	2000 1U...	0200 1U... 0800 1U... 1400 1U...
May 02 98	Fluconazole inj 200mg IVPB q24h verified Jeannie Chen PharmD jgchen May 02 98 2326	2200	2200 200mg...	
May 02 98	Ganciclovir inj 100mg IVPB q24h verified Jeannie Chen PharmD jgchen May 02 98 2326	2200	2200 100mg...	
May 02 98	Lansoprazole cap 30mg PO bid verified Jeannie Chen PharmD jgchen May 02 98 2326 same as prevacid Jeannie Chen PharmD jgchen May 02 98 2308	1000 2200	2200 30mg...	1000 30mg...
May 03 98	Linezolide inj 600mg IVPB q12h verified investigational drug infuse over 2 hrs protect from light	1000 2200	2200 600mg... 2200 600mg...	1000 600mg...
	Lipid 20% inj	0800		0800 500ml...

Tue May 05 98 1710

FIGURE 13.21. CareVue medication administration record (MAR) display. All medications are charted dose by dose in this system. (*Source:* M. Michael Shabot.)

In addition, many of the data logged in the chart are used for management and billing purposes (items 3 and 4 in Fig. 13.19). Many computer systems have ignored these requirements and thus have unwittingly forced the clinical staff to chart the same information in more than one place. Yet efficient management in hospitals is required, especially given the implementation of managed care strategies (see Chapter 19). Hospitals now have strong incentives to know the cost of procedures and to control these costs. As a result, it is necessary to know how sick the patient is, which in turn allows administrators to project nurse staffing needs and to account for the care of a patient by degree of illness. Communications (item 5 in Fig. 13.19) to other departments within the hospital is mandatory. Access from office or home to clinical and administrative information is a great convenience to physicians. Such communication is easier with a computer-based record. Because the computer-based ICU record is stored in the system, it is readily available for research purposes (item 6 in Fig. 13.19). Anyone who has tried to retrieve data from manual patient charts for research purposes will recognize the value of the computer's capability.

To meet the clinical management needs required by critically ill patients as well as to provide an adequate legal record, most patient data-management systems generate a variety of reports. At the LDS Hospital, in addition to the rounds report shown in Figure 13.1, there are a variety of other reports. Figure 13.22 shows a nursing shift report for a patient. The 12-hour report documents the physiological data and summarizes the laboratory data in its upper section. In the lower section, it displays a record of each drug given and each IV fluid administered. It lists the nurses who care for the patient; the nurses place their initials next to their names to indicate that they have verified the data. Total fluid-intake data are derived from the IV data, and fluid-output data are summarized as well. This allows a calculation of the net intake–output balance for the shift.

For the patient who is in the ICU for several days, a broader view of the course of the recovery process is essential. Thus, the system at LDS prepares weekly reports that summarize the data for each of the past seven 24-hour periods (Fig. 13.23). The data already are stored in the computer, so no additional data entry is required to generate the report. A program abstracts and formats the data.

Figure 13.24 shows a blood-gas report indicating the acid–base status of the patient's blood, as well as the blood's oxygen-carrying capacity. Note that, in addition to the numerical parameters for the blood, the patient's breathing status is indicated. Based on all these clinical data, the computer provides an interpretation. For life-threatening situations, the computer prompts the staff to take the necessary action

13.4.2 Calculation of Derived Variables

Increased sophistication of hemodynamic, renal, and pulmonary monitoring resulted in the need to calculate **derived parameters;** for the first time, ICU staff had to crunch numbers. At first, pocket calculators were used, with each step performed by a careful nurse. Then programmable calculators took over this task,

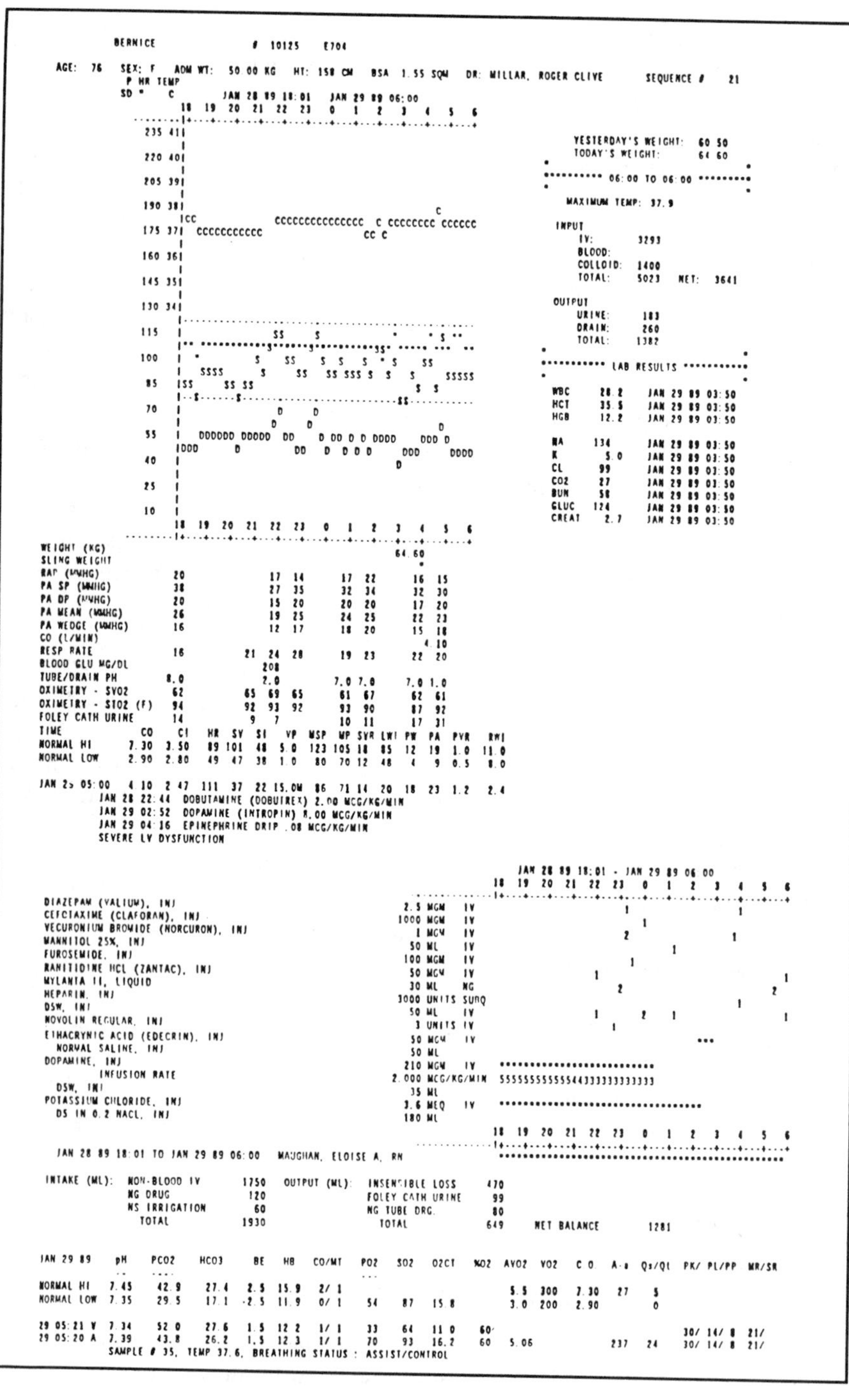

BERNICE # 10125 E704

AGE: 76 SEX: F ADM WT: 50.00 KG HT: 158 CM BSA 1.55 SQM DR: MILLAR, ROGER CLIVE SEQUENCE # 21

P HR TEMP
SD * C JAN 28 89 18:01 JAN 29 89 06:00

YESTERDAY'S WEIGHT: 60.50
TODAY'S WEIGHT: 64.60

********** 06:00 TO 06:00 **********

MAXIMUM TEMP: 37.9

INPUT
IV: 3293
BLOOD:
COLLOID: 1400
TOTAL: 5023 NET: 3641

OUTPUT
URINE: 183
DRAIN: 260
TOTAL: 1382

********** LAB RESULTS **********

WBC	28.2	JAN 29 89 03:50
HCT	35.5	JAN 29 89 03:50
HGB	12.2	JAN 29 89 03:50
NA	134	JAN 29 89 03:50
K	5.0	JAN 29 89 03:50
CL	99	JAN 29 89 03:50
CO2	27	JAN 29 89 03:50
BUN	58	JAN 29 89 03:50
GLUC	124	JAN 29 89 03:50
CREAT	2.7	JAN 29 89 03:50

	18	19	20	21	22	23	0	1	2	3	4	5	6
WEIGHT (KG)											64.60		
SLING WEIGHT													
RAP (MMHG)	20				17	14		17	22		16	15	
PA SP (MMHG)	38				27	35		32	34		32	30	
PA DP (MMHG)	20				15	20		20	20		17	20	
PA MEAN (MMHG)	26				19	25		24	25		22	23	
PA WEDGE (MMHG)	16				12	17		18	20		15	18	
CO (L/MIN)												4.10	
RESP RATE	16			21	24	28		19	23		22	20	
BLOOD GLU MG/DL					208								
TUBE/DRAIN PH	8.0				2.0			7.0	7.0		7.0	1.0	
OXIMETRY - SVO2	62			65	69	65		61	67		62	61	
OXIMETRY - STO2 (F)	94			92	93	92		93	90		87	92	
FOLEY CATH URINE	14			9	7			10	11		17	31	

TIME	CO	CI	HR	SV	SI	VP	MSP	MP	SVR	LWI	PW	PA	PVR	RWI
NORMAL HI	7.30	3.50	89	101	48	5.0	123	105	18	85	12	19	1.0	11.0
NORMAL LOW	2.90	2.80	49	47	38	1.0	80	70	12	48	4	9	0.5	8.0
JAN 29 05:00	4.10	2.47	111	37	22	15.0M	86	71	14	20	18	23	1.2	2.4

JAN 28 22:44 DOBUTAMINE (DOBUTREX) 2.00 MCG/KG/MIN
JAN 29 02:52 DOPAMINE (INTROPIN) 8.00 MCG/KG/MIN
JAN 29 04:16 EPINEPHRINE DRIP .08 MCG/KG/MIN
SEVERE LV DYSFUNCTION

JAN 28 89 18:01 - JAN 29 89 06:00

		18	19	20	21	22	23	0	1	2	3	4	5	6
DIAZEPAM (VALIUM), INJ	2.5 MGM IV						1					1		
CEFOTAXIME (CLAFORAN), INJ	1000 MGM IV							1						
VECURONIUM BROMIDE (NORCURON), INJ	1 MGM IV						2					1		
MANNITOL 25%, INJ	50 ML IV								1					
FUROSEMIDE, INJ	100 MGM IV						1							
RANITIDINE HCL (ZANTAC), INJ	50 MGM IV					1								1
MYLANTA II, LIQUID	30 ML NG						2						2	
HEPARIN, INJ	3000 UNITS SUBQ											1		
D5W, INJ	50 ML IV					1		2	1					1
NOVOLIN REGULAR, INJ	3 UNITS IV						1							
ETHACRYNIC ACID (EDECRIN), INJ	50 MGM IV									***				
NORMAL SALINE, INJ	50 ML													
DOPAMINE, INJ	210 MGM IV	************************												
INFUSION RATE	2.000 MCG/KG/MIN	5555555555554433333333333												
D5W, INJ	35 ML													
POTASSIUM CHLORIDE, INJ	3.6 MEQ IV	********************************												
D5 IN 0.2 NACL, INJ	180 ML													

JAN 28 89 18:01 TO JAN 29 89 06:00 MAUGHAN, ELOISE A, RN

INTAKE (ML):		OUTPUT (ML):	
NON-BLOOD IV	1750	INSENSIBLE LOSS	470
NG DRUG	120	FOLEY CATH URINE	99
NS IRRIGATION	60	NG TUBE DRG.	80
TOTAL	1930	TOTAL	649

NET BALANCE 1281

JAN 29 89	pH	PCO2	HCO3	BE	HB	CO/MT	PO2	SO2	O2CT	%O2	AVO2	VO2	C.O.	A-a	Qs/Qt	PK/ PL/PP	MR/SR
NORMAL HI	7.45	42.9	27.4	2.5	15.9	2/ 1					5.5	300	7.30	27	5		
NORMAL LOW	7.35	29.5	17.1	-2.5	11.9	0/ 1	54	87	15.8		3.0	200	2.90		0		
29 05:21 V	7.34	52.0	27.6	1.5	12.2	1/ 1	33	64	11.0	60						30/ 14/ 8	21/
29 05:20 A	7.39	43.8	26.2	1.5	12.3	1/ 1	70	93	16.2	60	5.06			237	24	30/ 14/ 8	21/

SAMPLE # 35, TEMP 37.6, BREATHING STATUS : ASSIST/CONTROL

FIGURE 13.22. Shift report for 12-hour ICU nursing shift at LDS Hospital. (*Source:* Courtesy of LDS Hospital.)

making the computation simpler, faster, and more accurate (Shabot, 1982; Shabot et al., 1977). Soon these devices were replaced by portable computers. Some of these systems also provided graphical plots and interpretations.

13.4.3 Decision-Making Assistance

One mark of a good physician is having the ability to make sound clinical judgments. Medical decision-making traditionally has been considered an intuitive, as well as a scientific, process. More recently, however, formal methods for decision- making have been applied to medical problem-solving (see Chapter 3), and computer-assisted medical decision-making has gained wider acceptance (see the discussions of decision-support systems in Chapter 16). We now have the opportunity to use the computer to assist staff in the complex task of medical decision-making in the ICU. For example, the HELP computer system at the LDS Hospital in Salt Lake City has been used effectively to assist in ICU decision-making (Evans et al., 1998; Garibaldi, 1998). The system collects and integrates data for the ICU patient from a wide variety of sources. The data are processed automatically by the HELP decision-making system to determine whether the new information, by itself or in combination with other data in the patient record (such as a laboratory result or a previously generated decision), leads to a new medical decision. These computer-generated medical decisions are based on predefined criteria stored in the system's knowledge base.

The HELP decision-making system has been used in the following areas:

- Interpretation of data; for example, interpretation of breathing status based on blood-gas reports and hemodynamic parameters
- Alerts; for example, notification that a drug is contraindicated at the time the drug is being ordered
- Diagnoses; for example, detection of hospital-acquired infections
- Treatment suggestions; for example, suggestions about the most effective antibiotics to order

The ICU component of HELP is one of the most mature of the system's clinical applications. The basic requirements for data acquisition, decision support, and information reporting are similar for patients in the ICU and on the general patient-care units of the LDS Hospital. The number of variables and the volume of observations that must be integrated, however, are much greater for patients in the ICU.

At Cedars-Sinai Medical Center, all laboratory and flowsheet data are continuously analyzed for critical laboratory results and adverse combinations of clinical (nonlaboratory) events. When such events are detected, they are transmitted to the responsible physician via an alphanumeric pager. Figure 13.25 shows a laboratory-value alert, and Figure 13.26 warns of a critical clinical event occurring over time (Shabot, 1995).

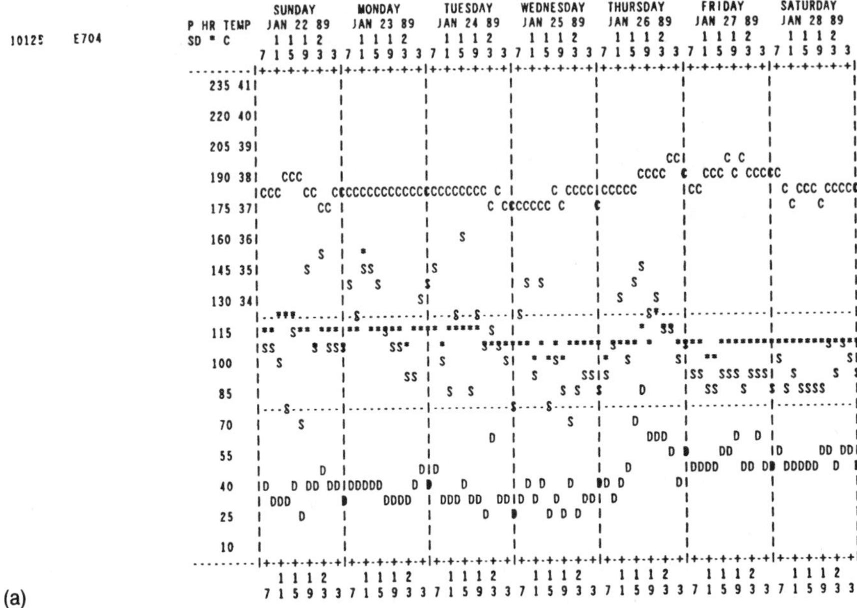

(a)

FIGURE 13.23. Two portions *(a, b)* of a weekly (7-day) ICU report, produced by the HELP system at LDS Hospital. The report provides a daily weight, fluid-balance, drug, and physiological-data summary for an individual patient. (*Source:* HELP System, LDS Hospital.)

13.4.4 Response by Nurses and Physicians

Currently, bedside terminals are functioning in all ICUs at LDS Hospital, and nurses use a computer-based system to create nursing care plans and to chart ICU data. The goals of automation were (1) to facilitate the acquisition of clinical data, (2) to improve the content and legibility of medical documentation, and (3) to increase the efficiency of the charting process so that nurses could devote more time to direct patient care. Studies have shown wide acceptance by nurses and physicians of the HELP system and its decision-support capabilities (Gardner & Lundsgaarde, 1994). Also, the content and quality of nursing charts has improved markedly (Bradshaw et al., 1988). To date, however, the studies have not shown improvements in the efficiency of information management by ICU nurses (time savings) that could be credited to use of the system.

The lack of demonstrable time savings may be due to several factors. First, the new system affected only selected aspects of the nursing process. For example, physiological and laboratory data were already acquired automatically, so the effects of these computer-based systems were not included in the analyses. Second, the computer-based charting system is not yet comprehensive; nurses still must perform some manual charting. Third, nurses do not always take advantage of the capabilities of the charting system. For example, they sometimes reenter vital signs that have already been stored in the computer. Fourth, the in-

			JAN 22	JAN 23	JAN 24	JAN 25	JAN 26	JAN 27	JAN 28
MORPHINE, INJ	MGM	IV	37.0	21.0	2.0			7.0	6.0
ACETAMINOPHEN, SUPP	MGM	RECT					1300	650	
DIAZEPAM (VALIUM), INJ	MGM	IV						10.0	5.0
CEFOTAXIME (CLAFORAN), INJ	MGM	IV							1000
GENTAMICIN, INJ	MGM	IV						60.0	60.0
CEFUROXIME (ZINACEF), INJ	MGM	IV	3000	3000	3000	3000	3000	3000	
DOBUTAMINE (DOBUTREX), INJ	MGM	IV	732	582	792	810	270	87	222
EPINEPHRINE DRIP, INJ	MGM	IV	22.20	11.46	3.96	0.00			1.53
VECURONIUM BROMIDE (NORCURON), INJ	MGM	IV	39	26	18	13	10	3	7
DOPAMINE, INJ	MGM	IV	648	492	420	396	522	864	738
METOLAZONE (ZAROXOLYN), TAB	MGM	NG					5.00		
NITROPRUSSIDE (NIPRIDE), INJ	MGM	IV	0						
AMRINONE (INOCOR), INJ	MGM	IV	0						
FUROSEMIDE, INJ	MGM	IV	80	80	80	80	120	80	280
MANNITOL 25%, INJ	ML	IV							50
ETHACRYNIC ACID (EDECRIN), INJ	MGM	IV							50
ACETAZOLAMIDE (DIAMOX), INJ	MGM	IV			250	250		250	
RANITIDINE HCL (ZANTAC), INJ	MGM	IV	150	100	150	150	150	150	150
MYLANTA II, LIQUID	ML	NG		60	30	120	90	60	180
MYLANTA, LIQUID	ML	NG			30	60			
HEPARIN, INJ	UNITS	SUBQ						3000	6000
HEPARIN FLUSH, INJ	UNITS	IV	400	300		300	500	200	100
ARTIFICAL TEARS (LACRIL), SOLUTION	GTTS	OPTH	6	4					
PLASMANATE 5%, INJ	ML	IV						250	1400
PACKED RBC	ML	IV					500		
ALBUMIN 25%, INJ	ML	IV	100	50	50	150			
PLATELETS (RANDOM DONOR)	ML	IV	400		150				
AMINOSYN 8.5%, INJ	ML	IV	311	621	472	529	608	1079	617
POTASSIUM	MEQ	IV	25.2	50.3	38.2	59.7	73.0	131.0	94.9
CALCIUM	MEQ	IV	3.1	6.2	4.7	5.3	5.7	9.9	5.8
MAGNESIUM	MEQ	IV	14.9	35.0	28.3	31.7	12.7	17.3	9.9
ZINC	MGM	IV	3.4	6.8	5.2	5.8	6.7	11.9	6.4
COPPER	MGM	IV	0.7	1.4	1.0	1.2	1.3	2.4	1.3
MANGANESE	MGM	IV	0.3	0.6	0.5	0.5	0.6	1.1	0.6
CHROMIUM	MCG	IV	6.8	13.7	10.4	11.6	13.4	23.7	12.7
CHLORIDE	MEQ	IV	20.8	41.6	31.6	35.4	35.0	50.6	47.5
ACETATE	MEQ	IV	24.9	49.7	37.8	42.3	41.5	69.7	52.2
PHOSPHATE	MEQ	IV	14.9	29.8	22.7	25.4	65.8	138.5	45.5
SULFATE	MEQ	IV	9.9	25.1	20.8	23.3	10.1	17.3	7.6
GLUCONATE	MEQ	IV	3.1	6.2	4.7	5.3	5.7	9.9	5.8
FAT EMULSION 10% (LIPOSYN), INJ	ML	IV							500
NORMAL SALINE, INJ	ML	IV	6	2		2	154	10	40
FAT EMULSION 20% (LIPOSYN), INJ	ML	IV	200	200	200	200	200	66	134
POTASSIUM CHLORIDE, INJ	MEQ	IV	67.9	78.0	183.7	51.9	51.6	104.3	17.6
D5W, INJ	ML	IV	410	215	25	150	5	10	
HETASTARCH (HESPAN), INJ	ML	IV				250	0		
MAGNESIUM SULFATE 50%, INJ	GM	IV	2.00						
NOVOLIN REGULAR, INJ	UNITS	IV	18	15					3
INTAKE (ML): BLOOD			400		150		500		
COLLOID			100	50	50	150		250	1400
NON-BLOOD IV			2783	3046	2707	2395	2254	3145	3293
NG DRUG				60	60	180	90	60	180
TOTAL			3313	3216	2967	2815	2874	3485	5023
OUTPUT (ML): INSENSIBLE LOSS			937	946	943	873	1016	1077	939
FOLEY CATH URINE			360	740	210	902	2950	895	183
NG TUBE DRG.			50	200	80	125	40	75	260
WATERSEAL DRG, 1			180	50					
TOTAL			3918	3936	4023	2512	5226	2470	1382
NET BALANCE (ML):			-605	-720	-1056	303	-2352	1015	3641
WEIGHT (KG)			61.2	61.4	60.8	62.2	60.4	60.5	64.6
NUTRITIONAL: NP ENERGY	KCAL (IV)		1468	2143	1784	1803	1953	2813	2395
TOTAL ENERGY	KCAL (IV)		1573	2354	1944	1982	2160	3181	2605
PROTEIN	GM		26	53	40	45	52	92	52
FAT	GM		40	40	40	40	40	13	77
CHO	GM		315	513	407	413	456	789	464
NP ENERGY/N2	KCAL/GM		367	238	254	257	244	200	266
N2 IN	GM		4	9	7	7	8	14	9

BERNICE # 1012[illegible] E704

TIME OUT: JAN 29 89 13:53 PROCESS TIME: 00:18

(END)

FIGURE 13.23. (Continued)

```
                    L D S   H O S P I T A L   B L O O D   G A S   R E P O R T


      STEVEN                                   NO.  10072     DR. STINSON, JAMES B.            RM E609
                               SEX: M  AGE: 43

JAN 05 89    pH    PCO2     HCO3     BE    HB    CO/MT   PO2   SO2   O2CT   %O2  AVO2  VO2   C.O.   A-a  Qs/Qt  PK/ PL/PP  MR/S
             --    ----                                  ---
NORMAL HI   7.45   40.6     25.9    2.5  17.7    2/ 1                              5.5   300   7.30    22    5
NORMAL LOW  7.35   27.2     15.7   -2.5  13.7    0/ 1     64    91   18.5          3.0   200   2.90          0

05 04:36 V  7.43   34.5     22.7    -.4  11.5    2/ 1     42    76   12.3    40                                   30/ 28/ 5  20/
05 04:35 A  7.48   29.3     21.7         11.6    2/ 1    128    96   15.9    40    3.43                 75   12   30/ 28/ 5  20/
            SAMPLE # 37, TEMP 37.3, BREATHING STATUS : ASSIST/CONTROL
            MILD ACID-BASE DISORDER
            MODERATELY REDUCED O2 CONTENT
            SUPRA-NORMAL PO2
            PULSE OXIMETER SO2  96.0

04 04:20 V  7.45   36.1     24.9    1.9  10.2    2/ 1     37    72   10.4    40                                   26/ 20/ 5  21/
04 04:19 A  7.49   31.6     24.0    2.0  10.2    2/ 1     90    95   13.7    40    3.36  353  10.50   111   18   26/ 20/ 5  21/
            SAMPLE # 36, TEMP 37.5, BREATHING STATUS : ASSIST/CONTROL
            MILD ACID-BASE DISORDER
            SEVERELY REDUCED O2 CONTENT (13.7) DUE TO ANEMIA (LOW HB)
            PULSE OXIMETER SO2  93.0

03 06:05 A  7.44   35.8     24.1    1.0  11.7    2/ 1     91    95   15.7    40                        105        26/ 22/ 5  23/
            SAMPLE # 35, TEMP 37.0, BREATHING STATUS : ASSIST/CONTROL
            NORMAL ARTERIAL ACID-BASE CHEMISTRY
            MODERATELY REDUCED O2 CONTENT
            PULSE OXIMETER SO2  93.0

02 04:16 V  7.46   37.4     26.4    3.4   9.1    1/ 1     35    71    9.1    40                                   32/ 25/10  20/
02 04:15 A  7.51   32.4     25.8    3.9   9.5    2/ 1     91    95   12.8    40    3.29  237   7.20   109   17   32/ 25/10  20/
            SAMPLE # 34, TEMP 37.1, BREATHING STATUS : ASSIST/CONTROL
            MODERATE METABOLIC ALKALOSIS
            SEVERELY REDUCED O2 CONTENT (12.8) DUE TO ANEMIA (LOW HB)
            PULSE OXIMETER SO2  95.0

01 10:53 A  7.47   37.0     26.8    4.0  11.1    1/ 1     77    94   14.7    60                        238        36/ 27/10  20/
            SAMPLE # 33, TEMP 37.7, BREATHING STATUS : ASSIST/CONTROL
            MILD ACID-BASE DISORDER
            MODERATELY REDUCED O2 CONTENT
            PULSE OXIMETER SO2  93.0

01 03:59 V  7.41   46.2     29.0    4.5  10.0    1/ 1     42    73   10.2    80                                     /   /12  20/
01 03:58 A  7.46   39.2     27.7    4.5   9.9    1/ 1    146    97   13.7    80    3.64  331   9.10   287   23     /   /12  20/
            SAMPLE # 32, TEMP 38.4, BREATHING STATUS : ASSIST/CONTROL
            MILD ACID-BASE DISORDER
            SEVERELY REDUCED O2 CONTENT (13.7) DUE TO ANEMIA (LOW HB)
            SUPRA-NORMAL PO2

01 00:39 A  7.44   42.2     28.4    4.7  10.0    1/ 1    104    95   13.5    90                        386          /   /10  20/
            SAMPLE # 31, TEMP 38.9, BREATHING STATUS : ASSIST/CONTROL
            MILD ACID-BASE DISORDER
            SEVERELY REDUCED O2 CONTENT (13.5) DUE TO ANEMIA (LOW HB)
            PULSE OXIMETER SO2  91.0

31 23:35 A  7.42   42.4     27.2    3.2  10.1    1/ 1     63    87   12.3    65                        276          /   / 5  20/
            SAMPLE # 30, TEMP 39.0, BREATHING STATUS : ASSIST/CONTROL
            MILD ACID-BASE DISORDER
            MODERATE HYPOXEMIA
            SEVERELY REDUCED O2 CONTENT (12.3) DUE TO ANEMIA (LOW HB)
            PULSE OXIMETER SO2  83.0

31 16:00 A  7.49   34.4     26.1    3.8   9.7    1/ 1     87    95   13.1    40                        111          /   / 5  21/
            SAMPLE # 29, TEMP 37.8, BREATHING STATUS : ASSIST/CONTROL
            MILD ACID-BASE DISORDER
            SEVERELY REDUCED O2 CONTENT (13.1) DUE TO ANEMIA (LOW HB)


PRELIMINARY INTERPRETATION -- BASED ONLY ON BLOOD GAS DATA.  ***(FINAL DIAGNOSIS REQUIRES CLINICAL CORRELATION)***
KEY: CO=CARBOXY HB, MT=MET HB, O2CT=O2 CONTENT, AVO2=ART VENOUS CONTENT DIFFERENCE (CALCULATED WITH AVERAGE OF A &V HB VALU
 VO2=OXYGEN CONSUMPTION, C.O.=CARDIAC OUTPUT, A-a=ALVEOLAR arterial O2 DIFFERENCE, Qs/Qt=SHUNT, PK=PEAK, PL=PLATEAU, PP=PEE
 MR=MACHINE RATE, SR=SPONTANEOUS RATE.        *** SPECIMEN IDENTIFICATION: BLOOD (A=ARTERIAL, V=VENOUS, C=CAPILLARY, W=WEDG
                                              FLUIDS (P=PLEURAL, J=JOINT, B=ABDOMINAL, S=ABSCESS); E=EXPIRED AIR;
                                              ECCo2R (I=INFLOW, M=MIDFLOW, O=OUTFLOW)

 KEEP FULL PAGE FOR RECORDS
(END)
```

FIGURE 13.24. Blood-gas report showing the patient's predicted values, as well as the measured values. The computer provides a decision-making interpretation and alerting facility. Note that this report summarizes, in reverse chronological order, the patient's blood-gas status over the course of 1 week. (*Source:* Courtesy of LDS Hospital.)

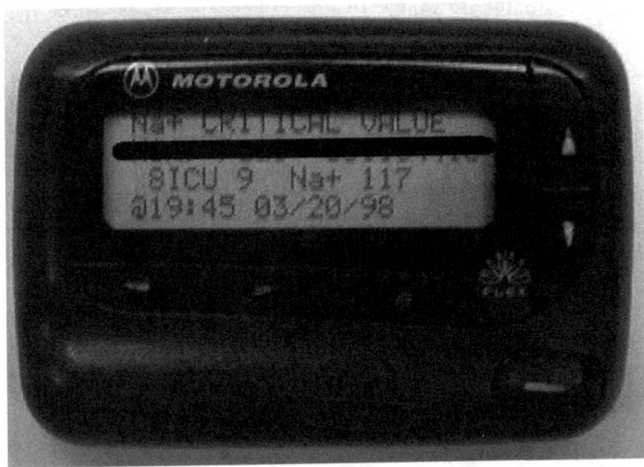

FIGURE 13.25. The alphanumeric pager displays a real-time alert message for a serum sodium level of 117 mg/dl. All laboratory data coming into CareVue is transferred to another computer system where it is run through a rules engine, which generates the pager alert messages.

tervals of time saved may have been too small to be measured using the work-sampling methods employed in the studies. Fifth, these small savings in time are easily absorbed into other activities. Despite the lack of widespread improvement in efficiency, the clinical staff at LDS Hospital are enthusiastic about using computers (Gardner & Lundsgaarde, 1994).

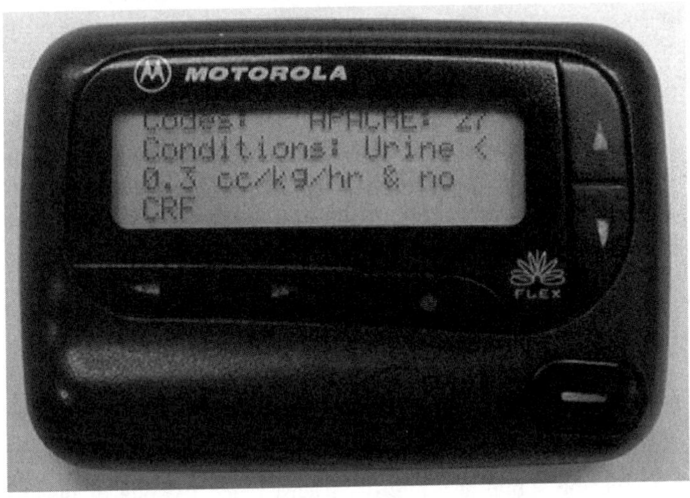

FIGURE 13.26. This pager alert is for low urine output, as defined by the following rule: urine output <0.3 cc/kg/hr for 3 hours and no history of renal failure on admission.

At Cedars-Sinai Medical Center, a national healthcare consulting firm was employed in 1989 to measure time savings associated with the computerized system in the surgical ICUs compared with the standard paper charting system in noncomputerized ICUs. The consultants drew their conclusions from observations of caregiver activities in both kinds of ICUs, as well as from detailed interviews. They concluded that the system saved about 20 percent of the nurses time spent in charting, about 25 percent of surgical residents' time reviewing data, and about 33 percent of attending surgeons' time reviewing data (Dorenfest and Associates, 1989, Chicago, IL, unpublished report).

13.5 Current Issues in Patient Monitoring

As more health services are shifted to outpatient settings, the acuity of hospitalized patients continues to increase; thus, the future of computer-based ICU monitoring systems is bright. Developments in bedside monitors have accelerated because of the availability of more powerful and affordable microcomputers. Nonetheless, some important areas of research in patient monitoring have not yet been addressed effectively.

13.5.1 Data Quality and Data Validation

There are still major problems with acquiring ICU data either automatically or manually (Gardner, 1997, p. 126). A system must provide feedback at various levels to verify correct operation, to carry out quality control, and to present intermediate and final results. As we discussed earlier, some **cross validation** between signals is possible, but this process is performed by few of the bedside monitors used today. An ICU study of early, standalone pulse oximetry monitors revealed that up to 46.5 percent of low saturation alarms were neither observed nor responded to by any caregiver in large part due to constant false alarms associated with such devices (Bentt et al., 1990). Some newer patient-monitoring devices, such as integrated pulse oximeters and direct pressure measuring systems, have built in noise-rejection algorithms to improve the quality of the data presented (Gardner et al., 1986). Data validation, however, is one area of patient monitoring that still offers much opportunity for technological development and improvement (Dalto et al., 1997; Strong et al., 1997; Young et al., 1997).

13.5.2 Continuous Versus Intermittent Monitoring

One of the persistent questions facing people who monitor patients is, Should I measure a parameter continuously, or is intermittent sampling enough? A related question is, How often do I make the measurement? These questions have no simple answer. If we are measuring the ECG and want to display it continuously, we must sample the signal at a rate of at least twice the rate of the maximum frequency of interest in the signal (the Nyquist frequency; see Chapter 4). Thus, for an ECG, the sampling rate should be at least 200 measurements per second.

To perform **intermittent monitoring**—periodic measurement of blood pH, for example—the overriding concerns in determining sampling rate are how rapidly the parameter can change, and how long before a dangerous change will result in irreversible damage. Sudden heart stoppage or severe dysrhythmias are the most frequent causes of sudden death. Therefore, heart-rate and rhythm monitors must function continuously and should sound alarms within 15 to 20 seconds after detecting a problem. Other physiological parameters are not as labile and can be monitored less frequently. For the most part, medical measurements are made intermittently, and even continuously measured parameters are displayed at intervals. For example, heart rate can change with each beat (by 0.35 to 1 second). To provide data that a human can interpret, however, a bedside monitor usually updates its display every 3 seconds.

13.5.3 Data Recording: Frequency and Quantity

In the past, because analog and early digital bedside monitors and central stations could not store continuous waveforms from all patients, it was acceptable for nurses to archive periodic strip chart recordings ("snapshots") in the patient's ICU chart. Most ICUs have policies and procedures for pasting waveform recordings during the nursing shift and for critical events. The newer central stations, however, record digitized waveforms to hard disk on a continuous basis, and theoretically these data could be archived with the patient's electronic chart or printed out for a paper chart. But must second-by-second waveform data be archived permanently? Will it improve the quality of patient care? Or will it simply increase the cost of care in the form of increased magnetic or optical storage media, paper usage, and material for lawyers to haggle over for years to come?

There is a worrisome precedent with fetal monitoring recordings: When it became possible to make a continuous record—first on paper and more recently on optical disk—it became mandatory for hospitals to do so. The fate of continuous recordings of routine ICU waveforms remains to be decided.

13.5.4 Invasive Versus Noninvasive Monitoring

Physiological and biochemical parameters commonly used in monitoring can be measured by instruments and devices that are either invasive (require breaking the skin or entering the body) or noninvasive. After several decades of development of **invasive techniques,** the recent trend has been to design **noninvasive methods.** Much of the development of noninvasive technology can be attributed to the availability of microcomputers and solid-state sensors.

The development of inexpensive light-emitting diodes (LED), small solid-state light detectors, and new computer methods made possible, for example, the development of the pulse oximeter, an exciting example of noninvasive monitoring technology. When alternately red and then infrared light is shined from the LEDs through a finger or an ear, the device can detect the pulsations of blood and determine arterial oxygen saturation and heart rate (Severinghaus & Astrup,

1986). Pulse oximetry is one of the most significant technological advances ever made in monitoring. The technology is reliable, yet inexpensive, and, because it is noninvasive, it does not subject the patient to the costs and risks of invasive techniques (e.g., infection and blood loss).

13.5.5 Integration of Patient-Monitoring Devices

Most bedside patient-support devices, such as IV pumps, ventilators, and physiological monitors, are microcomputer based. Each has its own display and, because each comes from a different manufacturer, each is designed as a standalone unit. As a result, it is common for a nurse or therapist to read a computer display from one of these devices and then to enter the data through a workstation into a different computer. The need to integrate the outputs of the myriad devices in the ICU is apparent. The absence of standards for medical-device communications has stymied the acceptance and success of automated clinical data management systems. Due to the large number and variety of medical devices available and to the peculiar data formats, it is impractical to interface the growing number of bedside devices to computers by building special software and hardware interfaces. For these reasons, an Institute of Electrical and Electronic Engineers (IEEE) **Medical Information Bus (MIB)** standards committee 1073 was established (Dalto et al., 1997; Kennelly & Gardner, 1997; Shabot, 1989; Wittenber & Shabot, 1990; Young et al., 1997). Automated data capture from bedside medical devices is now possible using the IEEE 1073 communications standards.[5] With these standards in place, it is possible for vendors and hospitals to implement "plug and play" interfaces to a wide variety of bedside medical devices such as bedside monitors, IV pumps, and ventilators.

Work at LDS Hospital (Gardner et al., 1992) and many other medical centers using the MIB has demonstrated that the use of a common bus system facilitates timely and accurate data acquisition from bedside devices such as pulse oximeters, ventilators, infusion pumps, pH meters, and mixed venous oxygen saturation monitoring systems. As a result of the standardization of MIB, it is much easier to establish communications with these devices in the ICU (Fig. 13.27). The larger information challenges in the ICU now include integration of patient-monitoring data and observations charted by clinicians within ICU management systems and subsequent integration of the critical-care records with the overall computerized patient record (Chapter 9).

13.5.6 Closed-Loop Therapy

The natural outcome from the remarkable developments noted above would seem to be **closed-loop control** of physiological processes. It can be argued that pacemakers in implantable defibrillators are such devices. In the ICU, however, precisely controlled intravenous pumps are available for drug infusions, and there

[5] http://ieee.org/groups/mib/index.html.

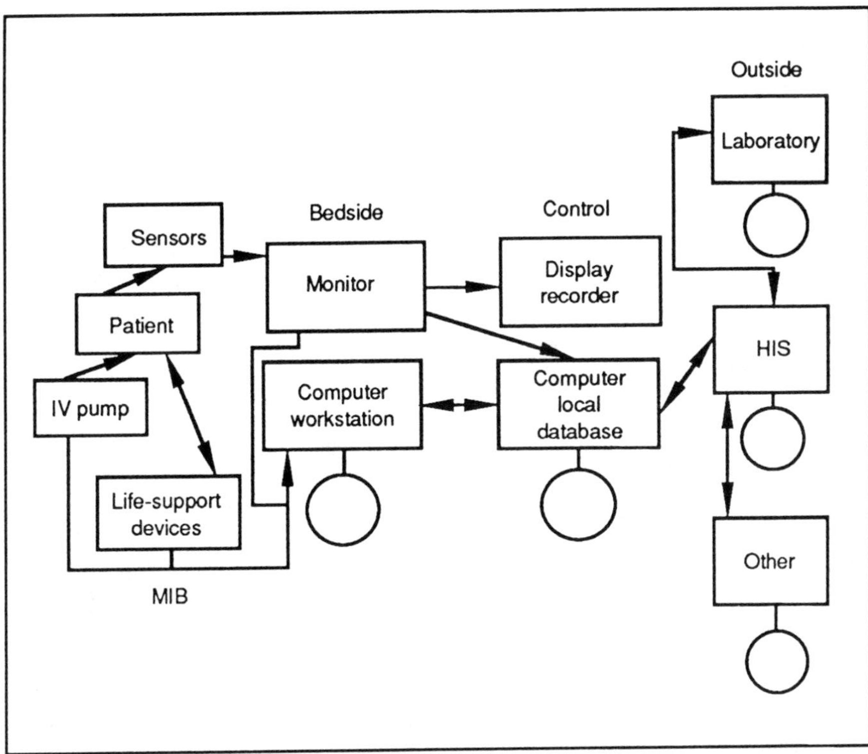

FIGURE 13.27. Block diagram of a distributed-database ICU system with networking. The database has been distributed to improve response time and reliability; the communications network has been implemented to enhance the integration function needed to care for the critically ill patient. MIB = medical information bus; HIS = hospital information system; IV = intravenous.

is no shortage of digitized physiological signals available at the bedside and on the monitoring network. Despite Sheppard and colleagues' pioneering work in automated blood infusion therapy after open-heart surgery over 30 years ago, however, very few examples exist of successful similar work. Although a closed-loop nitroprusside pump was marketed briefly a few years ago, no commercial products are available at this time. The major impediments include the difficulty of creating closed-loop systems with tolerance for the kind of artifacts and measurement errors seen in ICU patients and the difficult medicolegal environment in many industrialized countries.

13.5.7 Treatment Protocols

As in other areas of medical practice, there is considerable interest in developing standard treatment protocols to improve the consistency, quality, and cost effectiveness of critical-care settings. Two different examples will demonstrate the value of treatment protocols in the ICU. The first is an expert system for management of mechanical ventilation, and the second is a computer-assisted management program for antibiotics. Researchers at LDS Hospital initially implemented a program to manage the therapy of patients who have ARDS and who were enrolled in a controlled clinical trial (Sittig, 1987). More recently a broader set of protocols has been developed (East et al., 1992). These computerized protocols were developed to standardize therapy, ensure uniformity of care, provide equal intensity and frequency of monitoring, improve the consistency of decision-making strategies, and achieve common therapeutic goals. The HELP system automatically generates therapeutic instructions regarding ventilator management to healthcare providers based on data input by the laboratory and by physicians, nurses, and respiratory therapists. The system has been used successfully to manage complex patient trials with great success (Henderson et al., 1991).

In contrast, the **antibiotic-assistant program** developed by Evans and colleagues (1998) (also at LDS Hospital) acquires data from the rich coded database of the HELP system and provides "consultation" to physicians ordering antibiotics for patients who have or who are suspected of having an infection. The program is designed to fit into the work flow pattern of practitioners. It provides physicians with the latest pertinent information about individual patients. The computer provides decision support to suggest the appropriate antibiotic for the patient or even to indicate the lack of a need for such a medication. The program uses the patient's admission diagnosis, white-blood cell count, temperature, surgical-procedure data, chest radiograph interpretation (free text), and information from the pathology and microbiology laboratories to make its recommendations. The knowledge base used to drive the clinical recommendations was created from analysis of historical "antibiograms" and the knowledge of clinical and infectious disease experts. Physicians have been enthusiastic users of the system because it provides the relevant data in about 5 seconds, whereas it may take 15 minutes or more to acquire the same data from patient records. In addition, the system was shown to improve the quality of patient care and reduce costs (Evans et al., 1998).

13.5.8 Demonstrating the Efficacy of Care in the Intensive-Care Unit

Intensive-care-unit care is expensive. Given the current pressures to control healthcare spending (see Chapter 19), there is growing concern about the cost effectiveness of such care. In a 1984 study prepared for the Office of Technology Assessment, one researcher estimated that 15 to 20 percent of the nation's hospital budget, or almost 1 percent of the gross national product, was spent for ICU care (Berenson, 1984). Unfortunately, the problems of assessing the benefit of each element in the ICU are many; to date, no definitive studies have been performed. It is difficult to identify and isolate all the factors in the ICU setting that affect patient recovery and outcome. To this end, a Coalition of Critical Care Excellence of the Society of Critical Care Medicine recently reviewed the issues related to developing evidence about the safety and effectiveness of critical care monitoring devices and related interventions (Bone, 1995). Furthermore, the ethical implications of withholding potentially beneficial care from patients in the control group of a randomized clinical trial make such studies almost impossible to perform. As discussed in Section 13.5.7, a computer-assisted program for management of antibiotics at LDS Hospital was found to improve the quality of patient care while reducing associated costs (Evans et al., 1998).

At Cedar-Sinai Medical Center, physiological data, ICU utilization data, and measurable outcomes for specific subsets of ICU patients have been analyzed to determine which patients require care or observation that can only be performed in an ICU. Using these results, the medical center has developed guidelines and pathways for use of the ICU by similar patients. These guidelines have been approved by the various divisions of surgery. Intensive-care unit pathways, including guidelines for nonadmission to the ICU in some cases, are in place for elective craniotomy, thoracotomy, carotid endarterectomy, infrainguinal arterial surgery, ovarian cancer surgery, kidney transplantation, and liver transplantation. Use of these pathways and guidelines has reduced the average ICU cost of caring for these groups of patients, with no adverse changes in outcome (Amir et al., 1997; Chandra et al., 1995; Cunneen et al., 1998; McGrath et al., 1996; Shabot, 1997a). Figure 13.28 shows part of the pathway for infrainguinal arterial surgery,

Clinical Pathways | 8SICU 1 8246 | 1.83m2 150.01b | ? HELP

Actions | Print | Store... | S/O Data...

Pathway		Apr 01 96	Apr 02 96	Apr 03 96
1	1 INFRAINGUINL BYPASS GRAFT	Pathway Day 1	Pathway Day 2	Pathway Day 3 (Floor Care)
2	2 LEVEL OF CARE (B1)	1. Operating Room	1. SICU	
3		2. Recovery Room	2. Floor Care	
4		3. G2 - GUIDELINE FOR TRANSFER TO ICU VS. FLOOR CARE		
5	3 DIAGNOSTIC TESTS/PROCS (B1)		CBC + Chem I	
6			PT	
			PTT	
7	4 MEDICATIONS (B1)	Ancef q8h	Ancef q8h	
8		Heparin Drip	Heparin Drip	
		Pain Management (PCA)	Pain Management (PCA)	
LAB I/O SUMMARY	5 TREATMENTS (B1)	Intravenous line	D/C IV	
10		O2 PRN	D/C O2	
		Pulse Oximeter	D/C Pulse Oximeter	
11	6 ACTIVITY (B1)	Bedrest	OOB to chair	
12		Leg elevated	PT eval	
SICU MENU	7 NUTRITION (B1)	NPO	1. Start Clears	

ABG Results at 1815 Apr 01 96 Available | Mon Apr 01 96 1849

FIGURE 13.28. Cedars-Sinai pathway for managing infrainguinal bypass graft patient. Note the embedded guideline for ICU versus floor care after the Recovery Room (Pathway Day 1). (Source: Courtesy of Cedars-Sinai Medical Center.)

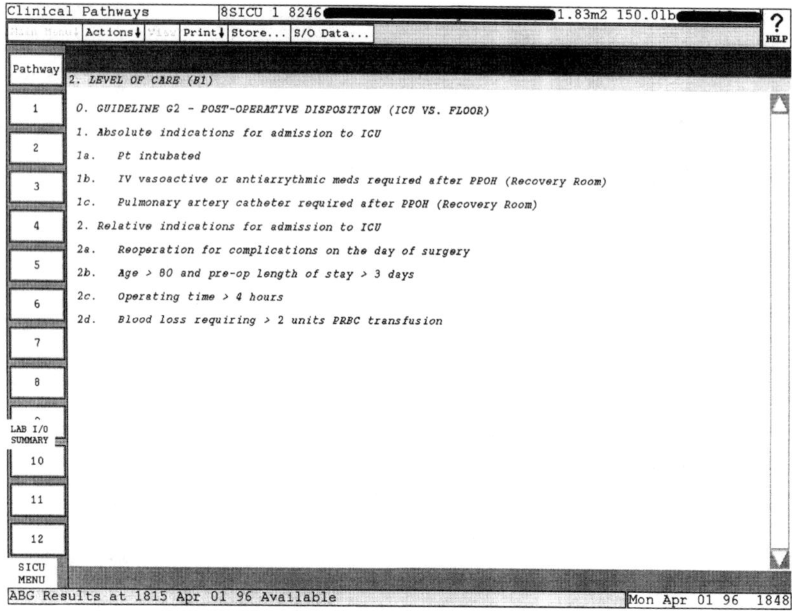

FIGURE 13.29. Pop-up guideline for admission to ICU versus floor care after infrainguinal bypass graft. The evidence-based criteria were derived from the actual ICU courses of hundreds of patients undergoing this operation at Cedars-Sinai. (*Source:* Courtesy of Cedars-Sinai Medical Center.)

and Figure 13.29 shows the pop-up guideline for ICU admission for these patients.

13.5.9 Responsible Use of Medical Software

Use of medical software has become ubiquitous, especially in the ICU. There is a growing literature documenting how computerized systems can improve healthcare delivery (Garibaldi, 1998). There are also concerns, however, about patient safety that must still be addressed. The Food and Drug Administration (FDA) has called for discussions about further regulating such software (Miller & Gardner, 1997a). The American Medical Informatics Association and others have made recommendations about how such software should be monitored and evaluated (Miller & Gardner, 1997b). See Chapter 7 for a discussion of legal issues in healthcare informatics and Chapter 8 for a detailed discussion of software evaluation.

13.5.10 Consensus Conference on Critical-Care Medicine

A global perspective on what should be done to improve critical-care patient-data management can be gained from a 1983 consensus conference organized by the National Institutes of Health (Ayers, 1983). Although formulated in the mid-

1980s, the conclusions of this conference concerning areas of improvement in treatment of critically ill patients remain pertinent today. Many of these problems are amenable to computer assistance. Technical difficulties, errors in data interpretation, and increasing interventions caused by continuous monitoring are potential nosocomial hazards for ICU patients. Based on the findings of the original conference, we identify eight areas in which computers can assist in the practice of critical-care medicine.

1. All ICUs should be capable of arrhythmia monitoring. Bedside physiological monitors with microcomputers now provide excellent arrhythmia monitoring.
2. Invasive monitoring should be performed safely. Computer-based charting of invasive events such as the insertion of an arterial catheter, analyzed in combination with data from the microbiology laboratory, can help to avoid infection (a major complication of invasive monitoring).
3. Generated data should be correct. The computer can check data as they are entered to verify that they are reasonable. In addition, data communications and calculation errors can be reduced or eliminated by letting the computer do the work.
4. Derived data should be interpreted properly. The computer can assist in the integration of data from multiple sources. In addition, the computer can derive parameters and also can provide prompt, accurate, and consistent interpretations and alerts. For example, note in Figure 13.24 that oxygen consumption (Vo_2) is calculated and displayed when data on arterial and venous blood gases and cardiac output are available (oxygen consumption was 353 ml/min on 4JAN89 at 04:19).
5. Therapy should be employed safely. The computer can assist physicians by suggesting therapy, calculating appropriate drug doses, and flagging combinations of interacting drugs.
6. Access to laboratory data should be rapid and comprehensive. Computer networking provides quick access to all laboratory data and can even interpret the results and provide alerts.
7. Enteral (tube-feeding) and parenteral (IV) nutritional-support services should be available. There are interactive computer programs that help physicians to prescribe care by assisting with the complex task of determining the appropriate volume and content of nutritional supplements.
8. Titrated[6] therapeutic interventions with infusion pumps should be available. In theory, closed-loop systems for controlling the administration of fluids and intravenous drugs could facilitate patient care. In reality, however, work to date in this area has proved unsuccessful.

The availability of microcomputers has greatly enhanced the ability to generate and process the physiological data used in patient monitoring. The use of com-

[6] Determination of the concentration of a dissolved substance. Titration is a method for adjusting the concentration of a drug to achieve a desired effect—for example, adjusting nitroprusside infusion to control blood pressure.

puters in the ICU is still an area of growth, however. Although advances in signal processing and ICU information systems have been significant, many challenges remain in the exploration of ways with which the computer can be used effectively to integrate, display results, evaluate, and simplify the complex data used in caring for critically ill patients.

Suggested Readings

Gardner R.M., Sittig D.F., Clemmer T.P. (1995). Computers in the intensive care unit: a match meant to be! In W.C. Shoemaker et al. (Eds.), *Textbook of Critical Care* (3rd ed., pp. 1757–1770). Philadelphia: W.B. Saunders.

This chapter summarizes the current status of medical practice in the ICU. Other chapters in the handbook will be of interest to the medical computer scientist who is exploring the use of computers in critical-care settings.

Ginzton L.E., Laks M.M. (1984). Computer aided ECG interpretation. *M.D. Computing,* 1:36.

This article summarizes the development of computer-based ECG interpretation systems, discusses the advantages and disadvantages of such systems, and describes the process by which a typical system obtains and processes ECG data.

Strong D.M., Lee Y.W., Wang R.T. (1997). 10 potholes in the road to information quality. *IEEE Computer,* 31:38–46.

This article provides an entertaining and thoughtful presentation of the problems we all face as we acquire data. Its use of a general strategy to discuss data-quality problems and relate them to the medical field is refreshing.

Wiederhold G., Clayton P.D. (1985). Processing biological data in real time. *M.D. Computing,* 2:16.

This article summarizes the logical elements of real-time data acquisition and analysis. It contains a detailed discussion of signal acquisition, sampling frequency, and analog-to-digital conversion.

Questions for Discussion

1. Describe how the integration of information from multiple bedside monitors, the pharmacy, and the clinical laboratory can help to improve the sensitivity and specificity of the alarm systems used in the ICU.
2. What factors must you consider when deciding when and how often a physiological, biochemical, or observational variable should be measured and stored in a computer's database?
3. You have been asked to design part of an electronic exercise bicycle. Sensors in the hand grips of the bicycle will be used to pick up transmitted electrical signals reflecting the rider's heart activity. Your system then will display the rider's heart rate numerically in a liquid crystal display (LCD).
   a. Describe the steps your system must take in converting the heart's electrical signals (essentially a single ECG lead) into the heart rate displayed on the LCD.
   b. Describe how computerized data acquisition can be more efficient and accurate than manual methods of data acquisition.

14
Imaging Systems

Robert A. Greenes and James F. Brinkley

After reading this chapter, you should know the answers to these questions:

- What six important roles do images play in health care?
- What are the history, methods, and issues of the four component areas of imaging informatics?
- What are spatial contrast and temporal resolution, the basic parameters that characterize digital medical images?
- What are imaging modalities, such as digital radiography, ultrasound, computed tomography, and magnetic resonance imaging, and how do they produce digital images?
- What are the four stages of image analysis, and which of them are difficult for the computer?
- What are the significant problems we face in managing medical images, and how are they being addressed?
- What methods have been used to integrate images with other information and for what purposes?

14.1 Imaging and Imaging Informatics

Visible light is the final common pathway for images rendered for human viewing, whether they are viewed in photographic form or on video screens. Yet the initial source of energy used to create the image may be the visible light spectrum, the X-ray spectrum, infrared, sound, or other energy. Just about every source of spectral energy is used for creating images, and various parts of the body lend themselves to being imaged with different modalities. Digital methods are being applied in all cases, so no discussion of the modalities is complete without a discussion of the informatics aspects of imaging. In this chapter, we discuss the use of information systems and networks to facilitate the acquisition, storage, transmission, processing, analysis, and management of medical images and to aid the integration of such images in the healthcare process.

14.1.1 Roles for Imaging in Health Care

Imaging is a central part of the healthcare process for diagnosis, treatment planning, image-guided treatment, assessment of response to treatment, and estimation of prognosis. In addition, it plays important roles in medical communication and education, as well as in research.

Diagnosis

One of the primary uses of images is for medical diagnostic purposes. This use includes images produced by *visible light*, as in ophthalmology, for example, to perform retinal photography; in dermatology, to view skin lesions; and in pathology, for gross specimen viewing and for light microscopy. The visible-light spectrum is also responsible for producing images seen endoscopically, rendered typically as video images or sequences. *Sound energy*, in the form of echos from internal structures, is used to form images in ultrasound, a modality used primarily in cardiac, abdominal, pelvic, breast, and obstetrical imaging, as well as in imaging of small parts, such as the thyroid and testes. In addition, Doppler shifts of sound frequency are used to evaluate blood flow in many organs and in major vessels. *X-ray energy* produces radiographic and **computed-tomography** (CT) images of most parts of the body: The differential absorption of X-rays by various tissues produces the varying densities that enable the images to characterize normal and abnormal structures. *Isotope emissions* of radioactive particles are used to produce nuclear-medicine images, which result from the differential concentration of radioactively tagged molecules in various tissues. **Magnetic-resonance imaging** (MRI) depicts *energy fluctuations* of certain atomic nuclei—primarily of hydrogen—when they are aligned in a magnetic field and then perturbed by an orthogonal radiofrequency pulse. Parameters such as proton density, rate at which the nuclei return to alignment, and rate of loss of phase coherence after the pulse can be measured in various combinations, depending on equipment configurations and pulse sequences. These quantities differ in various tissues due to differential concentrations of hydrogen atoms, thus enabling MRI to distinguish among them.

Assessment and Planning

In addition to being used for diagnosis, imaging is often used to assess a patient's health status in terms of progression of a disease process (such as determination of tumor stage), response to treatment, and estimation of prognosis. We can analyze cardiac status by assessing the heart's size and motion echographically. Similarly, we can use ultrasound to assess fetal size and growth, as well as development. Computed tomography is used frequently to determine approaches for surgery or for radiation therapy. In the latter case, precise calculations of radiation-beam configuration can be determined to maximize dose to the tumor while minimizing absorption of radiation by surrounding tissues. This calculation is often performed by simulating alternative radiation-beam configurations.

For surgical planning, three-dimensional volumes of CT or MRI data can be constructed and presented for viewing from different perspectives to facilitate determination of the most appropriate surgical approach.

Guidance of Procedures

Images can provide real-time guidance when virtual-reality methods are used to superimpose a surgeon's visual perspective on the appropriate image view in the projection that demonstrates the abnormality. With endoscopic and minimally invasive surgery, this kind of imaging can provide a localizing context for visualizing and orientating the endoscopic findings.

Although not practical currently, it is conceivable that such minimally invasive surgery could be conducted at a distance (see Chapter 20). Because the abnormality is viewed through a video monitor that displays the endoscopic field, the view can be physically remote, a technique called **telepresence**. Similarly, the manipulation of the endoscope itself could be controlled by a robotic device that reproduces the hand movements of a remote operator, a technique called **telerobotics**.

Communication

Medical decision-making, including diagnosis and treatment planning, is often aided by allowing clinicians to visualize images concurrently with textual reports and discussions of interpretations. Thus, we can consider imaging to be an important adjunct to communication and images to be a desirable component of a multimedia electronic medical record. Communicating digital images is essential to enable remote viewing, interpretation, and consultation, as in techniques such as teleradiology, telepathology, and teledermatology, collectively referred to as **telemedicine**.

Education and Training

Images, both still and in motion form, are an essential part of medical education and training, because so much of medical diagnosis and treatment depends on imaging and on the skills needed to interpret such images (see Chapter 17). Case libraries, tutorials, atlases, three-dimensional models, quiz libraries, and other resources using images can provide this kind of educational support.

Taking a history, performing a physical examination, and conducting medical procedures also demand appropriate visualization and observation skills. Training in these skills can be augmented by viewing images and video sequences, as well as through practice in simulated situations. An example of the latter is an approach to training individuals in endoscopy techniques by using a mannequin and video images in conjunction with tactile and visual feedback that correlate with the manipulations being carried out. An often-overlooked aspect of education that is aided by access to appropriate images is the provision of instructions and educational materials to patients—about their diseases, about procedures to be carried out, about follow-up care, and about healthy lifestyles.

Research

Imaging is, of course, also intimately involved in many aspects of research. An example is structural modeling of DNA and proteins, including their three-dimensional configurations (see Chapter 18). Another is the images obtained in cellular biology to follow the distributions of fluorescent or radioactively tagged molecules. The quantitative study of **morphometrics**, or growth and development, depends on the use of imaging methods. **Functional mapping**—for example, of the human brain—relates specific sites on images to particular functions.

14.1.2 The Radiologic Process and Its Interaction

In this chapter we concentrate on the subset of imaging that falls under the purview of **radiology**. Radiology departments are engaged in all aspects of the healthcare process, from diagnosis to treatment, and they illustrate well the many issues involved in acquiring and managing images, interpreting them, and communicating those interpretations. Space does not permit us to discuss the other imaging disciplines, but the processes involved and issues faced, which we discuss in the context of radiology, pertain to the other disciplines also. Occasionally, we intersperse examples from other areas, where we wish to emphasize a particular point, and imaging for educational purposes is discussed at length in Chapter 17.

The primary function of a radiology department is the acquisition and analysis of medical images. Through imaging, healthcare personnel obtain information that can help them to establish diagnoses, to plan therapy, and to follow the courses of diseases or therapies.

Diagnostic studies in the radiology department are provided at the request of referring clinicians, who then use the information for decision-making. The radiology department produces the images, and the radiologist provides the primary analysis and interpretation of the radiologic findings. Thus, radiologists play a direct role in clinical problem-solving and in diagnostic-work-up planning. **Interventional radiology** and image-guided surgery are activities in which the radiologist plays a primary role in treatment.

The radiologic process (Greenes, 1989) is characterized by seven kinds of tasks, each of which involves information exchange and which can be augmented and enhanced by information technology, as illustrated in Figure 14.1. The first five tasks occur in sequence, whereas the final two are ongoing and support the other five.

1. The process begins with an evaluation by a clinician of a clinical problem and determination of the need for an imaging procedure.
2. The procedure is requested and scheduled, the indication for the procedure is stated, and relevant clinical history is made available.

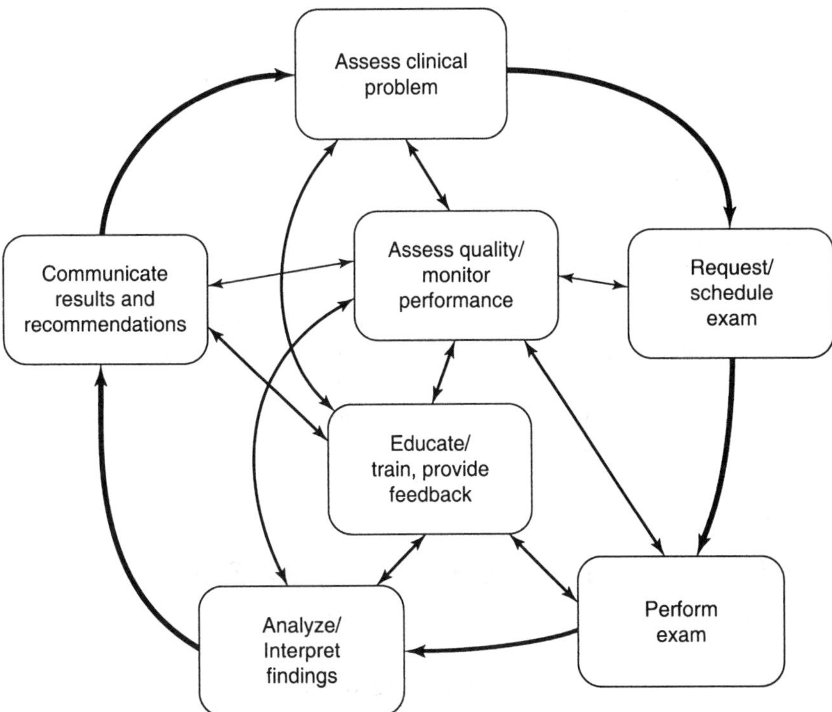

FIGURE 14.1. The radiologic process. The typical flow of activity begins when a clinician assesses a clinical problem and determines that an imaging procedure would be useful (topmost box). Subsequently, four classes of activities (moving clockwise around the circle) ensue, ending with a report to the clinician of the interpretation and possible recommendations for additional studies. The process may continue iteratively as needed. All these activities involve interaction between the clinical and imaging departments (e.g., performance of a particular imaging examination may require tailoring or special views, depending on the clinical question), and all depend on information exchange and information-technology support. The two classes of activity at the center of the diagram are not part of the workflow for individual procedures but are essential to maintaining quality and supporting the professional growth and development of participants; thus, ideally, they need to interact with all of the department-level workflow activities in the outer circle.

3. The imaging procedure is carried out, and images are acquired. The procedure may be tailored for particular clinical questions or patient status considerations.
4. The radiologist reviews the images in terms of the clinical history and questions to be answered and may manipulate the images. This task actually involves two subtasks: (a) perception of the relevant findings and (b) interpretation of those findings in terms of clinical significance.
5. The radiologist creates a report and may otherwise also directly communicate the results to the referring clinician, as well as frequently making suggestions

for further evaluation. The process may then be repeated if another procedure is considered to be helpful.

6. Quality control and monitoring are carried out, with the aim of improving the foregoing processes. Factors such as patient waiting times, workloads, numbers of exposures obtained per procedure, radiation dose, yields of procedures, and incidence of complications are measured and adjusted.
7. Continuing education and training are carried out through a variety of methods, including access to atlases, review materials, teaching-file cases, and feedback of subsequently confirmed diagnoses to interpreting radiologists.

All these tasks have been or will soon become computer assisted, and most of them involve images in some way. In fact, radiology is one branch of medicine in which even the basic data can be produced by computers and stored directly in computer memory. Radiology has also contributed strongly to advances in computer-aided instruction (see Chapter 17), in technology assessment (see Chapter 8), and in clinical decision support (see Chapter 16).

14.1.3 Imaging Informatics: Basis for a Subdiscipline

As is evident from the preceding sections, the use of images is pervasive throughout the healthcare enterprise, not only in radiology but also in such diverse areas as education and basic research. Because of the proliferation in the number and kind of images available, it has become imperative to find ways to organize and manage images. A new subdiscipline of medical informatics, called **imaging informatics**, has been proposed (Kulikowski, 1997) in recognition of the common issues that arise in all image modalities and applications once the images are converted to digital form. By trying to understand these common issues, we can develop general solutions that can be applied to all images, regardless of the source.

The common tasks addressed by imaging informatics can be roughly classified as image generation, image management, image manipulation, and image integration. **Image generation** is the process of generating the images and converting them to digital form if they are not intrinsically digital. **Image management** includes methods for storing, transmitting, displaying, retrieving, and organizing images. **Image manipulation** uses preprocessing and postprocessing methods to enhance, visualize, or analyze the images. **Image integration** is the combination of images with other information needed for interpretation, management, and other tasks. As such it overlaps many other subdisciplines of medical informatics, including **structural informatics**, which is the study of methods for organizing and managing diverse sources of information about the physical organization of the body and other physical structures (Brinkley, 1991).

In the following sections, we discuss each of these four areas separately, recognizing that there is considerable overlap among them but also that each area gives rise to unique problems.

14.2 Image Generation

The images of many radiologic studies are still recorded on film. This situation is rapidly changing, however: There are many intrinsically digital modalities, such as MRI or CT, and there is now widespread availability of devices for converting analog images to digital form. For these reasons, we can assume that most images of interest to the field of imaging informatics soon will be digital. This assumption provides a common basis for discussing all forms of images.

14.2.1 Basic Concepts in Image Generation

A **digital image** typically is represented in a computer by a two-dimensional array of numbers (a **bit map**). Each element of the array represents the intensity of a small square area of the picture, called a **pixel**. If we consider the image of a volume, then a three-dimensional array of numbers is required; each element of the array in this case represents a volume element, called a **voxel**.

We can store any image in a computer in this manner, either by converting it from an analog to a digital representation or by generating it directly in digital form. Once an image is in digital form, it can be handled just like all other data. It can be transmitted over communications networks, stored compactly in databases on magnetic or optical media, and displayed on graphics monitors. In addition, the use of computers has created an entirely new realm of capabilities for image generation and analysis; images can be *computed* rather than measured directly. Furthermore, digital images can be manipulated for display or analysis in ways not possible with film-based images.

All images can be characterized by several parameters of image quality. The most useful of these parameters are spatial resolution, contrast resolution, and temporal resolution. These parameters have been widely used to characterize traditional X-ray images; they also provide an objective means for comparing images formed by digital imaging modalities.

- **Spatial resolution** is related to the sharpness of the image; it is a measure of how well the imaging modality can distinguish points on the object that are close together. For a digital image, spatial resolution is determined by the number of pixels per image area.
- **Contrast resolution** is a measure of the ability to distinguish small differences in intensity, which in turn are related to differences in measurable parameters, such as X-ray attenuation. For digital images, the number of bits per pixel determines the contrast resolution of an image.
- **Temporal resolution** is a measure of the time needed to create an image. We consider an imaging procedure to be a *real-time* application if it can generate images at a rate of at least 30 per second. At this rate, it is possible to produce unblurred images of the beating heart.

Other parameters that are specifically relevant to medical imaging are the magnitude of risk to the patient, the degree of invasiveness, the dosage of **ionizing**

radiation, the degree of patient discomfort, the size (portability) of the instrument, the ability to depict physiologic function as well as anatomic structure, and the cost of the procedure.

A perfect imaging modality would produce images with high spatial, contrast, and temporal resolution; it would be low in cost, portable, free of risk, painless, and noninvasive; it would use nonionizing radiation; and it would depict physiological function as well as anatomic structure.

14.2.2 Historical Development of Imaging Modalities

The historical development of the various imaging modalities can be seen partly as a search for the perfect imaging modality; a primary reason for the proliferation of modalities is that no single modality satisfies all the desiderata. Another reason for the proliferation of image-generation methods is that progress has occurred in parallel in three main areas, and researchers have developed new methods quickly by combining elements from each of these areas. The three areas of development are energy source, reconstruction method, and higher dimensionality.

Energy Source

The earliest medical images used **light** to create photographs either of gross anatomic structures or, if a microscope was used, of histological specimens. Light is still an important source for creation of images. Visible light does not, however, allow us to see inside the body.

X-rays were first discovered in 1895 by Wilhelm Conrad Roentgen, who was awarded the 1901 Nobel Prize in Physics for this achievement. The discovery caused worldwide excitement, especially in the field of medicine; by 1900, there already were several medical radiological societies. Thus, the foundation was laid for a new branch of medicine devoted to imaging the structure and function of the body (Kevles, 1997).

Film-based **radiography** is the primary modality used in radiology departments today, although this emphasis is changing rapidly as digital or computed radiography services are installed. We produce a typical X-ray image by projecting an X-ray beam—one form of ionizing radiation—from an X-ray source through a patient's body (or other object) and onto an X-ray–sensitive film. Because an X-ray beam is differentially absorbed by the various body tissues, the X-rays produce shadows on the radiographic film. The resultant **shadowgraph** is a superposition of all the structures traversed by each beam. **Digital radiography** applies the same techniques, but nonfilm detectors are used (Fig. 14.2). In a technique known as **computed radiography**, a latent image is recorded on a specially coated cassette that is scanned by a computer to capture the image in digital form; in other techniques, detectors capture the data directly in digital form. Although the images obtained by these techniques may be printed subsequently on film, they do not need to be.

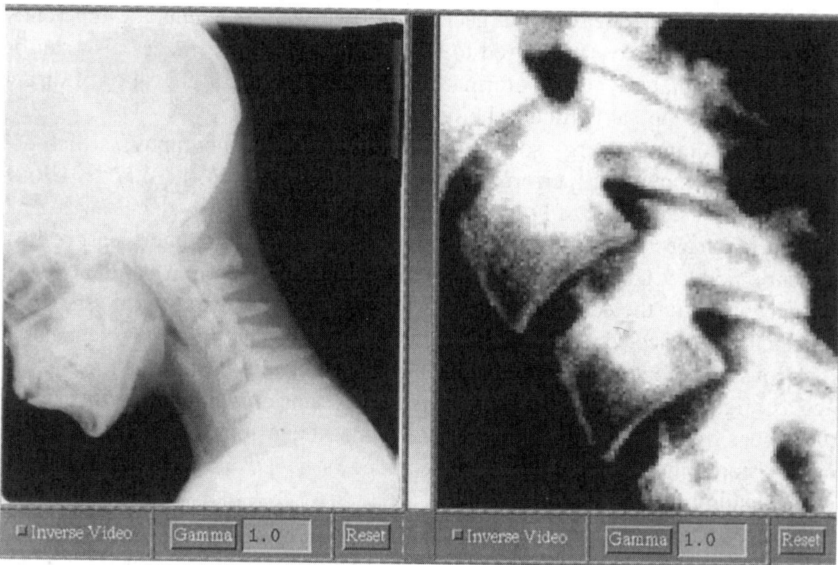

FIGURE 14.2. A digital X-ray image, displayed in an experimental Java applet. X-ray images are shadowgraphs, where each pixel value represents the attenuation of an X-ray beam along a line from the X-ray tube, passing through the object (in this case, the body), and ending at the pixel. Because the image is digital, it many be manipulated. The right-hand panel shows the result of a zoom and windowing operation. (*Source:* Courtesy of Andrew Barclay, Emory University; http://www.emory.edu/CRL/abb.)

Both film and fluoroscopic screens were used initially for recording X-ray images, but the fluoroscopic images were too faint to be used clinically. By the 1940s, however, television and image-intensifier technology were used to produce clear real-time fluorescent images. Today, a standard procedure for many types of examinations is to combine real-time television monitoring of X-ray images with the creation of selected higher resolution film images. Until the early 1970s, film and **fluoroscopy** were the only X-ray modalities available.

Traditional X-ray images have high spatial resolution and medium cost. Furthermore, they can be generated in real time (fluoroscopy) and can be produced using portable instruments. Their disadvantages are their relatively poor contrast resolution, their use of ionizing radiation, and their inability to depict physiological function. Alternate imaging principles have been applied to increase contrast resolution, to eliminate exposure to X-ray radiation, and so on. For example, in nuclear-medicine imaging, a **radioactive isotope** is chemically attached to a biologically active compound (such as iodine) and then is injected into the patient's peripheral circulation. The compound collects in the specific body compartments or organs (such as the thyroid), where it is stored or processed by the body. The isotope emits radiation locally, and the radiation is measured using a special detector. The resultant nuclear-medicine image depicts the level of radioactivity that was measured at each point. Because the counts are inherently digital, computers have been used to record them. Multiple images also can be processed to obtain dynamic information, such as the rate of arrival or of disappearance of isotope at particular body sites.

Another common energy source is **ultrasound** (echosonography), which developed out of research performed by the Navy during World War II. **Ultrasonography** uses pulses of high-frequency sound waves rather than ionizing radiation to image body structures. As each sound wave encounters tissues in a patient's body, a portion of the wave is reflected and a portion continues. The time required for the echo to return is proportional to the distance into the body at which it is reflected; the amplitude (intensity) of a returning echo depends on the acoustical properties of the tissues encountered and is represented in the image as brightness. The system constructs two-dimensional images by displaying the echoes from pulses of multiple adjacent one-dimensional paths. Such images can be stored in digital memories or recorded on videotape and then displayed as television (raster-display) images.

Creation of images from **magnetism** grew out of **nuclear magnetic resonance (NMR) spectroscopy**, a technique that has long been used in chemistry to characterize chemical compounds. Many atomic nuclei within the body have a net magnetic moment, so they act like tiny magnets. When a small chemical sample is placed in an intense, uniform magnetic field, these nuclei line up in the direction of the field, spinning around the axis of the field with a frequency dependent on the type of nucleus, on the surrounding environment, and on the strength of the magnetic field.

If a radio pulse of a particular frequency is applied at right angles to the stationary magnetic field, those nuclei with rotation frequency equal to that of the radiofrequency pulse resonate with the pulse and absorb energy. The higher energy state causes the nuclei to change their orientation with respect to the fixed magnetic field. When the radiofrequency pulse is removed, the nuclei return to their original aligned state, emitting a detectable radiofrequency signal as they do so. Characteristic parameters of this signal—such as intensity, duration, and frequency shift away from the original pulse—are dependent on the density and environment of the nuclei.

In the case of traditional NMR spectroscopy, different molecular environments cause different frequency shifts (called *chemical shifts*), which we can use to identify the particular compounds in a sample. In the original NMR method, however, the signal is not localized to a specific region of the sample, so it is not possible to create an image. Creation of images had to await the development of computer-based reconstruction techniques, which arguably represent the most spectacular application of computers in all of medicine.

Reconstruction Methods

Reconstruction techniques were first applied to X-ray images, growing out of the problem of superposition of structures. An X-ray image at a given point represents the total attenuation due to all the overlaid structures traversed by a beam as that beam passes through the body; shadows cast by surrounding structures may obscure the object that the clinician wishes to visualize. **Contrast radiography**—the use of radiopaque contrast material to highlight the areas of interest—was used as early as 1902 to address this problem. The first clinical experiments with **angiography**—imaging of blood vessels performed by the injection of opacifying agents into the bloodstream—were conducted in 1923.

The desire to separate superimposed structures also led to the development of a variety of analog tomographic techniques. In these methods, the X-ray source and detector were moved in opposite arcs, thereby causing a thin tomographic (planar) section to remain in focus while other planes were blurred. This method, however, exposes the patient to a relatively high X-ray dose because the blurred areas are exposed continuously.

Mathematical methods for reconstructing images from projections were first developed by Radon in 1917 and later were improved by other researchers. These methods were used in the 1950s and 1960s to solve scientific problems in many fields, including radio astronomy and electron microscopy. In the late 1960s, Cormack used the techniques to reconstruct phantoms (objects with known shape) using X-rays. In the early 1970s, Hounsfield led a team at the London-based EMI Corporation, which developed the first commercially viable CT scanner.

Instead of depicting a directly measurable parameter (the absorption of X-ray beams as they pass through the body), CT mathematically reconstructs an image from X-ray–attenuation values that have been measured from multiple angles. As a result, it is possible to view cross-sectional *slices* through the body rather than two-dimensional projections of superimposed structures. Thus, CT images provide a precise mapping of the internal structures of the body in three-dimensional space—a function not provided by standard X-ray images. They also greatly improve contrast resolution.

In the basic CT imaging technique, the patient is placed between an X-ray–sensitive detector and an X-ray source that produces a collimated (pencil-like) beam. The measured difference between the source and detector X-ray intensities represents the amount of X-ray attenuation due to the tissues traversed by the beam; this measured attenuation is a superposition, or **projection**, of the attenuations of all the individual tissue elements traversed by the beam. In the simplest reconstruction method, called **back-projection**, the measured intensity is distributed uniformly over all the pixels traversed by the beam. For example, if the measured attenuation is 20, and 10 pixels were traversed, then the CT number of each of the 10 pixels is incremented by 2 units.

The attenuation measured from a single projection is not sufficient to reconstruct an image. The same back-projection computation, however, can be applied to the attenuations measured from multiple projections. The source and detector are translated and rotated about the patient, and the X-ray attenuation is measured along each path. Because each pixel is traversed by multiple projection paths, its computed attenuation is the sum of the contributions from each path. The total sum provides a reasonable first approximation of the X-ray attenuation of the individual pixel. The image is further refined using a mathematical edge-enhancement technique called **convolution**. In effect, convolution removes shadows that result from the back projection, thus sharpening the blurry image.

The development of the CT scanner dramatically improved our ability to visualize adjacent structures; for the first time, physicians were able to see inside a living human being clearly, but noninvasively. This ability led to a revolution in medicine almost as great as the one occasioned by the invention of X-ray imaging. As a result, Cormack and Hounsfield were awarded the 1979 Nobel Prize in Medicine.

After the invention of the CT scanner, this basic method of reconstruction from projections was applied to other energy sources, including magnetism (MRI), ultrasound (ultrasound-transmission tomography), and variants of nuclear-medicine imaging called positron-emission tomography (PET) and single-photon-emission computed tomography (SPECT).

The most dramatic example of reconstruction from projections (other than CT) is MRI, which is based on NMR (Oldendorf & Oldendorf, 1991). As described in the previous section, NMR takes advantage of magnetic properties of nuclei to characterize the distribution and chemical environment of nuclei within a chemical sample. To create an image using these parameters, we need a way to restrict this sample to a small volume within a larger tissue. With this restriction, the parameters of the NMR signal from each small tissue volume can be mapped to voxel intensities depicting different tissue characteristics.

The restriction to a small sample volume was accomplished by taking advantage of the fact that the resonant frequency of atomic nuclei varies with the magnetic field. If the field can be made different for each small tissue volume, then a radiofrequency pulse with a given frequency will excite only those nuclei in the small volume that have the resonant frequency of that pulse. The basic method uses electromagnetic coils to superimpose a varying magnetic field on a large fixed magnetic field, thereby setting up a gradient in the magnetic field.

This gradient is changed electronically, setting the location of the sample volume. For example, we use one gradient to set the plane of section (the z direction, although the orientation of this section may be arbitrary with respect to the patient), and a second gradient sets a line within a single section (the x,y plane). As in CT, the signal detected along this line is a summation of the signals from all voxels along the line. Therefore, the x,y gradient is electronically rotated, rotating the plane of section and generating additional lines within a given plane. The same reconstruction techniques developed for CT then reconstruct the values for the individual voxels within the given plane. Because there are many different parameters that can be measured for each sampled voxel, many different types of images can be constructed, not all of which are yet available.

Higher Dimensionality

Most routine images in radiology are still two-dimensional. Because the body is a three-dimensional object that changes over time, however, there will always be a drive to create three-dimensional time-varying images. In recent years, advances in digital hardware have provided the storage and throughput to manage large time-varying voxel-based data sets. Reconstruction modalities—such as CT, PET, and MRI—all are either inherently three-dimensional or can be made three-dimensional by acquisition of a series of closely spaced parallel slices. Thus, the only drawbacks of these techniques are the time and expense required to acquire a series of parallel slices, both of which are becoming smaller.

Ultrasound images, on the other hand, cannot be acquired as parallel slices because sound does not pass through bone or air. For this reason, we usually obtain three-dimensional ultrasound information by attaching a three-dimensional locating device to the transducer. The locator gives the position and orientation of the slice plane in space. Before the availability of hardware that could store large numbers of volume data, the ultrasound images were first processed in two dimensions to *extract* relevant anatomy as two-dimensional contours or regions; the two-dimensional contours were converted to three-dimensional contours based on the location information and then were displayed with vector graphics (Brinkley et al., 1978). Such an approach was useful for quantitation, but did not provide a realistic three-dimensional view of the object.

14.2.3 Current Status of Image-Generation Methods

Table 14.1 compares imaging parameters for the most commonly used techniques in radiology today. Most imaging in radiology is still two dimensional, so Table 14.1 represents the common situation in a radiology department. For each of the

Table 14.1. Comparative imaging parameters for alternative imaging modalities.

	CR	MRI	CT	US	NM
Pixels per image	2,048 × 2,560	256 × 256	512 × 512	512 × 512	128 × 128
Bits per pixel	12	10	12	8	8
Typical number of images per study	2	100	60	30 (plus dynamic series)	30
Bytes per study[a]	20 million	12 million	30 million	7.5 million (for static images only)	0.5 million
Contrast resolution	Low	High	High	Low	Low
Spatial resolution	High	Low	Moderate	Moderate	Low
Temporal resolution	Low	Low	Moderate	High	High
Radiation	Moderate	None	Moderate	None	Moderate
Portability	Some	No	No	Yes	Yes
Physiological function	No	Yes	No	No	Yes
Cost	Moderate	High	High	Low	Moderate

CR = computed radiography; MRI = magnetic resonance imaging; CT = computed tomography; US = ultrasound; NM = nuclear medicine.

[a] We assume that 2 bytes are needed per pixel for images that have a pixel depth of 10 or 12 bits.

parameters, the values have improved gradually due primarily to advances in digital hardware and software.

In addition to improvements to these standard two-dimensional-imaging modalities, there are other new imaging modalities, many of which are or soon will be routinely available. Most of these new techniques can be seen as a combination of an energy source, a computer-based processing or reconstruction technique, and increased dimensionality due to advances in digital hardware. The remainder of this section describes examples of these techniques.

At the microscopic level the confocal microscope uses electronic focusing to move a two-dimensional slice plane through a three-dimensional tissue slice placed in a microscope. The result is a three-dimensional voxel array of a microscopic, or even submicroscopic, specimen (Paddock, 1994). At the gross anatomic level, **charge-coupled device (CCD) cameras** are used to convert existing film-based equipment to units that can produce images in digital form. Storage phosphor, or computed radiography (CR), systems replace film by substituting a reusable phosphor plate in a standard film cassette. The exposed plate is processed by a reader system that scans the image into digital form, erases the plate, and packages the cassette for reuse. An important advantage of CR systems is that the cassettes are of standard size, so they can be used in any equipment that holds film-based cassettes (Horii, 1996).

Ultrasound machines have essentially become specialized computers with attached peripherals. For example, one fairly recent machine by Advanced Technology Laboratories (the HDI-1000) is based on a personal-computer (PC) platform: Specialized modules plug into the expansion bus to acquire the ultrasound signal into central-processing unit (CPU) memory, after which software routines perform signal and image processing. The graphics display and input–output facilities of the PC are used for image display, archiving, and user control. Such an approach can reduce the cost of an ultrasound machine greatly, because off-the-shelf hardware and software are used. Newer machines may include a web server that allows images and patient reports to be transferred over the World Wide Web and can even send and receive electronic mail.

Another active area of development is three-dimensional ultrasound imaging. As in the past, a three-dimensional locating device is attached to the ultrasound transducer, but the data are now written directly into a three-dimensional array memory. As the transducer is swept throughout a volume by the human operator, the corresponding voxels are set. After enough of the volume has been imaged, the resulting three-dimensional voxel array can be displayed using standard rendering techniques (Fig. 14.3) (Ritchie et al., 1996).

Another trend is the development of methods for displaying *function*, as well as static anatomy. Nuclear medicine was the first technique to create such displays, but the images suffered the same superposition problem as X-ray images. Application of reconstruction techniques to radioisotope imaging led to PET images in which relatively low-spatial-resolution two-dimensional or three-dimensional arrays can be created to show uptake of radioisotopes by active tissues.

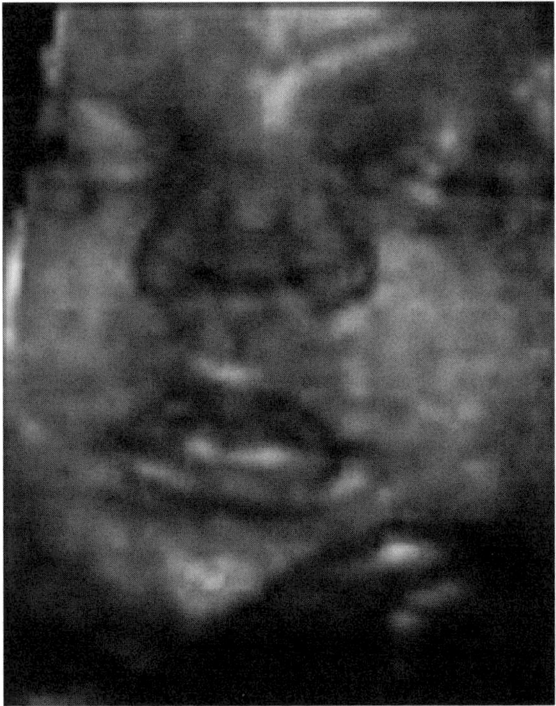

FIGURE 14.3. Volume-rendered image of a fetal face obtained from ultrasound. The beam of a volume tranducer was swept through the portion of the mother's uterus occupied by the fetal head, and the images were stored in a three-dimensional digital memory. Volume datasets such as these are now routine because of advances in computer hardware. (*Source:* Courtesy of Drs. TR Nelson and DH Pretorius, Department of Radiology, University of California at San Diego.)

MRI has probably undergone the most development in functional imaging. For example, functional MRI (fMRI) accomplishes a task similar to that of PET except that increased blood flow due to metabolic activity is measured by changes in MRI signals due to changes in the chemical environment of the tissue samples (Fig. 14.4) (Lee et al., 1996). fMRI has great potential because it does not require ionizing radiation and it provides higher spatial and temporal resolution than does PET.

Other applications of magnetic resonance include magnetic-resonance angiography (MRA) and magnetic-resonance venography (MRV), which employ special pulse sequences to image moving atoms, thereby providing contrast-enhanced images of vessels without requiring the injection of contrast material (Stringer, 1997). In addition, magnetic-resonance spectroscopy (MRS) extends traditional NMR spectroscopy by employing reconstruction techniques to localize the sample volume to a small volume in space, thereby allowing localized metabolic changes to be observed (Dager & Steen, 1992).

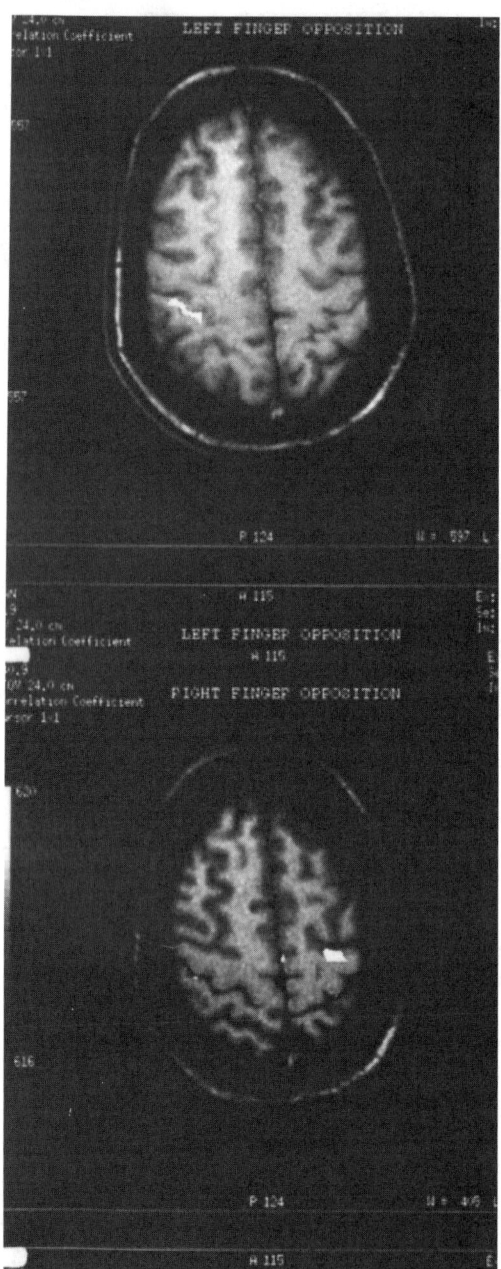

FIGURE 14.4. Functional magnetic-resonance imaging (fMRI), showing areas of brain activation in response to specific tasks. In this case, the volunteer performed a finger-tapping exercise, causing the motor cortex to be activated. *a,* Left-finger tapping, resulting in right-brain activation. *b,* Right-finger tapping, resulting in left-brain activation. Note that radiologists look at images from the perspective of standing at the patient's feet; thus right on the image is left in the body. (*Source:* Courtesy of Kenneth Maravilla, Department of Radiology, University of Washington.)

Another emerging trend in functional imaging is direct three-dimensional reconstruction of electrical activity in the brain by electroencephalography (EEG) and magnetoencephalography (MEG) (George et al., 1995). In these methods, reconstruction techniques process signals from an array of scalp sensors. The resulting three-dimensional volumes depict electrical activity within small regions of the brain. This method provides a measure of neuronal activity potentially more direct than PET or fMRI, because the latter two modalities measure increases in blood flow that are the result of neuronal activity rather than neuronal activity itself. MEG and EEG, however, require a good model of the underlying anatomy to localize the current sources with any precision, and the best such models arise from MRI. Thus, we obtain maximum information by combining several different techniques.

14.3 Image Management

One of the major burdens of the radiology department is the storage and retrieval of the images relating to specific examinations, which are required for interpretation by radiologists, for review by referring physicians, for consultation, for treatment planning, for education, and for research. As health-care delivery networks disperse geographically, the need for remote access to images increases. These factors create a strong push toward digital capture, storage, transmission, interpretation, and review of images.

14.3.1 Basic Concepts in Image Management

Although imaging modalities increasingly generate their images in digital form, many medical imaging studies are still primarily or secondarily recorded and stored on film. Even images produced by CT and MRI scans, which are inherently digital, are often transferred to film after the technologist has optimized them for viewing. Radiologists then place the filmed images on illuminated light boxes, where the films can be analyzed in comparison to previous and related studies. For certain procedures—for example, ultrasound and fluoroscopic studies—the images may be recorded on videotape or videodisk rather than on film.

Before widespread digital imaging, the management procedures have typically been as follows: Radiology personnel prepare a film folder for each examination (or type of examination), label it with patient-identification information, and file it with the patient's master film jacket in the film library. The staff must locate and retrieve the master jacket each time that the images are needed for review or for comparison with previous studies. If a clinician wishes to take a film out of the department, the staff must make a duplicate film or transact a loan.

Film storage requires a large amount of space. Typically, departments have the capacity to store films for only those patients whose studies were completed within the past 6 to 12 months. Older studies, usually retained for at least 7 years, are stored in a basement or warehouse. Film is also expensive; radiology departments typically sell film from outdated examinations for recycling of silver content.

Digital acquisition of images offers the exciting prospect of reducing the physical space requirements, material cost, and manual labor of traditional film-handling tasks through on-line digital archiving, rapid retrieval of images via querying of image databases, and high-speed transmission of images over communications networks. Researchers and industry have worked to develop systems that have such capabilities—**picture-archiving and communication systems** (PACS) (Fig. 14.5) (Dwyer, 1996). Many complex problems had to be solved for PACSs to be practical, including development of technology for high-resolution acquisition, high capacity storage, and high-speed networking; standardization of image-transmission and storage formats; development of storage-management schemes for enormous volumes of data; and design of workstations, or display consoles, that are as convenient and acceptable to radiologists for the interpretation of digital images as are the illuminated light boxes used for film-based interpretation. *Soft copy* interpretation—that is, by the radiologist viewing a study at a workstation—is done in the growing number of departments that have become *filmless*, and increasingly for interpretation of remotely acquired studies in the practice of *teleradiology*.

Image Acquisition

The primary requirement for PACS is that it must obtain images in digital form (Horii, 1996). As discussed in Section 14.2, most imaging modalities—even those traditionally done on film—are now capable of producing direct digital output, yet replacement of all imaging equipment with digital units is expensive and is proceeding sporadically as old equipment needs to be updated or as departments expand.

In departments in which traditional imaging devices are still being used for some modalities, the only option for achieving a full PACS is digital scanning of film. Such scanning is rarely done because it requires considerable manual handling, for transport and handling of examination folders and films, for operating the scanner, and for recording of the patient and examination identification information.

Storage Requirements

On-line digital archiving of image data for a busy radiology department requires vast amounts of storage. Image modalities differ substantially in their storage requirements, depending on the contrast and spatial resolution required, the number of images or the size of the data sets, whether raw or processed data are stored, and whether data-compression techniques are used.

Table 14.1 indicates typical raw-data storage requirements (that is, with no preprocessing or postprocessing and no compression) for examinations of a variety of image types. A CT image, for example, consists of a 512×512 array of pixels. If the full dynamic range of CT numbers is saved, each pixel is represented by 12 bits. Once the radiologist or technologist has determined the optimal brightness and contrast settings for displaying the region of interest, however, perhaps only 8 bits per pixel need to be saved. A typical CT examination consists of 40 to 80 cross-sectional slices. Additional slices are required if both precontrast and postcontrast images, or other special slices, are desired. Assuming that a CT examination consists of 60 images and that the full dynamic range is retained for each, then $60 \times 512 \times 512 \times 12$ bits, or approximately 180 mil-

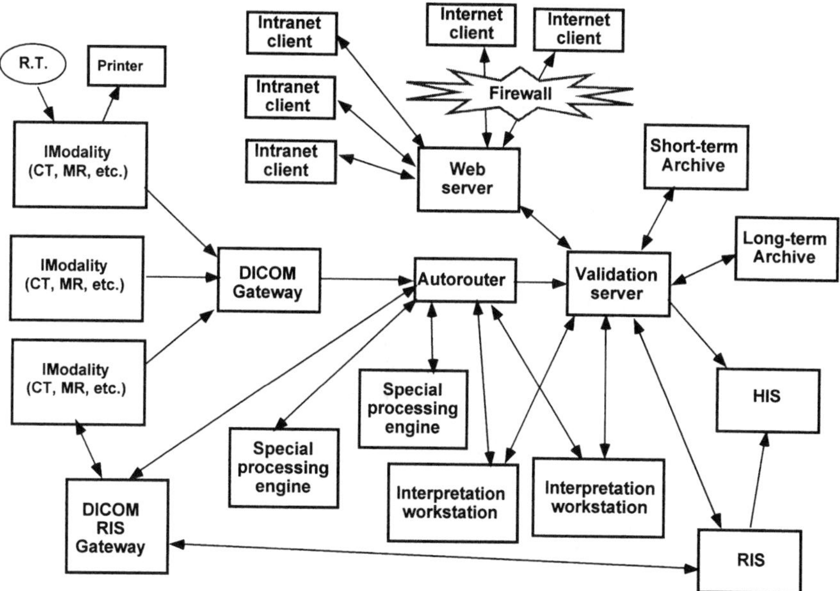

FIGURE 14.5. Architecture of a typical picture-archiving and communication system (PACS). Images are acquired by facilities specific to the various imaging modalities (such as computed radiography, CT, MRI, angiography, ultrasound, or nuclear medicine), and the facilities are operated largely by radiology (or imaging) technologists (denoted R.T.). Local printing of images on film or paper may be performed. Image procedures are scheduled through a radiology information system (RIS), and patient-identification and schedule information is transmitted to the modality workstation through a DICOM RIS gateway. Remote imaging centers operate in the same way.

The images produced are transmitted through a DICOM gateway to a server (autorouter), which is responsible for sending the images where they are needed and for managing workflow. The autorouter validates the linkage of images to the appropriate study (by interaction with a validation server) and distributes them according to rules (e.g., MRIs and CTs are sent to workstation x for interpretation).

Images can be viewed on interpretation workstations, both special purpose and generic, and manipulated by imaging professionals who use built-in workstation tools and invoke special processing functions through servers (e.g., for three-dimensional rendering, registration, and fusion of data from images obtained by two different modalities, for feature extraction, or for computer-aided detection).

Multiple images from a particular examination need to be associated, and both prior and other associated studies and reports may need to be available. This linkage is accomplished by the validation server, which is able to query for and retrieve information from the RIS or hospital information system (HIS), as well as from the PACS archives. The validation server is responsible for coordinating the association of image and non-image information. Referring physicians may access images at internal and Internet-based workstations, typically through a Web interface. Access from a browser through a Web server permits the user to obtain study information, including reports and images, through the validation server, which interacts with the PACS archive and with the HIS and RIS. (*Source:* Adapted from Brigham and Women's Hospital Department of Radiology internal document by William B. Hanlon.)

lion bits, must be saved. Because 12 bits of data typically are stored as 2 bytes, this storage requirement corresponds to 30 million bytes.

A single-view chest X-ray (or CR) image consists of 2,048 × 2,560 × 12 bits of data; therefore, a typical two-image (front and side views) examination contains about 120 million bits. A real-time ultrasound examination generates video images at 30 frames per second. Of these, a radiologist usually selects 30 to 40 frames for later analysis. Occasionally, dynamic sequences, such as those portraying a cardiac arrhythmia, are retained at the full rate of 30 images per second. Resolution per image is 512 × 512 pixels; about 8 bits per pixel are required to store the acoustical signal once the image has been postprocessed for optimal viewing. Nuclear-medicine images have lower resolution—typically, 128 × 128 × 8, or about 130,000 bits of data per image are sufficient. Magnetic resonance imaging has lower resolution but uses multiple images similar to CT except that data are available for a volume of the body rather than for single slices, and data on several parameters at each voxel are potentially useful.

Considering that a typical radiology department performs 250 examinations per day, and nominally assuming 10 megabytes per study, then, in an average day, approximately 2.5 gigabytes of data must be transmitted from the image-acquisition nodes to the image archive. Assuming 250 working days per year (ignoring weekends for simplicity), we estimate that the storage requirements per year for examination image data are on the order of 625 gigabytes.

In addition to the on-line maintenance of active images, an image-archiving system must provide for the storage of less current image data. Because of the large storage requirements, practical systems will use some form of hierarchical storage management, whereby the most current images are easily and rapidly accessible, and images that are less likely to be retrieved are stored in a less costly, less accessible form.

Magnetic disks and optical disks are the most promising media for on-line storage of image data. Magnetic disks currently available can store over 20 gigabytes for half-height drives. Cost per megabyte continues to drop dramatically. Optical write-once compact disks (CDs) are still only 650 megabytes, with long-awaited 4.6 gigabyte (or greater) digital video (DVD) drives still not available in writable form. Magneto-optical (MO) disks are 2.6 gigabytes, with 5.2 gigabyte drives expected soon. Magneto-optical media are expensive and have slow read and write times. Jukeboxes are available, however, in 150-, 500-, and 1,000-platter sizes. For archiving, dense media (such as tape) are still needed, so most departments must maintain an unattractive three-tiered storage scheme, using magnetic disks for active data, optical or MO disks for intermediate storage, and tape, optical disks, or laser cards for inactive storage.

An alternate strategy uses large magnetic disks of 500 gigabytes (0.5 terabytes), sufficient to store approximately 1 year's image data in a typical department; and a digital-tape library functioning for long-term storage, with **radiology information systems** (RISs) scheduling and pre-fetching to retrieve before-examination data before they are needed (see Section 14.5).

Data compression and prior selection or preprocessing of image data can reduce storage requirements considerably. Compression may be lossless or lossy (Dwyer, 1996; Woods, 1991). **Lossless compression** uses simple run-length encoding (RLE) or variations on other sequence coding schemes such as Huffman encoding, which assigns the shortest codes to most frequently occurring values. Maximum compression ratios achievable with lossless methods are on the order of 2:1 or 3:1.

Lossy compression uses methods to filter the image's frequency spectrum and to encode data selectively at various frequencies more compactly and to eliminate other frequencies, which primarily contain noise. A widely used method developed by the Joint Photographic Experts Group, is JPEG compression, which codes images for hue and saturation (or color and intensity). Because the eye is less sensitive to variations in hue than it is to variations in intensity, the hue values can be stored with lower resolution. Compression ratios as high as 20:1 can be obtained with JPEG compression, but with variable quality. Fractal compression is another method being explored.

Wavelet compression is becoming widely accepted as a superior method for image compression (Vetterli & Kovarevic, 1995). Wavelets are basis functions for representing discrete data or continuous functions; they operate more locally than the Fourier transform. They have compact support: There is no truncation error when finite signals, such as those for radiological images, are processed. Wavelet basis functions are orthonormal, meaning that the terms in a wavelet series are nonredundant. Wavelet series provide multiresolution representations for data, organizing them into a hierarchy according to spatial frequency and spatial position.

Compression at ratios as high as 80:1 for plain films such as mammograms are being evaluated. Wavelet compression may *enhance* image appearance by preferentially eliminating nonstructural noise, such as artifacts. Lower compression ratios are achievable for other modalities, depending on how much redundant information is present; for example, 20:1 to 30:1 is possible for chest X-ray images. CT scans may be less compressible, with ratios on the order of 6:1.

Another consideration in storage relates to speed of access. Storage on a local workstation provides fastest access from the point of view of responsiveness to user manipulations; storage on a server may be sufficient if the network speeds are sufficiently high. Images stored on a local workstation must be transmitted there in advance—for example, at off-peak network-traffic times. An examination may have multiple images, and the same image may need to be processed, enhanced, or viewed in multiple different ways (see Section 14.4), all of which require storage. After she completes the interpretation, the radiologist may indicate that only a few of the images contain clinically important information. It then may be practical to archive the other images on optical disk or on another slower access medium. After the examination is complete and has been reviewed by all relevant clinical practitioners, it can also be archived in toto. As a consequence, however, when a practitioner wants to compare an older study with a current study—for example, to evaluate progression of disease—the archived images must be retrieved from the slower access medium. Thus, hierarchies of storage and algorithms for deciding where to place image data based on patterns of expected use and network traffic are required for smooth functioning of a PACS.

Image Transmission

The integration of distributed viewing stations, on-line image databases, image-management systems, and broadband local-area networks (LANs) and wide-area networks (WANs) allows imaging data to be shared among health professionals at remote viewing sites. Furthermore, the data can be viewed at multiple locations simultaneously. Thus, health personnel throughout an institution or extended health-care enterprise can have timely and convenient access to medical images.

The principal media for image transmission and networking are broadband coaxial cable and fiberoptic cable (see Chapter 4). Coaxial cable, used in the cable-television industry, supports a variety of network topologies. Coaxial networks are relatively inexpensive, and they are reliable, although they are susceptible to electrical and radiofrequency interference. Fiberoptic networks offer a high degree of reliability without interference problems, but they are somewhat more limited with respect to the topologies that they can support and the ease with which connections can be added. Slow-speed connections using modems have maximum transmission rates of 56 kilobits per second (Kbps). Wide-area optical-network backbones can now transmit data at 2.4 gigabits per second (Gbps). Many options are available between these extremes, depending on cost limitations and distance requirements, and a network can be configured to combine different components via gateways. The network configuration and the capacity of each part must be planned in relation to considerations such as patterns of expected use and cost. Particular network topologies and protocols available for both LAN and WAN connectivity, and their influence on transmission speeds, are discussed in Chapter 4. Because of the large sizes of image files, image transmission times can vary from hours to seconds, depending on choice of network method and degree of compression.

Standardization of Formats

TCP/IP (see Chapter 4) is the dominant low-level protocol used in medical imaging. Transmission of data about a medical imaging procedure, however, including patient, examination, and image data, requires higher level messaging formats. Layered protocols are organized to build such messages. The seven-layer Open Standards Interconnect (OSI) protocol of the International Standards Organization (ISO) is a conceptual model that provides for application, presentation, session, transport, network, data link, and physical layers (see Chapter 4). In practice, higher level protocols at the application or presentation level tend to combine several of the layers of the OSI/ISO model.

For PACS to succeed, developers have needed to agree on a vendor-neutral format for patient demographic and clinical data, examination-specific data, and image-specific data to be stored, as well as on protocols for network communication of these data. The format, developed as an outgrowth of work by the American College of Radiology (ACR) and the National Equipment Manufacturers Association (NEMA), and known as Digital Imaging and Communications in Medicine (DICOM), has been adopted to a large extent worldwide for both radiological and other medical images (also see Chapter 6).

In DICOM, the higher level transmission protocol is loosely based on the OSI/ISO reference model but embraces traditional computer networks for the transport layer and below. DICOM is intended to ensure that a wide variety of equipment (acquisition devices, archive nodes, interpretation consoles, review workstations, servers doing special processing, and so on) can be interfaced with the network and that the data can be recognized and interpreted correctly by all the nodes on the network.

In contrast to the original ACR-NEMA standards, which dealt with only point-to-point transmission protocols, DICOM adopts an object-oriented model and consists of definitions of information objects, service classes (functions performed on or with objects), and network protocols. DICOM 3.0 is a complex multipart standard consisting of a potential for 13 parts, nine of which are defined at this time. The parts include object definitions, service-class specifications, data structures and encoding, data dictionary, network protocols, and media-storage and file-format specifications (Bidgood et al., 1997).

Display Capabilities

A major task of PACS researchers is to develop workstations on which users can view and interpret digital images. The design of image-viewing consoles that are suitable for interpretation of examinations by radiologists poses a host of technical and human engineering problems: Consoles must match the low cost, convenience, and flexibility of illuminated light boxes that radiologists use for interpreting film-based images.

Radiologists usually interpret an examination by comparing multiple images from both the current examination and previous or correlative studies. Flexibility is crucial as they organize and reorganize the images to display temporal sequence, to reflect anatomic organization, and to compare preintervention versus postintervention (e.g., images obtained before and after injection of a contrast medium). Furthermore, when radiologists analyze an image, their attention shifts rapidly between overview or general pattern-recognition modes of viewing and detailed inspection of specific areas. The ability to reshuffle images, to shift attention, to zoom in on a specific area, and to step back again to get an overview are all essential to the interpretive and analytic processes. These effects are easy to achieve with film, but are difficult to replicate on a viewing console (Fig. 14.6).

Experience with CT underscores the challenges of designing viewing consoles for image interpretation. Computed tomography is the quintessential digital imaging modality. Furthermore, viewing consoles are available to and operated by radiologists. Nonetheless, interpretation of CT scans still is often done on film. The

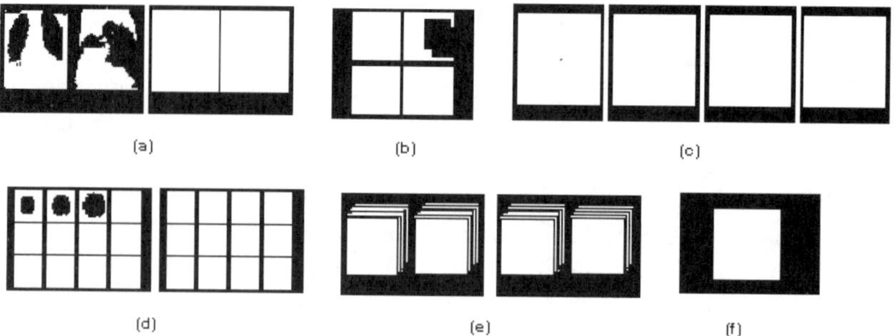

FIGURE 14.6. Workstation-display alternatives for multi-image data. Because most imaging studies involve more than one image per study, and because comparison with prior studies is frequently needed, a single monitor is almost never sufficient for viewing an entire study in full resolution.

Considering only gray scale modalities, most examinations produce images of more than 8 bits of data per pixel (more than 256 gray levels). Monitors are constrained to 8-bit pixel depth; however, brightness and contrast adjustment (window and level manipulation) are almost always needed so that the viewer can adapt the display to the particular kind of image and type of tissue or process being visualized. Horizontal and vertical dimensions of an image need to be considered, a task that involves many factors, including pixel dot resolution (how close pixels are to one another), physical size of monitor, typical viewing distance of user, and desired physical size of the image.

Examples *a–c* are three alternative views of chest X-rays (posteroanterior and lateral views of the current study compared with same two views of a previous study—four images in all). On either a 1,000 or 2,000 pixel-wide monitor, the images could be positioned in landscape mode (*a* and *b*) or in portrait mode (*c*). Whether or not reduced in size, areas of an image or an entire image can be zoomed to higher magnification as depicted by the inset in (*b*).

For studies with large numbers of images, such as CT and MRI studies, rather than proliferating monitors to view an entire study and comparisons, it is often preferable to link the current and previous study such that the viewer can compare similar portions of both studies—for example, by anatomic region, cross-sectional orientation, or window/level setting, as shown in *d*, where the entire study is not visible. The user can scroll through a study on each monitor independently, on both monitors as single continuous series, or simultaneously through subsets of images on both monitors (they are linked).

Alternatively, cross-sectional images can be viewed as linked volumes of stacked images, which are scrolled through, one slice at a time, either automatically (movie mode) or manually (*e*). Example *f* shows another way to view large numbers of slices that represent a volume: by reconstructing them as three-dimensional volumes.

Other factors to be determined in workstation design include luminance, orientation (landscape versus portrait), and nondisplay qualities such as kinds of controls (e.g., zoom, pan, measurement, enhancement), cost, quality of graphical user interface, and general ease of use, including degree to which functions are integrated into and facilitate workflow.

viewing console associated with a CT scanner permits the technologist to retrieve single images (slices) one at a time, to manipulate the image's gray scale for detailed inspection, and to perform limited analysis. Typically, however, it does not allow the operator to view all the images of a study concurrently, to rearrange them, or to zoom in rapidly on particular images for detailed inspection. For these reasons, the CT console is used only to determine whether patients have been positioned properly, to monitor the progress of studies, and to optimize the display if images are to be photographed onto sheets of film. Radiologists then do the interpretations from the film or from satellite workstations.

Interpretation consoles or workstations must support general image-manipulation operations (such as gray scale manipulation, histogram equalization, edge enhancement, image subtraction, and on-line measurement), and other operations that radiologists may need to perform while analyzing images (see Section 14.4). Significant issues concern size and number of display monitors to be used, resolution of the monitors, and design of the user interface to provide convenient and natural access to needed functionality (Lou et al., 1996).

The display of three-dimensional imaging data places even greater demands on consoles to calculate and redisplay oblique slices and rotated views rapidly (Vannier & Marsh, 1996). In addition, some interpretation requires image-specific processing capabilities; for example, a program may use mathematical models to calculate cardiac volume or fetal weight (Greenes, 1982).

It is not yet clear to what extent special capabilities can or should be incorporated in the design of generic viewing consoles. Such features might be associated more appropriately with the image-acquisition device itself or with image data servers, which are now feasible because of high-speed network connections. This idea is particularly relevant for MRI data manipulation because of the specialized nature of an MRI database. Magnetic resonance imaging data are inherently three dimensional. Each point typically is associated with multiple data values, the interpretations of which are also dependent on a variety of data acquisition and examination parameters. The design of practical image-interpretation workstations thus requires considerable human engineering and experimentation.

For distribution of images to referring clinicians, to enable them to review examinations that already have been preprocessed and interpreted, lower resolution may be required, as well as less processing and data-transmission volume and smaller local memory. Workstations for review and consultation, however, must be easily accessible and thus must be conveniently distributed throughout an institution, or throughout an extended integrated delivery network. Access via the World Wide Web provides a means for meeting this need.

Cost

Image management and PACS development were initially conceived as having significant benefits for radiology departments in terms of reductions in film-library space and personnel time, as well as immediacy of access to images. As noted, however, direct acquisition of high-quality digital images has taken longer than anticipated for some modalities—notably plain-film radiography and mammography. Secondary digitization by scanning from film is not cost-effective. As a result, some parts of radiology departments (such as the CT, MRI, ultrasound, and nuclear medicine sections, in which images are intrinsically digital) have been more amenable to PACS than other parts, giving rise to mini-PACS systems.

Furthermore, it is now recognized that much of the benefit of PACS accrues from the provision of image results to clinicians in a timely fashion to facilitate clinical management, the ability to conduct distant consultations, and the performance of teleradiology services (Goldberg, 1996). The push in those directions has shifted the emphasis in development. As a result, implementation of full-department PACS is often an evolutionary process in most places, concurrent with the evolution of the entire healthcare enterprise to a multimedia-capable environment suitable for image distribution. Interest is growing in distributing nonradiology image-based examination results (e.g., cardiology, pathology) as well (Siegel et al., 1997). Costs for the network infrastructure and for image acquisition, storage, and review thus eventually will be shared by the entire healthcare system rather than falling exclusively to radiology departments.

14.3.2 The Evolution of Image Management in Picture-Archiving and Communication Systems

Over the past 20 years, many researchers have worked to develop PACS implementations. Based on the experience of early projects in the 1980s, it became clear that researchers had to devote considerable work to building an infrastructure that would support (1) image acquisition from the various modalities; (2) storage of image data to accommodate both clinical use (short term) and archiving (long term); (3) transmission of image data within a LAN among the PACS acquisition, storage, and display nodes; (4) workstation display for interpretation and review; (5) integration with RISs and hospital information systems (HISs); and (6) generation of hard copy film recordings (Dwyer, 1996). Teleradiology uses WANs, but otherwise requires much of the same infrastructure.

Some early projects focused on one or two aspects of the overall PACS problem, whereas others attempted to incorporate all aspects of a PACS. A problem faced by early researchers was the rapid evolution of network, storage, and workstation technology, causing obsolescence of the initial systems. At the University of Kansas, Templeton and colleagues (1984) developed one of the earliest prototype systems to study the image-management requirements of a PACS-supported radiology department, investigating a hierarchical storage strategy and developing projections about network capacity and archival storage requirements. Blaine and colleagues (1983) at the Mallinckrodt Institute of Radiology in St. Louis developed a **PACS workbench**: a set of tools to study PACS design and to conduct experiments related to image acquisition, transmission, archiving, and viewing. Another prototype system developed by Arenson and colleagues (1988) at the Hospital of the University of Pennsylvania was designed to provide a comprehensive image database that could be used for image review and consultation, with an initial focus on the intensive-care unit. A fiberoptic network, in a star configuration, linked digital image-acquisition devices, image-archiving nodes, and image-review stations, with the central node of the network—the image manager—connected to the department's RIS. Nondigital images were scanned manually.

Progress since those early systems has been substantial on several fronts. Acquisition initially required hand-crafting of interfaces to proprietary imaging hardware. Gradually, DICOM has been adopted as the format for transmission of image, examination, and patient data from acquisition devices to storage devices. Storage of the huge volumes of data required for a typical radiology department's images was initially hampered by the cost and capacity limitations of disk storage systems. We have seen a marked expansion in disk capacities, dramatic decreases in costs, and the advent of read–write optical disks and jukebox units that provide multiple terabytes of storage. Hierarchical storage-management schemes schedule migration of image files from high-speed storage to slower media based on predictions of decreased likelihood of future access. Compression methods, such as the use of wavelet-transform encoding, can also greatly reduce storage requirements, although storage of only images compressed by lossy methods is not yet accepted as routine practice.

Workstation display also has greatly improved, with screens and image memory enabling 2,000 × 2,500 pixel resolution becoming relatively inexpensive. Workstation random-access memory (RAM) and video graphic board memory have increased, thus enabling local storage of image files at full resolution, with rapid selective display of reduced-size images, regions of interest, zoomed portions of images, and alterations in brightness or contrast characteristics. Luminance of a video monitor is one of the key factors enabling sufficient gray-scale range to be visualized; high-luminance monitors have appeared in recent years.

Workstation software enabling management of the images on the screen, in terms of placement, size, and sort sequence, as well as access to image-manipulation tools, has become progressively more user friendly, with brightness and contrast control, zoom, pan, various image enhancement methods, measurement, annotation, and methods of image processing (Lou et al., 1996). Higher end workstations permit three-dimensional reconstruction of images, rotations, exposure of arbitrary planes, and selective removal of specific anatomic structures that are identified by their imaging characteristics (Vannier & Marsh, 1996); these machines are used increasingly in surgical planning and image-guided therapy. For some image enhancement and for three-dimensional modeling, the computations involved are often performed by a networked server rather than at the workstation directly.

Network technology for the earliest systems was limited to slow-speed Ethernet. Fiber Distributed Data Interface (FDDI), asynchronous transfer mode (ATM), and fast Ethernet have all become widely available, and gateways among them have been developed for both LAN and WAN applications. Linkage of PACS with RISs and with HISs now has been accomplished in a number of ways by various commercial implementations. Such connection facilitates definitive patient identification, attachment of demographics, and association of radiology examination and report data with the relevant images, as discussed in Section 14.5.

As noted earlier, the initial PACS implementations were designed to support the all-digital, filmless radiology department. Although this goal has been achieved in a few noteworthy sites, the emphasis has largely shifted to image distribution and access to facilitate enterprise-wide communication and rapid result review, augmented by mini-PACS capabilities in those areas of the radiology department where modalities are already digital.

14.3.3 Current Status of Image Management

We are gradually developing digital methods for image acquisition, transmission, storage, and interpretation for most imaging modalities. The full integration of these capabilities is still realized at only a few sites, however, and the technology for accomplishing it is still in flux. In addition, the motivations for accomplishing such integration have shifted due to increased focus on enterprise-wide perspectives.

Picture Archiving and Communication Systems

The filmless radiology department is still limited today by the fact that plain-film radiography and mammography have not yet been supplanted by digital modalities to a significant extent. Mammography has the highest resolution demands (50 micron), and digital mammography has only recently become available commercially. Devices providing capture of other plain films (e.g., examinations of the chest, bone, and abdomen) are widely available, and units are being acquired gradually by radiology departments as new needs arise or as older film-based units are replaced.

Soft copy radiology interpretation at workstations is still somewhat hampered by technical difficulties and by user resistance. Interpretation of examinations—even those intrinsically in digital form—is still considered by some radiologists to be more conveniently done on film using illuminated light boxes, even given great improvements in workstation display software. One of the problems is the lack to date of full integration of images into the workflow of the department. An image workstation, for example, may allow viewing and manipulation of the images, but selection of a case to interpret and automatic identification of the header for either dictation or entry of a structured report are typically still separate steps supported by software on different computers. Available screen real estate to portray all relevant images does not exist without reduction of image size. Methods should ideally therefore exist for prescreening images to select regions that require further analysis, and the user interface should permit systematic scanning of the entire image at full resolution or the addition of other images designed to enhance detection of specific features (compounding the problem of screen real estate).

A popular misconception is that the barriers to soft copy interpretation will be removed by higher resolution display screens. If a 20-inch diagonal monitor can display 1,000 × 1,000 pixels, the question is whether it is inherently inferior to a 2,000 × 2,000 monitor or a 4,000 × 4,000 monitor, with a screen of the same 20-inch physical size. Clearly, each pixel in the 1,000 × 1,000 monitor is four times the area of an individual pixel on a 2,000 × 2,000 monitor and 16 times the area of a pixel on a 4,000 × 4,000 monitor. If individual pixels are sufficiently close together on a 1,000 × 1,000 monitor so that the eye cannot resolve them at normal viewing distance (as is the case), however, then the additional resolution of the 2,000 or 4,000 monitors will not improve perceived image quality.

Displaying a 4,000 × 4,000 image on a 1,000 × 1,000 monitor requires that each displayed pixel (of a 1,000 × 1,000 reduced image) summarizes the values in a corresponding 4 × 4 pixel area of the original image. How the value of that pixel is computed is the key determinant of image quality on the reduced image. Subsampling (e.g., every fourth pixel), or averaging, does not work well. A function that computes the brightness level that the eye would detect in that 4 × 4 area on a higher resolution monitor is the optimal way to determine the value of the single pixel on the lower resolution monitor. In fact, for certain classes of abnormalities (e.g., calcifications or masses on a mammogram) that are indicated by brighter areas, simply displaying the maximum pixel value in the 4 × 4 region is a satisfactory substitute. The question of optimal resolution for interpretation of most studies has not yet been satisfactorily answered. A few projects have assessed the adequacy of soft copy interpretation, but convincing receiver operating characteristic (ROC) studies (see Chapter 3) have generally not been done, except for specific kinds of abnormalities (e.g., a pneumothorax or interstitial disease on a chest X-ray image).

In a fairly recent worldwide survey (Bauman et al., 1996), the number of large-scale PACS had increased from 13 to 23 in a 15-month period. Only a small number handled soft copy interpretation; one of them was used at the Veteran's Administration Hospital in Baltimore, Maryland (Siegel et al., 1997). Many departments now have mini-PACS (both home-grown and commercial) installed in their departments, particularly in the CT, MRI, ultrasound, and nuclear-medicine divisions.

Teleradiology

Although some limitations remain, workstation suitability for interpretation, acquisition and transmission of radiological examinations over a distance is growing (Goldberg, 1996). It is now common for radiology departments to enable their radiologists to provide coverage from home, especially for interpretations of CT and MRI examinations obtained during nights or weekends and review of interpretations made by radiology residents before finalization of reports. **Teleradiology**—the provision of remote interpretations—is increasing as a mode of delivery of radiology services. Typically, a radiology center will offer these services to facilities that are generally understaffed or that seek coverage for specialized areas of interpretation. In the United States, expansion of teleradiology is still limited by the requirement that interpreting radiologists be licensed in the state in which the images are acquired.

Current work emphasizes enterprise-wide image distribution and access not only for radiology but also for other kinds of procedures—a major departure from the functionality of most clinical information systems, which have not traditionally been multimedia-capable. In addition to supporting the need for remote interpretation by imaging specialists, electronic distribution and access meet strong demands for review and consultation among clinicians, for surgical planning, and for teaching. To implement these capabilities, as well as to provide a variety of other functions for education and decision support, enterprises have developed intranet and Internet technologies, often using the World Wide Web. Client-based viewing applications are typically augmented by Java to provide needed user-interface features for image manipulation. At the back end of the systems is typically an image repository of images stored in a DICOM-compatible format. Patient-identification information permits linkage to an RIS or HIS, associating images with specific examinations and to reports (Khorasani et al., 1998).

Indexing and Image Retrieval

In a typical PACS system, images are archived on a file server. Identification data, usually obtained from the DICOM header, are stored in an associated relational database. Specific images are retrieved based on information that was entered in the database at the same time that the images were acquired, either directly or via linkage to an RIS. For routine radiology this information is usually sufficient, because current and previous images are retrieved mostly by patient identifier and imaging modality.

For research or education, however, it is often desirable to retrieve images that "look like this one"—for example, to show other examples of a particular disease process or to perform a retrospective research study. The standard approach to this task, for educational and research databases, is to index images manually according to keywords. The DICOM standard has provisions to include these keywords (Bidgood et al., 1997), and controlled vocabularies, such as the Systematized Nomenclature of Medicine (SNOMED) (Côté et al., 1993), Neuronames (Bowden & Martin, 1995), and the Digital Anatomist Symbolic Knowledge Base (Rosse et al., 1997) (all of which are part of the National Library of Medicine's Unified Medical Language system [UMLS] [Lindberg et al., 1993]), provide many of the needed source keywords (see Chapter 6).

In most routine cases, however, the relevant keywords will not have been entered, because it was not known ahead of time what the query would be. What is needed is *content-based* image retrieval, which allows the computer to index the images based on their content (Tagare et al., 1997). In the long run, such capabilities will require that the computer *understand* the image in the same way that the radiologist does.

As described in Section 14.4, image understanding is not likely to be available in the near future. Simpler methods have, however, been applied successfully in certain image domains. For example, color images can be indexed according to their relative percentages of red, green, and blue (Flickner et al., 1995). Asking for images with large amounts of blue from a collection of natural scenes will retrieve images showing a large amount of sea or sky. Of course most medical images are gray scale, so a color-based approach will not work. An alternative developed at Yale, called **qualitative arrangement** (Tagare et al., 1995), looks at the relative relationships of regions in the image, without trying to identify them, and retrieves images that have similar relationships. When applied to cardiac MRI images, this approach was able to retrieve images acquired in the same plane of section.

Although much more research is required before these kinds of techniques become widely used, the availability of digital images, PACS, and powerful display workstations will provide a good foundation on which to implement them.

14.4 Image Manipulation

One of the great advantages of digital images is that they can be manipulated just like any other kind of data. Although methods for processing images have been developed almost since the beginning of the computer, these methods were available only for large computers and were not relevant to clinical medicine. This situation is changing rapidly, however, as digital images become widely available through the image modalities themselves, PACS, and powerful desktop workstations. Even though there has been relatively little progress in the area of computer image understanding, there has been much progress in applying existing methods to aid the human as he or she analyzes the images.

14.4.1 Basic Concepts in Image Manipulation

Digital image manipulation, or **image processing**, generally involves the transformation of one or more input images either into one or more output images (which may be three-dimensional) or into some abstract representation of the contents of the input images. For example, a series of two-dimensional images can be combined to create a three-dimensional volume image, which in turn can be projected back onto a two-dimensional image that shows a different slice plane, or a set of terms (*pleural effusion*, *lung nodule*) can be attached to specific regions on a chest X-ray image.

Images can be enhanced to permit human viewing, to show views (such as three-dimensional reconstructions) not present in the original images, to flag suspicious areas for closer examination by the radiologist, to quantify the size and shape of an organ, and to prepare the images for integration with other information. Most of these applications require one or more of the four basic image-processing steps: global processing, segmentation, feature detection, and classi-

FIGURE 14.7. Image fusion. The figure shows magnetoencephalography (MEG) activation superimposed on a cutaway three-dimensional model of the brain and skull obtained with magnetic resonance imaging (MRI). No imaging modality provides all needed information, but multimodality displays such as this can greatly aid understanding. (*Source:* Courtesy of Cheryl Aine, John George, and Doug Ranken, Los Alamos National Laboratory.)

FIGURE 14.9. Several screens from a tool for radiation treatment planning. Computed tomography images from a patient are manually segmented to generate three-dimensional regions depicting the locations of tumors and of critical anatomical structures. Artificial intelligence techniques then configure a set of radiation beams to deliver maximum dosage to the tumor and minimum dosage to the critical structures. (*Source:* Courtesy of Ira Kalet, Department of Radiation Oncology, University of Washington.)

COLOR PLATE I

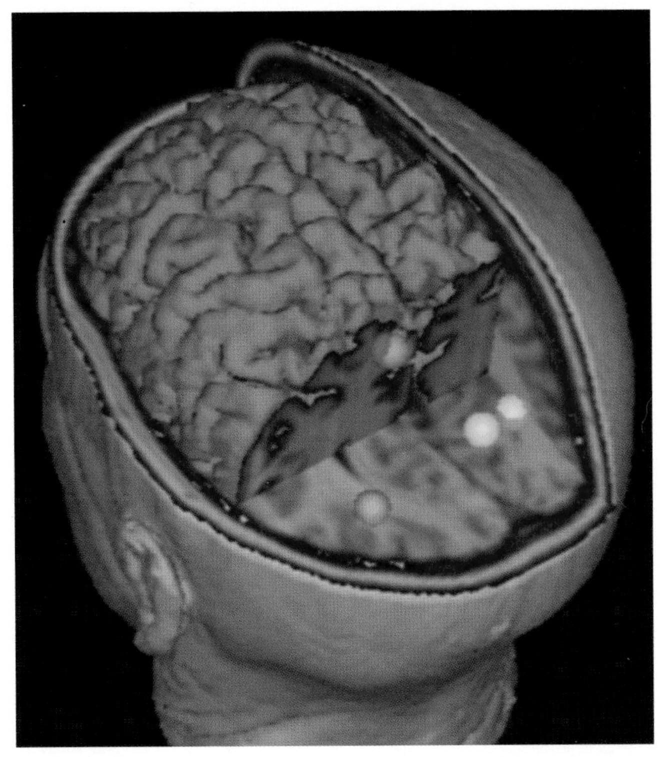

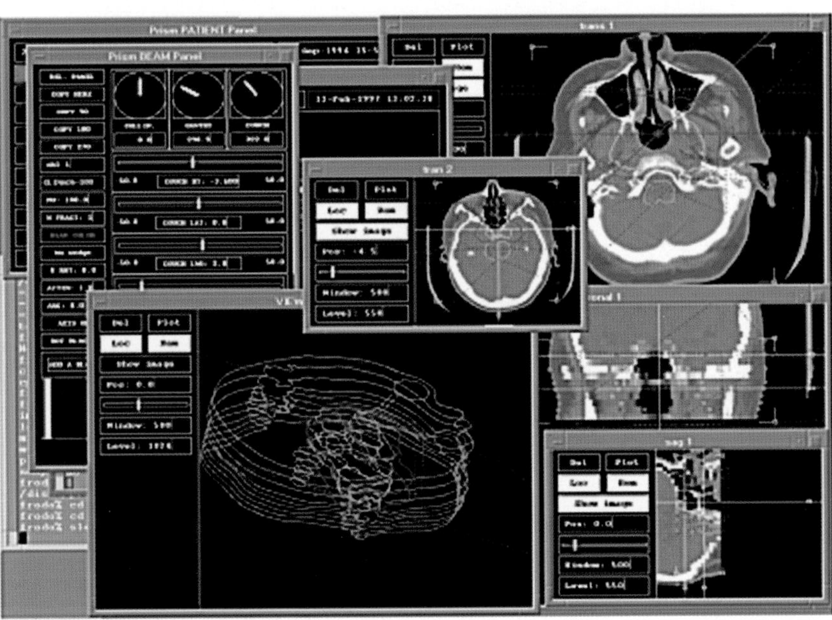

COLOR PLATE II

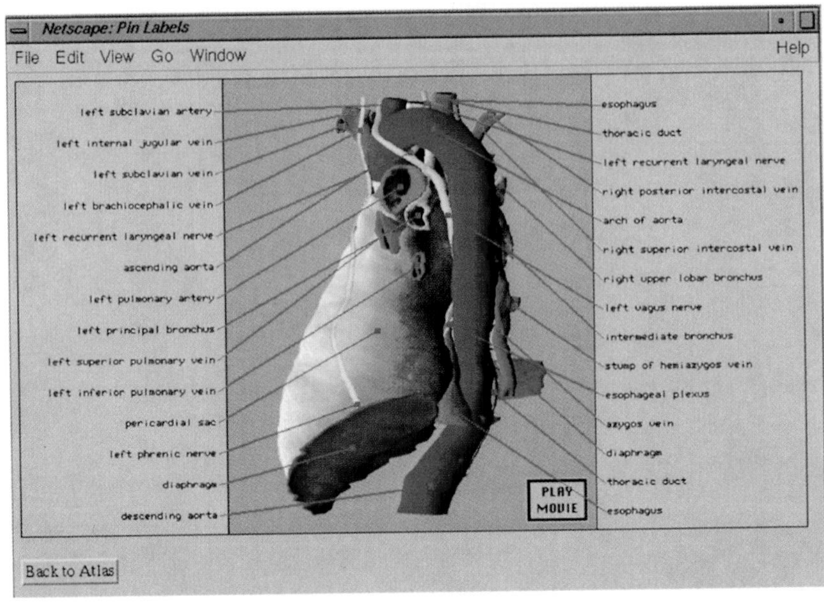

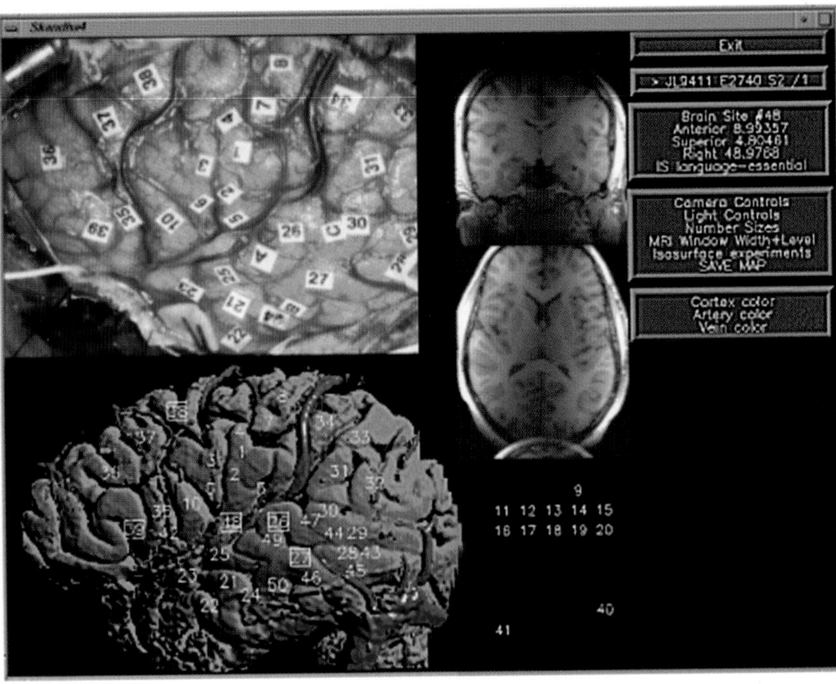

FIGURE 14.10. The Digital Anatomist interactive Web-based atlas, showing the integration of images with tools for anatomy education. Three-dimensional models were created from photographs of cadaver sections that were segmented and assembled into surface models. The models were rendered as static images, which were then annotated with anatomical names. Users can click on regions to obtain names, can take on-line quizzes, and can download saved animations. In this screenshot, the software has dynamically generated a labeled image from a set of annotated regions and labels, similar to pin diagrams often seen in anatomy textbooks. (*Source:* Courtesy of Cornelius Rosse, Department of Biological Structure, Universtiy of Washington.)

FIGURE 14.11. An interface for interactive brain mapping, showing the integration of photographic images of the exposed brain at neurosurgery, with MRI images and a three-dimensional surface model created from them. The model also includes veins and arteries imaged with MRV and MRA. The user visually matches the photograph with the model and then drags numbers onto the model to perform the mapping. The resulting three-dimensional coordinates, with the models and images, are saved in a Web-accessible multimedia database. (*Source:* Courtesy of James Brinkley, Department of Biological Structure, University of Washington.)

fication. These steps are generally performed in order, although later steps may feed back to earlier ones, and not all steps are required for each application. Most steps generalize from two-dimensional to three-dimensional images.

Global processing involves computations on the entire image, without regard to specific local content. The purpose is to enhance an image for human visualization or for further analysis by the computer. A simple but important example is *gray-scale windowing* of CT images. The CT scanner generates pixel values (CT numbers) in the range of −3,000 to +4,000. Humans, however, cannot distinguish more than about 100 shades of gray. To appreciate the full precision available with a CT image, the operator can adjust the midpoint and range of the displayed CT values. By changing the *level* and *width* (i.e., intercept and slope of the mapping between pixel value and displayed gray scale or, roughly, the brightness and contrast) of the display, radiologists enhance their ability to perceive small changes in contrast resolution within a subregion of interest.

Segmentation involves the extraction of regions of interest (ROIs) from the overall image. The ROIs usually correspond to anatomically meaningful structures, such as organs or parts of organs. The structures may be delineated by their borders, in which case **edge-detection techniques** (such as edge-following algorithms) are used, or by their composition on the image, in which case **region-detection techniques** (such as texture analysis) are used (Haralick & Shapiro, 1992). Neither of these techniques has been completely successful; regions often have discontinuous borders or nondistinctive internal composition. Furthermore, contiguous regions often overlap. These and other complications make segmentation the most difficult subtask of the medical image-analysis problem. Because segmentation is difficult for a computer, it is often performed manually by a human operator. It therefore remains a major bottleneck that prevents more widespread application of image processing techniques.

Feature detection is the process of extracting useful parameters from the segmented regions. These parameters may themselves be informative—for example, the volume of the heart or the size of the fetus. They also may be used as input into an automated **classification** procedure, which determines the type of object found. For example, small round regions on chest X-ray images might be classified as tumors, depending on such features as intensity, perimeter, and area.

Mathematical models often are used to aid in the performance of image-analysis subtasks. In classic pattern-recognition applications, the subtasks of global processing, segmentation, feature detection, and classification usually are performed sequentially. People, however, appear to perform pattern-recognition iteratively. For example, radiologists can perceive faint images and can trace discontinuous borders, in part because they know for which features they are searching. Many researchers have applied artificial-intelligence techniques to imitate such interaction among subtasks. The computer is programmed with some of the higher level anatomic knowledge that radiologists use when they interpret images. Thus, high-level organ models provide feedback to guide the lower level process of segmentation.

The nature of the application determines which of these subtasks is performed, the choice of technique for each subtask, and the relative order of the subtasks. Because image understanding is an unsolved problem, and because many applications are possible, there is a wealth of image processing techniques that can be applied to digital images.

14.4.2 Historical Perspective on Image Manipulation

Success in processing satellite and spacecraft images generated considerable interest in biomedical image processing, including automated image analysis for interpretation. Beginning in the 1960s, researchers devoted a large amount of work to this end, with the hope that eventually much of radiographic image analysis could be automated.

One of the first areas to receive attention was automated interpretation of chest X-ray images, because, previously, most patients admitted to a hospital were subjected to routine chest X-ray examinations. (This practice is no longer considered cost effective except for selected subgroups of patients.) Much of the work in automated interpretation was done at the University of California at Irvine, Nagoya University in Japan, the University of Southern California, and the University of Pittsburgh. Subsequent research, however, confirmed the difficulty of completely automating radiographic-image interpretation, and much of the initial enthusiasm has now worn off. Currently there is less emphasis on completely automatic interpretation and more on systems that aid the radiologist.

14.4.3 Current Status of Image-Analysis Systems

Although completely automated image-analysis systems are still in the future, the widespread availability of digital images, combined with PACS and powerful workstations, has led to many applications of image processing techniques. In general, routine techniques are available on the manufacturer's workstations (e.g., an MR console or an ultrasound machine), whereas more advanced image-processing algorithms are available as software packages that run on independent workstations.

The primary uses of image processing in the clinical environment are for image enhancement, screening, quantitation, three-dimensional visualization and display, and multimodality image fusion. Software for such image processing is primarily developed for use on independent workstations. Several journals are devoted to medical image processing (e.g., *IEEE Transactions on Medical Imaging, Journal of Digital Imaging, Neuroimage*), and the number of journal articles is rapidly increasing as digital images become more widely available. We describe just a few examples of image-processing techniques in the remainder of this section.

Image enhancement uses global processing to improve the appearance of the image either for human use or for subsequent processing by computer. All manufacturers' consoles and independent image-processing workstations provide some form of image enhancement. We have already mentioned CT windowing.

Another technique is **unsharp masking** in which a blurred image is subtracted from the original image to increase local contrast and to enhance the visibility of fine-detail (high-frequency) structures. **Histogram equalization** spreads the image gray levels throughout the visible range to maximize the visibility of those gray levels that are used frequently. **Temporal subtraction** subtracts a reference image from later images that are registered to the first. A common use of temporal subtraction is digital-subtraction angiography (DSA) in which a background image is subtracted from an image taken after the injection of contrast material.

Screening uses global processing, segmentation, feature detection, and classification to determine whether an image should be flagged for careful review by a radiologist or pathologist. In such an approach, the computer is allowed to flag a reasonable number of normal images (false positives) as long as it misses very few abnormal images (false negatives). If the number of flagged images is small compared with the total number of images, then automated screening procedures can be economically viable. Screening techniques have been applied successfully to mammography images for mass lesions, to chest X-rays for small cancerous nodules, and to Papanicolaou (Pap) smears for cancerous or precancerous cells (Giger & MacMahon, 1996), as well as to many other images. The huge potential cost savings to be realized by a screening procedure for the thousands of Pap smear images that are taken every day has resulted in the formation of a company, NeoPath, whose primary product, AutoPap, has been approved by the FDA for primary diagnostic Pap smear screening (Patten et al., 1996).

Quantitation uses global processing and segmentation to characterize meaningful regions of interest. For example, heart size, shape, and motion are subtle indicators of heart function and of the response of the heart to therapy (Clarysse et al., 1997). Similarly, fetal head size and femur length, as measured on ultrasound images, are valuable indicators of fetal well-being (Brinkley, 1993). Although the literature describes a wealth of automatic or semiautomatic techniques for segmenting images of the heart or of the fetus, the most common clinical scenario continues to be manual outlining by trained technicians. This situation should soon change, however, as semiautomatic techniques (those that let the user correct segmentation errors by the computer) become widely available on independent workstations that are custom tailored for particular applications.

Three-dimensional reconstruction and visualization generally uses global processing to enhance the images, followed often by segmentation. Modalities such as CT and MRI translate easily into three-dimensional voxel arrays because the images are acquired as closely spaced parallel slices. For this reason, almost all CT and MR manufacturers' consoles contain some form of three-dimensional reconstruction and visualization capabilities.

In these cases, the visualization technique is usually **volume rendering,** which projects a two-dimensional image directly from a three-dimensional voxel array by casting rays from the eye of the observer through the volume array to the image plane (Foley et al., 1990). Because each ray passes through many voxels, some form of segmentation (usually simple thresholding) often is used to remove obscuring structures. As workstation memory and processing power have advanced, volume rendering has become widely used to display all forms of three-dimensional voxel data—ranging from cell images produced by confocal microscopy, to three-dimensional ultrasound images, to brain images created from MRI or PET.

A visualization technique that provides an alternative to volume rendering is **surface rendering** (Foley et al., 1990). The primary technique used in computer graphics, surface rendering has been applied widely in the entertainment industry for movies such as *Toy Story*. Surface rendering requires that the surface of interest be segmented from the image volume, after which rendering speeds on standard workstations are much faster than those possible with volume rendering. In addition, the surface is available for three-dimensional quantitation or manipulation. Such capabilities are necessary for three-dimensional virtual reality and other applications to education, radiation treatment planning, and surgical treatment planning.

The most common method for three-dimensional surface segmentation is reconstruction from serial sections. In this case, manually or automatically segmented two-dimensional contours are stacked together, and then a surface (usually a polyhedral mesh) is **tiled** over these contours to create a continuous surface (Prothero & Prothero, 1986). Because automatic tiling is not yet foolproof, various interactive techniques have been developed to allow the user to correct errors.

An alternate approach to reconstruction from serial sections is the use of **deformable models**. In this case, a three-dimensional surface model that is close in shape to the organ of interest is deformed until it matches the imaged organ. The deformation is controlled by an optimization procedure that minimizes a cost function. The cost function usually includes both intrinsic factors to ensure smoothness and extrinsic factors to move the model surface toward surfaces in the image.

Deformable models arose out of the work of Kass and Terzopoulos (see Kass et al., 1987), who first applied these methods in two dimensions using a method called *Snakes*. Since the introduction of Snakes, this basic idea has been applied to many medical image segmentation problems, primarily in two dimensions but increasingly in three dimensions. In fact, a glance at any medical image-processing journal from the past few years shows that deformable models are now the primary paradigm for work in model-based segmentation.

The main application of these methods in three dimensions has been to images of the brain because the contrast between cortex and surrounding tissues usually is sufficient to permit simple cost functions to work. Current work in three-dimensional brain modeling is aimed not only at finding the general *envelope* of the brain shape but also allowing the model to extend itself into the detailed cortical gyri and sulci (Christensen et al., 1996; Thompson & Toga, 1996).

Application of deformable models to other tissues may be aided by addition to the model of shape knowledge. For example, a collection of local shape constraints generates a good approximation to the three-dimensional brain surface when incorporated in a constraint-propagation algorithm (Hinshaw & Brinkley,

1997), thereby letting the computer *hallucinate* organ boundaries where none are visible in the image.

Multimodality image fusion uses all these techniques to generate a composite visualization that combines images from more than one source (Fig. 14.7; see color insert). This approach has been particularly useful for brain imaging because each modality provides different information. For example, PET and MEG provide useful information about function, but they do not provide good localization with respect to the anatomy. Similarly, MRV and MRA show blood flow but do not provide the detailed anatomy visible with standard MRI. By combining images from these modalities with MRI, we can show functional images in terms of the underlying anatomy, thereby providing a common neuroanatomic framework.

The primary problems to solve in multimodality image fusion are **registration**—that is, the alignment of separately acquired image volumes—and visualization. In the simplest case, separate image volumes are acquired during a single sitting. The patient's head may be immobilized, and the information in the

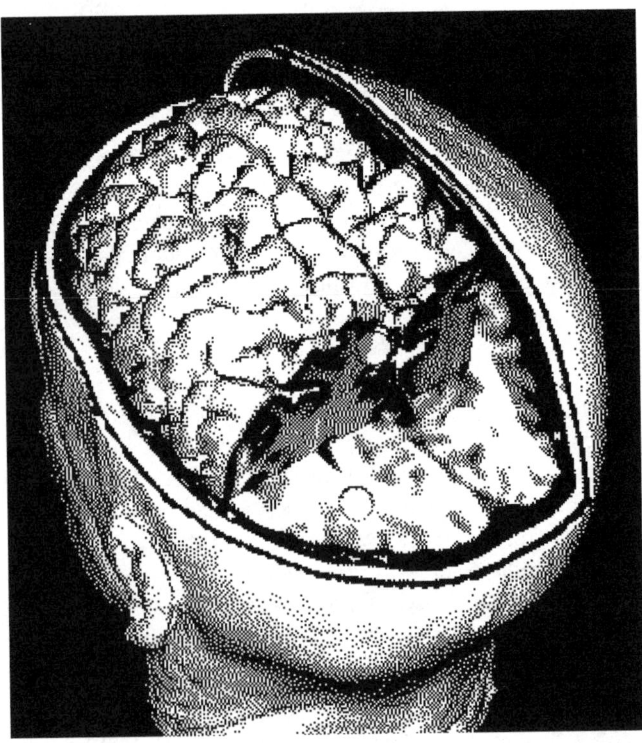

FIGURE **14.7.** Image fusion. The figure shows magnetoencephalography (MEG) activation superimposed on a cutaway three-dimensional model of the brain and skull obtained with magnetic resonance imaging (MRI). No imaging modality provides all needed information, but multimodality displays such as this can greatly aid understanding. (*Source:* Courtesy of John George, Los Alamos National Laboratory.) (See color insert.)

image headers may be used to rotate and resample the image volumes until all the voxels correspond. An example of this approach is superposition of veins and arteries taken with MRV and MRA onto a three-dimensional reconstruction taken from MRI (Modayur et al., 1997).

If the patient moves, or if examinations are acquired at different times, other registration methods are needed. A common approach is for the human operator to indicate corresponding landmarks on the image volumes to be aligned. The computer then calculates the best linear or nonlinear transform to maximize the overlap of these corresponding points (Bookstein, 1989). A potentially more robust approach is to compute the best transform based on a cost function that looks at the gray levels of all the voxels in the two images (Collins et al., 1994).

Given two registered volume data sets, segmentation may be necessary to extract the cortical anatomy and thus to remove overlying structures. The functional images may then be superimposed on this surface, with either volume-rendering or surface-rendering techniques. The resulting visualizations can provide spectacular insights into the functioning of the living brain.

14.5 Integration of Images with Other Healthcare Information

Health-care images are useful only to the extent that they are accessible to applications that make use of them. For clinical practice, images must be integrated with the data about them, including those indicating the examinations through which they were obtained and the patients to whom they relate. Radiological images and the associated data need to be available to interpreting radiologists as well as to clinicians. They need to be reviewed for diagnosis, treatment planning, and procedure guidance. Practitioners may need to consult about the images perhaps via a network. Images may also need to be shown to patients, with whom the findings are discussed.

Medical images arising from procedures carried out by specialists other than radiologists pose many of the same challenges. As health-care practice becomes increasingly distributed, the needs for image distribution and access become more varied, and timeliness of availability of the image, the associated report, and other relevant clinical information are key. In addition, uses of images in medical education and training, and in research, create further needs for image distribution and access. In this section, we discuss a variety of aspects of this challenge and approaches to fostering image integration.

14.5.1 Basic Concepts in Integration of Radiology Information

Healthcare information systems require both vertical and horizontal integration (Greenes & Deibel, 1996). Specialized functionality—such as for image manipulation or interpretation, for education, or for decision support—as well as more comprehensive capabilities embodied in HISs have tended to develop in relative isolation over many years or even decades. As a result, the software architectures of systems that implement these capabilities often are incompatible and frequently are inflexible with respect to ease of integration with one another. Newer systems approaches that rely on open architectures and distributed, component-based designs facilitate such integration (Deibel & Greenes, 1995) but often cannot simply replace existing legacy systems; instead, evolutionary strategies must be developed (also see Chapter 10).

Radiology Information Systems

The workings of a radiology department illustrate the many tasks in producing and managing clinical images. Management of work flow in a radiology department is a complex activity that involves not only maintenance of the film library (and digital archive) but also scheduling of examinations, registration of patients, performance of examinations, review and analysis of studies by radiologists, creation of interpretations, transcription of dictated reports (or generation of structured reports directly by radiologists), distribution of radiology reports to referring physicians, and billing for services. In addition, department managers must collect and analyze process-control and financial data to prepare budgets, to make appropriate informed decisions regarding staffing levels and the purchase of additional equipment, and to identify problems, such as overly large numbers of retakes of films, too many portable or urgent examination requests, excessive patient waiting times, and unacceptable delays in report transcription or signatures. Inventory control, quality assurance, radiation-exposure monitoring, and preventive-maintenance scheduling are other important managerial functions.

As noted in previous chapters, many information-intensive tasks yield readily to automation; computer-based RISs have been developed to handle almost the entire spectrum of information-management tasks in the radiology department. Radiology information systems have been implemented either as standalone systems or as components of total information systems. In either case, an RIS must be integrated with other information systems within an institution to allow reconciliation of patient data, to support examination scheduling and results reporting, and to facilitate patient billing.

Picture-archiving and communication system image-management functions must be integrated with RISs and HISs, as noted in Section 14.3. Because an RIS (or, in some cases, an HIS) keeps track of examinations and associates them with patients, and a PACS keeps track of images and associates them with examinations, the task is to provide coordination between the examination data on the two systems. Several different implementation approaches are possible. For example, the RIS (or HIS) can be augmented such that examination records indicate the presence of associated images. The path to the images can be stored directly with the examination record on the RIS (or HIS), or the examination data can be duplicated on the PACS, where pointers to the images for each examination are maintained. Alternatively, the PACS can be augmented with patient-lookup and examination-lookup capabilities and the databases from an RIS or HIS duplicated on it. Whenever a user application submits a query about images, the query is sent to a PACS server; queries about other clinical information are sent to the RIS or HIS.

Reporting Methodology

We consider the tasks of producing and distributing radiology reports separately because they pose unique challenges. Traditionally, most reporting of image interpretations has been done by means of dictation by the radiologist, with transcription by typists and editing and approval by the radiologist. In recent years, digital dictation systems have enabled retrieval of voice reports by referring physicians or even voice-report automatic distribution.

Considerable work has gone into voice-recognition systems; the user's voice may trigger canned phrases or complete prestructured templates, or it may add free-text comments. Until recently, these systems were cumbersome to use and did not have great success. The biggest impediment was the lack of ability to handle continuous speech—a hurdle that recent new systems have begun to overcome. Even with the best systems, if there is a non-negligible error rate, the radiologist must view the text as it is generated and correct the errors, causing a slowdown of the reporting process and thus reducing acceptability.

Reporting of interpretations using structured methods that encode findings in databases is desirable to facilitate retrieval for research studies. It also avoids the need for transcription. Structured reporting using computer interaction has been explored for many years. The idea here is that radiologists could compose reports by concatenating prestored phrases, augmenting the phrases by limited free-text keyboard or voice entry. They could use templates for certain classes of examinations that mimic typical report formats, which can then be tailored, or they could simply compose reports de novo through phrase selection from hierarchical or alphabetic menus. This approach has been used successfully in certain areas—for example, in fetal ultrasound (Greenes, 1982), where the entry of data on fetal size can be augmented by automatic calculation of gestational age, weight, and percentile; in ultrasound generally, where findings can be initially entered by technologists, for radiological review (Bell & Greenes, 1994); and in mammography, where the range of abnormalities is fairly limited and where a standardized vocabulary exists (BI-RADS, a mammography vocabulary standard developed by the American College of Radiology) (D'Orsi & Kopans, 1997).

Enterprise Integration

Beyond the integration of the HIS, RIS, and PACS, new challenges are posed by geographically distributed integrated delivery networks (IDNs) that have formed to deliver health care in a region more efficiently and effectively and to support the complete needs of patients in the networks. In an IDN environment, clinical data and images typically are obtained from multiple sources (hospitals, offices, imaging centers) and distributed for interpretation (to the imaging specialist) and for review (to the requesting clinician and other specialists). Multiway consultations can be carried out, with all parties concurrently viewing and perhaps annotating the images. Images from different sources may need to be fused or used in image-guided treatment.

Beyond the tasks of reconciling patient identification and of providing a consistent user interface to a virtual or real clinical repository (discussed in Chapter 10), IDNs must provide an information-technology infrastructure that supports multimedia-capable high-speed network connectivity among all participants to achieve enterprise-wide integration of images. The infrastructure must also provide the necessary servers for managing the imaging and clinical-data repositories and must ensure that these servers are readily available and able to handle the loads required. Client workstations must have the necessary hardware and software configurations to run the applications; in a distributed network with 10,000 or more workstations, as is not atypical, workstation management may require central resources for automatically checking client workstations and uploading software updates.

The multiple sources of image data and the diverse uses of data for clinical practice, education, and research all require an infrastructure that facilitates flexible integration of distributed software components, as opposed to design of comprehensive integrated, monolithic software packages (Deibel & Greenes, 1996). As demands become more complex, applications at a user workstation are increasingly functioning as the locus for integration of specialized services that are obtained over the network and for control of the **presentation layer**, or user interface. **Middleware** components are being developed that support access, processing, analysis, and composition of lower-level resources available through basic services, such as access to image data or clinical data (Fig. 14.8). The software architecture in some of these approaches permits middleware components to run either on workstations or on servers, thus enabling adaptation to workstation capacity, network speeds, traffic loads, and other factors that can affect performance.

14.5.2 Historical Perspective on Radiology Information Management

Information management for procedures associated with clinical-imaging activities had its origins in RISs. Over the years, similar information systems have been developed to handle the procedure flow in pathology, as well as in other departments that deal with images. In some cases, these services have been incorporated in the functionality of HISs; in other cases, they have been developed as separate systems that operate independently and have limited interface to an HIS. Gradually, as integrated delivery networks have forced the development of more highly modular and comprehensive software architectures, and as demands for both image and information access have spread enterprise-wide, a new level of integration is being developed among legacy systems and newer systems.

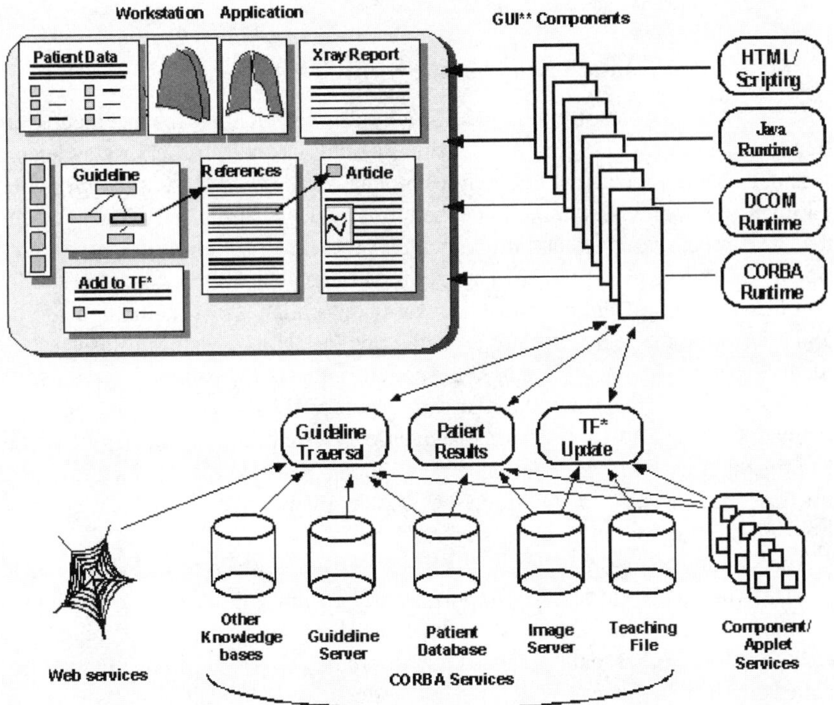

FIGURE 14.8. New architectures for imaging workstation applications. Workstations for both imaging specialists and clinicians should be able to bring together data, images, and knowledge resources of a variety of types, as required for a particular application. Consider a radiologist interpreting an examination, needing to retrieve the examination-request data, the images, and other relevant data about the patient and then creating a report (possibly through a voice-recognition interface). The radiologist may wish to review current guidelines for the clinical situation, including retrieval of pertinent references, before making a recommendation for further workup, to include in the report. Also, because the case had unusual findings, the radiologist may select relevant images for addition to a departmental teaching file, enter a brief description, and select diagnostic code terms.

The workstation must be able to assemble information from the HIS, the RIS, the PACS, a guideline library, and other knowledge bases and Web resources and to update the teaching file (TF). All of these resources may exist on separate hardware platforms, independent systems both old and new, and incompatible formats. A wide variety of capabilities must be integrated into the application, so complexity is managed by an approach in which each resource type responds to requests for services in a standard manner. That is, interfaces allow resources to be considered externally as well-defined components, independent of how they are implemented internally. They represent the message in a syntax and semantics understood by both sender and receiver and use a standard invocation and transport method. Evolving standards for messages include HL7 for clinical data and DICOM for image data. ActiveX/DCOM, CORBA, HTML, and Java provide alternative standards for invocation and transport of the messages. Note that the workstation does not need to perform all the work of integration. Components can be developed to do many of these tasks—an approach that is particularly desirable if there is likely to be a need to reuse that component in another application. As such *middleware* components proliferate, they can carry out increasingly sophisticated tasks, including invocation of other middleware components. Components may have client-side graphical-user-interface (GUI) responsibilities as well for visual display and interaction with the user.

Computer-Based Information Management Systems

The first applications of computers to radiology-information management were developed in the late 1960s. At that time, a study at the Massachusetts General Hospital (MGH) identified two major bottlenecks in the hospital's radiology department: (1) patient-examination scheduling and (2) film-library management. The researchers designed and implemented a system to automate these two functions (Bauman et al., 1975a,b). The examination-scheduling system checked for conflicting or duplicate examinations, assigned patients to examination rooms, and assisted in the registration of essential patient data. It produced flashcards to identify patients' imaging studies, generated requests for patients' master folders in the film library, and automatically produced daily worklists for each examination area. The film-library management system demonstrated one of the first medical uses of bar-code readers and labels; bar-code labels identified and tracked film jackets. In addition, the system maintained a database of film-library loan transactions.

The system was a precursor of today's RISs and evolved to include a variety of other functions. Particularly important was on-line transcription of radiology reports, including the capability for on-line editing and approval of reports by radiologists. Another feature, incorporated into the MGH system by Greenes and colleagues (1978), was a link to a computer-based surgical-pathology accessioning system. Radiologists had automated access to confirmed pathologic diagnoses and thus could receive automated feedback on their interpretations (Greenes et al., 1978). Links to other hospital systems were later incorporated.

With the development of new imaging techniques, the volume of and demand for radiologic studies grew, stressing existing manual systems for image and information handling. At the same time, radiology departments faced increasing pressures to control costs and to manage resources efficiently. Computer-based RISs rapidly became necessary to schedule equipment and examination rooms for maximum usage, to assist in film-library management, to track the locations of films, and to collect and analyze the data necessary for evaluation and planning decisions. A number of RISs currently exist. Some are one-of-a-kind systems that have been developed within a particular institution; others are available commercially.

Until the mid-1980s, one of the most comprehensive RISs in operation was that developed by Arenson and his associates at the Hospital of the University of Pennsylvania (HUP) (see Arenson, 1984). It was based on the MGH system but was expanded to support a wide range of department functions, including scheduling, patient tracking, film-library management, billing, and management reporting. Although the system provided essentially all of the functionality outlined, it was not commercially available. Under Arenson's leadership, however, a group of university-based radiology departments formed the Radiology Information Systems Consortium (RISC) in the early 1980s, which developed a comprehensive specification for an RIS, based in large part on the HUP experience (Arenson et al., 1982). Digital Equipment Corporation (DEC) was the vendor chosen to work with RISC to implement the system, known as DECRad. Since that time the product has changed hands and is now marketed and supported by IDX Corporation under the name IDXRad. Several other RISs are on the market, although IDXRad is the most widely installed.

Report Generation

Also in the late 1960s, several groups explored methods to allow radiologists to enter reports directly into computer-based systems rather than dictating reports for later transcription. The most elaborate was a system developed by Margulies and later enhanced by Wheeler at Johns Hopkins University Hospital (Margulies & Wheeler, 1972). Researchers created a set of large, graphically oriented displays on film. The displays could be selected randomly and back-projected onto a touch-sensitive screen. Radiologists were able to compose narrative reports by touching appropriate areas of the screen to select words, phrases, and even pictures. Branching from one display to another was controlled by the choices selected by the radiologist. SIREP, a commercial version of this system, marketed by Siemens, had limited acceptance; other companies explored reimplementations.

Bauman and colleagues at MGH also experimented with using branching hierarchical menus of displays as a means for entry of radiologic reports but abandoned this project because the approach did not seem to fit well with the radiologists' desire for freedom of expression when creating reports (Bauman et al., 1972). A similar menu-driven system, called CLIP, was developed by Leeming, Simon, and Bleich at Beth Israel Hospital in Boston (see Leeming & Simon, 1982). Radiologists chose from lists of statements by indicating the alphanumeric code for the desired phrase and then modified the selected statements by inserting appropriate adjectives and adverbs. A report-generation system developed in the late 1960s by Lehr and colleagues at the University of Missouri at Columbia allowed radiologists to compose reports by concatenating symbols that represented sentences or phrases. They could append free text to the report by typing it into the terminal. This system later added patient-registration, scheduling, and film-tracking capabilities, to become a full-function RIS known as MARS (Lehr et al., 1973). More recently, specialized systems—such as for obstetrical ultrasonography (Greenes, 1982) and for ultrasonography generally (Bell & Greenes, 1994)—have been successful in limited areas, but structured reporting has not progressed significantly, even with the improved graphical user interfaces now available.

In the 1980s, developers explored combining voice input with selection from screen-based menus (Robbins et al., 1988). Several such commercial systems were introduced, but success was limited because of the need for use of disconnected speech (e.g., enunciation of single words), persistent error rates of 2 to 5 percent, and awkward user interfaces. Recent improvements in the recognition of continuous speech have now made these systems easier to use and substantially reduced error rates.

14.5.3 *Current Status of Radiology Information Systems*

The radiology department provides examples of some of the most dramatic health-care computing applications to date. The use of computers in radiology has produced fundamental advances in image generation and image analysis, in addition to facilitating the communication and management of images and radiologic information. Radiology information systems (or incorporation of RIS functionality with HISs) are now widespread. Structured reporting using mouse and keyboard interaction has seen a few success stories but is not being widely adopted. Primary attention currently is focused on voice dictation systems some of which incorporate the new continous-speech recognizers.

Infrastructure is gradually shifting to a client–server, distributed-computing model, using the Internet, World Wide Web, Java for enhanced presentation layer, and Common Object Request Broker Architecture (CORBA) as the protocol for invoking remote distributed networked services. Progress is slow because of the investment in legacy systems, the size and diversity of IDNs, and the difficulty of creating the hardware and communications infrastructure necessary for integrating all the elements and connecting the various users.

Examples of Integrated Systems

In the following paragraphs, we provide examples of systems that integrate images with other information. We begin with radiology and then move to other areas that provide insight into the widespread uses of images within biomedicine.

PACS, RIS, and HIS Integration

The evolution of radiology at the Brigham and Women's Hospital is probably representative of that at many institutions. The Brigham is part of a growing IDN, the Partners HealthCare System, serving eastern Massachusetts. The Brigham has a large and successful HIS, known as BICS, and an IDXRad RIS. A homegrown PACS was developed for acquisition and archiving of the digital modalities. The HIS and RIS are interlinked for transfer of patient demographic, billing, and report information, and the RIS and PACS were interlinked to enable the RIS to keep track of images on the PACS associated with particular examinations (Hanlon et al., 1996). Ultrasound reports are generated by separate reporting modules (Bell & Greenes, 1994) and are integrated into the RIS through an HL7 interface (see Chapter 6). Other semi-independent reporting modules can be linked to the RIS in similar fashion. Voice-recognition systems for reporting have been introduced.

A major focus of PACS development at the Brigham has been distributing images to referring physicians and making them available in the homes of staff radiologists who are on call to residents and fellows. A Web interface to the RIS and PACS enables examinations to be retrieved based on a variety of search criteria (such as patient name or medical-record number, examination type, date, location, interpreting radiologist) (Khorasani et al., 1998). The reports can be reviewed and the images accessed if available. These files can be sent in different formats and image sizes, and gray scale can be modified. Images also can be selected by radiologists for storage as teaching-file cases. The system is now a combined home-grown and commercial effort.

Radiation treatment planning. Radiation therapy is the application of ionizing radiation to tumor treatment. The goal of a radiation-treatment-planning (RTP) system is to design an arrangement of radiation beams such that maximal dose is delivered to the tumor volume and minimal dose is delivered to surrounding tissues, particularly such critical structures as the spinal cord or liver. In the University of Washington PRISM RTP system (Kalet & Austin-Seymour, 1997), CT images are acquired and then are segmented to delineate the critical structures and tumor volume. Artificial-intelligence planning techniques are combined with manual techniques to design the optimum arrangement of beams. This arrangement is used to calculate an expected dosage, which is superimposed on the anatomic models, thereby allowing the dosimetrist to visualize and modify the adequacy of the beam arrangement. The final arrangement is then used to set up the actual radiation beams (Fig. 14.9; see color insert).

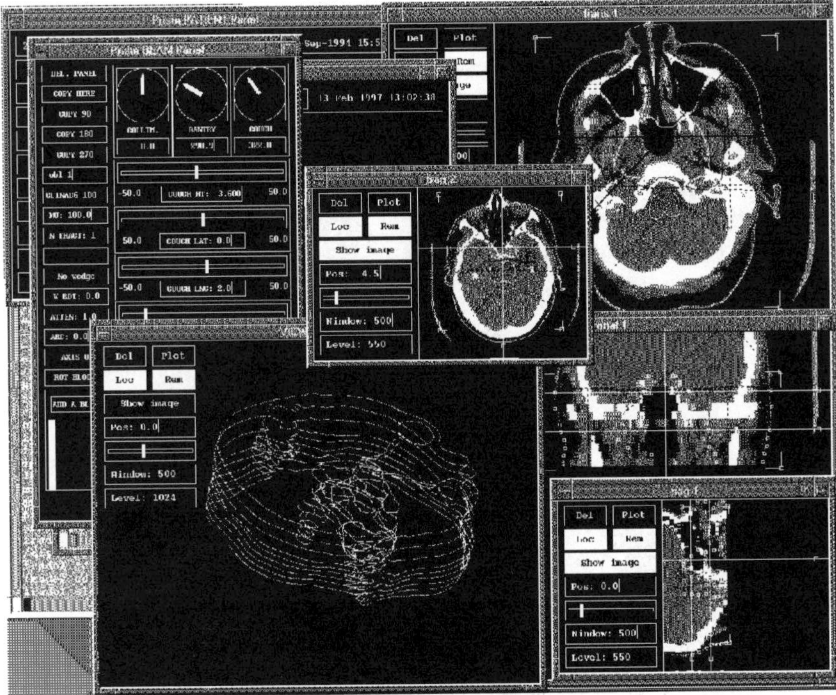

FIGURE 14.9. Several screens from a tool for radiation treatment planning. Computed tomography images from a patient are manually segmented to generate three-dimensional regions depicting the locations of tumors and of critical anatomical structures. Artificial-intelligence techniques then configure a set of radiation beams to deliver maximum dosage to the tumor and minimum dosage to the critical structures. (*Source:* Courtesy of Ira Kalet, Department of Radiation Oncology, University of Washington.) (See color insert.)

Telemedicine. As part of the national High Performance Computing and Communications Initiative (HPCC), the University of Washington (UW) is one of several medical centers developing a regional telemedicine network (Fuller, 1997). A DICOM Web server has been developed, which accepts images from CR, CT, MR, digital fluoroscopy (DF), and ultrasound scanners in radiology (Stewart et al., 1997). The images are then available for review by physicians through the MINDscape interface to the medical record (Tarczy-Hornuch et al., 1997), a locally developed World Wide Web interface that integrates diverse information sources available throughout the UW medical center and delivers them to authorized remote Internet users.

Surgical Planning and Image-Guided Therapy

A major revolution is occurring in the use of volumetric image data as an aid to surgery (Jolesz, 1997; Vannier & Marsh, 1996). Images can be modeled and reconstructed in a variety of projections, with certain layers removed and others enhanced or colored to enable abnormalities to be visualized clearly in context. The projections can be conformed to the exact perspective of a surgeon looking at an operating field by reconciling position on a head-mounted display with exact coordinates of the patient and superimposed on the operative field. Pioneering work at the Brigham and Women's Hospital (Jolesz, 1997) has integrated surgery and imaging more closely through use of an open MRI magnet that enables interventional procedures to be carried out directly while the patient is being imaged.

Augmented and Virtual Reality

Virtual reality and **augmented reality** refer to a collection of interface methods that simulate reality more closely than does the standard display monitor (Barfield & Furness, 1995). In virtual reality, users don head-mounted displays that track the motion of the head, changing a computer-generated scene as the head is moved. Input devices such as instrumented gloves track the position of the hands and then draw a computer-generated simulation of the position of the hands in the virtual world. Objects may be picked up and moved in the virtual world, and interactions may take place with other users who appear as three-dimensional *avatars* (Capin et al., 1997).

In augmented reality, a computer-generated scene is superimposed on the real world, usually by painting of the scene on semitransparent goggles that track the motion of the head. Augmented reality is increasingly being used for surgical planning and education (Pinciroli, 1995). A computer-generated reconstruction of the patient is superimposed on the operating field, using external or internal fiducials for registration. The surgeon can then visualize the location of the internal structures before any resection in order to plan the surgery.

Both augmented and virtual reality grew out of work in the military to provide better interfaces for fighter pilots. The military is very interested in applying these techniques to medical environments in order to provide better care for field personnel separated from central facilities. In all cases, both original and processed medical images are a major component of a virtual-reality environment.

An example of a virtual-reality environment is the Virtual Emergency Room being developed by the University of Washington Human Interface Technology Laboratory.[1] Photographs of the walls in a local hospital emergency room (ER) are texture-mapped onto three-dimensional models representing the walls and other surfaces. A model of the patient is present in the virtual ER, complete with relevant data, including ECG (see Chapter 13), X-ray, and CT images. The user dons a head-mounted display and can move about the virtual ER. He may grab X-rays and ECG strips from a virtual folder and place them on the virtual wall or pick up the CT images and place them in the virtual body at the orientation from which the images were obtained.

Although the routine use of such a virtual ER is still futuristic, these kinds of simulations hint at the possibilities when large amounts of information are accessed in a highly visual environment. Other similar applications are currently under development, many of which are presented at the annual conferences on Medicine Meets Virtual Reality sponsored by Aligned Management Associates, Inc., in conjunction with various leading medical schools.

Education

Medical images have always been an important part of medical education—many normal and pathologic functions can best be appreciated with images. An important use of images is the illustration of normal anatomy because anatomy provides a framework on which to organize most other medical information. Many CD-ROM products are available for learning anatomy; most of them integrate medical illustrations with terminology and other textual information. A popular example of this approach is the ADAM series of CD-ROMs (ADAM, 1995).

Three-dimensional images of anatomy are increasingly being incorporated into educational products (also see Chapter 17). The images are obtained from MRI or CT studies or directly from cadavers. A well-known example is the Visible Human male and female data sets, each of which is a series of parallel slices through a frozen cadaver. The developers obtained each slice by shaving off a thin section from the cadaver and then photographing the top of the remaining frozen block with a digital camera. The resulting slices form a high-spatial-resolution and high-contrast voxel array through the human body; they are available free to the public (Ackerman, 1991).

Most current uses of the Visible Human data provide either slice viewers or canned three-dimensional renderings of segmented organs. Use of the Visible Human will be maximized when the data sets have been completely segmented so that each voxel can be assigned to a well-defined structure. Several companies are segmenting the data; the Digital Anatomist Symbolic Knowledge Base

---

[1] See http://www.hitl.washington.edu/projects/medicine/limit.html.

in the UMLS will provide the necessary terminology. Eventually, it will be possible to develop educational and reference tools that integrate not only the image data but also symbolic knowledge that provides meaning to the individual voxels.

Two examples that illustrate the potential for this kind of integration are VoxelMan and the Digital Anatomist on-line atlas. VoxelMan (Honhe et al., 1995) is a series of three-dimensional voxel data sets (from the Visible Human, among others) in which every voxel is labeled with the name of a structure. A CD-ROM–based program, running on a Silicon Graphics workstation, accesses this data set to create three-dimensional renderings dynamically of selected structures within the dataset and to label them with corresponding names. An associated semantic net of anatomic terminology and relationships is used to select those structures to be displayed.

A similar approach is taken by the Digital Anatomist atlas (Brinkley & Rosse, 1997) except that three-dimensional renderings are precomputed and areas of interest are labeled separately from the extensive Digital Anatomist Symbolic Knowledge Base (Rosse et al., 1997). The user cannot create new three-dimensional scenes dynamically. The Digital Anatomist atlas is available to anyone who has a World Wide Web browser (Fig. 14.10; see color insert).

Both approaches will continue to evolve along with Internet and virtual-reality technology. Eventually we will be able to move through the virtual body, pointing to structures to obtain more information, much like fictional characters in the movie *Fantastic Voyage*.

Human Brain Project

As described in the previous examples on education, three-dimensional anatomic models are useful for teaching anatomy. Such models have also proved valuable as a means for organizing and visualizing functional information, especially for visualizing brain function. By imaging the brain with one or more functional imaging methods (PET, fMRI) while the subject is performing a defined mental task, we can visualize which parts of the brain are active during the task. Such imaging capabilities, which have allowed researchers to observe the thinking brain, have resulted in an explosion of new information about the human brain. The need to organize and integrate this information has led both to the national Human Brain Project to develop informatics tools for neuroscience and to a new subfield of medical informatics called **neuroinformatics** (Koslow & Huerta, 1997).

The University of Washington Human Brain Project provides an example of integration—in this case, between anatomic models obtained from MRI and functional language data obtained at the time of neurosurgery (Brinkley et al., 1997). The surgical data, which are obtained by application of electrical stimulation to the exposed brain of an awake patient, consist of small centimeter-sized regions on the brain surface that are found to be essential for language. MRI, MRA, and

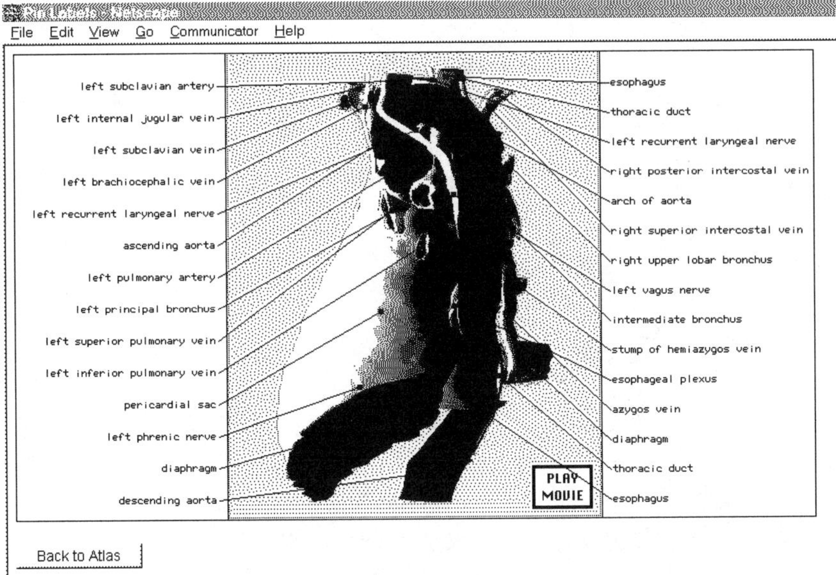

FIGURE 14.10. The Digital Anatomist interactive Web-based atlas, showing the integration of images with tools for anatomy education. Three-dimensional models were created from photographs of cadaver sections that were segmented and assembled into surface models. The models were rendered as static images, which were then annotated with anatomical names. Users can click on regions to obtain names, can take on-line quizzes, and can download saved animations. In this screenshot, the software has dynamically generated a labeled image from a set of annotated regions and labels, similar to pin diagrams often seen in anatomy textbooks. (*Source:* Courtesy of Cornelius Rosse, Department of Biological Structure, University of Washington.) (See color insert.)

MRV image volumes are taken of the patient before surgery and then are processed to create a composite surface rendering of the patient's own brain that shows veins and arteries superimposed on the anatomy. A software package, running on an independent workstation, integrates the rendering, the original images, and an intraoperative photograph of the language sites. The human user interactively clicks on the rendering to indicate the corresponding position of the language sites on the photograph and on the images (Fig. 14.11; see color insert) (Modayur et al., 1997). The three-dimensional coordinates of the sites are stored in an Internet-accessible database that permits individual patient data, as well as combined data from multiple patients, to be retrieved (Jakobovits et al., 1996). As these language-site data are integrated with other Human Brain Project sites available on the World Wide Web, the hope is that a distributed, structure-based information system for managing neuroscience data will emerge.

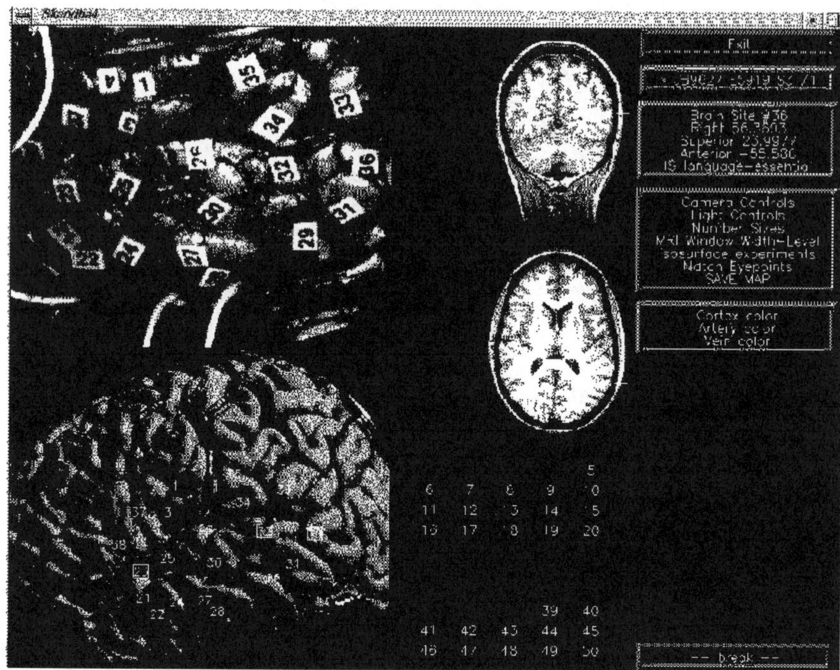

FIGURE 14.11. An interface for interactive brain mapping, showing the integration of photographic images of the exposed brain at neurosurgery, with MRI images and a three-dimensional surface model created from them. The model also includes veins and arteries imaged with MRV and MRA. The user visually matches the photograph with the model and then drags numbers onto the model to perform the mapping. The resulting three-dimensional coordinates, with the models and images, are saved in a Web-accessible multimedia database. (*Source:* Courtesy of James Brinkley, Department of Biological Structure, University of Washington.) (See color insert.)

14.6 Future Directions for Radiology Imaging Systems

It should be clear from this chapter's discussion that computers are an essential tool in radiology. As processing power and storage have become less expensive, newer, computationally intensive capabilities have been widely adopted. To date, this trend shows no signs of slowing.

The overall trend with respect to image generation is ever-increasing numbers of imaging modalities; almost every modality provides unique information, so most of them will remain available. For each modality, the trend is toward higher spatial, contrast, and temporal resolution, up to the physical limits. In addition, all modalities will continue the trend toward three-dimensional or four-dimensional data. New methods will continue to be found to image physiological function, and modalities will be combined to maximize the information content. Perhaps someday it will be possible to image the physiological activity of individual cells and even molecules within a living human body.

Widespread access to images and reports will be demanded throughout health-care delivery networks, as well as across wider geographic areas for teleradiology services. Methodology for meeting this demand probably will continue to build on the World Wide Web, augmented by Java for support of image-manipulation user interfaces. At the back end, systems will use distributed servers not only for storage and for connection to the patient's electronic medical record but also for various kinds of image manipulation. These systems will use the DICOM standard for format of image messages and HL7 for clinical-data exchange and will invoke functionality on the various servers through standardized distributed object management protocols, such as CORBA, in which the HL7 and DICOM messages will be layered.

Image retrieval for research and educational purposes will become much easier due to widespread use of controlled vocabularies such as the UMLS and to continued progress in content-based retrieval. Much of this progress will depend on research in image-manipulation techniques.

Images will be delivered via high-speed networks to increasingly powerful workstations equipped with commercially available software packages for image manipulation and visualization. These software packages will take advantage of advances that are now only at the research stage. Sophisticated user interfaces will be combined with high-level anatomical knowledge, often in the form of shape-based deformable models, to allow rapid creation of instantiations of the models to fit the image data for the given patient. Such three-dimensional instantiated models will provide a framework not only for visualizing and manipulating the three-dimensional anatomy and pathology of individual patients but also for superimposing nonimage information in a structure-based visual medical record.

Soft copy interpretation of radiology images will become common as user interfaces are improved and radiologists become comfortable with the process. For reporting, continuous-speech recognition offers the best hope for an acceptable automated method of capturing radiologist interpretations. Use of a combination of voice recognition for free text and for selecting phrases for structured reports will provide the best combination of methods, ultimately replacing dictation and transcription.

Enterprise integration will continue to occur in stages. As digital images replace analog images in the radiology department, PACSs will increasingly assume the functions of the film library. Databases of medical images, available for clinical and research purposes, will be indexed for retrieval by image, by case, by diagnosis, or by feature. The integration of RISs and PACSs will then allow coordination of all the major activities of the radiology department, from examination scheduling and patient registration; to image acquisition, storage, and retrieval; to report generation and distribution.

The radiology department systems in turn will be integrated with the enterprise health-information system of the IDN. Thus, health-care personnel throughout an enterprise will have on-line access to the images, in addition to radiologists' reports. At the same time, linkages between the RIS and patients' computer-based medical records will allow radiologists to access the clinical data that they need to interpret images and to obtain feedback on their work. Other imaging-based specialties will also be integrated increasingly into the enterprise network for distribution of their images and for teleconsulting.

We will see significant growth in image-guided surgery and advances in image-guided minimally invasive therapy as imaging is integrated in real time with the treatment process. Telesurgery will be feasible: Video images are currently used by endoscopists to guide their maneuvers, and techniques are improving to provide tactile feedback sensations to users as resistance is encountered by remote probes. Combining these techniques with the ability to visualize the anatomic context through real-time MR imaging of the body part could permit an expert interventionalist to conduct an endoscopic procedure entirely remotely, with only a lesser-trained individual on site to perform preprocedure and postprocedure tasks and to deal with problems, should they occur.

As we have described throughout this chapter, many parts of this future scenario already are operational or are well underway at different institutions. Key determinants of the pace of evolution of radiology-imaging systems include the adoption of software architectures that provide a distributed component infrastructure; the cost of computer processors, storage, displays, network servers, and other hardware; and continued advances in user interfaces and software functionality.

Suggested Readings

Aine C.J. (1995). A conceptual overview and critique of functional neuroimaging techniques in humans: I. MRI/fMRI and PET. *Critical Reviews in Neurobiology,* 9(2–3): 229–309.

This source provides a complete and detailed overview of the relatively new techniques that enable researchers to see the thinking brain. Good descriptions of MRI and PET principles are included.

Bauman R.A., Gell G., Dwyer S.J. 3rd. (1996). Large picture archiving and communication systems of the world, Part 2. *Journal of Digital Imaging,* 9(4):172–177.

This comprehensive survey describes the state of the art, in 1996, of operational PACS implementations.

D'Orsi C.J., Kopans D.B. (1997). Mammography interpretation: the BI-RADS method. *American Family Physician,* 55(5):1548–1550, 1997.

This article describes the use of the BI-RADS structured data encoding scheme, which was developed by the American College of Radiology for generating mammographic reports.

Greenes R.A., Bauman R.A. (Eds.) (1996). Imaging and information management: computer systems for a changing health care environment. *Radiology Clinics of North America,* 34(3):463–697.

This issue is an update of a 1986 survey on the use of computers in radiology, with more emphasis on image management and applications. Sections include image acquisition, PACS, networks, workstation design, three-dimensional imaging, image processing for diagnosis, reporting, decision aids, educational uses, telemedicine, and technology assessment.

Haralick R.M., Shapiro L.G. (1992). *Computer and Robot Vision*. Reading, MA: Addison-Wesley.

This volume is a general textbook on image processing. It describes most techniques used in medical image processing.

Jolesz F.A. (1997). 1996 RSNA Eugene P. Pendergrass New Horizons Lecture. Image-guided procedures and the operating room of the future. *Radiology*, 204(3), 601-612.

This article, by a leader in MRI-guided surgical planning and interventional procedures, describes major uses of imaging in treatment.

Koslow S.H., Huerta M.F. (1997). *Neuroinformatics: An Overview of the Human Brain Project*. Mahwah, NJ: Lawrence Erlbaum.

This book contains articles by most of the initial investigators. Many projects make heavy use of medical images.

Kulikowski C.A., Jaffe C.C. (Eds.) (1997). Focus on imaging informatics. *Journal of the American Medical Informatics Association,* 4(3):165–256.

This special issue introduces the field of medical imaging informatics. It includes articles on the Digital Anatomist, medical image databases, and DICOM.

Siegel E.L., Protopapas Z., Reiner B.I., Pomerantz S.M. (1997). Patterns of utilization of computer workstations in a filmless environment and implications for current and future picture archiving and communication systems. *Journal of Digital Imaging*, 10(3 Suppl 1):41–43.

This article describes one of the first and most comprehensive implementations of an all-digital, filmless radiology department, at the Baltimore Veterans Administration Medical Center.

Questions for Discussion

1. What is the general principle that underlies CT? What are three advantages of CT images over conventional X-ray images?
2. Explain the general principle underlying MRI. What are two advantages of this method compared with older methods of imaging?
3. Explain the differences among contrast, spatial, and temporal resolution.
4. Describe the four standard image-processing steps. Suggest how these steps might be applied by an image-analysis program that looks for small, round-appearing tumors on the chest X-ray image of a patient who is suspected of having lung cancer.
5. What is the segmentation step in image analysis? Why is it difficult to perform? Give two examples of ways by which current systems avoid the problem of automatic segmentation. Give an example of how knowledge about the problem to be solved (e.g., local anatomy) could be used in future systems to aid in automatic segmentation.
6. Why are most X-ray images currently stored in analog form? Describe the various factors that a planner must consider when estimating the storage requirements for image data in an all-digital radiology department. What are the

major factors that could reduce the volume of data that are maintained in on-line storage?

7. Refer to Table 14.1. How many bytes are needed to store a digitized chest X-ray image? How many bytes are needed to store a 15-image CT study? If you have a communication line that transmits 56,000 bits per second, how long will it take to transmit each of these images to the display workstations within the hospital? What are the implications of your answer for widespread transmission of image data?
8. What are the economic and technologic factors that will determine how quickly hospitals and clinics will adopt all-digital radiology departments?

15
Information-Retrieval Systems

William R. Hersh, William M. Detmer, and Mark E. Frisse

After reading this chapter, you should know the answers to these questions:

- What types of on-line content are available and useful to healthcare professionals?
- What are the three major steps in the information retrieval process?
- How do techniques differ for indexing bibliographic versus full-text information?
- How effectively do searchers utilize retrieval systems?
- What challenges do the Internet and World Wide Web pose for information-retrieval researchers?
- How will changes in technology affect the scientific, economic, and political aspects of medical publishing?

15.1 Evolution of Medical Information Retrieval

Information retrieval (IR) is the science and practice of identification and efficient use of recorded media. Although medical informatics has traditionally concentrated on the retrieval of text from the biomedical literature, the domain over which IR can be applied effectively has broadened considerably with the advent of multimedia publishing and vast storehouses of chemical structures, cartographic materials, gene and protein sequences, video clippings, and a wide range of other digital media of relevance to biomedical education, research, and patient care. As the ease with which information can be recorded and stored in digital form grows, the growth of biomedical knowledge, once spoken of primarily with reference to the biomedical literature, is now equally relevant to the retrieval of information from text within computer-based patient records, documents concerning the administration of medical care, supporting data for biomedical publications, and the literally tens of thousands of electronic-mail messages now sent and stored every day within personal and professional settings.

As has occurred in the the area covered by many chapters in this volume, IR has changed substantially since the first edition (Siegel et al., 1990). The name change alone (this chapter was previously titled "Bibliographic-Retrieval Systems") is telling, and the description of new content (full text and hypertext), methods (improved indexing, retrieval, and evaluation techniques), and technologies (CD-ROMs and the World Wide Web) shows that much progress has been made.

Although this chapter focuses on the use of computers to facilitate IR, methods for finding and retrieving information from medical sources have been in existence for over a century. In 1879, Dr. John Shaw Billings created ***Index Medicus*** to help medical professionals find relevant journal articles (DeBakey, 1991). Journal articles were indexed by author name and subject heading and then were aggregated in bound volumes. A scientist or practitioner seeking an article on a topic could manually search the index for the closest-matching subject heading and then be directed to citations of published articles.

The printed *Index Medicus* served as the main medical IR source until 1966, when the National Library of Medicine (NLM) developed an electronic version, the **Medical Literature Analysis and Retrieval System** (MEDLARS) (Miles, 1982). Because computing power and disk storage were tightly limited, MEDLARS, as well as the subsequent **MEDLARS Online (Medline)**, stored only abstracted information from each article, such as author names, article title, journal source, and publication date. In addition, the NLM assigned to each article a number of terms from its Medical Subject Heading (MeSH) thesaurus. Searchers could then retrieve articles on a topic by first identifying the most appropriate MeSH term for the topic, and then retrieving all articles from Medline that were indexed with that term.

As computing power grew and disk storage became less expensive in the 1980s, full-text databases began to emerge. These new databases allowed searching of the entire text of medical documents. Although lacking graphics, images, and tables from the original source, these databases made it possible for users to retrieve the full text of important documents quickly, as well as from remote locations. Advanced information-science methods that had been developed in the 1960s, such as vector-space and probabilistic retrieval techniques, could now be implemented on a large scale (Salton, 1983).

In the early 1990s, the pace of change in the IR field quickened. The advent of the World Wide Web and the exponentially increasing power of computers and networks enabled a world where vast quantities of medical information from multiple sources with various media extensions were now available over the global Internet (Berners-Lee et al., 1994). The result of these dramatic changes is that the scope over which IR technologies are relevant has become almost as broad as the scope of published biomedical thought.

15.2 The Information-Retrieval Process

How do we develop a framework for understanding a field that encompasses virtually all biomedical information recorded in digital format? One such framework comes from a modification of ideas advanced by one of the earliest pio-

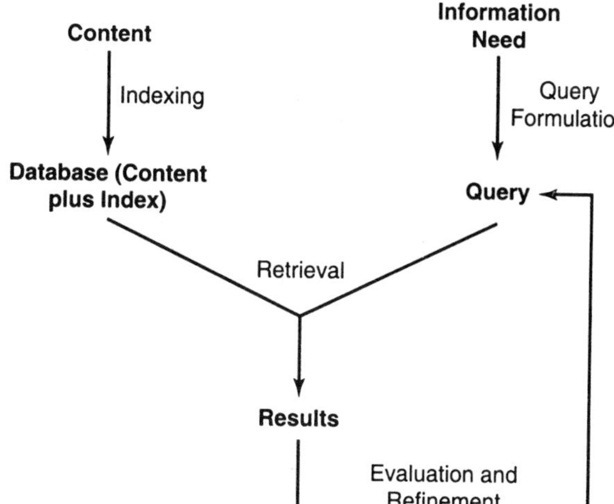

Figure 15.1. A graphic representation of the information retrieval process. The user retrieves content by formulating a query that contains index terms. The user may then modify the query to improve the results of the search.

neers in the field—Gerard Salton (Salton, 1983). A modified version of Salton's approach decomposes the problem of IR into four processes (Fig. 15.1): (1) indexing, (2) query formulation, (3) retrieval, and (4) evaluation and refinement.

The IR process starts with **indexing**, the process by which content (e.g., bibliographic information, full-text journal articles) is represented and stored in a computer database. An **IR database** typically contains both a shorthand representation of the content—an **index**—and the full original content. The index allows users to find relevant content rapidly; the full contents of the entries that the user selects are then displayed.

There are many types of indexes, the simplest being an **inverted index**, which consists of items and item attributes. For example, we might create an inverted index of journal articles that discuss heart disease (Table 15.1). All words found in the articles constitute the index items; the document numbers where the word appears constitute the item attributes. As we shall discuss, more complicated indexes are often created.

In parallel to indexing is **query formulation**: the process of stating information needs in terms of queries. An **information need** is the searcher's expres-

Table 15.1. An example of an inverted index that represents articles that discuss heart disease.

Item	Attribute (Document No.)
Aspirin	1,5,**6**,9
Attack	3,**6**,7,8
Heart	4,**6**,7,10
Prevention	1,2,**6**,9

sion, in her own language, of the information that she desires. For example, a physician examining a 55-year-old man might think, "Should middle-aged men be given a daily dose of aspirin to prevent heart attack?" Because most search systems do not efficiently process natural-language expressions, an information need often must be translated into a statement composed in the language of the index: a **query**. In our example, the query might be composed of individual items appearing in the index joined by combination operators: *aspirin AND prevention AND heart AND attack*.

Once an information need is represented in a query and content is represented in an index, the query can be compared against the index to produce results: a process, called **retrieval**, that includes matching queries against the index, ranking or sorting the output by some criteria, and displaying the results to the user. For instance, retrieval using our query *aspirin AND prevention AND heart AND attack* and our index of journal articles (see Table 15.1) would produce one document (6) as the result.

The final step in the IR process is **evaluation**. Results are inspected by the searcher and evaluated for relevance to the original information need. If the search results are inadequate, the searcher may attempt to reword the query and to rematch against the index in a process called **refinement**. The evaluation process also allows the comparison of different IR systems and techniques on the basis of a variety of metrics.

15.2.1 Content

Content can be defined as media developed to communicate information or knowledge. Content can be separated into two categories: original and synoptic. **Original content** (sometimes referred to as **primary literature**) is developed through new observations and analysis of the world. Medical journal articles that report original research are the most common type of original content. These articles are published after the authors' original findings are scrutinized by knowledgeable colleagues, a process called **peer review**. Original content is disseminated in venues other than journal publication, including conference proceedings, speeches, white papers, and personal communications; however, journal articles are the primary source of original content in health care. Consumers of original content are primarily researchers. This community both produces original content as a byproduct of its research and also uses original content to acquire detailed knowledge of others members' research. Increasingly, other participants in the healthcare process (clinicians, administrators, and even patients) are using original content to help them to make decisions.

In contrast, authors develop **synoptic content** by extracting important observations and principles from sources of original content, as well as from personal experience. These observations and principles are then synthesized and communicated in a form suitable for the intended audience. The classic example of synoptic content is the textbook, where experts, usually experts in their field, review and synthesize all available knowledge on a particular topic. Many other forms of synoptic content exist in health care, such as practice guidelines, drug monographs, and review articles. Consumers of medical synoptic content are primarily clinicians; most other healthcare participants also use synoptic content regularly. Patient information is another form of synoptic content, although it is usually written at a different level than professional-oriented content.

In addition to being classified on the original-to-synoptic spectrum, content can also be classified by the degree to which it represents the original source. **Bibliographic content** is information *abstracted* from the original source. As an example, bibliographic content derived from a collection of journal articles might include just the author names, article title, journal source, and publication date.

On the other hand, **full-text content** is the complete textual content of the source. As an example, full-text information from a collection of journal articles might include citation information (author, title, source, publication date) as well as the complete body text (article text, references, and footnotes). Until recently, it has typically not included nontextual information, such as graphics, images, and tables, but this is changing with the growth of the final class of information, **multimedia content**. Multimedia content encompasses all common computer-based forms of information: text, graphics, images, video, and sound. As an example, multimedia content to communicate new surgical techniques might include a textual description, graphics showing what to do, X-ray images from real patients, and video sequences with sounds of an operation.

Another classification is the extent to which content provides evidence for action in clinical care. In recent years, many people have advocated an approach called **evidence-based medicine** (EBM), where the best possible evidence from the medical literature is incorporated in decision-making (Sackett et al., 1997). In EBM, the clinician first phrases the question as one of four basic types: diagnosis, etiology, prognosis, or treatment/prevention. For each of these types of question, there are clinical studies that constitute the highest quality evidence; for example, the best studies for assessing therapeutic and preventive interventions are randomized controlled trials. Next, the clinician seeks and uses resources that locate this best evidence.

The EBM movement initially advocated exclusive use of original literature, with the clinician critically appraising each retrieved article, but this approach is impractical for the busy clinician. Gorman et al. (1994) have found that the original literature does contain answers to about one-half of the questions that arise in clinical practice; however, the time required to find the answers (e.g., 27 minutes for a skilled clinical librarian using Medline) makes the cost of this approach prohibitive. Many clinicians seek review articles, which are usually written by experts in their fields, to find the best evidence. This approach is problematic as well: Mulrow (1987) found, for example, that most review articles do not review the original literature exhaustively, state their methods explicitly, or apply appropriate statistical analysis (e.g., meta-analysis). **Systematic reviews** can provide more information. In the case of therapeutic interventions, systematic review aims to identify all clinical trials ever done, including those not published, and to perform a meta-analysis when appropriate (Chalmers & Altman, 1995).

The technique of meta-analysis does have its detractors (Feinstein, 1995), but few traditional review articles match systematic reviews in breadth of references and explicit phrasing of results. The largest producer of systematic reviews globally is the Cochrane Collaboration (Bero & Rennie, 1996); also, the U.S. Agency for Healthcare Research and Quality (AHRQ) has designated 12 Evidence-Based Practice Centers to develop systematic reviews.

15.2.2 Indexing

Now that we understand the different kinds of content, we can examine ways that content can be stored in IR databases. Recall that an IR database contains two components: (1) an index and (2) a complete copy of the content. The index is used to find matches with the user's query, and the complete content is used to display the results.

Basic Structure of an Index

The goal of indexing is to produce the smallest, most efficient representation of the original content that will facilitate high-quality retrieval. The basic structure of an index is a list of items and their attributes. **Index items** are units of information suitable for matching with a query. In some indexes, items are simply the words or phrases found in the collection of documents. In other indexes, items are terms assigned by humans or machines to represent the content.

In contrast, **index attributes** describe facets of the item, such as the document numbers where the item appears, the frequency with which the item appears in a document or collection, or the position where the item is found relative to other items. Attributes vary depending on the indexing method; for instance, the simple inverted index described earlier (see Table 15.1) has only one attribute: a list of documents in which the word appears. Index items and attributes are used in the IR process in the following way: queries are matched against index items and then index attributes are used to rank output or provide a pointer to the complete content. In our inverted-index example, queries are matched against the index items (words) and then the document-number attribute is used to locate the original content.

Capture of Content Structure with Indexes

For simplicity, we have assumed that an IR database is designed to contain a single index. This assumption might hold in the simplest of IR systems, but most modern systems contain multiple indexes. Developers create IR systems with multiple indexes to enable **content structuring**: the process by which distinct semantic regions of content are identified. Once identified, these regions can be labeled—a process called **markup**—and then used to create separate indexes. The benefit of content structuring is that users can focus their search in one particular semantic region of documents, often leading to better retrieval performance.

As an example, bibliographic information derived from a collection of journal articles usually contains author names, article title, source information, and publication date. The simplest structure for an IR database containing this content would have a single index representing all the bibliographic information: Author names, article titles, source information, and publication date would be placed in the same index. The advantage of this approach is that a searcher does not need to choose the index against which to match a query, given that there is only one index. The disadvantage—and it is a major one—is that each query is matched against all content. For instance, a search for *woods* would retrieve content written by the author *Woods* as well as content about forests found by the appearance of *woods* in an article's title.

To counter this problem, IR system developers often identify consistent semantic fields in content and then create separate indexes for the content found in each. This approach allows searchers to retrieve content with more precision—a search for *woods* in the author index will retrieve only articles written by authors of that name and will not retrieve articles that mention woods in other fields of the content.

We now look at specific examples of how different medical content is indexed and stored in IR databases.

Indexing of Bibliographic Information

Medline is the world's premiere bibliographic information source. Developed by the NLM, it contains references to 10 million biomedical journal articles published in 3,500 journals since 1966 (Wood, 1994). Medline is licensed to hospitals, medical schools, and information vendors. It is also available free of charge on the NLM's web site via two different interfaces, PubMed[1] and Internet Grateful Med.[2] Each implementation of Medline has its own IR database containing the Medline information; frequently, the indexing method and interface differ across implementations.

Medline is a highly structured source containing two types of information:

1. Information abstracted from the publication, such as the authors' names, article title, article source, publication date, and authors' abstract
2. Information added by a human indexer, such as subject headings and publication types (e.g., *editorial, randomized controlled trial*)

A sample Medline record is shown in Figure 15.2.

What distinguishes Medline from a simple catalog of journal article citations is human-assigned subject headings that indicate the topics covered in each article. These terms come from a tightly controlled, hierarchical vocabulary, called **Medical Subject Headings** (MeSH), that was developed by the NLM to represent important concepts in biomedicine. Medical Subject Headings is a collec-

---

[1] On the Internet, see http://www.ncbi.nlm.nih.gov/PubMed/.
[2] On the Internet, see http://igm.nlm.nih.gov.

Unique Identifier
98020545
Authors
Detmer WM. Barnett GO. Hersh WR.
Institution
Section on Medical Informatics, Stanford University School of Medicine, USA.
Title
MedWeaver: Integrating decision support, literature searching, and Web exploration using the UMLS Metathesaurus.
Source
Proceedings/AMIA Annual Fall Symposium.:490–4, 1997.
NLM Journal Code
cqw
Country of Publication
United States
MeSH Subject Headings
*Computer Communication Networks
*Diagnosis, Computer-Assisted
*Expert Systems
*Information Storage and Retrieval
MEDLINE Subject Headings
*Support, U.S. Government, P.H.S.
*Systems Integration
*Unified Medical Language System
*User-Computer Interface

Abstract

Integrating functions from disparate and widely distributed information systems has been an interest of the medical informatics community for some time. Barriers to progress have included the lack of network-accessible information sources, inadequate methods for intersystem messaging, and the lack of vocabulary-translation services. With the advent of the World Wide Web (WWW) and the evolution of the National Library of Medicine's Unified Medical Language System (UMLS), it is now possible to develop applications that integrate functions from diverse, distributed systems. In this paper, we describe one such system: MedWeaver, a WWW application that integrates functions from a decision-support application (DXplain), a literature searching system (WebMedline), and a clinical Web searching system (CliniWeb) using the UMLS Metathesaurus for vocabulary translation. This system demonstrates how application developers can design systems to meet anticipated clinical information needs, and then can meld the requisite content and functionality from diverse sources.
Publication Type
Journal Article
Language
English
Grant Numbers
LM-07033 (NLM)
Entry Month
9802

Figure 15.2. A sample MEDLINE record consisting of field names and their data. An asterisk before a subject heading connotes the concept is central to the article. (*Source*: Courtesy of the National Library of Medicine, Bethesda, MD.)

tion of over 18,000 **subject headings** grouped into one of 15 **trees** (Lowe & Barnett, 1994). Subject headings may have synonym forms, which are called **entry terms**. Each term is defined carefully, and its relationship to other terms is stated explicitly. For example, *Hypertension* is one of the *Vascular Diseases*, which in turn is one of the *Cardiovascular Diseases. Hypertension* also has more specific terms, such as *Hypertension, Malignant*. The full scope of the term hierarchy that includes the term *Hypertension* is shown in Figure 15.3.

Medical Subject Heading terms are assigned to a particular Medline record in the following manner: A human indexer with detailed knowledge of the MeSH

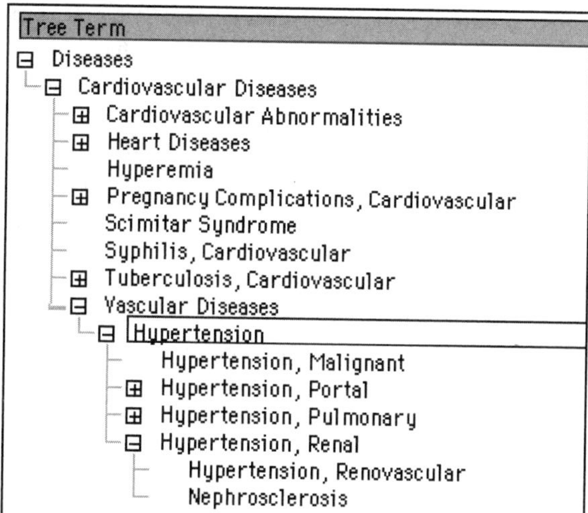

FIGURE 15.3. The MeSH hierarchy for the term *Hypertension*. Boxes that contain plus signs indicate MeSH terms that have hidden subordinate terms. (*Source*: Courtesy of Ovid Technologies, Inc., New York.)

vocabulary reads the complete text of an article and then assigns to the article up to a dozen MeSH terms that best represent the topics covered in the article (Bachrach & Charen, 1978). In addition, an indexer may apply to any MeSH term one or more subheadings; **MeSH subheadings** are qualifier terms that can be added to an MeSH entry term to specify the meaning further. For example, an article concerning the treatment of hypertension might be assigned the MeSH subheading *drug therapy*, to make the full MeSH entry *Hypertension/drug therapy*. Likewise, an article on diagnosis of hypertension would be assigned the subheading *diagnosis*, with the full MeSH entry being *Hypertension/diagnosis*. There are 76 subheadings used in MeSH; each subheading is associated with rules that prevent illogical combinations such as "diagnosis of aspirin."

The reason that Medline and other bibliographic information sources have manually assigned controlled-vocabulary terms is that bibliographic information—particularly information about the topic of a work—is sparse. For instance, the only places in a basic journal citation where topic information resides is the article title and the abstract provided by the author (the latter of which may not be available). The consequence of this paucity of information is that the main concepts contained in the original content may not be represented in the standard citation. A more thorough representation of the main concepts found in the work can be ensured if the appropriate terms are added from a controlled vocabulary, such as MeSH.

Another benefit of manual term assignment is that it facilitates retrieval by concept. For instance, if two articles discuss the treatment of heart attack, but one uses the medical phrase *myocardial infarction* whereas the other uses *heart attack*, only one will be retrieved when a user submits the search term *heart attack*. If both articles were assigned the MeSH term *myocardial infarction*, however, a search for that term would retrieve both articles.

An additional benefit to manual term assignment is the classification of **publication type**. As we noted, there is growing interest in using on-line resources to identify the highest quality evidence for making decisions. Practicing EBM requires finding studies containing the best evidence, such as randomized controlled trials in the case of therapeutic or preventive interventions. Beginning in 1991, the NLM began assigning more detailed publication types such as these to help searchers find such studies.

We have explained how the Medline information source is structured with citation information and MeSH terms. We now turn to how such information is made into an IR database suitable for searching. The most common way that Medline information is turned into an IR database is through the creation of separate word indexes for each semantic region. Thus, words found in the author, title, source, and other fields shown in Figure 15.2 are placed in separate indexes. If a searcher wishes to find articles written by a certain author, he searches for the author name in the author index. If he is interested in finding articles about *heart attack*, he might search for *myocardial infarction* in the index created for the article's MeSH terms. Thus, with these separate indexes, users can focus their searching to the region where the content is most likely to exist.

Indexing of Full-Text Information

Because full-text information contains all textual material from the original source, it permits different indexing techniques. Because full-text content contains many words that describe the content of the source, full-text indexes do not require terms assigned by an indexer; instead, they can contain words and phrases found in the original content. In addition, because important words will appear a number of times and places within the full content, term frequency and term location can be used in the indexing method.

Automated indexing is the most common method of full-text indexing. This approach was pioneered by Salton in the 1960s, but it did not achieve widespread use until the 1990s (Salton, 1983, 1991). It is sometimes called the **vector-space model**, because documents can be conceptualized as vectors of terms, with retrieval based on the cosine similarity of the angle between the query and document vectors. The first step in doing automated indexing is extracting all words from the document that will be used for indexing. High-frequency words that do not distinguish among documents, such as *the, and*, or *that*, are eliminated. Typically, all words on a **stop-word list** of 250 to 500 terms are eliminated. The remaining words are then **stemmed** to remove common suffixes, such as *s, es, ed, ing, al*, and *er*, and then are entered as items in the index. Stemming reduces word variants to a common form. For example, the words *cough, coughs, coughed*, and *coughing* are all reduced to *cough*.

After word stems are identified, they are assigned weights that are based on their ability to discriminate among documents. The term should help the system to differentiate relevant documents from nonrelevant documents in the database. Typically, words that are widely distributed across a database are not good discriminators, such as the words *diagnosis* or *treatment*. Word stems that occur in only a small number of documents, however, are usually good discriminators. For example, although the word *AIDS* is a poor indexing term in a collection of documents about AIDS (because most, if not all, of the documents will contain the word), *retinitis* should be helpful in distinguishing relevant articles on that topic in the same database, because it will likely occur infrequently.

A relatively simple weighting measure shown to be effective in a wide variety of databases is the **TF·IDF weighting**. It consists of two parameters, the first of which is the **inverse document frequency** (IDF):

$$\text{IDF}_i = \log\left(\frac{\text{number of documents}}{\text{number of documents with term } i}\right) + 1, \tag{1}$$

where IDF_i is the IDF for term i. The IDF measures how *in*frequently a term occurs in a document collection. The second parameter is the **term frequency** (TF):

$$\text{TF}_{ij} = \log(\text{frequency of term } i \text{ in document } j) + 1, \tag{2}$$

where TF_{ij} is the term frequency of term i in document j. The TF measures how frequently a term occurs in a document. Each term in each document therefore receives a weight:

$$\text{WEIGHT}_{ij} = \text{TF}_{ij} \cdot \text{IDF}_i, \tag{3}$$

where WEIGHT_{ij} is the weight of term i in document j. In general, TF·IDF weighting gives the highest weight to terms that occur often in a small number of documents. Salton (1983) dubbed these terms *discriminators*.

15.2.3 Information Needs

Query formulation is the process by which information needs are translated into queries suitable for searching (see Fig. 15.1). As background, we first describe common information needs encountered by health professionals.

The information needs of health professionals depend on a number of personal and professional characteristics. Perhaps the most important characteristic is the person's role in the healthcare process. For instance, medical researchers seek information primarily from original-content sources, such as journal articles. Clinicians, on the other hand, seek information that helps them to solve clinical problems, such as how to diagnose or treat a disease. This information is found most often in synoptic-content sources, such as textbooks or reference books. Information needs also depend on level of specialization: A generalist physician will often need basic information about a broad array of diseases and treatments, whereas a specialist might required detailed and late-breaking information about the areas in which she specializes. Many other characteristics play a role in a person's information needs, including practice location (rural versus urban), cognitive style (theoretical versus practical), and time of day (during practice hours versus nights or weekends).

Beyond these general characteristics, what specific information needs does a particular group have, and how frequently do they arise? In a classic study, Covell and colleagues (1985) tried to answer these questions. Observing 12 general practitioners and 35 specialist physicians in office practice settings in Los Angeles, California, they found that two information needs arose for every three patients seen. Of the questions, 40 percent were questions of fact ("What are the side effects of drug X"), 43 percent were questions of medical opinion ("How do you manage a patient who has disease Y"), and 17 percent were questions that sought nonmedical information ("How do you arrange home care for a patient"). In topic categories, 33 percent were about the treatment of a condition, 25 percent about diagnosis, and 14 percent about drugs. For the subspecialists, about one third of their questions related to their own specialties, and about two-thirds related to other subspecialties. Subsequent studies of physician information needs verified these findings (Gorman, 1995).

Understanding the information needs of users has two benefits for designers of IR systems. First, it helps designers to select content that is likely to answer common questions. For instance, knowing that the typical user will be a generalist clinician in a rural practice, a designer might acquire and index synoptic content targeted to answer basic questions about the diagnosis and treatment of a broad array of diseases. Second, it allows designers to develop interfaces that capture user's questions in a manner that facilitates successful translation. We talk about query-formulation interfaces in Section 15.2.4.

15.2.4 Query Formulation

The goal of query formulation is to translate an information need into a high-quality query. Historically, query formulation was performed not by the computer, but rather by the searcher. A searcher first learned the rules of the query language, such as what terms were legal and how relationships between terms were expressed. Then, the searcher translated his information need into a fully specified query and submitted the query to the computer. Today, query formulation is semiautomated, with some query specification performed by the searcher and some by the computer. Advances in interface design and retrieval methods may someday allow greater assistance by computers.

There are two major modes of query formulation, Boolean and natural language. The Boolean model has been the mainstay of commercial IR systems since their inception in the 1950s. The natural-language model, developed by Salton in the 1960s, did not achieve widespread use until recently.

Boolean Queries

We create Boolean queries by combining items found in the index with Boolean operators. The usual **Boolean operators** are AND, OR, and NOT: They are depicted graphically by Venn diagrams in Figure 15.4. The AND operator requires that both terms be present for a retrieval to occur, while the OR operator requires that only

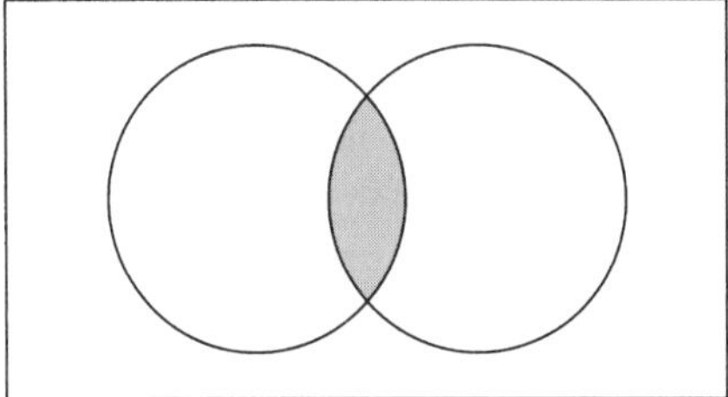
AND – Retrieve items common to both

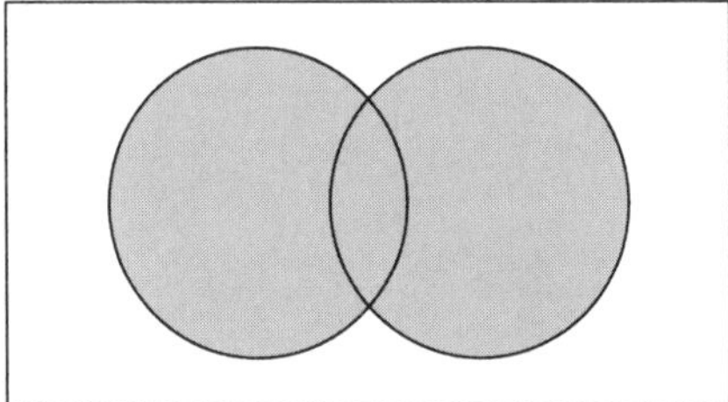
OR – Retrieve items in either

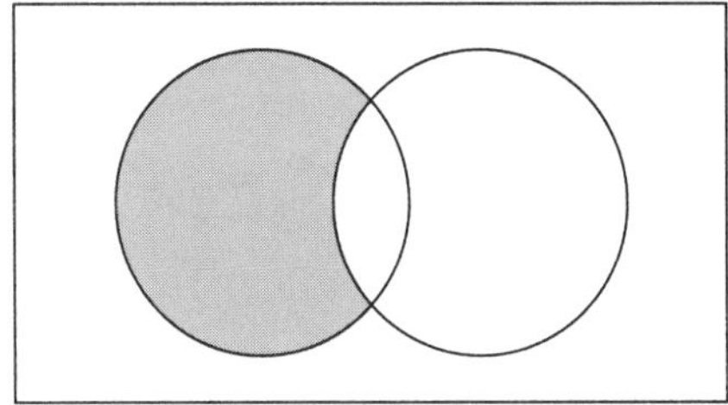
NOT – Retrieve items in one but not other

FIGURE 15.4. Venn diagrams depicting how query terms can be combined with the Boolean operators AND, OR, and NOT.

one of the terms be present. The NOT operator is generally used as a subtraction operator to exclude all items that contain the term listed after the NOT operator.

The simplest implementation of a Boolean query is that shown at the beginning of this chapter, where terms from a single index are combined with Boolean operators to create a query. As we mentioned earlier, however, most current IR databases contain multiple indexes. Thus, Boolean queries formulated for these databases require an additional step, **field qualification**: a designation of which index or field should be searched. Each IR system may have a slightly different method for specifying the index in which to search, but they all have some method of field qualification.

Boolean query formulation can also be aided by systems that take advantage of the hierarchical structure of the indexing vocabulary. As noted, MeSH is organized hierarchically into 15 trees (see Fig. 15.3). Sometimes, a user will want to search on a general topic, such as all types of hypertension or all drugs in the β-blocker category. Such general terms exist in MeSH, but because the indexer is instructed to assign terms at the most specific level (e.g., an article on malignant hypertension is indexed on *Hypertension, Malignant* but not on the more general *Hypertension*), just searching on the general term alone will not retrieve articles on the more specific topic. Most Medline systems thus allow term **explosion**, where a general term and the more specific terms beneath it in the hierarchy are combined with the OR operator.

Most IR systems also have other features that assist the user in Boolean query formulation. All modern Medline systems, for example, allow **text-word searching**, where the user can search on text words in the title and abstract. Such words can be combined with other field-qualified indexing terms. Most systems also allow **wildcard characters** to be used with text words. These characters allow

```
SS 1 /C?
USER:
Aids

PROG:
SS (1) PSTG (9393)

SS 2 /C?
USER:
zidovudine/ae

PROG:
SS (2) PSTG (222)

SS 3 /C?
USER:
1 and 2 and leukopenia

PROG:
*NONE-

SS 3 /C?
USER:
1 and 2 and exp leukopenia

PROG:
SS (3) PSTG (8)

SS 4 /C?
USER:
Prt

PROG:

1
UI - 94180309
AU - Bozzette SA
AU - Parker R
AU - Hay J
TI - A cost analysis of approved antiretroviral strategies in persons
     with advanced human immunodeficiency virus disease and zidovudine
     intolerance [published erratum appears in J Acquir Immune Defic
     Syndr 1994 Nov;7(11):1212]
SO - J Acquir Immune Defic Syndr 1994 Apr;7(4):355-62

     ;;; 7 additional documents follow
```

FIGURE 15.5. A command-line search of the NLM ELHILL system for the adverse effects of zidovudine in AIDS.

single-character or multiple-character expansion at the end of a word. In the NLM's Medline system, the character for the former is # and for the latter is :. Thus, the query term *cough*: will retrieve all articles that begin with *cough: coughs, coughing*, and so on.

Early IR systems required that the searcher be responsible for the entire query-formulation process. For instance, the NLM's ELHILL online system, developed in the 1960s, required searchers to translate an information need into a complete, field-qualified, Boolean query. Figure 15.5 shows an example of a query submitted to ELHILL that requests documents about the *adverse effects of zidovudine in AIDS*. To retrieve meaningful results, the searcher—at that time commonly a medical librarian—would need to know what indexes were available, what terms were found in each index, and how to combine terms with Boolean operators.

Evaluation studies have shown that many novice users get confused about or misuse Boolean operators (Kirby & Miller, 1986; Sewell & Teitelbaum, 1986), leading system designers to create systems that assist in Boolean query formulation. Interface conventions such as entry boxes for each index and checkboxes that add common terms to the query help searchers to express an information need.

An example of such a system is **WebMedline**, the first World Wide Web interface developed for Medline (Fig. 15.6) (Detmer & Shortliffe, 1995). In WebMedline, searchers enter text into predefined fields, such as Author, Title, Journal, and Keyword. In addition, they can choose to constrain the search by standard limiters such as *English, Human Subjects*, and *Publication Type*.

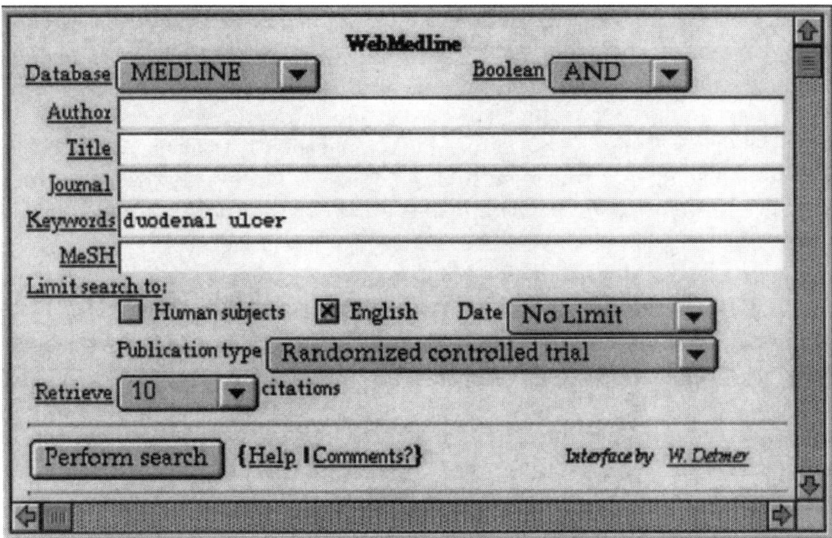

FIGURE 15.6. WebMedline, an example of a World Wide Web interface to MEDLINE that assists users in formulating field-qualified, Boolean queries. See text for explanation.

Table 15.2. The most accurate search strategies for obtaining MEDLINE references of high methodologic quality since 1991.

Question type	Search terms[a]
Etiology	Cohort Studies or Exp Risk or Odds (tw) and Ratio: (tw) or Case (tw) and Control: (tw)
Prognosis	Survival Rate or Survival Analysis or Follow-up Studies or Prognos: (tw) or Clinical (tw) and Course (tw)
Diagnosis	Exp Sensitivity and Specificity or Diagnosis (sh) or Diagnostic Use (sh) or Specificity (tw) or Predictive (tw) and Value: (tw)
Treatment	Randomized Controlled Trial (pt) or Random: (tw)

[a]Terms are MeSH unless specified as text words by (tw), subheadings (sh), or publication types (pt). Exp denotes explosion; # and : denote single-letter and multiple-letter wildcard characters, respectively.

(*Source:* Haynes R.B., Wilczynski N., McKibbon K.A., Walker C.J., Sinclair J.C. (1994). Developing optimal search strategies for detecting clinically sound studies in MEDLINE. *Journal of the American Medical Informatics Association,* 1(6):447–458.

WebMedline formulates queries by assuming an OR between words in a particular field and an AND between fields. As an example, if a searcher enters *duodenal ulcer* in the WebMedline keyword field, checks the box *English,* and selects *randomized controlled trial* from the publication-type menu, WebMedline will formulate the field-qualified Boolean query *duodenal ulcer [title, abstract, MeSH]* AND *english [MeSH]* AND *randomized controlled trial [publication type],* where the labels in brackets are the names of different indexes.

Another method for optimizing Medline queries is to use strategies that facilitate retrieval of the highest quality evidence. As noted, the EBM approach identifies four general categories of questions—diagnosis, etiology, prognosis, and treatment/prevention—and the types of studies that provide the best evidence for answering each. Haynes and colleagues (1994) have identified strategies that retrieve the best evidence for each of these questions; these strategies are shown in Table 15.2.

Natural-Language Queries

Although field-qualified Boolean queries can specify an information need in great detail, they are often complex to formulate and require training. Because they have not received training, most healthcare professionals have difficulty using search systems effectively. For this reason, researchers are investigating systems that permit **natural-language queries**. Such systems allow searchers to enter sentences of any length without any special syntax. An example of a natural-language query is, *Is carotid endarterectomy effective for prevention of stroke?* (Fig. 15.7).

Because natural-language queries are not field qualified and do not specify explicitly the relationships among words, they are frequently processed before being matched against the index. Processing steps can be divided into two categories: (1) **syntactic**, or relating to the structure of words, phrases, or sentences; and (2) **semantic**, or relating to the meaning of the words and phrases. Common syntactic processing steps include removal of stop words, identification of each word's part of speech, identification of common phrases, and stemming of words to their roots. Semantic processing may include identifying a word's semantic type (such as "diagnosis" or "treatment"), expanding the query to include synonyms of the entered terms, and identifying indexes in which individual words should be searched. Although each natural-language IR system processes the

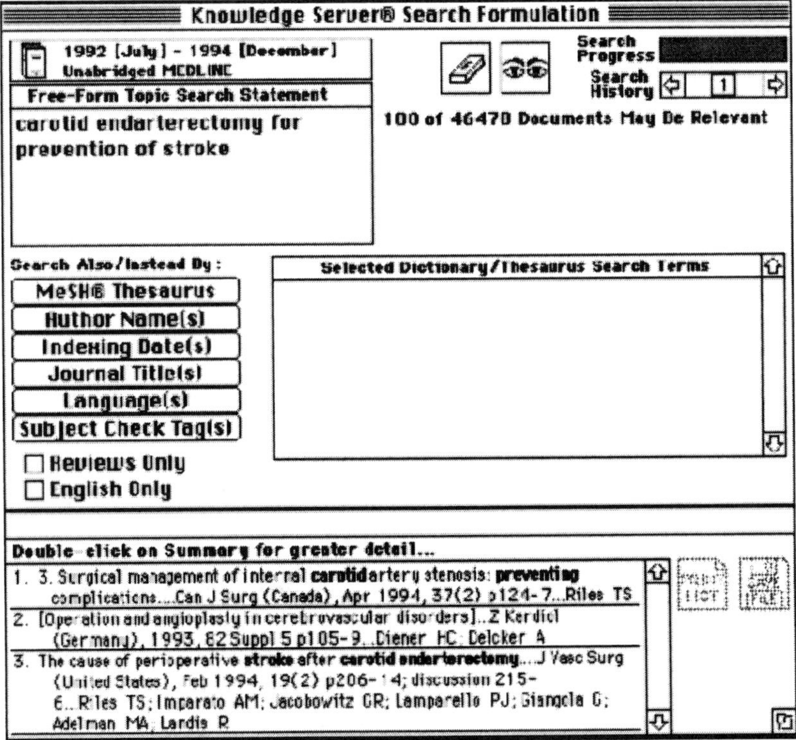

FIGURE 15.7. Knowledge Finder, an IR system that allows natural-language formulation of queries. (*Source*: Courtesy of Aries Systems, North Andover, MA.)

query differently, the output of the query-processing step is a more detailed representation of the user's original input.

15.2.5 *Retrieval*

We have discussed the two components of the general IR framework that are required for retrieval to take place: indexing of content and formulation of queries. We now turn to **retrieval**, in which queries are compared against the index to create results.

The retrieval process comprises matching, ranking, and display. During **matching**, queries are compared against the index, and a result set is created. In **ranking**, the original result set is sorted or ranked by criteria. In the **display**, the final result set is shown to the user. Although each of these steps is not always strictly implemented in an IR system, we look at each to illustrate the process of retrieval.

Matching

In many IR systems—particularly Boolean systems—matching a query with an index is straightforward. An algorithm to perform simple matching takes a term from the query and looks up that term in an index. If there is a match between a query and an index item, the index attributes for the match are stored for later manipulation. As an example, if the Boolean query *heart* AND *attack* was submitted to an IR system containing our simple inverted index (see Table 15.1), the matching algorithm looks for the appearance of both *heart* and *attack* in the index. If it finds both, then it compares the index attributes for each (in this case, document numbers) to find documents in which both words appear. In natural-language systems, matching and ranking are performed together as one process.

Ranking

In the ranking process, the system ranks or sorts preliminary results by criteria to produce an ordered list of results. The purpose of this ranking is to help users find the most relevant information quickly. In many IR systems, the main ranking criterion is **chronology**; that is, the most recent entries are output first. In most Medline systems, for instance, results are ranked by the date of publication, with the most recently published records appearing first.

In addition to chronological ranking, **alphabetic ranking** is common: For a particular field in the IR database, results are ranked based on the order of the field's first word in the alphabet. In some Medline implementations, for instance, users can choose alphabetical ranking of records based on the author's last name.

Although chronology and alphabetic order can help users to find relevant information, these ranking criteria are somewhat limited. Most healthcare professionals, when they examine information in day-to-day practice, use a more complex set of ranking criteria, which may include the authority of the source, the relevance of the source to the user's profession, the relevance of the output to the stated need, and the currency of the output. Although not all of these criteria are modeled and used in current IR systems, there is a trend toward understanding users' ranking criteria and thus developing systems that use these criteria.

Of the criteria just discussed, **relevance ranking**, or the degree to which the results are relevant to the information need, has received the most study (Salton, 1991). Relevance ranking is most commonly used in natural-language IR systems. In this approach, the search results are ranked by presumed relevance to the query. The system usually operationalizes the ranking by calculating a score based on the frequency of terms from the query in the document. Those documents with the highest number, or highest frequency, of query terms are ranked at the top of the list of retrieved documents.

This approach also allows for **relevance feedback**, a process that allows a searcher to obtain more relevant documents by designating retrieved documents as relevant and adding terms from them into a new query (Salton & Buckley, 1990). This technique is based on the assumption that relevant documents have similar indexing terms. In relevance feedback, new terms from the designated relevant documents are added while the weights of existing terms are modified: Weights are increased when the terms occur in relevant documents and are decreased when the terms occur in nonrelevant documents.

Display

The final step in the retrieval process is the display of ranked output to the user. The entire content or parts thereof, rather than items or attributes from the index, usually is displayed.

The most common display in medical IR systems is summary textual output. Often, a portion of the most important information in the full content is displayed, and some mechanism for retrieving the full content is provided. An increasingly popular way of displaying results is with **hypertext**: text that contains highlighted portions that users can traverse to retrieve additional information.

As an example, WebMedline displays for each citation result the author names, article title, article source, and publication date (Fig. 15.8). In addition, it displays hyperlinks to other views of the content including the article's abstract, the complete Medline citation, or the full text of the article.

There are new, experimental techniques to summarize results in a more compact, graphical manner. The goal of such systems it to give users more information about the relationships among results than is provided by a linear display of text. One experimental technique is the three-dimensional cone-tree representation (Fig. 15.9). Each cone represents results that are conceptually related to one another. Users navigate the results by selecting cone elements; this action leads to rearrangement of the display such that the relationships to the target term are displayed. Once a desired cone element is found, detailed textual results can be displayed.

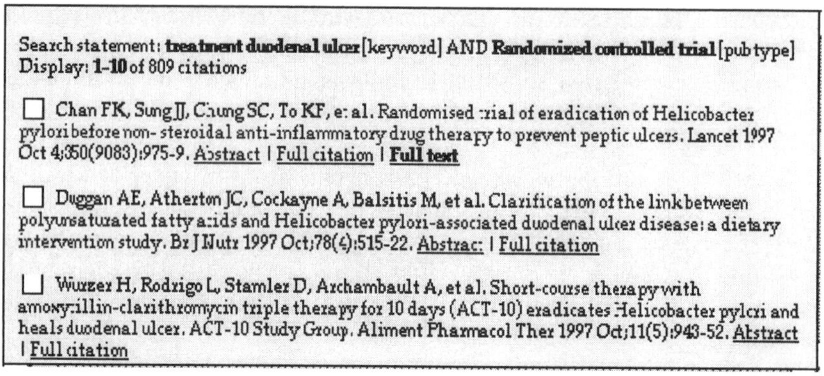

Search statement: **treatment duodenal ulcer** [keyword] AND **Randomized controlled trial** [pub type]
Display: **1-10** of 809 citations

☐ Chan FK, Sung JJ, Chung SC, To KF, et al. Randomised trial of eradication of Helicobacter pylori before non-steroidal anti-inflammatory drug therapy to prevent peptic ulcers. Lancet 1997 Oct 4;350(9083):975-9. Abstract | Full citation | **Full text**

☐ Duggan AE, Atherton JC, Cockayne A, Balsitis M, et al. Clarification of the link between polyunsaturated fatty acids and Helicobacter pylori-associated duodenal ulcer disease: a dietary intervention study. Br J Nutr 1997 Oct;78(4):515-22. Abstract | Full citation

☐ Wurzer H, Rodrigo L, Stamler D, Archambault A, et al. Short-course therapy with amoxycillin-clarithromycin triple therapy for 10 days (ACT-10) eradicates Helicobacter pylori and heals duodenal ulcer. ACT-10 Study Group. Aliment Pharmacol Ther 1997 Oct;11(5):943-52. Abstract | Full citation

FIGURE 15.8. A WebMedline hypertext display of MEDLINE search results.

15.2.6 Evaluation

Evaluation of IR systems is important not only for users who must judge the utility of their searching but also for system developers and researchers who want to better understand how to make them more effective. A variety of questions can be asked: Do they provide access to relevant information? Do they do it in a timely fashion? Is the database being searched the appropriate one for the question at hand? Although there are many useful and important intermediate mea-

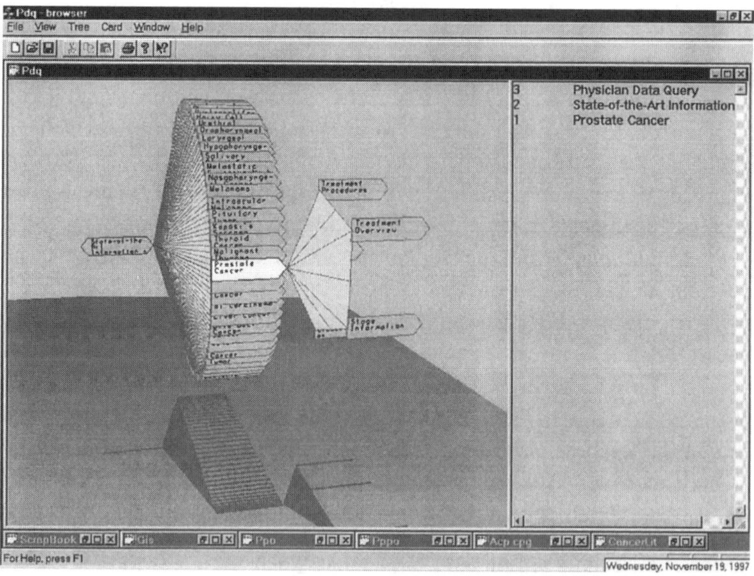

FIGURE 15.9. Cone-tree representation of search results. (*Source*: Courtesy of Xerox Corp., Palo Alto, CA.)

sures of evaluation, it has been difficult to develop comprehensive measures of the outcome of the user's interaction with the IR system.

One simple approach to evaluation has been to measure whether and to what extent systems are used. In a review of studies assessing use of IR systems in actual clinical settings, Hersh and colleagues (1996b) found that system users performed searches only a few times per month. Remember that physicians are known to generate, in the course of care, two questions for every three patients, and it is clear that the physicians were not using the system to answer all their questions (Covell et al., 1985; Gorman & Helfand, 1995). Other studies have also demonstrated that physicians tend to rely on colleagues and tertiary sources of literature, which often are outdated. These observations imply that clinicians cannot search the literature, let alone retrieve or critically appraise articles, in busy practice settings.

The bulk of evaluation in IR, however, has focused on measuring the retrieval of relevant documents. This component does meaure the ultimate utility of the system: whether useful information is retrieved and whether users benefit from the system. The measures used for these characteristics are recall and precision. **Recall** is defined as the ratio of relevant documents retrieved to the total number of relevant documents in a database:

$$\text{Recall} = \frac{\text{number of documents retrieved and relevant}}{\text{number of relevant documents in database}} \qquad (4)$$

Precision is the ratio of relevant documents retrieved to the total number of documents retrieved:

$$\text{Precision} = \frac{\text{number of documents retrieved and relevant}}{\text{number of documents retrieved}} \qquad (5)$$

For example, consider a text database with 100 articles on a specific topic. If the user retrieves 90 of these documents, the recall is 0.9 (or 90 percent). If the total number of documents displayed during the interaction is 180, the precision is 0.5 (or 50 percent). Recall, then, is like the sensitivity of a diagnostic test (see Chapter 3); it measures the recorded "positives" as a fraction of all "true positives" in the population. Precision, in this context, is like the positive predictive value; it measures the "true positives" in proportion to the "total positive tests" recorded.

The same concepts of test characterization apply to the field of IR. If a relatively small database has a high "prevalence" of desired items, even a low-precision search will afford an ample number of documents, and the proportion of desired documents to all retrieved documents will be high. If, on the other hand, the database of documents is huge and the number of desirable documents is small, we can expect to get the same number of overall desired documents from a query, but we will also retrieve many more irrelevant items. This fundamental characteristic of IR systems explains why searches become more frustrating to conduct as the size of a digital library or a collection of Internet web pages grows.

The first comprehensive study of Medline searching performance in clinical settings was carried out at McMaster University (Haynes et al., 1990). Novice searchers in a clinical setting used Grateful Med, a PC-based front end for accessing the NLM's ELHILL system; then, the same searches were performed by medical librarians and clinicians experienced with MEDLINE (Table 15.3). The experienced users retrieved documents with 20% to 40% better precision and twice the recall compared with novices, indicating that experience was helpful in retrieving more relevant documents. This study yielded two other interesting findings. First, there was minimal overlap of articles retrieved by different searchers on the same topic, suggesting that different query strategies lead to different retrieved sets, all of which contain some relevant articles. Second, the original novice searchers tended to be satisfied with their search results, even though the experts were able to retrieve twice as many relevant articles. This showed that either the novices were able to meet their information needs effectively with the smaller amount of relevant articles retrieved or that they were just unaware that the other relevant articles existed.

Hersh and Hickam (1994) compared novice searchers using the Knowledge Finder Medline system (Aries Systems, North Andover, MA), which implements the natural-language querying described in section 15.2.4, with more experienced searchers using the NLM's ELHILL system. They also compared the experienced searchers' use of text-word searching of the title, abstract, and MeSH fields versus regular Medline searching that included the use of MeSH headings, subheadings, explosions, and text words. As in the study of Haynes and colleagues (1990), experienced clinician searchers and librarians searched for answers to the same questions as novice searchers. The novice searchers had much larger retrieval sets due to Knowledge Finder's natural-language and relevance-ranking approach to retrieval, at a price of significantly lower precision. When the retrieval-set size was adjusted to that of the other searchers, the novice searchers still had comparable recall and somewhat lower precision. The experienced searchers did not have any significant difference in recall and precision using text words only or the full Medline feature set. This study showed that natural-language searching allowed novice users to search Medline nearly as effectively as those more experienced.

Researchers also have evaluated full-text retrieval systems. McKinin and colleagues (1991) assessed the performance of searching full-text journal databases

Table 15.3. Recall and precision of clinician searchers at McMaster University.

User	% Recall	% Precision
Novice clinicians	27	38
Experienced clinicians	48	49
Medical librarians	49	58

Source: Haynes R.B., McKibbon K.A., Walker C.J., Ryan N., Fitzgerald D. Ramsden M.F. (1990). Online access to MEDLINE in clinical settings. *Annals of Internal Medicine,* 112(1):78–84.

compared with Medline searching over the same references. The full-text searching resulted in higher recall and lower precision, reflecting the fact that full-text articles have a larger quantity of words to match against than Medline references. This indicates that users must adapt their queries accordingly when searching on full-text databases versus Medline references only.

Why do users not achieve 100 percent recall and precision? There are reasons related to both indexing and retrieval. Human indexers are not consistent. In a study of 700 Medline references indexed in duplicate, the consistency of main-subject-heading indexing was only 68 percent and that for heading-subheading combinations was significantly less (Funk et al., 1983). Word-based indexing also suffers from numerous problems:

- *Context:* Words' meaning are affected by the meaning of other words around them. For example, the relatively common words *high, blood*, and *pressure*, take on added meaning when occurring together in the phrase *high blood pressure* as opposed to in the sentence, low *pressure* at *high* altitudes increases red *blood* cell count.
- *Polysemy*: The same word may have several different senses. For example, the word *lead* can represent the verb *to lead*, the chemical *lead*, or the electrocardiogram (ECG) machine *lead* that is connected to the patient.
- *Synonymy*: Different words may have the same meaning, such as *high* and *elevated*. This ambiguity may extend to phrases that have no words in common, such as the synonyms *hypertension* and *high blood pressure*.
- *Granularity*: Queries and documents may describe concepts at different levels of a hierarchy. For example, a user might query for *antibiotics* to determine which of these drugs to use to treat a specific infection, whereas the documents might describe specific antibiotics themselves, such as *penicillin*.
- *Content*: Words in a document may not be the focus of a subject. For example, an article describing *hypertension* may mention in passing *congestive heart failure*.

Searching success is also hampered by problems related to retrieval. Whether MeSH terms or text words are used, query terms connected by Boolean operators cannot create the exact context of a user's search, especially if the context is complex. Furthermore, many users—especially novices—have difficulty applying Boolean operators (Kirby & Miller, 1986; Sewell & Teitelbaum, 1986). The most common error is to use ANDs in excess, resulting in empty retrieval sets. An analysis of searches logged at the NLM found that 27 percent had zero documents retrieved, usually a result of excess ANDs (Kingsland et al., 1993).

With the emphasis on the use of recall and precision in evaluation studies, researchers have been criticized for overreliance on these measures (Hersh, 1994; Saracevic, 1991). Critics have noted, for example, that recall may be of minor consequence when the user has found a single document that answers her question. Also, in both of the major Medline searching studies described (Haynes et al., 1990; Hersh & Hickam, 1994), there was considerable disagreement by those judging relevance of the retrieved documents regarding which documents were relevant to a given query. These problems with recall and precision have spawned other approaches to evaluating system effectiveness, such as task-oriented methods that measure how well the user is able to perform specified tasks (Egan et al., 1989; Hersh et al., 1995, 1996b; Whitely et al., 1994).

15.3 Trends in Medical Information Retrieval

The pace of change in IR has increased substantially, mostly due to advances in technology and a standard platform of distribution, the World Wide Web, both of which have allowed hypermedia content to be distributed across networks. Additional advances have occurred in vocabulary standardization and aggregation of content.

15.3.1 Distributed Hypermedia

One of the most exciting developments has been the evolution of the Internet and the advent of the World Wide Web. Whereas the Internet was initially used by researchers to communicate via electronic mail, it has evolved to be the conduit through which media of all types (text, graphics, images, audio, and video) are integrated, interlinked, and delivered to all corners of the globe (see Chapter 4). The web's support of such **network-based hypermedia** has advanced knowledge dissemination and communication in all fields. In this section, we discuss the benefits and challenges of these advances for medical IR.

The Internet and the web provide a robust infrastructure and protocol for global knowledge dissemination and communication in health care. The Internet, with its millions of host computers around the globe connected via physical networks, allows medical centers, hospitals, government agencies, publishers, and professional societies to reside on a common network. Moreover, the web, with its shared document-markup language (hypertext-markup language, HTML), retrieval protocol (hypertext-transfer protocol, HTTP), and cross-platform viewing applications (web browsers) allows these same organizations to publish, interlink, and retrieve health information over the Internet.

The Internet and the web, however, pose several significant challenges for health professionals and IR researchers. First, most content on the web is not health related, and most of the health-related material is not suited for professionals. For example, a search of the web for *heart attack* using one of the general search systems will retrieve mostly documents that are written for health consumers. Thus, searches for professional health information in the "mass media" information space of the web often produces results with low precision.

A related concern about the web is whether the information is trustworthy or authoritative (also see Chapter 11). Unlike the journal literature, which is tightly peer reviewed, the Internet allows anyone with access to a server to become a publisher on the web. Although this freedom may have benefits in furthering a democratic society, it is potentially problematic in a professional area such as health care, where quality of evidence is important and the incentives for misrepresentation can be powerful. Silberg and colleagues (1997) have defined elements for web pages to enable users of clinical web sites to determine qualifications and disclosure of conflicts of interest:

- *Authorship*: Names, affiliations, and credentials of content creators
- *Attribution*: References, sources, and (where appropriate) copyright of information presented
- *Disclosure*: Statement of potential and real conflicts of interest
- *Currency*: Dates content posted and updated

A second challenge posed by the web is that documents are usually loosely and irregularly structured. Whereas a searcher can perform a high-precision search in a bibliographic database such as Medline, field-qualified searches are generally not possible on the web. The result of this loose document structuring is reduced retrieval performance. Finally, early web technology has not permitted some search functionality that was previously available in older search applications. Capabilities such as saving of state information (e.g., queuing results throughout a session) and interactive display of results (e.g., hierarchy of controlled vocabulary terms or results) have been difficult to implement in HTML-based systems.

Many people have worked to overcome these problems with the web. Several techniques have been used to carve out from the vast information space of the web the portion relevant to health professionals. The most common of these techniques is to develop authoritative health-information web sites, backed by organizations that already have significant standing in the healthcare community. Using this approach, medical schools, hospitals, government agencies, health publishers, and professional societies have set up their own web sites (Table 15.4 lists some examples). The goals for many of these sites are to provide access to their own content and to serve as another communication channel between the organization and its constituents.

A second approach to providing professional health information on the Web is to aggregate content from multiple sources in one service. The goals of this approach are to give users a single interface to a variety of health information and to provide linkages among sources that may not have been part of the original content. Table 15.5 contains examples of current aggregation services.

A third approach to providing access to professional health content on the web is to create searchable compendia of pointers to useful clinical resources (see Table 15.6 for examples). Most such compendia (e.g., Medical Matrix or MedWeb) catalog health sites by subject area and are useful for browsing and for finding organizations that may have relevant content. Because they compile resources at the organization level, however, they do not help a user to find a particular document that would answer a specific question.

Other systems catalog resources at the document or topic level. One such system is CliniWeb (Hersh et al., 1996a). Human indexers trained in medicine explore the Web, select high-quality medical pages, assign to them appropriate

Table 15.4. A sampling of the many established health-care organizations that disseminate medical information via the web.

Organization	Content	URL
Professional societies		
American Medical Association	Electronic versions of journal articles	www.ama-assn.org
American College of Physicians–American Society of Internal Medicine	Electronic information for internists	www.acponline.org
American Medical Informatics Association	Electronic information about medical informatics	www.amia.org
Government agencies		
Centers for Disease Control and Prevention	Health information for travelers; MMWR, a public health journal	www.cdc.gov
National Library of Medicine	MEDLINE and other NLM databases; Visible-Human project	www.nlm.nih.gov
Agency for Healthcare & Quality Research	Clinical guidelines; evidence-based practice summaries; technology assessments	www.ahrq.gov

MMWR = *Morbidity and Mortality Weekly Report*; URL = uniform resource locator.

MeSH anatomy and disease terms, and enter the pages and indexing terms into a database. This database enables two access methods: a browsing interface that presents the MeSH hierarchy with all the clinical resources associated with each term (Fig. 15.10) and a searching interface that assists users in mapping natural-language queries to MeSH terms and then viewing associated Web resources.

Table 15.5. A sampling of medical content aggregators.

Organization	Content	URL
HighWire Press	Aggregation of leading science journals	www.highwire.org
MD Consult	Online service that includes MEDLINE, textbooks, drug information, and medical news	www.mdconsult.com
Ovid Technologies	Aggregation of bibliographic databases (e.g., MEDLINE), leading biomedical journals, evidence-based medicine reviews, and textbooks	www.ovid.com
Medscape	Online service that includes MEDLINE, electronic mail, discussion groups, and continuing medical education	www.medscape.com

URL = uniform resource locator.

TABLE 15.6. Searchable compendia of pointers to useful clinical content on the web.

Organization	Content	URL
CliniWeb	Catalog of clinically oriented Web pages indexed by MeSH terms	www.ohsu.edu/cliniweb
Medical Matrix	Catalog of clinically oriented Web sites	www.medmatrix.org
MedWeb	Catalog of clinically oriented Web sites	www.cc.emory.edu/WHSCL/medweb.html

URL = uniform resource locator.

Although these three techniques hold promise for harnessing the Internet and the web for the dissemination of medical information, they by no means solve the information problems facing health professionals. Further advances are required before these technologies will affect health care profoundly. Among the needed advances are improvement of network infrastructure in health-care organizations, improvement in web-based software capabilities (such as those provided by Java), institution of intellectual-property controls, changes in production to make content more usable in electronic form, and better integration of knowledge systems with medical records and other data systems.

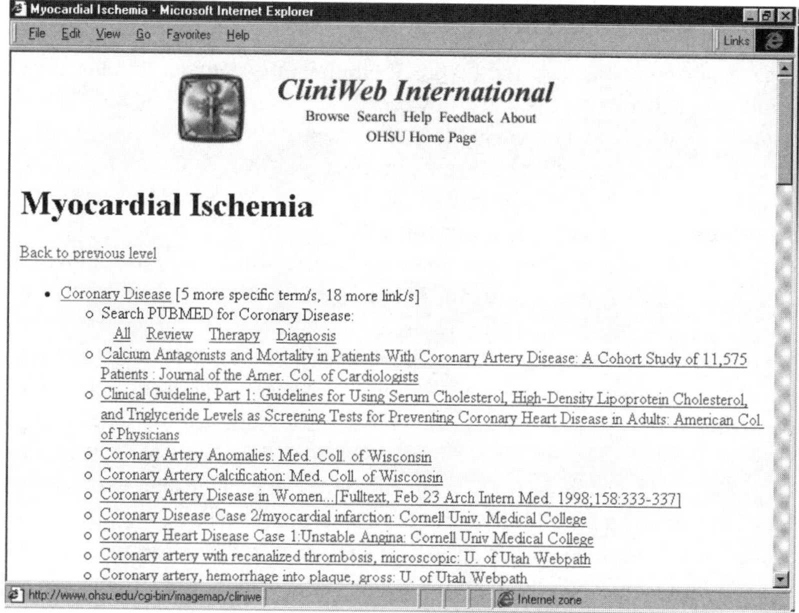

FIGURE 15.10. Browsing interface to CliniWeb (Hersh et al., 1996a). This screen shows Internet resources for the MeSH term *Myocardial Infarction*. Each resource has been found by a human indexer to have clinically relevant and substantial content.

15.3.2 The Need for a Common Medical Vocabulary—the Unified Medical Language System

As noted in Chapter 6, there is a growing desire for a common clinical vocabulary. That vocabulary is needed in IR not only to normalize terms within databases but also to allow systems to interact with other applications, such as intelligent electronic medical records that can retrieve and display pertinent knowledge in the proper context of care. There are several initiatives designed to foster common vocabularies; the largest and most pertinent to IR is the NLM's **Unified Medical Language System** (UMLS) project.

The UMLS is an ongoing initiative by the NLM to improve access to electronic medical information (Lindberg et al., 1993). It was initially spurred by the proliferation of different medical vocabularies that was impeding integration of medical computing applications. There are many coding schemes in medicine, unlinked and therefore unusable in cross-application programs (see Chapter 6). For example, there is MeSH for indexing literature, ICD-9 for diagnostic coding, SNOMED for coding clinical information, and CPT-4 for coding procedures. Many specialized decision-support applications (e.g., QMR, DXplain, Iliad; see Chapter 16) have their own vocabularies and cannot take data directly from sources other than user input. These disparate vocabularies make applications unable to communicate with one another, impeding the next level of clinical applications where, for example, an electronic medical record might feed clinical information into a decision-support system, or a literature search might be generated from the patient's ICD-9 diagnostic code (Cimino et al., 1992).

The major component of the UMLS is the **Metathesaurus**. Initially containing linkages between MeSH and a few other vocabularies (e.g., SNOMED, ICD-9, and CPT), it has now expanded to include some or all of the terms from several dozen other vocabularies (Lindberg et al., 1993). Table 15.7 depicts the concept *atrial fibrillation*, and shows how each string (or lexical variant) of each term relates to the same underlying concept.

The Metathesaurus is designed not to replace existing vocabularies but rather to serve as a bridge between them. It thus has several limitations, such as allowing only one-to-one mapping (thereby not allowing multiple simple terms from one vocabulary to map into single complex terms from another) and not allowing decomposition or extension of terms. The Metathesaurus also does not have its own hierarchy but rather contains the hierarchy from a term's original source vocabulary. Despite these limitations, the Metathesaurus has generated several unique applications, such as an automated indexing program that exploits the breadth of concepts and diversity of synonyms (Hersh, 1991), and a system to generate literature queries from patient diagnosis codes (Cimino et al., 1992) and from electronic medical records (Miller et al., 1992).

Another component of the UMLS is the **Information Sources Map** (ISM) (Masys, 1992). Sometimes, a query fails not because of poor indexing or a bad search strategy but rather because the user looks in the wrong database. The ISM

TABLE 15.7. The UMLS Metathesaurus term *atrial fibrillation*.

Concepts	Terms	Strings
C0004238	L0004238	S0016668
(preferred)	(preferred)	(preferred)
Atrial Fibrillation	Atrial Fibrillation	Atrial Fibrillation
Atrial Fibrillations	Atrial Fibrillations	
Auricular Fibrillation		S0016669
	L0004327	Atrial Fibrillation
	(synonym)	
	Auricular Fibrillation	S0016899
	Auricular Fibrillations	(preferred)
		Auricular Fibrillation
		S0016900
		(plural variant)
		Auricular Fibrillations

Source: Courtesy of National Library of Medicine, Bethesda, MD.

is designed to help users choose the correct database. For example, there are more documents on health administration in the HEALTH database, whereas documents on ethics are more likely to be in BIOETHICSLINE. There are also many specialty databases of which users may be unaware, such as PDQ for cancer-treatment protocols. The ISM is a database of databases, indexed by terms in the Metathesaurus. Several researchers have developed searching interfaces that first help users to find the most relevant database to search and then connect them to that database.

15.3.3 Aggregation of Content

We have looked at IR systems that deliver a specific kind of content and that do not communicate with other IR systems: Indeed, until recently, all IR systems were created to fulfill a specific purpose using limited content. With advances in information-science methods, content, and technology, however, systems are now able to **aggregate content** from many different sources. For instance, clinicians are now able to view textbook information, drug-manufacturer information, and Medline records using one IR interface. The main advantage of aggregation is that it gives users access to a variety of content sources, but presents the information using a consistent interface. In addition, aggregation facilitates the creation of linkages between information sources—a feature that did not exist in the original content and that speeds users' traversal of information.

Another, more powerful type of aggregation is **systems aggregation**. In this type of aggregation, functions from disparate and widely distributed information systems can be brought together in one application. In the past, barriers to progress in this area have included the lack of network-accessible information sources, inadequate methods for intersystem messaging, and lack of vocabulary-translation services. With the advent of the web and the evolution of the UMLS, it is now possible to develop applications that integrate functions from diverse, distributed systems.

An example is **MedWeaver**, a Web application that integrates functions from a decision-support application (DXplain) (Barnett et al., 1987), a literature-search system (WebMedline) (Detmer & Shortliffe, 1995), and a clinical Web-search system (CliniWeb) (Hersh et al., 1996a) using the UMLS Metathesaurus for vocabulary translation (Detmer et al., 1997). This system demonstrates how application developers can design systems to meet anticipated clinical information needs and then can draw together the needed content and functionality from diverse sources.

The three standalone systems are each useful to clinicians, but they are limited because they perform only a specific task: diagnosis of a patient, search of the literature, or search of the web. In contrast, MedWeaver aggregates all three functions so that a user can develop a differential diagnosis and then receive assistance in formulating a medical literature search or in searching the Web for medical content.

The user begins a MedWeaver session by entering a patient's clinical findings. MedWeaver uses DXplain functions to map these findings to controlled vocabulary terms and then to produce a ranked list of possible diagnoses (Fig. 15.11).

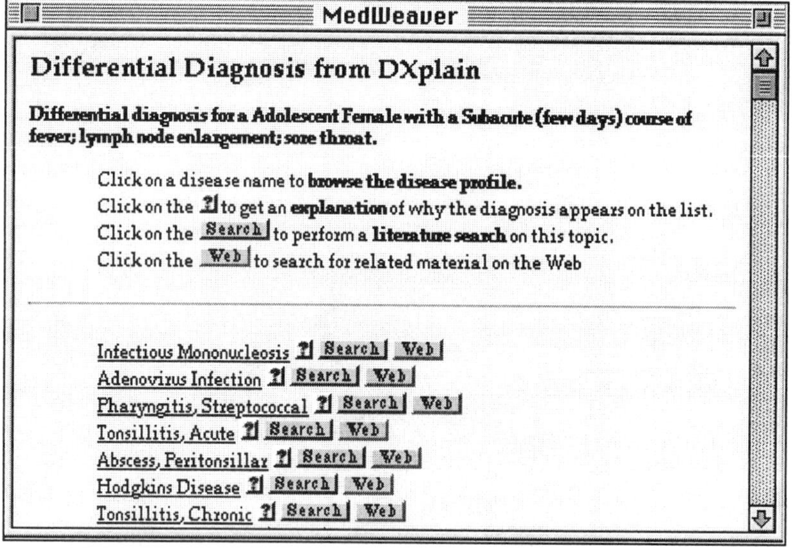

FIGURE 15.11. MedWeaver's aggregation of functions from three systems. MedWeaver uses a DXplain function to retrieve a list of possible diagnoses for the clinical findings *adolescent female, subacute (few days), fever, lymph node enlargement*, and *sore throat*. From this page, users can retrieve a disease profile (a DXplain function), view an explanation of why the diagnosis is on the list (a DXplain function), perform an assisted search of the medical literature (a WebMedline function), or retrieve a list of related Web resources (a CliniWeb function).

It then displays, for any diagnosis on the list, (1) a summary description of that disease (a DXplain function), (2) an explanation of why the diagnosis appears on the list (a DXplain function), (3) an assisted search of the medical literature (a WebMedline function), or (4) a list of clinically relevant Internet sites (a CliniWeb function).

MedWeaver takes the output from one information system, transforms it into an intelligent query of another system, manages the interaction with the remote system, and displays the results in a way that anticipates the user's current and future information needs. A major obstacle to this integration is the translation of one system's vocabulary to another. MedWeaver uses translation functions that were developed with the UMLS Metathesaurus to map one vocabulary to another. For instance, MedWeaver can query the Metathesaurus with a DXplain disease name and retrieve the closest matching term from the MeSH vocabulary. MedWeaver then uses this MeSH term to retrieve bibliographic citations from WebMedline or to identify Internet resources from CliniWeb.

One of the advantages of aggregated applications that draw from diverse information sources is that they allow needs-based, as opposed to source-based, design. In the past, developers created applications by taking an existing information source (e.g., Medline) or by creating a new source (e.g., DXplain) and then developing functionality that maximized that individual source's potential. Now, with the advent of network-accessible information servers and aggregation technology, developers can design systems to meet the information needs of users and then use aggregation technology to retrieve the needed content and to deliver the content at the appropriate point during the interaction with the user.

Another advantage of this approach is that content creation and maintenance are distributed across institutions. Individual organizations have limited resources and talent for producing and maintaining medical content and thus are unlikely to produce the vast libraries of information that may be required to meet users' information needs. Tying together distributed content using aggregation technology offers a parsimonious approach to maintaining content yet meeting users' diverse information needs.

15.4 Future Challenges in Medical Information Retrieval

The new world of IR generates significant challenges for all people who use, archive, and produce information. Many authors have compared the profundity of its arrival to that of the printing press. The web, or what it evolves to be, probably will serve as the platform for delivery of clinical information to users in the future. It has the capacity to realize the trends in information content described in Section 15.2.1. As problems of intellectual property protection and electronic commerce are solved, linkage of various resources (e.g., systematic reviews, primary literature, and textbooks) will emerge. Likewise, as solutions to bandwidth limitations emerge (e.g., ATM and other technologies described in Chapter 4), greater multimedia capabilities will become available.

The web also poses problems for people who archive information. On the web, documents no longer need to be static entities like journal papers; instead, they can be dynamic resources that change as evidence changes. This dynamic potential has profound implications for archiving of scientific information. For example, should outdated versions of the same dynamic document be archived or deleted? There are also questions related to content ownership. The traditional library buys books and journals to make them available to patrons. On the web, however, information is maintained on servers owned by the producers. The library no longer "owns" the information that it may want to make available to patrons.

The web also has the capacity to affect information producers—both the authors (typically academicians who receive little if any direct remuneration for their work) and publishers. Authors now have the ability to bypass traditional publishers and to publish their work directly on the web. Although they have done so to a much greater degree in other scientific fields, authors still rarely self-publish in medicine, most likely due to respect for the peer-review process. The whole idea of electronic publications may lead to rethinking of academic promotion and tenure policies, which are geared toward counting specific numbers of (peer-reviewed) publications. Few medical schools have policies regarding electronic publication at present, and it is likely that fewer recognize the ongoing commitment that maintaining an electronic information resource, such as a systematic review, requires (Bader, 1993).

Publishers face challenges on all fronts, from users who want easier and less expensive access to content to authors who want their work published as quickly and widely as possible. Many medical publications come from specialty societies, which fund other important activities from revenues that derive from print publications, these revenues coming from both dues and subscription fees as well as advertisements. Loss of this revenue could affect their ability to provide services to their members. Even for some commercial publishers, many books and journals are produced with low profit margins such that electronic publications could tip the scales from profitability to bankruptcy.

The Internet and the World Wide Web have laid the foundation for ubiquitous access to electronic medical information. As we have shown in this chapter, there are still significant challenges to all who use, archive, and produce such information. First, even though information is more accessible than ever, clinicians still need high-quality, trusted information that they can use in the delivery of health care. Second, that information must be organized and indexed effectively for easy retrieval. Third, it must be delivered on a platform that is convenient and reliable.

Suggested Readings

Detmer W.M., Shortliffe E.H. (1997). Using the Internet to improve knowledge diffusion in medicine. *Communications of the ACM*, 40:101–108.

This paper describes the use of the Internet in health care. The authors emphasize linkage of different types of information resources, from "legacy"databases to innovative hypertext collections.

Frakes W.B., Baeza-Yates R. (1992). *Information Retrieval: Data Structures and Algorithms*. Englewood Cliffs, NJ: Prentice-Hall.

This textbook on implementation of information-retrieval systems covers all the major data structures and algorithms, including inverted files, ranking algorithms, stopword lists, and stemming. There are plentiful examples of code in the C programming language.

Frisse M.E., Braude R.M., Florance V., Fuller, S. (1995). Informatics and medical libraries: changing needs and changing roles. *Academic Medicine*, 70(1):30–35.

This article describes the changes taking place in modern medical libraries.

Hersh W.R. (1996). *Information Retrieval, A Health Care Perspective*. New York: Springer-Verlag.

This textbook on information retrieval systems in the health-care domain covers state-of-the-art, as well as research, systems.

Lindberg D.A., Humphreys B.L., McCray, A.T. (1993). The Unified Medical Language System project. *Methods of Information in Medicine*, 32(4):281–291.

This paper describes the rationale for and implementation of the National Library of Medicine's Unified Medical Language System.

Miles W.D. (1982). *A History of the National Library of Medicine*. Bethesda, MD: U.S. Dept. of Health & Human Services.

This comprehensive history of the National Library of Medicine and its forerunners covers the story of Dr. John Shaw Billings and his founding of *Index Medicus* to the modern implementation of MEDLINE.

Sackett D.L., Richardson W.S., Rosenberg W., Haynes R.B. (1997). *Evidence-Based Medicine: How to Practice and Teach EBM*. New York: Churchhill Livingstone.

This overview describes the techniques needed to practice evidence-based medicine.

Salton G. (1991). Developments in automatic text retrieval. *Science*, 253:974–980.

This paper is the most recent succinct exposition of word-statistical retrieval systems, written by the person who originated the approach.

Williams R.M., Baker L.M., Marshall, J.G. (1992). *Information Searching*. Thorofare, NJ: Slack.

One of best how-to manuals on searching the medical literature, this book is primarily concerned with bibliographic databases but does cover evidence-based techniques well.

Questions for Discussion

1. Indicate whether each of the following is original or synoptic content:
   a. A textbook chapter that describes the clinical trials assessing the use of spinal manipulation for low-back pain
   b. A study that compares the use of two new drugs in the treatment of hypertension
   c. A meta-analysis of surgical procedures for gastroesophogeal reflux
   d. A bibliography of journal articles on human immunodeficiency virus diagnostic tests

2. Identify a bibliographic database to which you can obtain access. List the content, indexing method(s), and retrieval methods for this database.
3. Describe the two major types of indexing used in bibliographic databases. Discuss several advantages and disadvantages of each.
4. Describe in general the effect on recall and precision of MEDLINE subheadings and explosions.
5. What are the limitations of recall and precision as evaluation measures? What alternatives would have fewer constraints?
6. Describe the tenets of evidence-based medicine. Describe how you would maximize the accuracy of searches for the best evidence.
7. Select a concept that appears in two or more clinical vocabularies. Demonstrate how it would be combined into a record in the UMLS Metathesaurus.
8. Describe two benefits and two limitations of the Internet and the World Wide Web platforms for clinical information-retrieval systems.

16
Clinical Decision-Support Systems

MARK A. MUSEN, YUVAL SHAHAR, AND EDWARD H. SHORTLIFFE

After reading this chapter, you should know the answers to these questions:

- What are three requirements for an excellent decision-making system?
- What are three decision-support roles for computers in clinical medicine?
- How has the use of computers for clinical decision support evolved since the late 1950s?
- What is a knowledge-based system?
- What influences account for the gradual improvement in professional attitudes toward use of computers for clinical decision support?
- What are the five dimensions that characterize clinical decision-support tools?
- What are the principal scientific challenges in building useful and acceptable clinical decision-support tools?
- What legal and regulatory barriers could affect distribution of clinical decision-support technologies?

16.1 The Nature of Clinical Decision-Making

If you ask people what the phrase "computers in medicine" means, they often describe a computer program that helps physicians to make diagnoses. Although computers play numerous important medical roles, from the earliest days of computing people have recognized that computers might support physicians by helping these people to sift through the vast collection of possible diseases and symptoms. This idea has been echoed in futuristic works of science fiction. In *Star Trek*, for example, medical workers routinely point devices at injured crew members to determine instantly what is the problem and how serious is the damage. The prevalence of such expectations, coupled with a general societal concern about the influence of computers on interpersonal relationships and on job security, has naturally raised questions among health workers. Just what can computers do today to support clinical decision-making? How soon will diagnostic tools be generally available? How good will they be? What will their effects be on the practice of medicine, on medical education, and on relationships among colleagues or between physicians and patients?

We can view the contents of this entire book as addressing medical data and decision-making. In Chapter 2, we discussed the central role of accurate, complete, and relevant data in supporting the decisions that confront clinicians and other healthcare workers. In Chapter 3, we described the nature of good decisions and the need for clinicians to understand the proper use of information if they are to be effective and efficient decision-makers. Subsequent chapters have mentioned many real or potential uses of computers to assist with such decision-making. Medical practice *is* medical decision-making, so most applications of computers in medical care are intended to have a direct or tangential effect on the quality of healthcare decisions. In this chapter, we bring together these themes by concentrating on systems that have been developed specifically to assist health workers in making decisions.

16.1.1 Types of Decisions

By now, you are familiar with the range of clinical decisions. The classic problem of **diagnosis** (analyzing available data to determine the pathophysiologic explanation for a patient's symptoms) is only one of these. Equally challenging, as emphasized in Chapter 3, is the **diagnostic process**—deciding which questions to ask, tests to order, or procedures to perform and determining the value of the results relative to associated risks or financial costs. Thus, diagnosis involves not only deciding what is true about a patient but also what data are needed to determine what is true. Even when the diagnosis is known, there often are challenging **management** decisions that test the physician's knowledge and experience: Should I treat the patient or allow the process to resolve on its own? If treatment is indicated, what should it be? How should I use the patient's response to therapy to guide me in determining whether an alternate approach should be tried or, in some cases, to question whether my initial diagnosis was incorrect after all?

Biomedicine is also replete with decision tasks that do not involve specific patients or their diseases. Consider, for example, the biomedical scientist who is using laboratory data to help with the design of her next experiment or the hospital administrator who uses management data to guide decisions about resource allocation in his hospital. Although we focus on systems to assist with clinical decisions in this chapter, we emphasize that the concepts discussed generalize to many other problem areas as well. In Chapter 19, for example, we examine the need for formal decision techniques and tools in creating health policies. The requirements for excellent decision-making fall into three principal categories: (1) accurate data, (2) pertinent knowledge, and (3) appropriate problem-solving skills.

The data about a case must be adequate for making an informed decision, but they must not be excessive. Indeed, a major challenge occurs when decision-makers are bombarded with so much information that they cannot process and synthesize the information intelligently and rapidly. Thus, it is important to know when additional data will confuse rather than clarify and when it is imperative to use tools (computational or otherwise) that permit data to be summarized for easier cognitive management. The operating room and intensive-care units are classic settings for this problem; patients are monitored extensively, numerous data are collected, and decisions often have to be made on an emergent basis. Equally important is the *quality* of the available data. In Chapter 2, we discussed imprecision in terminology, illegibility and inaccessibility of records, and other opportunities for misinterpretation of data. Similarly, measurement instruments or recorded data may simply be erroneous; use of faulty data can have serious adverse effects on patient-care decisions. Thus, clinical data often need to be *validated*. Even good data are useless if we do not have the basic knowledge necessary to apply them properly. Decision-makers must have broad knowledge of medicine, in-depth familiarity with their area of expertise, and access to information resources that provide pertinent additional information. Their knowledge must be accurate, with areas of controversy well understood and questions of personal choice well distinguished from topics where a dogmatic approach is appropriate. Their knowledge must also be current; in the rapidly changing world of medicine, facts decay just as certainly as dead tissue does.

Good data and an extensive factual knowledge base still do not guarantee a good decision; good problem-solving skills are equally important. Decision-makers must know how to set appropriate goals for a task, how to reason about each goal, and how to make explicit the trade-offs between costs and benefits of diagnostic procedures or therapeutic maneuvers. The skilled clinician draws extensively on personal experience, and new physicians soon realize that good clinical judgment is based as much on an ability to reason effectively and appropriately about what to do as it is on formal knowledge of the field or access to high-quality patient data. Thus, clinicians must develop a strategic approach to test selection and interpretation, understand ideas of sensitivity and specificity, and be able to assess the urgency of a situation. Awareness of biases (see Chapter 3) and of the ways that they can creep into problem-solving also are crucial. This brief review of issues central to clinical decision-making serves as a fitting introduction to the topic of computer-assisted decision-making: Precisely the same topics are pertinent when we develop a computational tool for clinical problem-solving. The programs must have access to good data, they must have extensive background knowledge encoded for the clinical domain in question, and they must embody an intelligent approach to problem-solving that is sensitive to requirements for proper analysis, appropriate cost–benefit trade-offs, and efficiency.

16.1.2 The Role of Computers in Decision Support

A **clinical decision-support system** is any computer program designed to help health professionals make clinical decisions. In a sense, any computer system that deals with clinical data or medical knowledge is intended to provide decision support. It is accordingly useful to consider three types of decision-support functions, ranging from generalized to patient specific.

Tools for Information Management

Health-care information systems (Chapter 10) and information-retrieval systems (Chapter 15) are tools that manage information. Specialized knowledge-management workstations are under development in research settings; these workstations provide sophisticated environments for storing and retrieving clinical knowledge, browsing through that knowledge much as we might page through a textbook, and augmenting it with personal notes and information that we may need later for clinical problem-solving. Information-management tools provide the data and knowledge needed by the clinician, but they generally do not help her to *apply* that information to a particular decision task. Interpretation is left to the clinician, as is the decision about what information is needed to resolve the clinical problem.

Tools for Focusing Attention

Clinical-laboratory systems that flag abnormal values or that provide lists of possible explanations for those abnormalities and pharmacy systems that alert providers to possible drug interactions (Evans et al., 1986; Tatro et al., 1975) are tools that focus the user's attention. Such programs are designed to remind the user of diagnoses or problems that might otherwise have been overlooked. Typically, they use simple logics, displaying fixed lists or paragraphs as a standard response to a definite or potential abnormality.

Tools for Providing Patient-Specific Recommendations

Such programs provide custom-tailored assessments or advice based on sets of patient-specific data. They may follow simple logics (such as algorithms), may be based on decision theory and cost–benefit analysis, or may use numerical approaches only as an adjunct to symbolic problem solving. Some diagnostic assistants (such as DXplain [Barnett et al., 1987] or QMR [Miller et al., 1986]) suggest differential diagnoses or indicate additional information that would help to narrow the range of etiologic possibilities. Other systems (such as the original Internist-1 program [Miller et al., 1982], from which QMR was derived) suggest a single best explanation for a patient's symptomatology. Other systems interpret and summarize the patient's record over time in a manner sensitive to the clinical context (Shahar & Musen, 1996). Still other systems provide therapy advice rather than diagnostic assistance (Musen et al., 1996).

The boundaries among these three categories are not crisp, but the distinctions are useful in defining the range of capabilities that computers can provide to assist clinicians with making decisions. Systems of the first two types are discussed elsewhere in this book. For example, Chapters 9 through 14 describe systems that contain and manipulate patient data that are of importance in reaching good clinical decisions. Chapters 15 and 17 discuss methods for accessing information, knowledge, and the accumulated experience of other professionals. In this chapter, we focus on the third category: patient-specific systems.

16.2 Historical Perspective

Since the earliest days of computers, health professionals have anticipated the time when machines would assist them in the diagnostic process. The first articles dealing with this possibility appeared in the late 1950s (Ledley & Lusted, 1959), and experimental prototypes appeared within a few years (Warner et al., 1964). Many problems prevented the widespread introduction of such systems, however, ranging from the limitations of the scientific underpinnings to the logistical difficulties that developers encountered when encouraging clinicians to use and accept systems that were not well integrated into the practitioners' usual workflow.

Three advisory systems from the 1970s provide a useful overview of the origin of work on clinical decision-support systems: deDombal's Leeds abdominal pain system for diagnosis of abdominal pain (de Dombal et al., 1972), Shortliffe's MYCIN system for selection of antibiotic therapy (Shortliffe, 1976), and the HELP system for delivery of inpatient medical alerts (Kuperman et al., 1991; Warner, 1979).

16.2.1 Leeds Abdominal Pain System

Starting in the late 1960s, F.T. deDombal and his associates at the University of Leeds studied the diagnostic process and developed computer-based decision aids using Bayesian probability theory (see Chapter 3). Using surgical or pathologic diagnoses as the gold standard, they emphasized the importance of deriving the conditional probabilities used in Bayesian reasoning from high-quality data that they gathered by collecting information on thousands of patients (Adams et al., 1986). Their system, the Leeds abdominal pain system, used sensitivity, specificity, and disease-prevalence data for various signs, symptoms, and test results to calculate, using Bayes' theorem, the probability of seven possible explanations for acute abdominal pain (appendicitis, diverticulitis, perforated ulcer, cholecystitis, small-bowel obstruction, pancreatitis, and nonspecific abdominal pain). To keep the Bayesian computations manageable, the program made the assumptions of (1) conditional independence of the findings for the various diagnoses and (2) mutual exclusivity of the seven diagnoses (see Chapter 3).

In one system evaluation (de Dombal et al., 1972), physicians filled out data sheets summarizing clinical and laboratory findings for 304 patients who came to the emergency room with abdominal pain of sudden onset. The data from these sheets became the attributes that were analyzed using Bayes' rule. Thus, the Bayesian formulation assumed that each patient had one of the seven conditions and selected the most likely one on the basis of the recorded observations. Had the program been used directly by emergency-room physicians, results could have been available, on average, within 5 minutes after the data form was completed. During the study, however, the cases were run in batch mode; the computer-generated diagnoses were saved for later comparison to (1) the diagnoses reached by the attending clinicians and (2) the ultimate diagnosis verified during surgery or through appropriate tests.

In contrast to the clinicians' diagnoses, which were correct in only 65 to 80 percent of the 304 cases (with accuracy depending on the individual clinician's training and experience), the program's diagnoses were correct in 91.8 percent of cases. Furthermore, in six of the seven disease categories, the computer was more likely to assign the patients to the correct disease category than was the senior clinician in charge of the case. Of particular interest was the program's accuracy regarding appendicitis—a diagnosis that is often made incorrectly (or, less often, is missed or at least delayed). In no cases of appendicitis did the computer fail to make the correct diagnosis, and in only six cases were patients with nonspecific abdominal pain incorrectly classified as having appendicitis. Based on the actual clinical decisions, however, more than 20 patients with nonspecific abdominal pain underwent unnecessary surgery for an incorrect diagnosis of appendicitis, and six patients who did have appendicitis were observed for more than 8 hours before they were finally taken to the operating room.

With the introduction of personal computers, deDombal's system began to achieve widespread use—from emergency departments in other countries to the British submarine fleet. Surprisingly, the system has never obtained the same degree of diagnostic accuracy in other settings that it did in Leeds—even when adjustments were made for differences in prior probabilities of disease. There are several reasons possible for this discrepancy. The most likely explanation is that there may be considerable variation in the way that clinicians *interpret* the data that must be entered into the computer. For example, physicians with different training or from different cultures may not agree on the criteria for identification of certain patient findings on physical examination, such as "rebound tenderness." Another possible explanation is that there are different probabilistic relationships between findings and diagnoses in different patient populations.

16.2.2 MYCIN

A different approach to computer-assisted decision support was embodied in the **MYCIN** program, a consultation system that de-emphasized diagnosis to concentrate on appropriate management of patients who have infections (Shortliffe, 1976). MYCIN's developers believed that straightforward algorithms or statistical approaches were inadequate for this clinical problem in which the nature of expertise was poorly understood and even the experts often disagreed about how best to manage specific patients, especially before definitive culture results became available. As a result, the researchers were drawn to the field of **artificial intelligence** (AI), a subfield of computer science that has focused on manipulation of abstract symbols rather than on numerical calculations.

Knowledge of infectious diseases in MYCIN was represented as production rules, each containing a "packet" of knowledge derived from discussions with collaborating experts (Fig. 16.1). A **production rule** is simply a conditional state-

Rule507		
IF:	1)	The infection which requires therapy is meningitis,
	2)	Organisms were not seen on the stain of the culture,
	3)	The type of infection is bacterial,
	4)	The patient does not have a head injury defect, and
	5)	The age of the patient is between 15 years and 55 years
THEN:		The organisms that might be causing the infection are diplococcus-pneumoniae and neisseria-meningitidis

FIGURE **16.1.** A typical rule from the MYCIN system. Rules are conditional statements that indicate what conclusions can be reached or actions taken *if* a specified set of conditions is found to be true. In this rule, MYCIN is able to conclude probable bacterial causes of infection if the five conditions in the premise are all found to be true for a specific patient. Not shown are the measures of uncertainty that are also associated with inference in the MYCIN system.

ment that relates observations to associated inferences that can be drawn. MYCIN's power was derived from such rules in a variety of ways:

- The MYCIN program determined which rules to use and how to chain them together to make decisions about a specific case.
- The rules often formed a coherent explanation of MYCIN's reasoning—those that applied to the current decision were displayed in response to users' questions (Fig. 16.2). Although rules were stored in a machine-readable format, English translations could be displayed.
- By removing, altering, or adding rules, system developers could modify the program's knowledge structures rapidly, without explicitly reprogramming or restructuring other parts of the knowledge base. (Making such changes, however, could lead to unintended side effects.)

The developers evaluated MYCIN's performance on therapy selection for patients with blood-borne bacterial infections (Yu 1979b), and for those with meningitis (Yu et al., 1979a]. In the latter study, MYCIN gave advice that compared favorably with that offered by experts in infectious diseases. MYCIN, however, is best viewed as an early exploration of methods for capturing and applying ill-structured expert knowledge to solve important medical problems. Although the program was never used clinically, it paved the way for a great deal of research and development in the 1980s. In fact, the development of **knowledge-based systems**, and the commercialization of the rule-based approach in a variety of nonmedical fields during the early 1980s, evolved from MYCIN and from related systems developed during the 1970s (Hayes-Roth et al., 1983).

16.2.3 HELP

You have already learned about the HELP system, the integrated hospital information system developed at LDS Hospital in Salt Lake City over the past 3

```
     In this series, how many of the cutures were positive of the e.coli            (typical system prompt)
     (ORGANISM-1)?

     ** WHY                                  (request from user to determine motivation for question)

[i.e. WHY is it important to determine the number of cultures which were       (system's rephrasing of the WHY
positive for the organism?]                                                          question, and answer)

[1.0] This will help to determine whether there is significant disease
associated with this occurrence of the organism.
    It has already been established that
        [1.1] the culture was taken from a sterile source
        [1.2] the number of cultures in the series is greater than 2
    Therefore, if
        [1.3] the number of cultures which were positive for ORGANISM-1
              is greater than 2
    Then there is suggestive evidence (.5) that there is significant disease
            associated with this occurrence of the e.coli (ORGANISM-1).
        [RULE049]
        ** WHY                          (repeated WHY to determine relevance of previous explanation)

[i.e. WHY is it important to determine if there is significant disease
associated with this occurrence of the organism?]

[2.0] This will help to determine a diagnosis for which the infection should
be treated.
    It has already been established that
        [2.1] the infection is not one of: primary bacteremia, meningitis
        [2.2] for some current culture of the patient it is true that the site
              of the culture is blood
    Therefore, if
        [2.3] there is significant disease associated with this occurrence of
              the organism
    Then
        It is definite (1.0) that the diagnosis for which the infection should
        be treated is secondary-bacterimia
        [RULE103]
```

FIGURE 16.2. Two examples of MYCIN's explanation capabilities. User input is shown in boldface capital letters and follows the double asterisks. The system expands each ["WHY"] question (enclosed in square brackets) to ensure that the user is aware of its interpretation of the query.

decades. In Chapter 9, you learned about its ability to generate alerts when abnormalities in the patient record are noted. In Chapter 10, HELP was again described, in comparison with other hospital information systems, and its internal organization was outlined. Indeed, HELP could have been mentioned in almost any chapter in this book, because it has incorporated applications and methodologies that span nearly the full range of activities in medical informatics (Kuperman et al., 1991).

You will recall that HELP adds to a conventional medical-record system a monitoring program and a mechanism for storing decision logic in "HELP sectors" or logic modules. Thus, patient data are available to users who wish to request specific information, and the usual reports and schedules are automatically printed or otherwise communicated by the system. In addition, there is a mechanism for *event-driven* generation of specialized warnings, alerts, and reports. HELP's developers originally created a specialized language named PAL for writing medical knowledge in HELP sectors. Beginning in the 1990s, workers at LDS Hospital and elsewhere created and adopted a standard formalism for encoding decision rules known as the **Arden syntax**—a programming language that provides a canonical means for writing rules that relate specific patient situations to appropriate actions for practitioners to follow (Hripcsak et al., 1994). The Arden syntax incorporates many of the features of PAL, as well as those of other frameworks for writing clinical decision rules that other research groups developed during the 1970s and 1980s. In the Arden syntax, each decision rule, or **HELP sector**, is called a **medical logic module** (MLM). Figure 16.3 shows one such MLM and its representation in the Arden syntax.

Whenever new data about a patient become available, regardless of the source, the HELP system checks to see whether the data match the criteria for invoking an MLM. If they do, the system evaluates the MLM to see whether that MLM

```
penicillin_order :=
    event {medication_order
                where class = penicillin};
  /* find allergies */
  penicillin_allergy :=
    read last {allergy
            where agent_class = penicillin};
  ;;
  evoke: penicillin_order ;;
  logic:
  If exist (penicillin_allergy) then conclude true;
  endif;
  ;;
  action:
  write
  "Caution, the patient has the following allergy to penicillin documented:"
  || penicillin_allergy ;;
```

FIGURE 16.3. This medical logic module (MLM), written in the Arden syntax, prints a warning for healthcare workers whenever a patient who reportedly is allergic to penicillin receives a prescription for a drug in the penicillin class. The **evoke** slot defines a situation that causes the rule to be triggered; the **logic** slot encodes the decision logic of the rule; the **action** slot defines the procedure to follow if the logic slot reaches a positive conclusion.

is relevant for the specific patient. The logic in these MLMs has been developed by clinical experts working with medical information scientists. The output generated by successful MLMs includes, for example, alerts regarding untoward drug actions, interpretations of laboratory tests, or calculations of the likelihood of diseases. This output result is communicated to the appropriate people through the hospital information system's terminals or on written reports, depending on the urgency of the output message and the location and functions of the person for whom the report is intended.

Since the 1970s, HELP has served as a superb example of how the integration of decision support with other system functions can heighten a program's acceptance and encourage its use. Several studies (e.g., Evans et al., 1986) have demonstrated the beneficial effect of HELP's decision logic on clinical measurements at LDS Hospital. Alerts and warnings are produced through the normal collection of patient data; transcription of data for reuse in secondary settings is avoided through the full integration of the computing environment. As discussed in Chapter 10, HELP and other systems are evolving toward more distributed architectures, with either microcomputers or network computers serving as workstations and data being shared over local-area networks. This large project at the University of Utah has served as an important model of how decision support through integrated data monitoring can bypass many of the traditional barriers to the use of computers for clinical decision support.

16.2.4 Lessons from Early Decision-Support Systems

The Leeds abdominal pain system was an important exemplar of the clinical value of Bayesian diagnostic systems. More recent Bayesian systems, such as the **Pathfinder** system for diagnosis of lymph-node pathology (Heckerman et al., 1989), build solidly on the foundation laid by deDombal and his co-workers. Similarly, rule-based approaches to clinical decision-making, as pioneered in systems such as MYCIN and HELP, have led to more recent frameworks for representing medical knowledge, such as the Arden syntax. The early decision-support systems demonstrated the feasibility of encoding medical knowledge so that it could be processed by computers. They also have helped researchers in medical informatics to clarify both the strengths and limitations of alternative knowledge-representation approaches.

Although the HELP system is a notable exception, most decision-support tools developed in the 1970s were rarely used by health personnel and were viewed with skepticism. The subsequent evolution in attitudes has been due in large part to four influences: (1) the emergence of microcomputers and easy-to-use software, with a concomitant demystification of computers and a general sense in society that such machines are manageable and useful; (2) the increasing recognition on the part of technology developers that computer systems must meld transparently with the work practices of groups that are asked to adopt new technologies; (3) the growing distress among health professionals and managed-care organizations regarding the amount of information that practitioners need to practice medicine well; and (4) the increasing fiscal pressure to practice cost-effective medicine, which leads practitioners to consider carefully the clinical utility and reliability of tests, procedures, and therapies—especially when the latter are expensive or risky.

Gradual changes in attitudes and increasing acceptance of the *ideas* of computer-based decision tools for healthcare professionals are of course not in themselves adequate to ensure developmental progress and the adoption of new information-management facilities. Current enthusiasm will sour rapidly if the products of research are not responsive to real-world needs and sensitive to the logistical requirements of the practice settings in which clinicians work.

16.3 A Structure for Characterizing Clinical Decision-Support Systems

If we are to assess adequately any new clinical decision-support tool or to understand the range of issues that can affect the chances for successful implementation, we must have an organizing framework for considering such programs. One approach is to characterize decision-support systems along five dimensions: (1) the system's intended function, (2) the mode by which advice is offered, (3) the consultation style, (4) the underlying decision-making process, and (5) the factors related to human–computer interaction. As this spectrum of considerations suggests, excellent decision-making capabilities alone do not guarantee system utility or acceptance.

16.3.1 System Function

Decision-support programs generally fall into two categories: those that assist healthcare workers with determining *what is true* about a patient (usually what the correct diagnosis is—as in the Leeds abdominal-pain system) and those that assist with decisions about *what to do* for the patient (usually what test to order, whether to treat, or what therapy plan to institute—as in MYCIN). Many systems assist clinicians with both activities (e.g., diagnostic programs often help physicians to decide what additional information would be most useful in narrowing the differential diagnosis for a given case), but the distinction is important because advice about what to do for a patient cannot be formulated without balancing of the costs and benefits of action. Determination of what is true about a patient, based on a fixed set of data that are already available, can theoretically be made without consideration of cost and risk. Thus, a "pure" diagnostic program leaves to the user the task of deciding what data to gather or requires a fixed set of data for all patients. As all practitioners know, however, it is unrealistic to view making a diagnosis as separable from the process of choosing from the available options for data collection and therapy. Moreover, many physicians believe that the majority of questions about which they seek consultation deal with what they should *do* rather than with what is true about a patient given a fixed data set.

16.3.2 The Mode for Giving Advice

Like the abdominal pain program and MYCIN, most decision-support programs have assumed a passive role in giving advice to clinicians (Reggia & Turhim, 1985). Under this model, the practitioner must recognize when advice would be useful and then must make an explicit effort to access the computer program; the decision-support system waits for the user to come to it. The clinician then describes a case by entering data and requests a diagnostic or therapeutic assessment.

There are also technologies, such as the HELP system, that play a more active role, providing decision support as a byproduct of monitoring or of data-management activities; such systems do not wait for physicians or other health workers specifically to ask for assistance. A great appeal of such systems is their ability to give assistance to healthcare workers without requiring laborious data entry by the clinicians themselves. Such capabilities are possible only because the system's decision logic is integrated with a comprehensive database of patient information that is already being gathered from diverse sources within the healthcare institution. Because practitioners generally do not request assistance from such systems, but instead receive it whenever monitored patient data warrant it, one challenge is to avoid generating excessive numbers of warnings for minor problems already likely to be understood. Otherwise, such "false-positive" advisory reports can generate antagonistic responses from users and can blunt the usefulness of those warnings that have greater clinical significance.

16.3.3 Style of Communication

Decision-support systems have tended to operate under one of two styles of interaction: the *consulting model* or the *critiquing model*. In the **consulting model**, the program serves as an advisor, accepting patient-specific data, asking questions, and generating advice for the user about diagnosis or management. For example, MYCIN was an early example of a program that adopted the consulting approach. In the **critiquing model**, on the other hand, the clinician has a preconceived idea of what is happening with a patient or what management plan would be appropriate. The computer then acts as a sounding board for the user's own ideas, expressing agreement or suggesting reasoned alternatives. A pioneering example of a critiquing system was **ATTENDING**, a standalone program that critiqued a patient-specific plan for anesthetic selection, induction, and administration after that plan had been proposed by the anesthesiologist who would be managing the case (Miller, 1986). Such critiquing systems meet many physicians' desires to formulate plans on their own but to have those plans double-checked occasionally before acting on them. In the critiquing style, the program focuses more directly on the plan in which the physician is interested.

The critiquing model also can be applied in an active monitoring setting. For example, the HELP system monitors physicians' drug-therapy decisions and can suggest alternate approaches that may be preferable (Evans et al., 1986). Similarly, the HyperCritic system (van der Lei & Musen, 1991) can offer suggestions regarding how primary-care physicians might improve their management of patients with hypertension by performing a behind-the-scenes analysis of the patients' computer-based record at the time of each clinic visit.

16.3.4 Underlying Decision-Making Process

A wide variety of techniques has been used in the design and implementation of decision-support systems. The simplest logics have involved problem-specific flowcharts designed by clinicians and then encoded for use by a computer. Although such algorithms have been useful for triage purposes and as a didactic technique used in journals and books where an overview for a problem's management has been appropriate, they have been largely rejected by physicians as too simplistic for routine use (Grimm et al., 1975). In addition, the advantage of their implementation on computers has not been clear; the use of simple printed copies of the algorithms generally has proved adequate (Komaroff et al., 1974). A noteworthy exception is a large computer program first described in the early 1970s at the Beth Israel Hospital in Boston (Bleich, 1972); it uses a detailed algorithmic logic to provide advice regarding the diagnosis and management of acid–base and electrolyte disorders. Although additional techniques—such as mathematical modeling, pattern recognition, and statistical analysis of large databases—have been used in experimental decision-support systems (Shortliffe et al., 1979), the predominant methods have been drawn from Bayesian modeling, decision analysis, artificial neural networks, and AI.

Because computers were traditionally viewed as numerical calculating machines, people had recognized by the 1960s that they could be used to compute the pertinent probabilities based on observations of patient-specific parameters (as long as each had a known statistical relationship to the possible disease etiologies). Large numbers of **Bayesian diagnosis programs** have been developed in the intervening years, many of which have been shown to be accurate in selecting among competing explanations of a patient's disease state (Heckerman & Nathwani, 1992). As we mentioned earlier, among the largest experiments have been those of deDombal and associates (1972) in England, who adopted a simple Bayesian model that assumed that there are no conditional dependencies among findings (e.g., that the presence of a finding such as *fever* never affects the likelihood of the presence of a finding such as *chills*). More recent work on the use of **belief networks** for automated decision-making has demonstrated that it is practical to develop more expressive Bayesian systems in which conditional dependencies can be modeled explicitly rather than ignored. (Belief networks are described in Chapter 3.)

Because making most decisions in medicine requires weighing the costs and benefits of actions that could be taken in diagnosing or managing a patient's illness, researchers also have developed tools that draw on the methods of decision analysis (Sox et al., 1988; Weinstein & Fineberg, 1980). **Decision analysis** adds to Bayesian reasoning the idea of explicit *decisions* and of **utilities** associated with the various outcomes that could occur in response to those decisions (see Chapter 3). One class of programs is designed for use by the analysts themselves; such programs assume a detailed knowledge of decision analysis and would be of little use to the average clinician (Pauker & Kassirer, 1981). A second class of programs uses decision-analysis concepts within systems designed to advise physicians who are not trained in these techniques. In such programs, the underlying decision models generally have been prespecified—either as decision trees that enumerate all possible decisions and all possible ramifications of those decisions or as belief networks in which explicit decision and utility nodes are added, called **influence diagrams**.

In recent years, there has been considerable interest in the use of artificial neural networks as the basis for automated medical diagnosis. **Artificial neural networks** are computer programs that perform classification, taking as input a set of findings that describe a given case and generating as output a set of numbers, where each output corresponds to the likelihood of a particular classification that could explain the findings. The program performs this function by propagating carefully calculated **weights** through a network of several layers of nodes. The structure of the network is uniform for any class of decision problem; the weights associated with each of the nodes, however, are tuned so that the network tends to generate the correct classification for any set of inputs. The values for the weights are determined in incremental fashion when a network is trained on a large collection of previously classified examples during a period of **supervised learning**. Like statistical pattern-recognition methods, artificial neural networks translate a set of findings into a set of weighted classifications consistent with those findings. Unfortunately, there is no way that an observer can directly understand why an artificial neural network might reach a particular conclusion. Artificial neural networks may have significant advantages, however, when the correct diagnosis may depend on interactions among the findings that are difficult to predict.

Since the early 1970s, a growing body of researchers have been applying AI techniques to the development of diagnostic and therapy-management systems (Clancey, 1984; Miller, 1988; Szolovits, 1982). We have already discussed the MYCIN system, an important early example of work in this area. Artificial intelligence is closely tied to psychology and to the modeling of logical processes by computer. Psychological studies of how medical experts perform problem-solving (Elstein et al., 1978; Kupiers & Kassirer, 1984) therefore have been influential in much research in medical AI. Of particular pertinence to the development of decision-support systems is the subfield of AI research that is concerned with knowledge-based systems. A **knowledge-based system** is a program that symbolically encodes concepts derived from experts in a field—in a **knowledge base**—and that uses that knowledge base to provide the kind of problem analysis and advice that the expert might provide.

Clinical decision-making often requires reasoning under uncertainty. Knowledge-based systems in medicine have consequently incorporated either Bayesian or ad hoc schemes for dealing with partial evidence and with uncertainty regarding the effects of proposed interventions. What is most characteristic of a knowledge-based system, however, is that the knowledge base encodes a non-numeric, **qualitative model** of how inferences are related to reach abstract conclusions about a case (e.g., the diseases that a patient might have, the therapy that should be administered, the laboratory tests that should be ordered) (Clancey, 1989). Thus, instead of modeling the relationships among patient findings and possible diagnoses purely in terms of statistical associations or mathematical equations, knowledge-based systems might represent those relationships in terms of qualitative, symbolic structures. Production rules such as those in MYCIN (see Fig. 16.1) often have been used to build knowledge-based systems, as have many other approaches (David et al., 1993). The knowledge in a knowledge-based system may include probabilistic relations, such as between symptoms and underlying diseases. Typically, such relations are augmented by qualitative relations, such as causality and temporal relations.

16.3.5 Human–Computer Interaction

There is perhaps no omission that accounts more fully for the impracticality of many clinical decision tools than the failure of developers to deal adequately with the logistical, mechanical, and psychological aspects of system use. Often, system builders have concentrated primarily on creating computer programs that can reach good decisions. Yet researchers have shown repeatedly that an ability to make correct diagnoses, or to suggest therapy similar to that recommended by human consultants, is only one part of the formula for system success. Fortunately, there is increasing recognition that decision-support systems should, at the very least, present interfaces to their users that are uncluttered and intuitive, where users can predict in advance the consequences of their actions (and undo those actions, if necessary). At best, the decision-support element should be embedded within some larger computer system that is already part of the users' professional routine—thus making decision support a byproduct of the practitioners' ordinary work practices.

Many potential users of clinical decision-support tools have found their early enthusiasm dampened by programs that are cumbersome to access, slow to perform, and difficult to learn to use. Systems can fail, for example, if they require that a practitioner interrupt the normal pattern of patient care to walk down the hall to a workstation or to follow complex, time-consuming startup procedures. Lengthy interactions, or ones that fail to convey the logic of what is happening on the screen, also discourage use of the program. Health professionals are likely to be particularly frustrated if the decision tool requires the manual reentry of information available on other computers. Solutions to such problems require sensitivity during the design process and, frequently, resolution of inadequacies at the institutional level. For example, linking computers to one another so that they can share data requires implementation of an overall networking strategy for the hospital or clinic. The advent of wireless networks that allow users to roam about a hospital or clinic, writing directly onto a computer tablet with a pen-based interface, offers solutions for both clinical computing in general and for access to decision-support systems in particular. Similarly, novel human–computer interfaces based on speech, gestures, and virtual reality offer new dimensions to the ways in which healthcare workers can interact with decision-support systems.

16.4 Construction of Decision-Support Tools

Despite significant research progress since the idea of computer-based medical decision-support systems first emerged, several barriers continue to impede the effective implementation of such tools in clinical settings. As we implied earlier, these obstacles include unresolved questions of both science and logistics.

16.4.1 Acquisition and Validation of Patient Data

As emphasized in Chapter 2, few problems are more challenging than the development of effective techniques for capturing patient data accurately, completely, and efficiently. You have read in this book about a wide variety of techniques for data entry, ranging from keyboard entry, to speech input, to methods that separate the clinician from the computer (such as scannable forms, real-time data monitoring, and intermediaries who transcribe written data for use by computers). All these methods have limitations, and healthcare workers frequently state that their use of computers will be limited unless they are freed of the task of data entry and can concentrate instead on data review and information retrieval (Shortliffe, 1989). Even if computers could accept unrestricted speech input, there would be serious challenges associated with properly structuring and encoding what was said. Otherwise, spoken input becomes a large free-text database that defies semantic interpretation. Many workers believe that some combination of speech and graphics, coupled with integrated data-management environments that will prevent the need for redundant entry of the same information into multiple computer systems within a hospital or clinic, are the key advances that will attract busy clinicians and other health workers to use computer-based tools.

The problems of data acquisition go beyond entry of the data themselves, however. A primary obstacle is that we lack standardized ways of expressing most clinical situations in a form that computers can interpret. There are several controlled medical terminologies that healthcare workers use to specify precise diagnostic evaluations (e.g., the International Classification of Diseases and SNOMED International), clinical procedures (e.g., Current Procedural Terminology), and so on (see Chapter 6). Still, there is no controlled terminology that captures the nuances of a patient's history of present illness or findings on physical examination. There is no coding system that can reflect all the details of physicians' or nurses' progress notes. Given that much of the information in the medical record that we would like to use to drive decision support is not available in a structured, machine-understandable form, there are clear limitations on the data that can be used to assist clinician decision-making. Nevertheless, even when computer-based patient records store substantial information only as free-text entries, those data that are available in coded form (typically, diagnosis codes and prescription data) can be used to significant advantage (van der Lei et al., 1991). Finally, even full electronic medical records may not include *all* of the relevant patient-specific data (e.g., professional and marital problems) and thus should be viewed realistically as an incomplete source of information.

16.4.2 Modeling of Medical Knowledge

People who have attempted to acquire the knowledge for a medical decision-support system by reading a textbook or several journal articles and by trying to encode the implied knowledge in some program can attest to the complexity of translating from the usual text approach for communicating knowledge to a structure appropriate for the logical application of that knowledge by a computer. The problem is not unlike that of identifying what you as a reader need to do to interpret, internalize, and apply properly the wealth of information in a book such as this. Creation of a computer-based decision-support system thus requires substantial **modeling** activity: deciding what clinical distinctions and patient data are relevant, identifying the concepts and relationships among concepts that bear on the decision-making task, and ascertaining a problem-solving strategy that can use the relevant clinical knowledge to reach appropriate conclusions.

You cannot glean any of this information simply by reading a textbook; clinical experts themselves may not be able to verbalize the knowledge needed to solve even routine cases (Johnson, 1983). Consequently, construction of any decision-support system—regardless of the underlying decision-making methodology—entails development of a model of both the required problem-solving behavior and the clinical knowledge that will inform that problem-solving. Considerable work in medical informatics currently concentrates on the design of frameworks that allow system builders to model the knowledge that ultimately will be captured within decision-support tools. Abstract modeling methodologies such as KADS (Schreiber et al., 1993) have been widely adopted by commercial developers of decision-support systems, particularly in Europe. Development of computer-based tools that can assist in the modeling of clinical knowledge remains an active area of investigation (Eriksson et al., 1995; Musen et al., 1995; van Heijst et al., 1995).

16.4.3 Elicitation of Medical Knowledge

Researchers are devising methods that will facilitate the development and maintenance of medical knowledge bases (Musen, 1993). The rapid evolution of medical knowledge makes knowledge-base maintenance a particularly important problem. In the past decade, investigators have developed a variety of computer programs that acquire the knowledge base for a decision-support program by interacting directly with the expert, the goal being to avoid the need for a computer programmer to serve as intermediary (Eriksson & Musen, 1993; Lanzola et al., 1995; Musen et al., 1987). In all these approaches, analysts must first work with clinical experts to model the relevant application area.

For example, researchers used a special-purpose tool known as **OPAL** (Musen et al., 1987) (Fig. 16.4) to enter and maintain the knowledge base of the cancer-chemotherapy advisor **ONCOCIN** (Shortliffe, 1986); the developers of OPAL built into the tool a comprehensive model of cancer-chemotherapy administration, allowing OPAL to transform the process of knowledge elicitation for ONCOCIN into a matter of filling in the blanks of structured forms and of drawing flowchart diagrams on the computer screen. When creating domain-specific knowledge-elicitation tools such as OPAL, developers create their model of the intended application area for the target decision-support system and then either program that model by hand into the tool (as they did in the case of building the original OPAL program) or enter the model into a **meta-tool** (Eriksson & Musen, 1993), which then generates automatically a special-purpose knowledge-elicitation tool based on that model. **Protégé** (see Section 16.5.2) is a meta-tool that many developers have used to create automatically domain-specific knowledge-elicitation tools like OPAL by taking as input analysts' models of the relevant application areas (Musen, 1998; Musen et al., 1995).

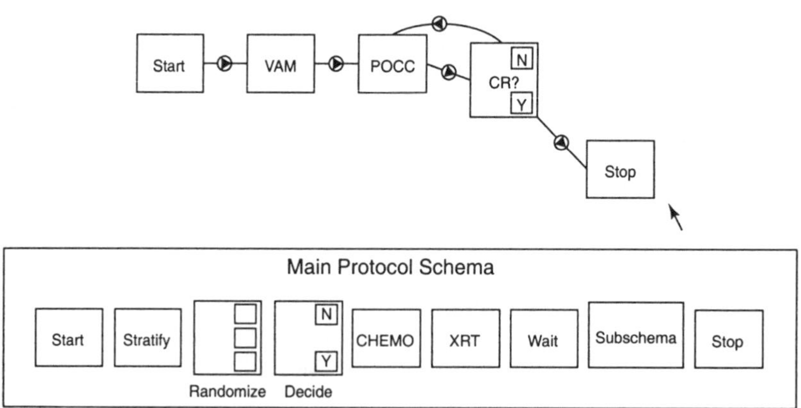

FIGURE 16.4. A clinical researcher can use OPAL to describe the overall schema of an ONCOCIN cancer-treatment plan using the graphical environment shown here. She creates the individual boxes by making selections from the palette of choices at the bottom of the screen and then positions and joins them as desired. The model of cancer chemotherapy built into OPAL determines that possible selections include chemotherapy (CHEMO in the diagram), X-ray therapy (XRT), as well as the idea of randomization and stratification of patients enrolled in clinical trials. The figure shows a relatively simple protocol in which patients are treated with a three-drug chemotherapy called VAM, followed by a four-drug chemotherapy called POCC, until there is complete response (CR).

16.4.4 Representation of and Reasoning About Medical Knowledge

Among the ongoing research challenges is the need to refine the computational techniques for encoding the wide range of knowledge used in problem-solving by medical experts. Although well-established techniques such as the use of *frames* or *rules* exist for storing factual or inferential knowledge, several complex challenges remain. For example, physicians use mental models of the three-dimensional relationships among body parts and organs when they are interpreting data or planning therapy. Representing such anatomical knowledge and performing spatial reasoning by computer have proved to be particularly challenging. Similarly, human beings have a remarkable ability to interpret changes in data over time, assessing temporal trends and developing models of disease progression or the response of disease to past therapies. Researchers continue to develop computer-based methods for modeling such tasks.

Another kind of expertise, often poorly recognized but clearly important to optimal knowledge management by computer-based tools, is the human skill inherent in knowing how to use what is known. In medicine, we often call this skill "good clinical judgment," and we properly distinguish it from the memorization of factual knowledge or data from the literature. It is similarly clear that simply giving computers lots of factual knowledge will not make them skilled in a field unless they also are expert in the proper application of that knowledge. It is in this area particularly that improved understanding of the psychology of human problem-solving is helping researchers to develop decision-support tools that more closely simulate the process by which expert clinicians move from observations to diagnoses or management plans.

16.4.5 Validation of System Performance

Many observers are horrified when they imagine what they might have to do to validate and maintain the currency of large clinical knowledge bases. After all, medical knowledge is advancing at a rapid pace, and an advisory system that uses yesterday's knowledge may fail to provide the best advice available for a patient's problem. Although researchers with limited goals have been willing to take on responsibility for short-term knowledge-base maintenance in support of their scholarly activities, it is likely that professional organizations or other national bodies will in time need to assume responsibility for the currency and integrity of large clinical knowledge bases.

When a knowledge base is well validated, developers still face challenges in determining how best to evaluate the performance of the decision-support tools that use the knowledge. When a gold standard of performance exists, formal studies can compare the program's advice with that accepted standard of "correctness." This technique is especially pertinent for diagnostic tools, where biopsy, surgery, or autopsy data can be used as an appropriate gold standard. In the case of therapy-advice systems, however, the gold standard is more difficult to define. Even experts may disagree about the proper way to treat a specific patient, and there can seldom be a realistic controlled trial that attempts to show which approach is right in any absolute sense. For this reason, workers have experimented with techniques that compare the recommendations of a therapy-management program with those of experts (see Chapter 8). With proper controls, such studies can be useful, although they have shown that even experts in a field generally do not receive perfect marks when assessed by their peers. The problem of evaluation remains a ripe area for further research (Friedman & Wyatt, 1997a).

16.4.6 Integration of Decision-Support Tools

As we have emphasized in discussing many of the computer applications described in this book, the successful introduction of decision-support tools is likely to be tied to these tools' effective integration with routine clinical tasks. We need more innovative research on how best to tie knowledge-based computer tools to programs designed to store, manipulate, and retrieve patient-specific information. We explained how the HELP system includes decision-support functions that are triggered to generate warnings or reports whenever an internally specified set of conditions holds for a given patient. As hospitals and clinics increasingly use multiple small machines optimized for different tasks, however, the challenges of integration are inherently tied to issues of networking and systems interfaces. It is in the electronic linking of multiple machines with overlapping functions and data needs that the potential of distributed but integrated patient data processing will be realized.

16.5 Illustrative Examples of Clinical Decision-Support Systems

To illustrate the status of current systems and the ways in which new technologies have affected the evolution of decision-support tools, we shall discuss selected features of two well-known decision-support systems. Quick Medical Reference (like its predecessor, Internist-1) supports diagnostic problem solving in general internal medicine. The EON system, on the other hand, provides therapeutic recommendations for treatment in accordance with predefined protocols. Quick Medical Reference is used primarily as a standalone system, whereas EON comprises a set of software components that are designed to be integrated within larger clinical information systems.

16.5.1 Diagnosis: The Internist-1/QMR Project

Internist-1 was a large diagnostic program that was developed at the University of Pittsburgh School of Medicine in the 1970s (Miller et al., 1982; Pople, 1982). The Internist-1 program subsequently grew into a decision-support system known as **Quick Medical Reference** (QMR). Quick Medical Reference is now marketed commercially and is used by a large community of practitioners and students.

The goal of the original Internist-1 project was to model diagnosis in general internal medicine. Internist-1 contained knowledge of almost 600 diseases and of nearly 4,500 interrelated *findings*, or *disease manifestations* (signs, symptoms, and other patient characteristics). On average, each disease was associated with between 75 and 100 findings. The task of diagnosis would be straightforward if each disease were associated with a unique set of findings. Most findings, however, such as fever, are associated with multiple disease processes, often with varying levels of likelihood for each disease. Clinicians have long recognized that it is not feasible to perform simple pattern matching to make difficult diagnoses. On the other hand, it is impractical to estimate conditional probabilities (such as those used by the Leeds abdominal pain system) for all the diseases and findings in Internist-1's knowledge base—particularly because many of the 600 disease syndromes are rare and thus are not well described in the clinical literature. For these reasons, the developers of Internist-1 chose to create an ad hoc scoring scheme to encode the relationships between specific findings and diseases.

To construct the Internist-1 knowledge base, the senior physician on the project (a clinician who had over 50 years of practice experience), other physicians, and medical students worked together, considering each of the encoded diseases. Through careful literature review and case discussions, they determined the list of pertinent findings associated with each disease. For each of these findings, they assigned a **frequency weight** (FW) and an **evoking strength** (ES), two numbers that reflect the strength of the relationship between the disease and the finding (Fig. 16.5). The FW is a number between 1 and 5, where 1 means that the

Disease profile for

ECHINOCOCCAL CYST<S> OF LIVER

ES	FW	
1	2	CHEST PERCUSSION DIAPHRAGM ELEVATED UNILATERAL
1	2	COUGH
1	1	FECES LIGHT COLORED
0	2	FEVER
1	3	HEPATOMEGALY PRESENT
1	2	JAUNDICE
1	2	LIVER CONTAINING LARGE PALPABLE MASS<ES>
1	1	LIVER CONTAINING LARGE PALPABLE MASS<ES> FLUCTUANT
1	1	LIVER DISTORTED OR ASYMMETRICAL
1	1	LIVER ENLARGED MASSIVE
1	2	LIVER ENLARGED MODERATE
1	2	LIVER ENLARGED SLIGHT
1	2	LIVER TENDER ON PALPATION
1	1	PRESSURE ARTERIAL DIASTOLIC LESS THAN 60
1	1	PRESSURE ARTERIAL DIASTOLIC LESS THAN 90
1	1	RHONCHI DIFFUSE

FIGURE 16.5. A sample disease profile from Internist-1. The numbers beside the findings represent the evoking strength ([ES] ranging from 0 [nonspecific] to 5 [pathognomonic]) and the frequency weight ([FW] ranging from 1 [rare] to 5 [always seen]). Only an excerpt from the disease profile for echinococcal cysts is shown here.

TABLE 16.1. Interpretation of frequency weights.

Frequency weight	Interpretation
1	Listed manifestation occurs rarely in the disease
2	Listed manifestation occurs in a substantial minority of cases of the disease
3	Listed manifestation occurs in roughly one-half of the cases
4	Listed manifestation occurs in the substantial majority of cases
5	Listed manifestation occurs in essentially all cases—that is, it is a prerequisite for the diagnosis

Source: Miller, R.A., Pople, H.E., Myers, J.D. Internist-1: an experimental computer-based diagnostic consultant for general internal medicine. *New England Journal of Medicine*, 307:468.

finding is seldom seen in the disease and 5 means it is essentially always seen (Table 16.1). The ES reflects the likelihood that a patient with the finding has the disease in question and that the disease is the cause of the finding (Table 16.2). An ES of 0 means that the disease would never be considered as a diagnosis on the basis of this finding alone, whereas an ES of 5 means that the finding is **pathognomonic** for the disease (i.e., *all* patients with the finding have the disease).

In addition, each finding in the knowledge base is associated with a third number, an **import number** that has a value between 1 and 5 (Table 16.3). The import number captures the idea that some abnormalities have serious implications and must be explained, whereas others may be safely ignored. Internist-1 uses the import number to handle red herrings (minor problems that are not explained by the current disease process). This familiar clinical-diagnosis problem is not handled well by formal statistical approaches.

Based on these simple measurements, Internist-1 then uses a scoring scheme that is similar to the hypothetico-deductive approach described in Chapter 2. The physician-user enters an initial set of findings, and then the program determines an initial differential diagnosis. Based on the current set of hypotheses, the program selects appropriate questions to ask, choosing from several strategies, depending on how many diseases are under consideration and how closely matched

TABLE 16.2. Interpretation of evoking strengths.

Evoking strength	Interpretation
0	Nonspecific—manifestation occurs too commonly to be used to construct a differential diagnosis
1	Diagnosis is a rare or unusual cause of listed manifestation
2	Diagnosis causes a substantial minority of instances of listed manifestation
3	Diagnosis is the most common, but not the overwhelming, cause of listed manifestation
4	Diagnosis is the overwhelming cause of listed manifestation
5	Listed manifestation is pathognomonic for the diagnosis

Source: Miller, R.A., Pople, H.E., Myers, J.D. Internist-1: an experimental computer-based diagnostic consultant for general internal medicine. *New England Journal of Medicine*, 307:468.

TABLE 16.3. Interpretation of import values.

Import	Interpretation
1	Manifestation is usually unimportant, occurs commonly in normal persons, and is easily disregarded
2	Manifestation may be of importance but can often be ignored; context is important
3	Manifestation is of moderate importance but may be an unreliable indicator of any specific disease
4	Manifestation is of high importance and can only rarely be disregarded (as, for example, a false-positive result)
5	Manifestation absolutely must be explained by one of the final diagnoses

Source: Miller, R.A., Pople, H.E., Myers, J.D. Internist-1: an experimental computer-based diagnostic consultant for general internal medicine. *New England Journal of Medicine*, 307:468.

they are to the available patient data. The program considers the cost and risks of tests, as well as the benefits, and asks for simple historical and physical-examination data before recommending laboratory tests or invasive diagnostic procedures. An important feature, not previously implemented in diagnostic programs, is Internist-1's ability to set aside some of the findings not well explained by the current differential diagnosis and to return to them later after making an initial diagnosis. Thus, Internist-1 can diagnose multiple coexistent diseases and does not make the assumptions of mutual exclusivity and completeness that have characterized most Bayesian diagnostic programs.

Using these simple knowledge structures and weighting schemes, Internist-1 demonstrates impressive diagnostic performance. In one study, the developers tested the program on 19 difficult diagnostic cases taken from a major clinical journal (Miller et al., 1982). The 19 patients had a total of 43 diagnoses, of which Internist-1 correctly identified 25. By comparison, the physicians who had cared for the patients in a major teaching hospital made 28 correct diagnoses, and the expert discussants who presented the cases before a large audience before the publication of each case in the journal correctly identified 35 diagnoses. Although Internist-1 missed several of the difficult cases (as did the physicians and discussants), the test patients had problems that were drawn broadly from across all problems in general internal medicine—no other diagnostic program would have been able to deal effectively with more than a small subset of these cases.

Internist-1 was created to run on only large, mainframe computers and therefore is not suited for widespread use by practitioners. In the 1980s, the program was adapted to run on personal computers as QMR (Quick Medical Reference) (Miller et al., 1986). Unlike Internist-1, which was developed to provide only patient-specific diagnostic advice, QMR can serve health professionals in three modes. In its basic mode, QMR is an expert consultation system that provides advice much as Internist-1 did (using essentially the same knowledge base and scoring scheme). Quick Medical Reference can also be used as an **electronic textbook**, listing the patient characteristics reported to occur in a given disease or, conversely, reporting which of its 600 diseases can be associated with a given characteristic. Third, as a **medical spreadsheet**, it can combine a few characteristics or diseases and determine the implications. For example, the user can specify two apparently unrelated medical problems and obtain suggestions about how coexisting diseases could, under the right circumstances, give rise to both problems (Fig. 16.6).

The developers of QMR argue that the system's use as an electronic reference is far more important than its use as a consultation program to help a clinician to clinch a particularly difficult diagnosis (Miller & Masarie, 1990). In fact, in the current version of QMR, many of the consultation features of Internist-1 have been removed. For example, QMR does not ask questions directly of the user in order to pursue a diagnosis and does not attempt to evaluate whether more than one disease might be present at a given time.

16.5.2 Patient Management: The EON System

Quick Medical Reference, like most computer programs that provide decision support, is a standalone system that resides on a workstation or personal computer. Healthcare workers interact directly with the computer and explore challenging clinical cases by entering data into the system and observing how QMR responds. As we have already seen, decision-support elements can be built into advanced clinical information systems (such as HELP), monitoring patient data as they are entered into a central database and providing alerts and reminders in response to changes in the clinical situation. Such **reminder systems** have been particularly effective in helping practitioners to follow desired practice guidelines and policies. Because the clinician does not need to enter data into the computer expressly for the purpose of receiving decision support, the computer is able to work efficiently behind the scenes, alerting the clinician to aberrant patient situations or to the need to consider alternative treatment interventions only when necessary.

Developers often encode the knowledge needed to provide such decision support for patient management as **situation–action rules**, such as the rule in Figure 16.3. A **rule interpreter** processes such rules—scanning the patient database for situations that trigger relevant rules, evaluating whether the condition part of the rule holds, and, if it does, taking whatever action the rule might specify. Although such rule-based approaches for representing knowledge have been used successfully since the time of MYCIN, development and maintenance of large rule bases can be difficult. Interactions among rules may have unanticipated side effects, leading to unexpected system behaviors when rules are added to or deleted from a previously debugged knowledge base (Bachant & McDermott, 1984; Clancey, 1984; Heckerman & Horvitz, 1986). Furthermore, treatment of patients often involves more than following a single relevant rule; rather, applying and following through a coherent plan is called for. Designers of second-generation knowledge-based systems consequently have sought new ways to define more clearly the knowledge that a decision-support system contains and to make distinct separations between the knowledge in the system and the problem-solving procedures that operate on that knowledge (David et al., 1993).

Pulmonary Disease and DIARRHEA Chronic

Pairs of diseases consistent with Entered Finding and Topic

Atelectasis
caused-by Carcinoid Syndrome Secondary to Bronchial Neoplasm

Eosinophilic Pneumonia Acute <LOEFFLER>
caused-by Hookworm Disease

Pulmonary Legionellosis
predisposed-to-by Immune Deficiency Syndrome Acquired <AIDS>

Pleural Effusion Exudative
caused-by Pancreatic Pseudocyst

Pneumoccoccal Pneumonia
predisposed-to-by Immune Deficiency Syndrome Acquired <AIDS>

Pulmonary Hypertension Secondary
caused-by Progressive Systemic Sclerosis
or co-occurring-with Schistosomiasis Chronic Hepatic

Pulmonary Infarction
predisposed-to-by Carcinoma of Body or Tail of Pancreas
or predisposed-to-by Carcinoma of Head of Pancreas
or caused-by Hepatic Vein Obstruction

Pulmonary Lymphoma
coinciding-with Lymphoma of Colon
or coinciding-with Small Intestinal Lymphoma

FIGURE 16.6. A sample associations list from QMR, a system that permits the physician to request exploratory searches of the knowledge base for associations that might be clinically relevant. For example, as shown here, the physician has asked for pulmonary diseases that may also be associated with chronic diarrhea. The resulting lists, which QMR generates dynamically, can be useful memory joggers for physicians who might otherwise overlook the suggested relationships.

Developed at Stanford University, EON is a second-generation knowledge-based system that aids practitioners in the care of patients who are being treated in accordance with **protocols** and guidelines (Musen, 1998; Musen et al., 1996). Unlike systems such as MYCIN or QMR, EON cannot be run by itself. Instead, EON constitutes a set of software components that must be embedded within some clinical information systems that healthcare workers use to enter and browse patient-related data. Figure 16.7 shows the major components of EON, which are the following:

- **Problem solvers** each address specific tasks (Eriksson et al., 1995), such as (1) determining the treatment that should be given at a particular time if a patient is to receive therapy in accordance with a predefined clinical protocol and (2) determining, for a given patient, whether there are any protocols for which the patient might be eligible.
- **Knowledge bases** encode descriptions of clinical protocols in a way that all the problem solvers in EON can examine a shared, coherent representation of protocol knowledge, thus using the protocol knowledge bases to solve their particular task. The EON therapy-planning component accesses the protocol knowledge base to identify what are the potential clinical interventions that might

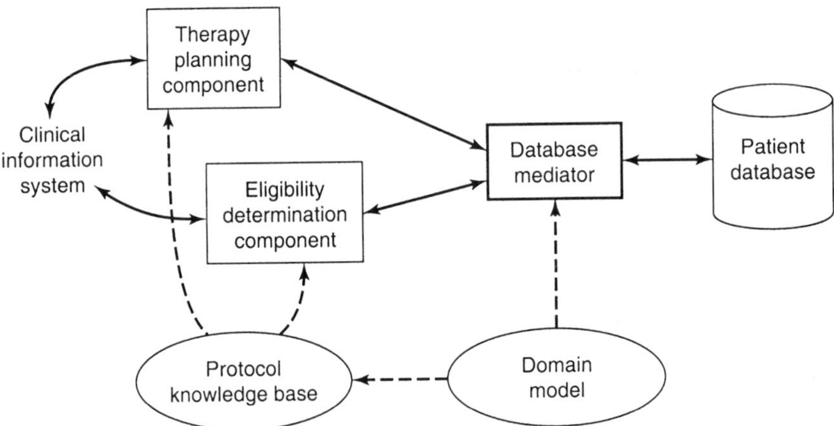

Figure 16.7. The EON architecture. EON consists of a number of problem-solving components (e.g., programs that plan protocol-based therapy and that determine whether a patient potentially is eligible for protocols) that share a common knowledge base of protocol descriptions. The protocol domain model, created with the Proégé system, defines the format of the protocol knowledge base. The same model also defines the schema for the database mediator, a system that channels the flow of patient data between the problem-solving components and an archival relational database. The entire architecture is embedded within a clinical information system.

be administered to a given patient and what knowledge is needed to determine precisely what treatment is appropriate; the EON eligibility-determination component consults the same knowledge base to identify the factors that establish when a given protocol is appropriate and then accesses patient data to see whether the protocol might be a good match.

- A **database mediator** serves as a conduit between all the problem solvers in EON and the database that stores all the patient data (Nguyen et al., 1997). The mediator insulates all the EON problem solvers from many of the logistical problems of querying patient data and making sense out of various time-dependent relationships among the data (e.g., querying the data for the existence of certain trends or patterns). The mediator includes within it a problem solver that addresses the specific task of abstraction of time-oriented patient data into higher-level concepts, the RÉSUMÉ system (Shahar & Musen, 1996). Thus, queries such as "Did the patient have more than 2 weeks of bone-marrow toxicity grade II (in a specific context)" can be answered by the mediator directly. The method underlying the RÉSUMÉ solver is the knowledge-based temporal-abstraction method (Shahar, 1997).

The components in EON are designed such that they can be mixed and matched to create different decision-support functionalities. For example, EON's therapy-planning component (Tu et al., 1995) and eligibility-determination component (Tu et al., 1993), plus knowledge bases for protocol-based care of AIDS and HIV-related diseases, formed the decision-support elements of a system known as THERAPY-HELPER (or T-HELPER for short) (Musen et al., 1992). T-HELPER contained an electronic patient record with which practitioners could enter patient information at the time of each visit to an outpatient clinic specializing in the care of people with AIDS. T-HELPER would then invoke the EON components to generate specific recommendations regarding patient therapy. If the patient was not currently enrolled in applicable protocols, the T-HELPER system would indicate those protocols for which the patient potentially was eligible. For those protocols in which the patient was already enrolled, the system would indicate what therapy should be administered, given the protocol requirements, the patient's current stage of therapy, and the patient's clinical situation.

In other experiments, the same therapy-planning component and eligibility-determination component were used in conjunction with a knowledge base of breast-cancer protocols (Musen et al., 1996). The EON architecture made it possible to simply "plug in" these previously developed modules and to use them in conjunction with the new breast-cancer knowledge bases. Again, the EON components did not run as a standalone system but were embedded within a computer-based patient-record system that could invoke the EON decision-support components when appropriate.

The EON architecture also makes it relatively straightforward to add new problem-solving components in addition to new knowledge bases. For example, developers might design a new problem solver that analyzed the electronic patient record retrospectively to determine whether past treatment was consistent with protocol guidelines. (A specific design for such a problem solver has, in fact, been suggested [Shahar et al., 1988].) Although such a quality-assurance problem solver has not yet been implemented, it would be simple to add such a module to the suite of problem solvers already in EON. The new module would then be driven by the same shared knowledge bases used by the other components in EON.

Although it may be easy to apply the EON components to new kinds of protocol knowledge bases, creating such knowledge bases in the first place can be a complex task. Fortunately, knowledge-acquisition for the EON system is greatly facilitated by a knowledge-base-development environment known as Protégé (Musen, 1998; Musen et al., 1995). Protégé provides a set of tools and a principled methodology for building knowledge-based systems. Use of Protégé begins when developers create an abstract model of the application area for which knowledge-based systems are to be built. As shown in Figure 16.7, there is a common model for all the clinical-protocol knowledge bases processed by EON (Tu & Musen, 1996). This protocol model, or **ontology**, specifies the concepts necessary to define clinical protocols in a given domain of medicine. For example, construction of the T-HELPER system required creation of a model that defined the concepts common among protocols for AIDS and HIV-related diseases (drug therapy, laboratory tests, and so on); analogously, construction of the decision-support system for breast-cancer protocols required creation of a somewhat similar model that defined the concepts common among protocols for breast cancer (including concepts such as surgery, radiotherapy, and so on). The terms and relationships of such models when entered into Protégé do more than define the concepts that form the structure of clinical protocols in machine-understandable form: The models serve as the starting point for generation of special-purpose computer-based tools that assist developers in the construction and maintenance of detailed protocol knowledge bases (Musen, 1998; Tu et al., 1995).

In the Protégé approach, developers first create a general model of the concepts and relationships that characterize a particular application area. For example, the model shown in Figure 16.8 represents a small subset of the concepts needed to define clinical protocols. A module in the Protégé system takes as input such a model and generates as output a custom-tailored tool based on that model that developers can use to enter detailed knowledge bases (Eriksson et al., 1994). Protégé thus processes the model for clinical protocols (see Fig. 16.8) to construct a tool that knowledge-base authors can use for entry and review of specific protocol descriptions (Fig. 16.9). This tool—because it reflects the predefined model of clinical protocols—can be used by medical experts themselves. Because the tool is produced directly from the protocol model, developers can update and enhance the model and then generate a new knowledge-acquisition tool that reflects the corresponding changes. At the same time, developers can modify their abstract protocol models to reflect modalities of clinical care in new areas of medicine and then generate knowledge-acquisition tools that healthcare

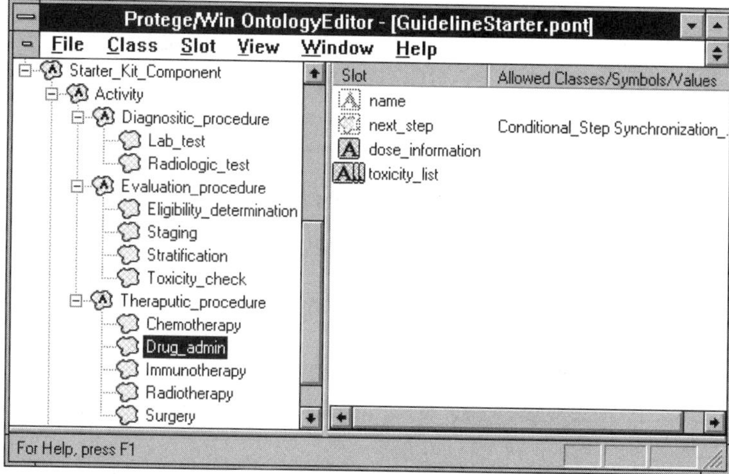

FIGURE 16.8. A small portion of a generic model of clinical guidelines entered into the PROTÉGÉ system. The hierarchy of entries on the left includes concepts that constitute a *starter kit* that may be used as building blocks to construct guideline descriptions. The panel on the right shows the attributes of whatever concept is highlighted on the left. Here, *dose-information* and *toxicity list*, for example, are attributes of the concept *Drug-administration*. The domain model entered into Protégé reflects concepts common to all guidelines, but does not include specifications for any guidelines in particular. The complete domain model is used to generate automatically a graphical knowledge-acquisition tool, such as the one shown in Figure 16.9.

workers can use to enter new protocol specifications for these new clinical disciplines.

Although the EON architecture currently is in use only experimentally, the approach demonstrates several dimensions of modern clinical decision-support systems. EON shows how decision-support systems can be embedded within larger clinical information systems. The architecture also exemplifies the use of emerging standards for network-based communication among software modules—a trend in software engineering that will become increasingly important in the years ahead (see Chapter 4). The coupling between the EON decision-support architecture and the Protégé knowledge-acquisition framework exemplifies the use of special-purpose tools for entering and maintaining protocol knowledge bases. As work in the development of clinical decision-support systems evolves, there will be expanding expectations that decision-makers themselves be able to review and modify the electronic knowledge bases that codify an institution's decision-making policies. As demonstrated by EON, that kind of direct involvement of clinical personnel in knowledge-base management will require increasing use of systems such as Protégé, which can simplify the creation and modification of the necessary knowledge-editing tools.

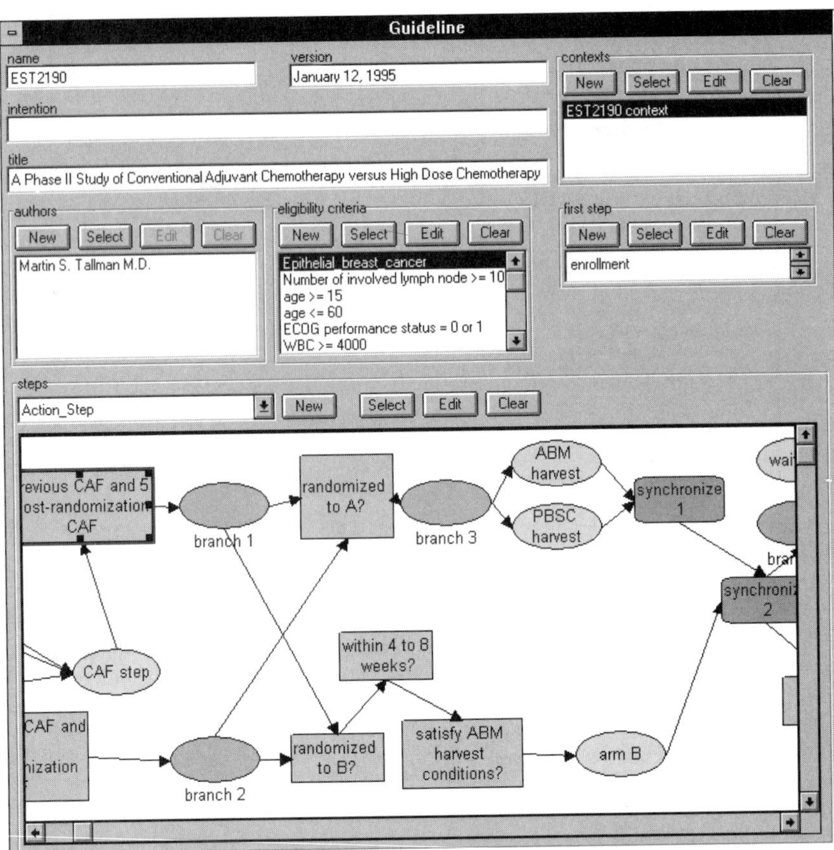

FIGURE 16.9. A screen from a Protégé-generated knowledge-acquisition tool for entry of breast cancer protocols. This tool is generated automatically from a domain model, part of which appears in Figure 16.8. The protocol depicted specifies the knowledge required to carry out a clinical trial that compares the effects of conventional adjuvant chemotherapy with those of high-dose chemotherapy followed by bone-marrow transplantation.

16.6 Decision Support in the Decade to Come

After more than three decades of research on medical decision-support systems, investigators have learned a great deal about the difficulties inherent in the task and about the complex barriers to successful implementation of programs. In the 1970s and 1980s, researchers made major progress in tackling the scientific questions of computer-based decision support. Technological advances in knowledge representation, knowledge acquisition, and automated reasoning led to significant new insights related to the modeling, encoding, and dissemination of human expertise in a machine-processable form. Although early workers in medical informatics frequently raised concerns that clinicians might always be reluctant to interact with computer-based decision-support systems, the landscape changed radically in the 1990s.

The advent of managed health care in the United States and growing concerns about the cost and quality of patient care globally have altered the practice of medicine in profound ways (see Chapter 19). Clinical practice guidelines based on empirical medical evidence are now advocated by government, by payers, by medical professional societies, and by healthcare institutions as essential mechanisms to guarantee the quality of care. These treatment protocols attempt to define best practices for managing groups of patients who present with stereotypical problems.

Practitioners often are highly motivated to follow such guidelines: Not only do physicians inherently want to offer their patients the best care possible based on available evidence in the literature, but often physicians' remuneration and even their medical malpractice premiums depend on their ability to follow predefined guidelines. In an era when there is increasing emphasis on continuous quality improvement via instruments such as clinical practice guidelines, computers are assuming a central role in communicating guideline-based advice to all healthcare workers.

As healthcare organizations were undergoing radical change in the 1990s, computing technology was making an equally radical advance. The advent of the World Wide Web and of new approaches for distributed computing based on Hypertext Markup Language (HTML) and the Java programming language popularized computers in new ways. The World Wide Web demystified computers for many new users while providing connections among distributed processors that had not been imagined just a few year earlier. The Web provided a basis for inexpensive network computers that could use a common browser to access a diverse collection of information resources in a uniform manner. Suddenly, it was almost trivial to bring a rich collection of programs directly to the point of care, greatly simplifying access to a variety of information sources and decision-support systems.

The educational potential of decision-support systems has long been recognized (Association of American Medical Colleges, 1986). New pressures to learn best practices coupled with the ubiquity of information technology, however, have greatly encouraged the use of computer-based decision aids in health-professional schools around the world. For the next generation of health-care workers, the use of information technology in most aspects of patient care probably will be taken for granted—much as it is in *Star Trek*.

16.6.1 Legal and Regulatory Questions

It may already have occurred to you that there are legal implications inherent in the development and use of such innovations. As mentioned in Chapter 7, formal legal precedents for dealing with clinical decision-support systems are lacking at present. Several observers have noted that a pivotal concern is whether the courts will view the systems under negligence law or product liability law (Miller et al., 1985). Under **negligence law** (which governs medical malpractice), a product or activity must meet reasonable expectations for safety. The principle of **strict liability**, on the other hand, states that a product must not be harmful. Because it is unrealistic to require that decision-support programs make correct assessments under all circumstances—we do not apply such standards to physicians themselves—the determination of which legal principle to apply will have important implications for the dissemination and acceptance of such tools. A related question is the potential liability borne by physicians who could have accessed such a program, and who chose not to do so, and who made an incorrect decision when the system would have suggested the correct one. As with other medical technologies, precedents suggest that physicians will be liable in such circumstances if the use of consultant programs has become the *standard of care* in the community (see Chapter 7). Several guidelines have been suggested for assigning legal liability to builders of knowledge-based medical decision-support systems or to the physicians using them [Allaërt & Dusserne, 1992].

Questions have also arisen regarding the validation of decision-support tools before their release (see Chapter 8). The evaluation of complex decision-support tools is challenging; it is difficult to determine acceptable levels of performance when there may be disagreement even among experts with similar training and experience. There is often no such thing as *the* correct answer to a clinical question. Moreover, component-based architectures such as EON may comprise multiple (potentially fallible) problem-solvers, each of which addresses different clinical problems and which shares a common (potentially fallible) set of knowledge bases. The objective then becomes to isolate the cause of possible errors and to make appropriate modifications to the system overall. Evaluations of medical decision-support tools have suggested a variety of methods for assessing the adequacy of clinical knowledge bases and problem-solving components before such software is introduced for routine use (Friedman & Wyatt, 1997a).

What then should be the role of government in prerelease regulation of medical software? Current policy of the Food and Drug Administration (FDA) in the United States indicates that such tools will not be subject to federal regulation if a trained practitioner is assessing the program's advice and making the final determination of care (Young, 1987). This policy is subject to ongoing reevaluation, however (see Chapter 7). Programs that make decisions directly controlling the patient's treatment (e.g., closed-loop systems that administer insulin or that adjust intravenous infusion rates or respirator settings; see Chapter 13) are viewed as medical devices subject to FDA regulation.

Additional problems arise when considering suggestions to enable access to electronic patient records through the World Wide Web, such as privacy and security. Ease of access versus data security will always constitute a trade-off in medical information systems.

16.6.2 Future Directions for Clinical Decision-Support Systems

Trends for decision-support research and development in the decade ahead are becoming evident. As already mentioned, the World Wide Web will continue to expand the influence of computers in all aspects of society, and the Internet and numerous intranets will link information technologies throughout large healthcare organizations and communities of patients. The Internet will bring decision-support systems designed for patient use directly into those patients' homes and will provide more effective communication among all participants in the healthcare system (see Chapter 11). We already see many communities of patients with illnesses such as coronary-artery disease, AIDS, and breast cancer turning to the Internet to seek out the latest available information and to converse electronically both with healthcare personnel and with other patients.

Research laboratories will continue to explore how new Internet-based media can assist in clinical decision-making and how cyberspace affects both patient and provider information access and use. For example, it is unknown whether many of the information resources available on-line lead to more informed decision-making on the part of patients or whether these resources cause increased confusion and potential patient anxiety about the complexity of clinical problems.

The emerging ubiquity of the Internet in modern culture will affect the underlying technology with which decision-support systems are developed. Many research laboratories already are studying ways in which decision-support software can be assembled from previously created, tested, and debugged components—much like the software components in the EON system. In the future, repositories of such components will be stored in libraries accessible over the Internet. Such libraries will contain, for example, reusable problem-solving modules for tasks such as diagnosis and planning that developers will apply to the construction of new decision aids. Internet-based libraries will contain standard, controlled terminologies, as well as knowledge bases of commonly needed concepts (e.g., anatomical relationships, temporal properties of clinical data, and frequently prescribed medications and their indications and side effects). Construction of clinical decision aids will involve searching the Internet-based libraries for appropriate reusable components and configuring those components into useful problem-solvers. There will be a need for a new kind of information-retrieval technology—one that can help system builders to locate and configure appropriate decision-support software components from the diverse component libraries that research laboratories, healthcare organizations, and a new industry of component vendors will make available.

Considerations of whether specific components happen to use pattern-recognition methods, Bayesian reasoning, or AI techniques will become less important, as researchers create new approaches for combining different reasoning methods to meet the specific requirements of increasingly complex decision-making tasks.

Thus, by mixing and matching components, developers will be able to use Bayesian reasoners for performing probabilistic classification, AI techniques for tasks such as planning or constraint satisfaction, and mathematical models for solving problems that can be best understood in terms of systems of equations. There will be enhanced emphasis on modeling the overall task that a decision-support system performs (e.g., tasks such as therapy planning, differential diagnosis, and simulation of surgical interventions). These task models will then inform the selection of appropriate problem-solving components from various libraries.

Concomitantly, heightened understanding of organizational behavior and of clinical workflow will stimulate a new generation of clinical information systems that will integrate smoothly into the practices of healthcare workers of all kinds. Most important, these new information systems will become the vehicles for delivery of decision-support technology in the decade ahead. The very concept of a *decision-support system* itself will fade away, as intelligent assistants that can enhance the judgment of healthcare workers blend into the infrastructure of healthcare delivery. Automated decision support will take place with every practitioner's routine access to clinical data in a manner that is unobtrusive, transparent, and tailored to the specific patient situation.

16.6.3 Conclusions

The future of clinical decision-support systems inherently depends on progress in developing useful programs and in reducing logistical barriers to implementation. Although ubiquitous computer-based decision aids that routinely assist physicians in most aspects of clinical practice are currently the stuff of science fiction, progress has been real and the potential remains inspiring. Early predictions about the effects such innovations will have on medical education and practice have not yet come to pass (Schwartz, 1970), but growing successes support an optimistic view of what technology will eventually do to assist practitioners with processing of complex data and knowledge. The research challenges have been identified much more clearly, and the implications for health-science education are much better understood. The basic computer literacy of health professional students can be generally assumed, but health-science educators now must teach the conceptual foundations of medical informatics if their graduates are to be prepared for the technologically sophisticated world that lies ahead.

Equally important, we have learned much about what is *not* likely to happen. The more investigators understand the complex and changing nature of medical knowledge, the clearer it becomes that trained practitioners will always be required as elements in a cooperative relationship between physician and computer-based decision tool. There is no evidence that machine capabilities will ever equal the human mind's ability to deal with unexpected situations, to integrate visual and auditory data that reveal subtleties of a patient's problem, or to deal with social and ethical issues that are often key determinants of proper medical decisions. Considerations such as these will always be important to the humane practice of medicine, and practitioners will always have access to information that is meaningless to the machine. Such observations argue cogently for the discretion of physicians in the proper use of decision-support tools.

Suggested Readings

Berg M. (1997). *Rationalizing Medical Work: Decision Support Techniques and Medical Practices*. Cambridge, MA: MIT Press.

This book, written by a physician who also is a sociologist, examines the difficulty of incorporating decision-support systems into clinical workflow from an organizational perspective. The book analyzes the failures of early automated decision aids and suggests new principles for decision-system design and integration.

David J.M., Krivine J.P., Simmons R. (Eds.). (1993). *Second Generation Expert Systems*. Berlin: Springer-Verlag.

This excellent collection of articles provides a broad overview of work on the development of knowledge-based systems.

Ledley R., Lusted, L. (1959). Reasoning foundations of medical diagnosis. *Science*, 130:9–21.

This classic article provided the first influential description of how computers might be used to assist with the diagnostic process. The flurry of activity applying Bayesian methods to computer-assisted diagnosis during the 1960s was largely inspired by this provocative article.

Musen M. (1997). Modeling for decision support. In van Bemmel J., Musen M. (Eds.), *Handbook of Medical Informatics* (pp. 431–448). Heidelberg: Springer-Verlag.

This chapter provides a general discussion of current modeling approaches for building decision-support systems. It emphasizes the principles of creating a structured model of domain concepts and of linking those concepts to well-defined problem-solving methods that can carry out the necessary reasoning tasks.

Schwartz W. (1970). Medicine and the computer: the promise and problems of change. *New England Journal of Medicine*, 283(23):1257–1264.

A senior clinician from Boston wrote this frequently cited article, which assessed the growing role of computers in health care. Thirty years later, many of the developments anticipated by Schwartz had come to pass, although the rate of change was slower than he predicted.

Shortliffe E.H. (1989). Testing reality: the introduction of decision-support technologies for physicians. *Methods of Information in Medicine*, 28:1–5.

This editorial summarizes the historical reasons for physicians' resistance to the introduction of computing technologies in general and of decision-support tools in particular. The discussion is based on a market-research study from the 1980s in which physicians' opinions were solicited.

Questions for Discussion

1. Researchers in medical AI have argued that there is a need for more expert knowledge in medical decision-support systems, but developers of Bayesian systems have argued that expert estimates of likelihoods are inherently flawed and that advice programs must be based on solid data. How do you account

for the apparent difference between these views? Which view is valid? Explain your answer.

2. Explain the meaning of Internist-1/QMR's frequency weights and evoking strengths. What does it mean for a finding to have a frequency weight of 4 and an evoking strength of 2? How do these parameters relate to the concepts of sensitivity, specificity, and predictive value that were introduced in Chapters 2 and 3?
3. Let us consider how deDombal and other developers of Bayesian systems have used patient-care experience to guide the collection of statistics that they need. For example, consider the database in the following table, which shows the relationship between two findings (f_1 and f_2) and a disease (D) for 10 patients.

Patient	f_1	f_2	D	$\sim D$
1	0	1	0	1
2	0	1	1	0
3	0	1	0	1
4	1	1	1	0
5	1	1	1	0
6	1	1	0	1
7	1	0	1	0
8	1	1	1	0
9	1	0	0	1
10	1	1	1	0

In the table, $\sim D$ signifies the absence of disease D. A 0 indicates the absence of a finding or disease, and a 1 indicates the presence of a finding or disease. For example, based on the above database, the probability of finding f_1 in this population is 7/10 = 70 percent.

Refer back to Chapters 2 and 3 as necessary in answering the following questions:

a. What are the sensitivity and specificity of each of f_1 and f_2 for the disease D? What is the prevalence of D in this 10-person population?
b. Use the database to calculate the following probabilities:
   - $p[f_1|D]$
   - $p[f_1|\sim D]$
   - $p[f_2|D]$
   - $p[f_2|\sim D]$
   - $p[D]$
   - $p[\sim D]$
c. Use the database to calculate $p[D|f_1$ and $f_2]$.
d. Use the probabilities determined in b to calculate $p[D|f_1$ and $\sim f_2]$ using a heuristic method that assumes that findings f_1 and f_2 are conditionally independent given a disease and the absence of a disease. Why is this result different from the one in c? Why has it generally been necessary to make this heuristic approximation in Bayesian programs?

4. In an evaluation study, the decision-support system ONCOCIN provided advice concerning cancer therapy that was approved by experts in only 79 percent of cases (Hickam et al., 1985b). Do you believe that this performance is adequate for a computational tool that is designed to help physicians to make decisions regarding patient care? What safeguards, if any, would you suggest to ensure the proper use of such a system? Would you be willing to visit a particular physician if you knew in advance that she made decisions regarding treatment that were approved by expert colleagues less than 80 percent of the time? If you would not, what level of performance would you consider adequate? Justify your answers.
5. A large international organization once proposed to establish an independent laboratory—much like Underwriters Laboratory in the United States—that would test medical decision-support systems from all vendors and research laboratories, certifying the effectiveness and accuracy of those systems before they might be put into clinical use. What are the possible dimensions along which such a laboratory might evaluate decision-support systems? What kinds of problems might such a laboratory encounter in attempting to institute such a certification process? In the absence of such a credentialling system for decision-support systems, how can health-care workers feel confident in using a clinical decision aid?

17
Computers in Medical Education

Parvati Dev, Edward P. Hoffer, and G. Octo Barnett

After reading this chapter, you should know the answers to these questions:

- What are the advantages of computer-aided instruction over traditional lecture-style instruction in medical education?
- What are the different learning methods that can be implemented in computer-based education?
- How can computer-based simulations supplement students' exposure to clinical practice?
- What are the issues to be considered when developing computer-based educational programs?
- What are the significant barriers to widespread integration of computer-aided instruction into the medical curriculum?

17.1 The Role of Computers in Medical Education

The goals of medical education are to provide students and graduate clinicians specific facts and information, to teach strategies for applying this knowledge appropriately to the situations that arise in medical practice, and to encourage development of skills necessary to acquire new knowledge over a lifetime of practice. Students must learn about physiological processes and must understand the relationships between their observations and these underlying processes. They must learn to perform medical procedures, and they must understand the effects of different interventions on health outcomes. Medical school faculty employ a variety of strategies for teaching, ranging from the one-way, lecture-based transmission of information to the interactive, Socratic method of instruction. In general, we can view the teaching process as the presentation of a situation or a body of facts that contains the essential knowledge that students should learn; the explanations of what the important concepts and relationships are, how they can be derived, and why they are important; and the strategy for guiding interaction with a patient.

As has been discussed throughout this book, information technology is an increasingly important tool for accessing and managing medical information—both patient-specific and more general scientific knowledge. Medical educators are aware of the need for all medical students to learn to use information technology effectively. Computers also can play a direct role in the education process; students may interact with educational computer programs to acquire factual information and to learn and practice medical problem-solving techniques. In addition, practicing physicians may use computers to expand and reinforce their professional skills throughout their careers. The application of computer technology to education is often referred to as **computer-assisted learning**, **computer-based education** (CBE), or **computer-aided instruction** (CAI).

In this chapter, we present basic concepts that people should consider when they plan the use of computers in medical education.[1] We begin by reviewing the historical use of computers in medical education, describing various modes of computer-based teaching, and giving examples of teaching programs for preclinical students, clinical students, medical professionals, and the lay public. We then present questions and discuss methodologies to consider in the design and development of teaching programs. In closing, we describe evaluation studies that investigate how these programs are used, as well as the efficiency of computer-based education.

17.1.1 Advantages of Using Computers in Medical Education

A computer can be used to augment, enhance, or replace traditional teaching strategies to provide new methods of learning. With its vast storage capacity, a computer can be an extension of the student's memory, providing quick access to reference and new content. Multimedia capabilities allow the computer to present rapidly a much larger number of images than can be accessed through a book or an atlas and to supplement the static images with sounds, video clips, and interactive teaching modules. Immersive interfaces, which present three-dimensional worlds and allow touch and force feedback through a joystick or instrumented glove, promise to support the training environment of tomorrow.

A computer, properly used, can approach the Socratic ideal of a teacher sitting at one end of a log and a student at the other. In contrast to traditional fact-based, lecture-oriented, mass broadcasting of information, computers can support personalized one-on-one education, delivering material appropriate for learners' needs and interests. "Any time, any place, any pace" learning becomes practical. In traditional education, the learner goes to the lecture, which is held at a specific time and location. If it is not possible for the learner to attend the lecture, or if the location is difficult or expensive to reach, the potential experience may be lost. Computer-based learning can take place at the time and location best suited to the needs of the learner. It can also be individualized and in-

---

[1]Although the focus of this chapter is *medical* education, the underlying concepts and issues apply equally to nursing and health-sciences education.

teractive; the learner is able to proceed at his or her own pace, independent of the larger group. By placing the student in simulated clinical situations, or in a simulated examination, a computer-based teaching program can exercise the student's knowledge and decision-making capabilities in a nonthreatening environment. Finally, well-constructed computer-based learning can be enjoyable and engaging, maintaining the interest of the student.

17.1.2 A Historical Look at the Use of Computers in Medical Education

Despite the many advantages, computer-assisted learning programs initially experienced slow growth before gaining acceptance. Piemme (1988) traced the early development of computer-assisted learning in medicine and discussed reasons for the slow acceptance of this technology. Today, computer-assisted learning has become widely available in the medical field.

Pioneering research in computer-assisted learning was conducted in the late 1960s at three primary locations in the United States: Ohio State University (OSU), Massachusetts General Hospital (MGH), and the University of Illinois. Earlier attempts to use computers in medical instruction were hindered by the difficulty of developing programs using low-level languages and the inconvenience and expense of running programs on batch-oriented mainframe computers. With the availability of time-sharing computers, these institutions were able to develop interactive programs that were accessible to users from terminals via telephone lines.

Computer-based education research began at OSU in 1967 with the development of Tutorial Evaluation System (TES). Tutorial Evaluation System programs typically posed true–false, multiple-choice, matching, or ranking questions and then immediately evaluated the student's responses. The programs rewarded correct answers with positive feedback. Incorrect answers triggered corrective feedback, and, in some cases, students were given another opportunity to respond to the question. If a student was not doing well, the computer might suggest additional study assignments or direct the student to review related materials.

In 1969, TES was incorporated into the evolving Independent Study Program, an experimental program that covered the entire preclinical curriculum and was designed to teach basic medical-science concepts to medical students (Weinberg, 1973). Although the program did not use CBE in a primary instructional role, students in the program relied heavily on a variety of self-study aids and used the computer intensively for self-evaluation. The use of COURSEWRITER III, a high-level authoring language, facilitated rapid development of programs. By the mid-1970s, TES had a library of over 350 interactive hours worth of instructional programs.

Beginning in 1970, Barnett and colleagues at the MGH Laboratory of Computer Science developed CBE programs to simulate clinical encounters (Hoffer & Barnett, 1986). The most common simulations were case-management programs that allowed students to formulate hypotheses, to decide which information to collect, to interpret data, and to practice problem-solving skills in diagnosis and therapy planning. By the mid-1970s, MGH had developed more than 30 case-management simulations, including programs for evaluation of comatose patients, for workup of patients with abdominal pain, and for evaluation and therapy management in areas such as anemia, bleeding disorders, meningitis, dyspnea, secondary hypertension, thyroid disease, joint pain, and pediatric cough and fever.

The MGH laboratory also developed several programs that used mathematical or qualitative models to simulate underlying physiological processes and thus to simulate changes in patient state over time and in response to students' therapeutic decisions. The first simulation modeled the effects of warfarin (an anticoagulant drug) and its effects on blood clotting. The system challenged the user to maintain a therapeutic degree of anticoagulation by prescribing daily doses of warfarin to a patient who had a series of complications and who was taking medications that interacted with warfarin. Subsequently, researchers developed a more complex simulation model to emulate a diabetic patient's reaction to therapeutic interventions.

About the same time, Harless and researchers (1971) at the University of Illinois were developing a system called Computer-Aided Simulation of the Clinical Encounter (CASE), which simulated clinical encounters between physician and patient. The computer assumed the role of a patient; the student, acting in the role of practicing physician, managed the patient's disease from onset of symptoms through final treatment. Initially, the computer presented a brief description of the patient, and then the student interacted with the program using natural-language queries and commands. The program was able to provide logical responses to most student requests. This feature added greatly to the realism of the interaction, and CASE programs were received enthusiastically by students. The TIME system, later developed by Harless and researchers (1986) at the National Library of Medicine (NLM), extended CASE's approach to incorporate videodisc technology.

Computer-based education programs proliferated on a variety of hardware, using a Babel of languages. A 1974 survey of the status of medical CAI identified 362 programs written in 23 different computer languages, ranging from BASIC, FORTRAN, and MUMPS to COURSEWRITER III and PLATO (Brigham & Kamp, 1974). Little sharing of programs among institutions was possible because the task of transferring programs was typically as large as writing the material de novo. Thus, there was little opportunity to share the substantial costs of developing new CAI programs. The lack of portability of systems and the extreme expense of system development and testing served as barriers to the widespread use of CAI.

The establishment of an NLM-sponsored, nationwide network in 1972 was a significant event in the development of CBE in medicine because it allowed users throughout the country to access computer-based educational programs easily and relatively inexpensively. Previously, the programs created at OSU, MGH, and the University of Illinois were available to users in selected regions over voice-grade telephone lines. Poor quality of transmission and high costs, however, combined to limit access to CBE programs by distant users. Acting on the recommendation of a committee of the Association of American Medical Colleges, the NLM's Lister Hill Center for Biomedical Communications funded an experimental CBE network. Beginning in July 1972, the CBE programs developed at the MGH, OSU, and the University of Illinois Medical College were made available from these institutions' host computers over the NLM network. During the first 2 years of operation, 80 institutions used the programs of one of the three hosts. The high demand for network use prompted the NLM to institute an hourly usage charge, but use continued to rise. Having exhausted the funds set aside for this experiment, the NLM discontinued financial support for the network in 1975.

As a testimony to the value placed on the educational network by its users, MGH and OSU continued to operate the network as an entirely user-supported activity. Beginning in 1983, the MGH programs were offered as the continuing medical education (CME) component of the American Medical Association's Medical Information Network (AMA/NET). AMA/NET provided a variety of services to subscribing physicians in addition to the CME programs, including access to information databases, to the clinical and biomedical literature, to the DXplain diagnostic decision-support tool, and to electronic-mail services. By the mid-1980s, approximately 100,000 physicians, medical students, nurses, and other people had used the MGH CBE programs over a network, with about 150,000 total contact hours.

During the early 1970s, medical schools around the country began to conduct research in CBE. One of the most interesting programs was the PLATO system (Programmed Logic for Automated Teaching Operations) developed at the University of Illinois. PLATO used a unique plasma-display terminal that allowed presentation of text, graphics, and photographs, singly or in combination. An electrically excitable gas was used to brighten individual points on the screen selectively. The system also included TUTOR, an early authoring language, to facilitate program development. By 1981, authors had created 12,000 hours of instruction in 150 subject areas. The programs received heavy use at the University of Illinois; some of them also were used at other institutions that had access to the system. The high cost of PLATO and the need for specialized terminals and other computer hardware, however, limited the widespread dissemination of the system.

Research on medical applications of artificial intelligence (AI) stimulated the development of systems based on models of the clinical reasoning of experts. The explanations generated by computer-based consultation systems (e.g., why a particular diagnosis or course of management is recommended) can be used in computer-assisted learning to guide and evaluate students' performance in running patient simulations. The GUIDON system was one of the most interesting examples of such an intelligent tutoring system. GUIDON used a set of teaching strategy rules, which interacted with an augmented set of diagnostic rules from the MYCIN expert system (see Chapter 16), to teach students about infectious diseases (Clancey, 1986).

Researchers at the University of Wisconsin applied a different approach to the simulation of clinical reasoning. Their system was used to assess the efficiency of a student's workup by estimating the cost of the diagnostic evaluation (Friedman et al., 1978). In one of the few successful field studies that demonstrated the clinical significance of a simulated diagnosis problem, Friedman (1973) found significant levels of agreement between physicians' performance on simulated cases and actual practice patterns.

As we discuss in Section 17.4, the development of personal computers (PCs), authoring systems, and network technology removed many of the barriers to program development and dissemination, and CBE software proliferated. Personal computers provide an affordable and relatively standard environment for development, and CBE programs are now widely available via Internet, CD-ROM, and other media. Section 17.3 describes just a few of the many CBE applications now available.

17.2 Modes of Computer-Based Learning

To practice medicine effectively, physicians must have rapid access to the contents of a large and complex medical knowledge base, and they must know how to apply these facts and heuristics to form diagnostic hypotheses and to plan and evaluate therapies. Thus, among the goals of medical education are to convey a body of specific medical facts, to teach strategies for applying this information in medical practice situations, and to assist students in developing skills for lifelong learning. Computers can be used for a wide range of learning methods, from drilling students on a fixed curriculum to allowing students to explore a body of material using methods best suited to their own learning styles.

17.2.1 Drill and Practice

Drill and practice was the first widespread use of computer-based learning, developed almost as soon as computers became available. Teaching material is presented to the student, and the student is evaluated immediately via multiple-choice questions. The computer grades the selected answers and, based on the accuracy of the response, repeats the teaching material or allows the student to progress to new material (Fig. 17.1).

Although it can be tedious, drill and practice still has a role in teaching factual material. It allows the educational system to manage the wide variation in ability of students to assimilate material and frees up instructors for more one-on-one interaction where that technique is most effective. It also allows the instructor to concentrate on more advanced material while the computer deals with presenting the routine factual information. Studies at the elementary school level have found that it is the poorest students who benefit most from computer-based learning, primarily from drill-and-practice work that lets them catch up to their peers (Piemme, 1988).

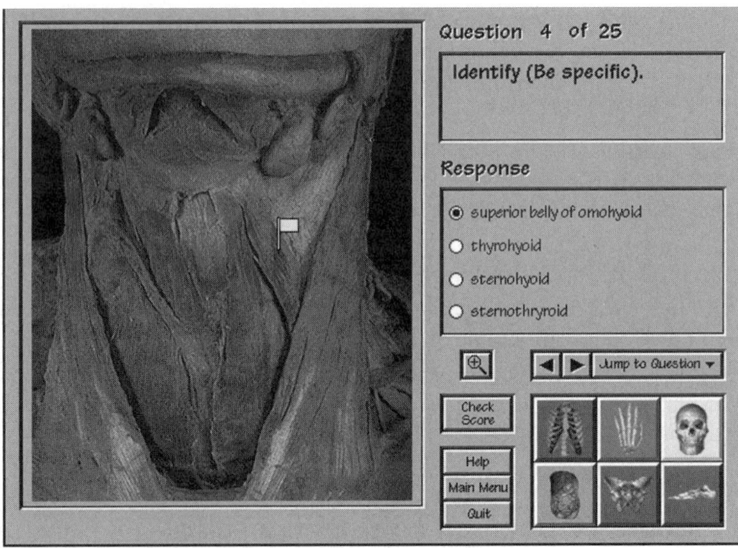

FIGURE 17.1. Drill and practice. In this image-based quiz, the student is presented with a dissected part and is asked to identify the structure marked with a flag. The question is presented in a multiple-choice format. If she wishes, the student can switch to the more difficult option of typing in a textual answer. In typical use, students will use the multiple choice option while learning the material and the free-text option when evaluating themselves. (*Source:* © 1994, Stanford University, and D. Kim et al. Screen shot from Kim et al., 1995.)

17.2.2 Didactic: The Lecture

Although much of the focus of computer-based teaching is on the more innovative uses of computers to expand the teaching format, computers can be employed usefully to deliver didactic material, with the advantage of the removal of time and space limitations. A professor can choose to record a lecture and to store, on the computer, the digitized video of the lecture as well as the related slides or other teaching material. This approach has the advantage that relevant background or remedial material can also be made available through links at specific points in the lecture. The disadvantage, of course, is that the professor may not be available to answer questions when the student reviews the lecture (Fig. 17.2).

Another use of this method could be the immediate availability on the Internet of presentations from national conferences for interested health students and professionals unable to attend the meetings. With media reports of news from medical meetings often reaching patients the next day as newspaper headlines, physicians can now access the details of the reported news on the Web rather than waiting for published reports, which may lag many months behind the presentations.

An excellent example of how computer-based learning can go beyond the traditional lecture is the Howard Hughes Medical Institute website on teaching ge-

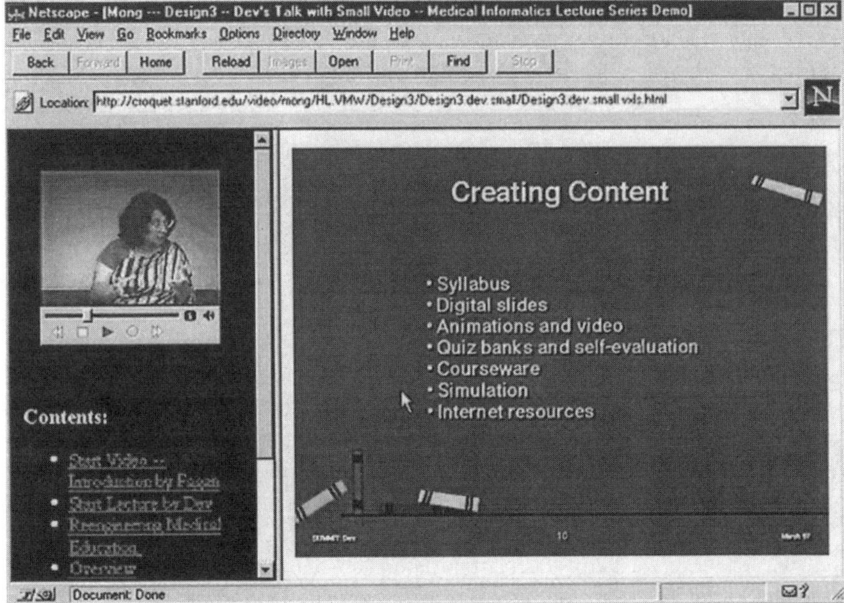

FIGURE 17.2. Didactic teaching. A digital video lecture is presented within a browser for the World Wide Web. The video image in the upper left is augmented with a listing of the lecture contents in the lower left and with high-resolution images of the lecture slides on the right. Because the whole is presented within a web browser, additional information, such as links to other web sites or to study material, could have been added to the web page. (*Source:* © 1997, Stanford University. Screen shot of a digital video lecture.)

netics.[2] This multimedia textbook of genetics uses graphics, hot links, and photographs along with text to present a lively and entertaining series of lectures on genetic disease.

17.2.3 Discrimination Learning

Many clinical situations require the practitioner to differentiate between two apparently similar sets of clinical findings, where subtle differences lead to different diagnoses. **Discrimination learning** is the process that teaches the student to differentiate between the different clinical manifestations. A computer program, through a series of examples of increasing complexity, can train the student to detect the subtle differences. An example is a dermatologic lesion that comprises red rash and inflammation. A rash of the same appearance on different parts of the body can imply different diagnoses. The computer program be-

[2]Howard Hughes Medical Institute website on teaching genetics. http://www.hhmi.org/GeneticTrail/.

gins with the differences between a few standard presentations of this lesion and, as the student learns to discriminate between these, presents additional types (Sanford et al., 1996).

17.2.4 Exploration Versus Structured Interaction

Teaching programs differ by the degree to which they impose structure on a teaching session. In general, drill-and-practice systems are highly structured. The system's responses to students' choices are specified in advance; students cannot control the course of an interaction directly. In contrast, other programs create an exploratory environment in which students can experiment without guidance or interference. For example, a neuroanatomy teaching program may provide a student with a fixed series of images and lessons on the brainstem, or it may allow a student to select a brain structure of interest, such as a tract, and to follow the structure up and down the brainstem, moving from image to image, observing how the location and size of the structure changes.

Each of these approaches has advantages and disadvantages. Drill-and-practice programs usually teach important facts and concepts but do not allow students to deviate from the prescribed course or to explore areas of special interest. Conversely, programs that provide an exploratory environment and that allow students to choose any actions in any order, encourage experimentation and self-discovery. Without structure or guidance, however, students may waste time following unproductive paths and may fail to learn important material, the result being inefficient learning.

17.2.5 Constrained Versus Unconstrained Response

The mechanism for communication between a student and a teaching program can take one of several basic forms. At one extreme, a student, working with a simulation of a patient encounter, may select from a constrained list of responses that are valid in the current situation. The use of a predefined set of responses has two disadvantages: It cues the student (suggests ideas that otherwise might not have occurred to him), and it detracts from the realism of the simulation. On the other hand, simulations that provide students with a list of actions that are allowable and reasonable in a particular situation are easier to write, because the authors do not need to anticipate all responses.

At the opposite extreme, students are free to query the program and to specify actions using unconstrained natural language. Computer recognition of such natural language, however, is just beginning to be feasible. An intermediate approach is to provide a single, comprehensive menu of possible actions, thus constraining choices in a program-specific, but not a situation-specific, manner. The use of a list of actions and a constrained vocabulary is less frustrating to those students who may have difficulty formulating valid interactions.

17.2.6 Construction

One of the most effective—but extremely difficult to implement on the computer—ways to teach is the **constructive** approach to learning. A relatively simple example is learning anatomy through reconstructing the human body either by putting together the separated body parts or by placing cross sections at the correct location in the body.

17.2.7 Simulation

Many advanced teaching programs use **simulations** to engage the learner. Learning takes place most effectively when the learner is engaged and actively involved in decision-making. The use of a simulated patient presented by the computer can approximate the real-world experience of patient care and concentrates the learner's attention on the subject being presented.

Simulation programs may be either **static** or **dynamic**. Figure 17.3 illustrates an interaction between a student and a simulated patient. Under the static simulation model, each case presents a patient who has a predefined problem and set of characteristics. At any point in the interaction, the student can interrupt data

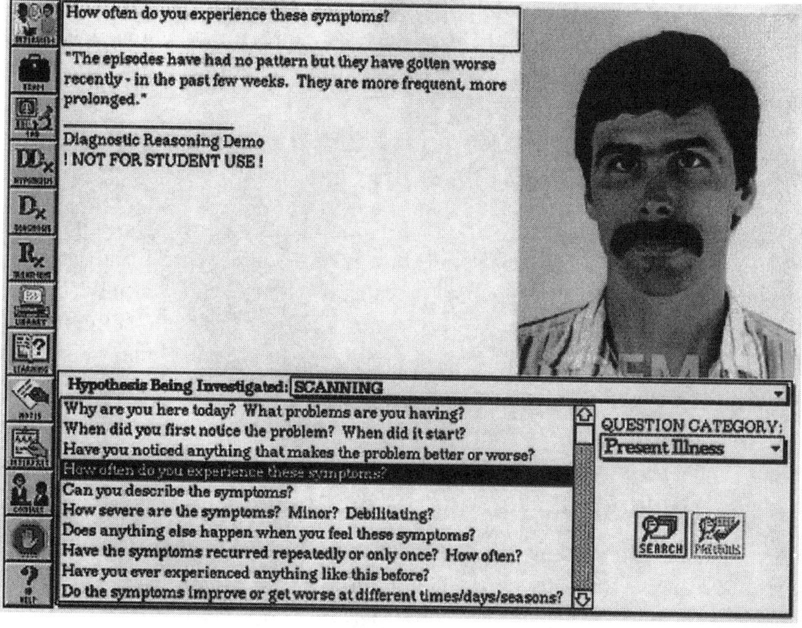

FIGURE 17.3. A typical interaction screen in a sequential diagnosis problem with a simulated patient. The user interrogates the computer about history, physical findings, and laboratory-test results of a simulated patient to reach a diagnosis. (*Source:* © 1993, Diagnostic Reasoning, Illinois. Screen shot from the Diagnostic Reasoning program.)

collection to ask the computer consultant to display the differential diagnosis (given the information that has been collected so far) or to recommend a data-collection strategy. The underlying case, however, remains static. Dynamic simulation programs, in contrast, simulate changes in patient state over time and in response to students' therapeutic decisions. Thus, unlike those in static simulations, the clinical manifestations of a dynamic simulation can be programmed to evolve as the student works through them. These programs help students to understand the relationships between actions (or inactions) and patients' clinical outcomes. To simulate a patient's response to intervention, the programs may explicitly model underlying physiological processes and may use mathematical models.

Immersive simulated environments have emerged as a new method of teaching, particularly in the teaching of surgical skills. This technology is still under development, and it is extremely demanding of computer and graphic performance. Early examples have focused on endoscopic surgery and laparoscopic surgery in which the surgeon manipulates tools and a camera inserted into the patient through a small incision. In the simulated environment, the surgeon manipulates the same tool controls, but these tools control simulated instruments that act on computer-graphic renderings of the operative field. Feedback systems inside the tools return pressure and other haptic sensations to the surgeon's hands, further increasing the realism of the surgical experience. Simulated environments will become increasingly useful for all levels of surgery, beginning with training in the basic operations of incision and suturing and going all the way to complete surgical operations.

17.2.8 Feedback and Guidance

Closely related to the structure of an interaction is the degree to which a teaching program provides **feedback** and **guidance** to students. Virtually all systems provide some form of feedback—for example, they may supply short explanations of why answers are correct or incorrect, present summaries of important aspects of cases, or provide references to related materials. Many systems provide an interactive help facility that allows students to ask for hints and advice.

17.2.9 Intelligent Tutoring Systems

More sophisticated systems allow students to take independent action but may intervene if the student strays down an unproductive path or acts in a way that suggests a misconception of fact or inference. Such **mixed-initiative systems** allow students freedom but provide a framework that constrains the interaction and thus helps students to learn more efficiently. Some researchers make a distinction between **coaching** systems and **tutoring** systems. The less proactive coaching systems monitor the session and intervene only when the student requests help or makes serious mistakes. Tutoring systems, on the other hand, guide a session aggressively by asking questions that test a student's understanding of the material and that expose errors and gaps in the student's knowledge. Mixed-initiative systems are difficult to create because they must have models both of the student and of the problem to be solved (Eliot et al., 1996).

17.3 Current Applications

Computer-based learning has been developed for the beginning medical student and the experienced practitioner, for the lay person and the medical expert. In this section, we present examples of actual programs that are being used to support medical education for each of these categories of learners.

17.3.1 Preclinical Applications

Traditional teaching in the preclinical years has been through lectures to large groups and laboratory exercises. With increasing laboratory costs and increasing amounts of information to be imparted to students, the individual, hands-on component of learning has decreased. Computer-based learning has the promise to return the student to individualized, interactive learning while reducing the need to teach in the lecture setting. Teaching programs have been developed for most subjects and using all styles of pedagogy. We describe here a few interesting programs for preclinical learning.

BrainStorm, developed at Stanford University, is an interactive atlas of neuroanatomy, with images of dissections and cross sections, diagrams, and extensive supporting text (Hsu, 1996). The unit of knowledge is a brain structure, such as nucleus, tract, vessel, or subsystem. Each unit has references to three modes of information presentation—image, diagram, and text—each of which contains representations of many structures, the result being a richly connected network of information. When compared with hyperlinks on web pages, which may lead the student astray from the original learning goal, a named link, such as a cross-reference to an image, contains information that helps the student to decide whether to follow that link and to retrieve the expected information. Multiple-choice quizzes on every image provide thousands of questions for self-evaluation. Animated simulations teach the basics of skills such as performing an examination for a cranial-nerve lesion.

The Digital Anatomist, at the University of Washington, Seattle, uses three-dimensional models of brain and anatomic structures to teach about anatomic structure and localization. A unique aspect of this program is its accessibility over the Internet. Using a client program, the student requests new views of the models. Rotations of the model are performed on the powerful server at the university, and the resulting images are sent to the student for viewing on the client program (Rosse et al, 1998).

The Visible Human male and female are an extraordinary resource available through the National Library of Medicine.[3] Thousands of cross sections represent the entire bodies of two humans. These data have been licensed freely by numerous sites that then use these images for teaching, for annotation of anatomic structures, for reconstruction of three-dimensional anatomy, for research on image processing and object segmentation, and for research on the development of large image databases.

Developed by researchers at the Harvard Medical School, HeartLab is a simulation program designed to teach medical students to interpret the results of auscultation of (listening to) the heart, a skill that requires regular practice on a variety of patient cases (Bergeron & Greenes, 1989). Physicians can diagnose many cardiac disorders by listening to the sounds made by the movement of the heart valves and the movement of blood in the heart chambers and vessels. HeartLab provides an interactive environment for listening to heart sounds as an alternative to the common practice of listening to audio tapes. A student wearing headphones can compare and contrast similar-sounding abnormalities and can hear the changes in sounds brought on by changes in patient position (sitting versus lying down) and by physician maneuvers (such as changing the location of the stethoscope).

17.3.2 Clinical Teaching Applications

For many years, teaching hospitals usually had numerous patients with diagnostic problems such as unexplained weight loss or fever of unknown origin. This environment allowed for thoughtful "visit rounds," at which the attending could tutor the students and house staff, who could then go to the library to research the subject. A patient might be in the hospital for weeks, as testing was pursued and the illness evolved. In the modern era of Medicare's system of lump-sum payment for diagnosis-related groups (DRGs) and of managed care, such a system appears as distant as professors in morning coats. The typical patient in today's teaching hospital is very sick, usually elderly, and commonly acutely ill. The emphasis is on short stays, with diagnostic problems handled on an outpatient basis and diseases evolving at home or in chronic-care facilities. Thus, the medical student is faced with few "diagnostic problems" and has little opportunity to see the evolution of a patient's illness over time.

One response of medical educators has been to try to move teaching to the outpatient setting; another has been to use computer-modeled patients. Simulated patients allow rare diseases to be presented and allow the learner to follow the course of an illness over any appropriate time period. Faculty can decide what clinical material must be seen and can use the computer to ensure that this core curriculum is achieved. Moreover, with the use of an indestructible patient, the learner can take full responsibility for decision-making, without concern over

---

[3]The Visible Human project: http://www.nlm.nih.gov/research/visible/visible_human.html.

harming an actual patient by making mistakes. Finally, cases developed at one institution can be shared easily with other organizations. Case libraries are available on the Internet; examples include the Short Rounds from Stanford[4] and geriatric cases from the University of Florida.[5]

Clinical reasoning tools—such as DXplain, Iliad, and Quick Medical Reference (QMR)—are discussed in Chapter 16. Although not typically thought of as educational in the traditional sense, such diagnostic-support systems can provide the ideal educational experience of giving aid to a physician or student when she is involved with a real case and thus is most receptive to learning. Literature searching (Chapter 15) confers the same advantages.

The National Board of Medical Examiners (NBME) has had a longstanding interest in using computer-based case simulations for their examinations. These simulations include cost as well as time considerations. The NBME plans to use these cases in their computer-based examination of medical students.

17.3.3 Continuing Medical Education

Medical education does not stop after the completion of medical school and formal residency training. The science of medicine advances at such a rapid rate that much of what is taught becomes outmoded, and it has become obligatory for physicians to be lifelong learners both for their own satisfaction and, increasingly, as a formal government requirement to maintain licensure.

Although the physician practicing at a major medical center usually has no problem obtaining the required hours of accredited CME, physicians who practice in rural areas or other more isolated locations may face considerable obstacles. Physician CME has become a large industry and is widely available, but often the course fees are high, and attendance also incurs the direct costs of lodging and transportation and the indirect costs of time lost from practice. The cost of CBE is often much lower.

With increasing specialization and subspecialization has come an added difficulty. Traditional lecture-based CME must aim at a broad audience. Therefore, many listeners know as much or more about the topic than the speaker; many others find the material too difficult or of little relevance. A pure subspecialist—even one at a major medical center—may find the majority of CME offerings irrelevant to his practice. The ideal form of CME for many physicians would be a preceptorship with a mentor in the same discipline, but the costs of providing such an experience on a wide scale would be prohibitive. With the increasing amount of computer-based material available, including self-assessment examinations from specialty societies, specialists can select topics that are of interest to them.

---

[4]Stanford University website for Short Rounds: http://summit.stanford.edu/shortrounds.
[5]University of Florida website on clinical teaching cases:
http://www.medinfo.ufl.edu/cme/geri/.

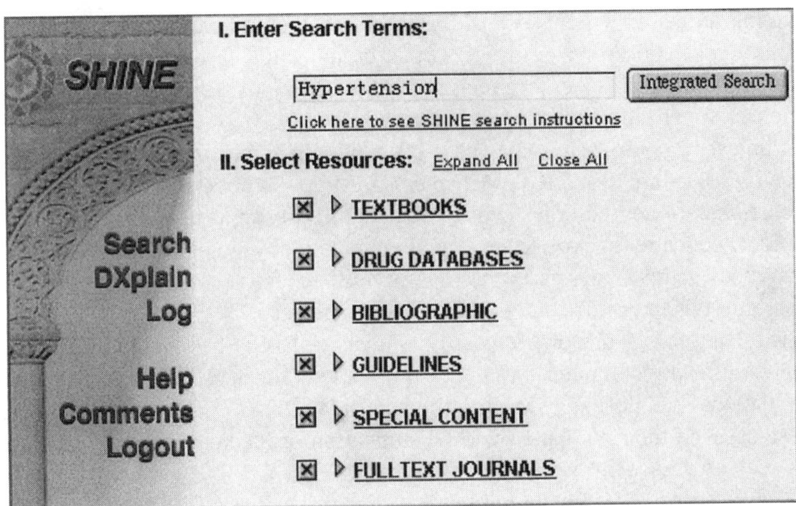

FIGURE 17.4. The SHINE CME system.This search screen allows the user to enter a query and to select the resources to be searched. This unified query method makes it unnecessary for the student to learn the peculiarities of the search system for each resource. (*Source:* © 1997, Stanford University. Screen shot of the SHINE program.)

Both literature searching (Chapter 15) and use of diagnostic-support systems (Chapter 16) are an important part of a physician's continuing education. These aids to the diagnosis and management of complex patient problems reach the physician when she is most receptive to learning new material.

The SHINE project at Stanford is an example of point-of-need support, which provides student-specific continuing education (Fig. 17.4). This experimental system allows the primary-care physician to enter queries in short phrases. Multiple content collections are searched in parallel, including some standard medical texts, a drug database, guidelines and consensus reports from national agencies and professional groups, the Medline bibliographic database, and locally generated teaching material. Query responses can be read immediately or can be perused later at the user's leisure. The system maintains a log of student actions from which a curriculum can be generated that is custom tailored to the student (Hubbs et al, 1997; Strasberg et al, 1999).

17.3.4 Consumer Health Education

Today's patients have become health-care consumers; they often bring to the health-care provider a mass of health-related information (and misinformation) gathered from the media. Medical topics are widely discussed in general-interest magazines, in newspapers, on television, and over the Internet. Patients may use the Internet to join disease-focused or symptom-focused chat groups or to search for information about their own conditions. At the same time that patients have become more sophisticated in their requests for information, practitioners have become increasingly pressed for time under the demands of managed care. Shorter visits allow less time to educate patients. Computers can be used to print information about medications, illnesses, and symptoms so that patients leave the office with a personalized hand-out that they can read at home. Personal risk profiling can be performed with widely available software, often free from pharmaceutical firms. This type of software clearly illustrates for the patient how such factors as lack of exercise, smoking, or untreated hypertension or hyperlipidemia can reduce life expectation and how changing them can prolong it.

A torrent of consumer-oriented health sites has flowed onto the Web. As we discussed in Chapter 11, one problem that complicates the use of any information site on the Internet is lack of control. Consumers are not readily able to distinguish factual information from hype and snake oil. An important role for the health-care provider today is to suggest high-quality websites that can be trusted to provide valid information. Many such sites are available from the various branches of the National Institutes of Health (NIH) and from medical professional organizations. The American Medical Association maintains a website[6] that includes validated information about such topics as migraine, asthma, human immunodeficiency virus and acquired immune deficiency syndrome (HIV/AIDS), depression, high blood pressure, and breast cancer. The National Institute of Diabetes and Digestive and Kidney Diseases of the NIH has extensive consumer-oriented material[7] which can be directly accessed by patients. Alternatively, physicians can use the site to print material for distribution to their patients. Most national disease-oriented organizations such as the American Heart Association and the American Diabetes Association now maintain websites that can be recommended with confidence. These sites provide additional links to numerous websites that have been evaluated for and found to meet a minimum level of quality.

17.3.5 Distance Learning

The Internet, and in particular the World Wide Web, has radically changed the way that we access information. It is now possible to earn university degrees from home at every level from bachelor's to doctorate. Physician CME credit is increasingly available in the same way, in many instances free with pharmaceutical company sponsorship or at modest cost.

A widely used example is Medscape.[8] In 1997, this website provided on-line coverage of the November 1997 American Heart Association's annual meeting. A physician could read synopses of papers from the meeting and get 1 hour of CME credit for every three papers read by writing summaries of the articles and

---

[6]American Medical Association website: http://www.ama-assn.org/.
[7]National Institute of Diabetes and Digestive and Kidney Diseases website: http://www.niddk.nih.gov/.
[8]Medscape website: http://www.medscape.com/.

submitting an evaluation form. In 1998, Medscape charged $50 for up to 20 hours of CME credit.

Numerous Internet sites offer a teaching experience along with CME credit. Helix,[9] sponsored by GlaxoWellcome, but without obvious commercial bias, offers articles on nutrition, exercise, and fitness, each of which provides 1 or 1.5 hours of credit after the student completes a test. Grand Rounds on Frontiers in Biomedicine from the George Washington University School of Medicine is also available, in either text or video format. The Marshall University School of Medicine offers the Interactive Patient,[10] a simulated case with which a physician can earn 1 hour of CME credit for a fee of $15. A good source of pointers to on-line medical education is maintained at the Meducation website.[11] This site provides a listing of Web educational resources at multiple levels, from those written for children through consumer-education materials, medical school resources, online journals, and CME.

As we begin a new century, the Internet shows great promise for supporting distance education, but it still has many problems. The challenges facing a physician or other health-care provider who is seeking education via the Internet are similar to those of any other user. Technical problems still abound, and the regular user of the Internet is subject to being disconnected in miduse for no apparent reason. Those people who most need distance learning, such as rural practitioners, are least likely to have high-speed connections, and so are faced with very slow downloading of programs that make extensive use of graphics. In addition to technical problems, the anarchic nature of the Internet means that the environment still dictates caveat emptor. There is no way of telling in advance whether a listed CME program is of high quality, although restricting use to sites that offer AMA Category 1 credit provides some assurance of worthwhile content. Students must also be prepared to find that sites listed in reference guides no longer exist or have changed from the description in the reference guide.

17.4 Design, Development, and Technology

Creation of computer-based learning material requires a systematic process of design and implementation, using technologies appropriate to learning goals. We present some of the issues that arise in this process.

17.4.1 Design of Computer-Based Learning Applications

In the past, each university or group developed its own approach to the design and implementation of its learning software. Developers at each site climbed a

[9]GlaxoWellcome's Helix website: http://www.helix.com/.
[10]Marshall University School of Medicine's "Interactive Patient" website: http://medicus.marshall.edu/medicus.htm.
[11]Meducation website: http://www.meducation.com/.

learning curve as they determined appropriate designs for pedagogy on the computer and the associated structuring of information. Although no broadly accepted method of design yet exists, a four-level approach to program design appears to be emerging independently at many sites. The four levels are structured content; query, retrieval, and indexing; authoring and presentation; and analysis and reasoning.

Structured Content

The authoring tools used for teaching programs, such as HyperCard and ToolBook, contributed to a development approach in which the learning content, both text and media, was embedded inside the program, along with the code that presented the content and allowed navigation through the program. This intuitive approach to development had the beneficial result that engaging courseware was developed by numerous content experts who did not need to know complex programming languages. On the negative side, these programs were difficult to maintain, expand, or modify. Because the content was distributed throughout the program, and intermixed with the code, locating a specific sentence or image could not be achieved through a simple search process. Understanding the functionality of a segment of code was also complicated because its operation might depend on many other segments scattered throughout the program. It is therefore desirable that content should be maintained external to the code or program. Once content is externalized, it is necessary that the content be formatted in a predictable structure such that it can be read and correctly linked by a computer program.

Structured content is different from narrative text. A paragraph of text in a clinical report is narrative text. When the paragraph is broken into subsections, each subsection representing a coherent concept, with the name of the concept used as a tag or keyword to label that subsection, the paragraph has been converted to structured text. The concept of structured content exists in domains other than computer-based learning. A database record, with fields, is a structured item. We can perform computations on a structured item other than simply displaying it. For example, a database can be searched for all occurrences of a specific type of content within a specified field. A more text-oriented approach to structured content is seen in the document layout languages Standardized General Markup Language (SGML) and HyperText Markup Language (HTML).

Structured content requires more than structuring for layout. It adds labels or tags for semantic structuring (Fig. 17.5). The Digital Library Project (Fox & Marchionini, 1998) has developed sample document models and semantic tags for numerous domains, such as environmental engineering and computer-science technical reports. Tags that indicate the title of an article, its author, and its date of publication are examples of semantic tags. In clinical material, tags can be developed at many different levels of specificity. A single tag may be used to indicate an entire section on physical examination of the patient. Alternatively, a tag could be used for each step of the examination. Careful design of semantic

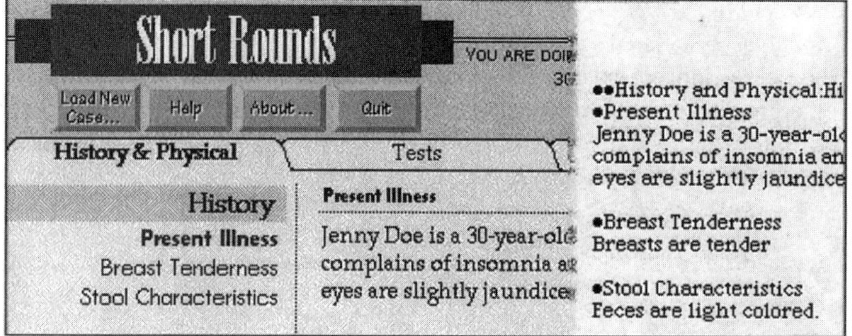

FIGURE 17.5. Comparison of the final presentation of some clinical content (on the left) with the structured text (on the right) that generated the final view. Simple markup tags (· and ··) are used to indicate header elements and individual feature or findings elements. The program that creates the presentation detects these markup tags and positions the corresponding content appropriately on the page or screen. (*Source:* © 1998, Stanford University. A composite screen shot of the Short Rounds program and of the text file used in the program.)

tags may allow content created for one learning purpose to be reused in other programs.

Query, Retrieval, and Indexing

The second level of design of teaching programs is providing the ability for users to index into and retrieve desired content. Query and retrieval capabilities are rarely used in teaching programs, but indexing is often available. This difference is significant. An **index** is developed by the author either manually or automatically and is stored along with the program. The student can access only the terms and links made available by the author. Segments of the content that are not indexed cannot be accessed by the student through the index.

In **query and retrieval**, the terms are selected by the student. They can be matched against a predetermined index or, preferably, against a thesaurus that searches for synonyms, more global concepts, and more specific concepts. The system searches the content using the student's terms and any other terms selected through the thesaurus. The entire searchable content can be accessed through this method. Queries that were not conceived of by the program's author, such as one involving an unexpected combination of terms, can be executed by the student.

In unstructured content, searches are executed on the full text. If the content is structured, searches can be applied specifically to certain categories of information. This technique has the potential to increase the specificity of the search because the content is searched in the context (category) specified by the student.

Authoring and Presentation

The third level of teaching-program design is programming for author support and for presentation. The ability of subject-matter experts to develop courseware within a reasonable time frame depends on the availability of good authoring systems. The ability of the student to understand the program and to make good use of its content depends on the presentation of the content.

An **authoring system** allows the expert to focus on the content of the teaching program and to be unconcerned with the details of writing a computer program. Early teaching programs, using multimedia and hyperlinks, had their content and code intermixed. The content author was also the person programming the navigation and presentation of the content. She had to do both even if the programming was at a high level, such as creating flow diagrams for content navigation. An authoring system is based on the recognition that a content domain has a predictable structure—then the author is provided with a template that represents this structure. Content is entered into the template through familiar operations such as typing or importing a digital image. In microbiology, for example, a category of microbes is *bacteria*. For almost every type of bacteria, the following categories are required: description, pathogenesis, laboratory tests, clinical syndromes caused, and other bacteria that can also cause these syndromes. Similarly, every description of a patient's case includes categories such as history, physical examination, tests and procedures, diagnosis, and treatment. Not only does a template based on domain structure provide a framework for authoring, but also it allows multiple authors to create content in parallel, greatly speeding the authoring process.

The *presentation* includes the graphic design of the screen, the location and appearance of the content, the selection of the content to be presented, and the navigation to other content. Although there are numerous resources for guidance in graphic design and content presentation, little is known about how presentation affects the process of learning or the use of the content. Studying the use of the richly linked program for neuroanatomy, BrainStorm, described in Section 17.3.1, Hsu (1996) observed that students who were reviewing the subject made extensive use of annotated cross-section images and the related quizzes. On the other hand, students who were engaged in primary learning made significant use of the many textual resources in the program. The presentation was the same in both cases, but the users' objectives differed, leading to different uses of the program. A further question that has not been studied is whether manipulation of the presentation could have altered the usage. For example, if the program had detected significant study of brainstem nuclei and had prompted the student about the availability of diagrams that had not been examined, would a large number of students have chosen to examine these diagrams?

Teaching content available on the Web is characterized by a large number of links, many leading to material that is distracting for the serious learner. The value of these links lies in making available a large range of content. The student is often, however, unable to judge the quality and value of the content reachable by these links. Navigation-support information that indicates the nature of the linked content could increase greatly the value of each such link.

Content-driven automated presentation systems are based on the use of structured content. The selection of content, the layout of the presentation, and the availability of linked information all can be driven by structured content. Figure

17.5 shows the contents of a text file containing structured content and the resulting multimedia presentation. On the one hand, the display program reads and parses the structured content, determining the text and links that will be displayed and the layout that will accommodate the necessary content. On the other hand, because the display is created anew each time, the author has the flexibility to use any terms desired to represent the findings to be displayed. For example, the author may choose to add a finding under the label "Diet," remove the "Stool Characteristics" finding, and change the name of a finding from "Present Illness" to "Chief Complaint." The presentation program will read this file of structured content and will delete the button "Stool Characteristics," add a button for "Diet," and change the name of the "Present Illness" button. The appropriate text will get linked to the new Diet button.

Analysis and Reasoning

The fourth level of design, analysis and reasoning, frequently is not included in a teaching program. A program with built-in automated assessment of students would have analysis capability. A program that observed the student's use of it and identified relevant missed material would be reasoning about the student's possible needs. Intelligent tutoring systems, discussed in Section 17.2.9, have this capability.

17.4.2 *Application Development*

The process for development of computer-based teaching material is similar to the process for almost any other software project (see Chapter 5). The process begins with identification of a need and a definition of what that need is. This step is followed by a system design and prototyping stage, accompanied by a formative evaluation process. Once the design of the software has been clarified, the software is implemented in the programming language of choice, and the teaching content is entered. The software is then integrated into the teaching process and is evaluated in use. Throughout, the design is guided by available standards for software design as well as for design of content structure.

Definition of the Need

Because the development process for teaching programs is labor intensive and time consuming, appropriate planning is essential. Defining the need for computer-based teaching in the curriculum is the first step. Are there difficult concepts that could be explained well through an interactive animated presentation? Is there a need for an image collection that exceeds that which is presented in the context of the lecture? Does the laboratory need support in the form of a guided tour through a library of digitized cross-section images? Could a quantitative concept be explained clearly through a simulation of the physiological or biochemical process, with the student being able to vary the important parameters? Is there a need for a chat group or a newsgroup to supplement the lectures or discussion sections? Would a central repository for course handouts reduce the load on departmental staff?

Assessment of the Resources

The availability and commitment of a content and teaching expert is an obvious necessity. The rich multimedia nature of most computer-based teaching programs implies that graphic, video, and audio media resources must be acquired or be available. Slides or video that are used in the classroom are supplemented by comments from the lecturer, which compensate for their deficiencies. These materials must stand on their own in a software program. Therefore, acquiring media of sufficient quality and comprehensiveness, along with the necessary release of rights, is an important next step in development. Supporting staff for the development process and the necessary funds are additional resources that must be considered.

Prototyping and Formative Evaluation

Significant scholarly work is needed in **prototyping** and **evaluation**, because so little is known about how technology can support medical teaching. Anecdotal results suggest that market-research focus groups and small discussion groups with a facilitator can lead to significant useful design changes in the early stages of development. Participatory development can clarify the focus of the project and modify it so as to make the tool more useful to students (Dev et al., 1998).

Formative evaluation is conducted during the evolution of a project, sometimes at many stages: as the idea is being developed, after the first storyboards are prepared (storyboards are sketches of typical screens, with the interactive behavior indicated), during examination of comparable software, and as segments of the software are developed. During formative evaluation, developers must be prepared to make major changes in direction if such changes will increase the value of the project while retaining the overall goal and keeping the budget within the available resources.

Production

Prototyping determines the form of the teaching program, its goals, the levels of media inclusion and interactivity, the nature of the feedback, and other design parameters. **Production** is the process of executing this design for the entire range of content determined earlier. The requirements during production differ from those of prototyping. Adequate funding and staffing resources must be available at all times. Media must be acquired and processed to the specified standard, and content must be written. Because simultaneous authoring may be needed for different segments and multiple authors may need to review the same section, a method of content collection and version control must be set up. Regular integration of the content into the overall program is required so that any problems of scaling or compatibility will be determined early. Production should be embarked on only if it is very clear that the project is needed and that the resources for completion will be available.

Integration in the Curriculum

An important aspect of courseware development that is often overlooked is the integration of computer-based materials with the curriculum. Currently, most computer-based materials are treated as supplementary material; they are placed in libraries and are used by students or physicians on these users' own initiative. This use is valid, and the programs serve as valuable resources for the students who use them; however, an educator can use such materials more effectively by integrating them into the standard curriculum. For example, programs might be assigned as laboratory exercises or used as the basis of a class discussion.

One of the barriers to integration is the initial high cost of acquiring sufficient computing resources. The cost of the computer equipment has fallen drastically in recent years; even so, the cost of purchasing and supporting enough computers for a whole school to use would be a major item in the curriculum budget of a school. This consideration will grow less important as more students purchase their own computers. A second, and important, barrier is the reluctance of faculty to modify their teaching to include references to computer-based material or to operate these programs in the context of their teaching. One of the most effective uses of these programs has been as a lead-in to small-group discussion, such as the presentation of a clinical case on the computer, with students choosing the questions to ask the computer.

Maintenance and Upgrades

Changes in content and changes in the computer operating system or hardware, as well as the discovery of problems with the program, necessitate regular maintenance and upgrades. At the same time, good design requires that any major change in teaching method should trigger iteration through the entire design cycle.

Standards

Maintaining a balance between evolution and standards is difficult but necessary. It is particularly difficult because the publicly acknowledged standards themselves change so rapidly. The standards that apply to teaching programs have to do with the **metacontent**: the information that describes the content and thus adds structure to the content. Understanding of metacontent is in its infancy and is fertile ground for scholarly research.

A simple example is that of annotation of images. Many groups collect and annotate images for their teaching programs. Each has its unique method for representing and storing this information. Some use the representations provided in the authoring programs they use; typically, these representations are proprietary and cannot be used by other programs. Others develop their own representations.

To the extent that they publicize their representations, as well as the methods or programs to read, display, and modify this information, their systems are open, although still proprietary. A useful representation is one that is easily converted to other representations and that is widely available.

An important value of standardization for sharing among groups is that content created by one group of developers or authors is available for use by a later group of authors. Another result of standardization is that development of display or editing programs can continue in parallel with content creation done with older authoring programs. Furthermore, if the standard is upgraded, or if new features are added, programs can be created to convert automatically all the material from the old standard to the new.

17.4.3 Technology Considerations

Technology considerations determine the cost and availability of the final teaching product. For example, a program can be delivered on a Web client, or the software designer can choose between developing for the Windows or Macintosh operating system. True platform independence is a myth, but it is possible to restrict development to a subset of features such that the teaching program has a high probability of running on most computers. The choice of operating over the Internet versus processing on a local machine is a decision that is dependent on the source of the learning content and the performance requirements of the program. Teaching programs that draw on content at many locations on the Internet—such as image collections, digital video, and text reference material—will be restricted by the constraints of a Web client, including a restricted number of display and interaction features. On the other hand, Internet access is more desirable if the program accesses rapidly changing content or bibliographic sources such as Medline.

A need for high performance, or for very large volumes of content, will restrict usage to a local machine. In some cases, such as the use of three-dimensional models in the Virtual Reality Modeling Language (VRML), the model is obtained from a site on the Internet but is then manipulated and displayed locally. The availability of high-capacity storage devices, such as digital video disk (DVD), will make it possible to distribute large quantities of material, with the Internet used for updates, extension of content, and links to additional content.

17.5 Evaluation

Evaluation of a new teaching or training method can measure numerous attributes of success: Four levels of evaluation are commonly accepted. The first is the reaction of the student population to the new teaching method and how well the method is assimilated into the existing process of teaching. These measure the *acceptability* of the method. The second level of evaluation is the *usability* of the teaching program. The third level of evaluation measures whether the new teaching method actually had any impact on what the students learned. Here *knowledge acquisition* is measured. The fourth level measures whether the new method results in *behavioral change* because, in the final analysis, content and procedures learned by students should affect how they practice medicine.

17.5.1 Reaction and Assimilation

Many evaluation studies focus on the acceptability of a teaching program to teachers and students. This information is collected through questionnaires, subjective reports, and measurement of actual usage. Without this baseline information, interpretation of more sophisticated analysis may be difficult. These measures do not, however, inform the developer about the effectiveness of a teaching program.

17.5.2 Usability and Cognitive Evaluation

If we wish to measure whether the student understands the operation and capabilities of the program, numerous methods are available. Two complementary methods are the use of the videotaped encounter with the program and the use of the automatically generated log of the student's interaction with the program.

The videotape encounter typically records the actions and words of the student as well as the events on the screen, often presented for analysis in a picture-in-picture format. The video transcript is then segmented into individual events or items. Subsequently, these items are categorized in terms of their cognitive aspects, such as "searching for button" or "selects link to additional information." The researchers use the resultant list of cognitive transactions to identify major categories of usage, sources of success and frustration, and typical information-seeking patterns.

A computer-generated log file can be created if the teaching program is instrumented to record the student's interaction with the program. It may be desirable to be able to select which types of interactions will be recorded. In an analysis of BrainStorm usage (Hsu, 1996), the granularity of recorded information ranged from detecting transfers between pages of information to detecting the selection of every click on a highly detailed annotated image. A computer-generated log file of student interactions can be processed automatically to detect frequency and patterns of usage. Figure 17.6 shows the pattern of transitions between four different types of information in BrainStorm. The students clearly preferred to study the cross-sectional images over all other types of information. A drawback of the automated log is the lack of any information about the student's motives for the interactions. Researchers can gather such information by interrupting selected interactions and requesting the student to type in a comment, but this method is intrusive and breaks the process of information acquisition.

17.5.3 Knowledge Acquisition

Evaluation of knowledge acquisition includes the question that is asked most often of developers: Is this computer program more effective than traditional meth-

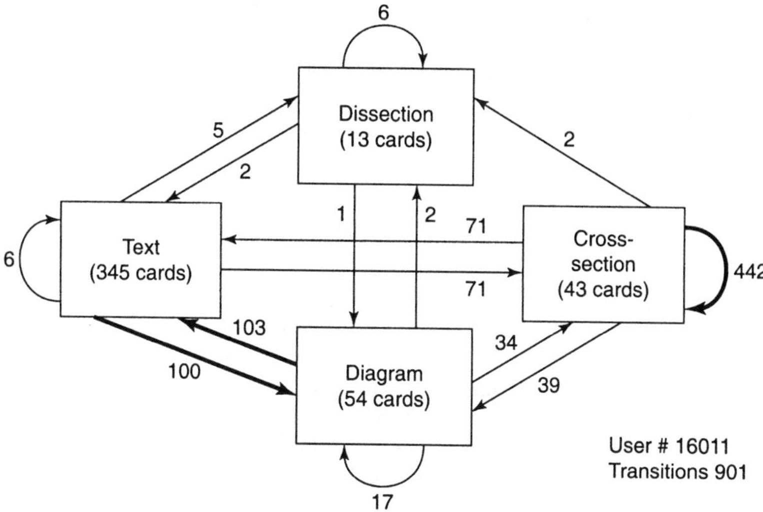

FIGURE 17.6. Transition graph showing how one student moved between different types of information in the neuroanatomy program BrainStorm. Of the 900 transitions, almost one-half were from one cross-sectional image to another. Even though there were a large number (345) of text screens, with many available hyperlinks between the screens, there was little movement from one text screen to another. Analyses such as these clarify usage and suggest program design strategies. (*Source:* © 1996, Hsu. Adapted from Hsu, 1996.)

ods of teaching the same material? This question has proved difficult to answer because of the many changes introduced when computer-based teaching is used. One of the most important confounding factors is the renewed attention that the professor pays to preparing teaching material because the course is to be taught in a new format. Perhaps the most interesting evaluation questions are, In what ways is computer-based learning *different from* traditional methods of learning? Can computers enable learning in ways never before possible? Going further, can computers perform evaluations of knowledge acquisition that would be impossible using traditional written or oral examination techniques?

An example of computer-based evaluation is the evaluation of nonverbal knowledge of spatial location in anatomy (Friedman et al., 1993). The rationale was that the better a person knows anatomy, the more accurately she will recognize and localize an image of a cross section of the human body. The authors developed a computer game in which the examinee was given an outline of a cross section, with no internal structures displayed, and was asked to position it on a drawing of the human body. The examinee could request additional clues, the clues being pictures of organs in the cross section. After each clue, the examinee was asked to make an attempt to position the slice in the body. Requesting too many clues resulted in a penalty that reduced the maximum possible score. The final score was based on the accuracy of the placement and the number of clues requested. The test differentiated between first-year medical students, fourth-year medical students, and anatomy faculty in their mastery of anatomic knowledge.

17.5.4 *Problem Solving and Behavioral Change*

The ultimate goal of medical knowledge acquisition is to improve a student's ability to solve problems through application of that knowledge. In some cases, particularly in skill acquisition, such as insertion of an intravenous line, or in interpersonal interaction, such as history taking, the measure is not problem-solving ability but rather behavioral change.

17.6 Conclusion

Computer-based educational systems have the potential to help students to master subject matter and to develop problem-solving skills. Properly integrated into the medical-school curriculum and into the information systems that serve health-care institutions and the greater medical community, computer-based teaching can become part of a comprehensive system for lifelong education. The challenge to researchers in computer-based teaching is to develop this potential. The barriers to success are both technical and practical. To overcome them, we require both dedication of support and resources within institutions and a commitment to cooperation among institutions.

Suggested Readings

Kirkpatrick D.L. (1994). *Evaluating Training Programs*. San Francisco: Berrett-Koehler Publishers.

This book presents a multilevel system for evaluating training programs.

Lyon H.C., Healy J.C., Bell J.R., O'Donnell J.F., Shultz E.K., Moore-West M., Wigton R.S., Hirai F., Beck J.R. (1992). PlanAlyzer, an interactive computer-assisted program to teach clinical problem solving in diagnosing anemia and coronary artery disease. *Academic Medicine*, 67(12):821–828.

The authors describe their clinical teaching program and present a thoughtful evaluation of its efficacy in learning.

Rosse C., Mejino J.L., Modayur B.R., Jakobovits R., Hinshaw K.P., Brinkley J.F. (1998). Motivation and organizational principles for anatomical knowledge representation: the digital anatomist symbolic knowledge base. *Journal of the American Medical Informatics Association*, 5(1):17–40.

Rosse's group has developed one of the more comprehensive representations of a domain, in their case, anatomy. Such domain knowledge representation will be necessary for the next generation of educational software systems.

Vosniadou S., DeCorte, E., Glaser, R., Mandl, H. (1996). *International Perspectives on the Design of Technology-Supported Learning Environments*. Mahwah, NJ: L. Erlbaum Associates.

This is a collection of research articles presenting many different aspects of development and assessment in technology-supported learning environments.

Westwood J.D., Hoffman H.M., Stredney D., Weghorst S.J. (1998). *Medicine Meets Virtual Reality*. Amsterdam: IOS Press.

This volume is one in a series of conference proceedings on the emerging area of virtual environments in training and education.

Questions for Discussion

1. What are two advantages and two limitations of including visual material in the following teaching programs:
   a. A simulated case of a patient who is admitted to the emergency unit with a gunshot wound
   b. A lecture-style program on the anatomy of the pelvis
   c. A reference resource on bacteria and fungi
2. You have decided to write a computer-based simulation to teach students about the management of chest pain.
   a. Discuss the relative advantages and disadvantages of the following styles of presentation: (1) a sequence of multiple choice questions, (2) a simulation in which the patient's condition changes over time and in response to therapy, and (3) a program that allows the student to enter free-text requests for information and that provides responses.
   b. Discuss at least four problems that you would expect to arise during the process of developing and testing the program.
   c. For each approach, discuss how you might develop a model that you could use to evaluate the student's performance in clinical problem-solving.
3. Examine two clinical simulation programs. How do they differ in their presentation of history-taking or physical examination of the patient?
4. Select a topic in physiology with which you are familiar, such as arterial blood-gas exchange or filtration in the kidney, and construct a representation of the domain in terms of the concepts and subconcepts that should be taught for that topic. Using this representation, design a teaching program using one of the following methods: (1) a didactic approach, (2) a simulation approach, or (3) an exploration approach.
5. Describe at least three challenges you can foresee in dissemination of computer-based medical education programs from one institution to another.
6. Discuss the relative merits and problems of placing the computer in control of the teaching environment, with the student essentially responding to computer inquiries, versus having the student be in control, with a much larger range of alternative courses of action.

18
Bioinformatics

Russ B. Altman

After reading this chapter, you should know the answers to these questions:

- Why is sequence, structure, and biological pathway information relevant to medicine?
- Where on the Internet should you look for a DNA sequence, a protein sequence, or a protein structure?
- What are two problems encountered in analyzing biological sequence, structure, and function?
- What two changes should we anticipate in the medical record as a result of these new information sources?
- What are two computational challenges in bioinformatics for the future?

18.1 The Problem of Handling Biological Information

Bioinformatics is the study of how information is represented and transmitted in biological systems, starting at the molecular level. Whereas clinical informatics deals with the management of information related to the delivery of health care, bioinformatics focuses on the management of information related to the underlying basic biological sciences. As such, the two disciplines are closely related—more so than generally appreciated (see Chapter 1). Bioinformatics and clinical informatics share a concentration on systems that are inherently uncertain, difficult to measure, and the result of complicated interactions among multiple complex components. Both deal with living systems that generally lack straight edges and right angles. Although reductionist approaches to studying these systems can provide valuable lessons, it is often necessary to analyze them using integrative models that are not based solely on first principles. Nonetheless, the two disciplines approach the patient from opposite directions. Whereas applications within clinical informatics usually are concerned with the social systems of medicine, the cognitive processes of medicine, and the technologies required to understand human physiology, bioinformatics is concerned with understanding how basic biological systems conspire to create molecules, organelles, living cells, organs, and entire organisms. Remarkably, however, the two disciplines share significant methodological elements, so an understanding of the issues in bioinformatics can be valuable for the student of clinical informatics.

The discipline of bioinformatics is currently in a period of rapid growth, because the needs for information storage, retrieval, and analysis in biology—particularly in molecular biology—have increased dramatically in the past decade. History has shown that scientific developments within the basic sciences tend to lag about a decade before their influence on clinical medicine is fully appreciated. The types of information being gathered by biologists today will drastically alter the types of information and technologies available to the healthcare workers of tomorrow.

18.1.1 Sources of Information Explosion

There are three sources of information that are revolutionizing our understanding of human biology and that are creating significant challenges for computational processing. The most dominant new type of information is the sequence information being produced by the **Human Genome Project**, an international undertaking intended to determine the complete sequence of human deoxyribonucleic acid (DNA) as it is encoded in each of the 23 chromosomes.[1] Essentially the entire set of events from conception through embryonic development, childhood, adulthood, and aging are encoded by the DNA blueprints within most human cells. Given a complete knowledge of these DNA sequences, we will be in a position to understand these processes at a fundamental level and to consider the possible use of DNA sequences for diagnosing and treating disease.

While we are studying the human genome, a second set of concurrent projects is studying the genomes of numerous other biological organisms, including important experimental animal systems (such as mouse, rat, and yeast) as well as important human pathogens (such as *Mycobacterium tuberculosis* or *Haemophilus influenzae*). Some of these genomes have already been completely determined by sequencing experiments and thus allow two important types of analysis: the analysis of mechanisms of pathogenicity and the analysis of animal models for human disease. In both cases, the functions encoded by genomes can be studied, classified, and categorized, allowing us to begin to understand how genomes work in human health and disease.

These ambitious scientific projects not only are proceeding at a furious pace but also are accompanied in many cases by a new approach to biology, which produces a third new source of biomedical information. In addition to small, relatively focused experimental studies aimed at particular molecules thought to be important for disease, large-scale experimental methodologies are used to collect data on thousands or millions of molecules simultaneously. Scientists apply these methodologies longitudinally over time and across a wide variety of organisms

[1]http://www.nhgri.nih.gov/HGP/.

or (within an organism) organs to watch the evolution of various physiological phenomena. New technologies give us the abilities to follow the production and degradation of molecules on **DNA arrays**[2] (Lashkari et al., 1997), to study the association of large numbers of proteins with one another (Bai & Elledge, 1997), and to create multiple variations on a genetic theme to explore the implications of various mutations on the biological function (Spee et al., 1993). All these technologies, along with the genome-sequencing projects, are conspiring to produce a volume of biological information that at once contains secrets to age-old questions about health and disease and threatens to overwhelm our current capabilities of data analysis. Thus, bioinformatics is becoming critical for medicine in the twenty-first century.

18.1.2 Implications for Clinical Informatics

The effects of this new biological information on clinical medicine and clinical informatics are difficult to predict precisely. It is already clear, however, that some major changes to medicine will have to be accommodated.

1. *Sequence information in the medical record.* It is likely that, once the first set of human genomes is available, it will become cost effective to consider sequencing at least sections of many other genomes. The sequence of a gene involved in disease may provide the critical information that we need to select appropriate treatments. For example, the set of genes that produces essential hypertension may be understood at a level sufficient to allow us to target antihypertensive medications based on the precise configuration of these genes. It is possible that clinical trials may use information about genetic sequence to define precisely the population of patients who would benefit from a new therapeutic agent. Finally, clinicians may learn the sequences of infectious agents (such as of the *Escherichia coli* that causes recurrent urinary-tract infections) and store them in a patient's record to record the precise pathogenicity and drug susceptability observed during an episode of illness. In any case, it is likely that genetic information will need to be included in the medical record—and will introduce special problems. Raw sequence information is meaningless without context and thus is not well suited to a printed medical record. Like images, it can come in high information density and must be presented to the clinician in novel ways. As there are for laboratory tests, there may be a set of nondisease (or normal) values to use as comparisons, and there may be difficulties in interpreting abnormal values. Fortunately, most of the human genome is shared and identical among individuals; less than 1 percent of the genome seems to be unique to individuals. Nonetheless, the effects of sequence information on clinical databases will be significant.

[2]These are small glass plates onto which specific DNA fragments can be affixed and then used to detect other DNA fragments present in a cell extract.

2. *New diagnostic and prognostic information sources.* One of the main contributions of the genome-sequencing projects (and of the associated biological innovations) is that we are likely to have unprecedented access to new diagnostic and prognostic tools. Diagnostically, the sequences of a patient with an autoimmune disease, or of an infectious pathogen within a patient, will be highly specific and sensitive indicators of the subtype of disease and of that subtype's probable responsiveness to different therapeutic agents. In general, diagnostic tools based on the gene sequences within a patient are likely to increase greatly the number and variety of tests available to the physician. Physicians will not be able to manage these tests without significant computational assistance. Moreover, genetic information will be available to provide more accurate prognostic information to patients. What is the standard course for this disease? How does it respond to these medications? Over time, we will be able to answer these questions with increasing precision, and will develop computational systems to manage this information.
3. *Ethical considerations.* One of the critical questions facing the genome-sequencing projects is "Can genetic information be misused?" The answer is certainly yes. With knowledge of a complete genome for an individual, it may be possible in the future to predict the types of disease for which that individual is at risk years before the disease actually develops. If this information fell into the hands of unscrupulous employers or insurance companies, the individual might be denied employment or coverage due to the likelihood of future disease, however distant. There is even debate about whether such information should be released to a patient even if it could be kept confidential. Should a patient be informed that she is likely to get a disease for which there is no treatment? This is a matter of intense debate, and such questions have significant implications for what information is collected and for how and to whom that information is disclosed (Durfy, 1993).

18.2 The Impetus for Bioinformatics

A brief review of the biological basis of medicine will bring into focus the magnitude of the revolution in molecular biology and the tasks that are created for the discipline of bioinformatics.

The genetic material that we inherit from our parents, that we use for the structures and processes of life, and that we pass to our children is contained in a sequence of chemicals known as **deoxyribonucleic acid** (DNA).[3] The total collection of DNA for a single person or organism is referred to as the **genome**. Deoxyribonucleic acid is a long polymer chemical made of four basic subunits.

[3]If you are not familiar with the basic terminology of molecular biology and genetics, reference to an introductory textbook in the area would be helpful before you read the rest of this chapter.

The sequence in which these subunits occur in the polymer distinguishes one DNA molecule from another, and the sequence of DNA subunits in turn directs a cell's production of proteins and all other basic cellular processes. The Human Genome Project is an international endeavor with the goal of determining the sequence of DNA for a human being to facilitate the use of genetic information in medical settings. Since the inception of the Human Genome Project in the early 1990s, *Science* magazine has devoted an entire issue annually to reporting the progress made on this project (Science, 1997). In the United States, the two agencies with the greatest interest in this project are the National Institutes of Health (NIH) and the Department of Energy (DOE);[4] together they allocate hundreds of millions of dollars annually for this project.[5]

The benefit to medicine of the Human Genome Project is both short and long term. The short-term benefits lie principally in diagnosis: The availability of sequences of normal and abnormal human genes will allow for the rapid identification of these genes in any patient (e.g., Babior & Matzner, 1997). The long-term benefits will include a greater understanding of the proteins produced from the genome: how the proteins interact with drugs; how they malfunction in disease states; and how they participate in the control of development, aging, and responses to disease.

18.2.1 The Importance of Sequences in Biology

Sequence information (including DNA sequences, RNA sequences, and protein sequences) is critical in biology: DNA, RNA, and protein can be represented as a set of sequences of basic building blocks (bases for DNA and RNA, amino acids for proteins). Computer systems within bioinformatics thus must be able to handle biological sequence information effectively and efficiently.

One major difficulty within bioinformatics is that standard database models, such as relational database systems, are not well suited to sequence information. The basic problem is that sequences are important both as a set of elements grouped together and treated in a uniform manner and as individual elements, with their relative locations and functions. Any given position in a sequence can be important because of its own identity, because it is part of a larger subsequence, or perhaps because it is part of a large set of overlapping subsequences, all of which have different significance. It is necessary to support queries such as, "What sequence motifs are present in this sequence?" It is often difficult to represent these multiple, nested relationships within a standard relational database schema. In addition, the neighbors of a sequence element are also critical, and it is important to be able to perform queries such as, "What sequence ele-

[4]For more information, see http://www.ornl.gov/TechResources/Human_Genome/project/hgp.html.

[5]The Department of Energy supports such research in part because of its interest in understanding the effects of energy (e.g., radiation) on animal and plant life and especially on human cellular processes.

ments are seen 20 elements to the left of this element?" For these reasons, researchers in bioinformatics are developing object-oriented databases in which a sequence can be queried in different ways, depending on the needs of the user.

18.2.2 The Importance of Structures in Biology

The sequence information mentioned in the previous section is rapidly becoming inexpensive to obtain and easy to store. On the other hand, the **three-dimensional–structure information** about the proteins that are produced from the DNA sequences is much more difficult and expensive to obtain and presents a separate set of analysis challenges. Currently, only about 10,000 three-dimensional structures of biological macromolecules are known. These models are incredibly valuable resources, however, because an understanding of structure often yields detailed insights about how the biological function follows. In the end, it is the physical forces between molecules that determine what happens within a cell. In particular, understanding the physical properties of therapeutic agents is the key to understanding how agents interact with their targets within the cell (or within an invading organism). These are the key questions for structural biology within bioinformatics:

1. How can we analyze the structures of molecules to understand how molecules produce their associated function? Approaches range from detailed molecular simulations (Levitt, 1983) to statistical analyses of the structural features that may be important for function. (Wei & Altman, 1998)
2. How can we extend the limited structural data by using information in the sequence databases about closely related proteins from different organisms (or within the same organism, but performing a slightly different function)? These are significant unanswered questions about how to extract maximal value from a relatively small set of examples.
3. How should structures be grouped for the purposes of classification? The choices range from purely functional criteria ("these proteins all digest proteins") to purely structural criteria ("these proteins all have a toroidal shape"), with mixed criteria in between. One interesting resource available today is the **Systematic Classification of Proteins** (SCOP),[6] which classifies proteins based on shape and function.

18.3 Roots of Modern Bioinformatics

Practitioners of bioinformatics have come from many backgrounds, including medicine, molecular biology, chemistry, physics, mathematics, engineering, and computer science. It is difficult to define precisely the ways in which this discipline emerged. There are, however, two main developments that have created

---

[6]See http://scop.mrc-lmb.cam.ac.uk/scop/.

opportunities for the use of information technologies in biology. The first is the progress in our understanding of how biological molecules are constructed and how they perform their functions, dating back to the elucidation of the structure of DNA in the 1950s and the subsequent sequence of discoveries in the relationships among DNA, RNA, and protein structure. The second development has been the parallel increase in the availability of computing power. Starting with mainframe computer applications in the 1950s and moving to modern workstations, there have been hosts of biological problems addressed with computational methods.

18.3.1 Early Work in Sequence and Structure Analysis

As it became clear that the information from DNA and protein sequences would be voluminous and difficult to analyze manually, algorithms began to appear for automating the analysis of sequence information. The first requirement was to have a reliable way to align sequences so that their detailed similarities and distances could be examined directly. Needleman and Wunsch (1970) published an elegant method for using dynamic programming techniques to align sequences in time related to the cube of the number of elements in the sequences. Smith and Waterman (1981) published refinements of these algorithms that allowed for searching both the best global alignment of two sequences (aligning all the elements of the two sequences) and the best local alignment (searching for areas in which there are segments of high similarity surrounded by regions of low similarity). A key input for these algorithms is a matrix that encodes the similarity or substitutability of sequence elements: When there is an inexact match between two elements in an alignment of sequences, it specifies how much "partial credit" we should give the overall alignment based on the similarity of the elements, even though they may not be identical. Looking at a set of evolutionarily related proteins, Dayhoff et al. (1974) published one of the first matrices derived from a detailed analysis of which amino acids (elements) tend to substitute for others.

Within structural biology, the vast computational requirements of the experimental methods (such as X-ray crystallography and nuclear magnetic resonance) for determining the structure of biological molecules drove the development of powerful structural-analysis tools. In addition to software for analyzing experimental data, graphical display algorithms allowed biologists to visualize these molecules in great detail and facilitated the manual analysis of structural principles (Langridge, 1974; Richardson, 1981). At the same time, methods were developed for simulating the forces within these molecules as they rotate and vibrate (Gibson & Scheraga, 1967; Karplus & Weaver, 1976; Levitt, 1983).

The most important development to support the emergence of bioinformatics, however, has been the creation of databases with biological information. In the 1970s, structural biologists, using the techniques of X-ray crystallography, set up the Protein Data Bank (PDB) of the Cartesian coordinates of the structures that they elucidated (as well as associated experimental details) and made PDB publically available. The first release, in 1977, contained 77 structures: The growth of the database is chronicled on the World Wide Web.[7] The PDB now has over 6,000 detailed atomic structures and is the primary source of information about the relationship between protein sequence and protein structure. Similarly, as the ability to obtain the sequence of DNA molecules became widespread, the need for a database of these sequences arose. In the mid-1980s, the GENBANK database was formed as a repository of sequence information. Starting with 606 sequences and 680,000 bases in 1982, the GENBANK has grown to much more than 2 million sequences and 5 billion bases. The GENBANK database of DNA sequence information supports the experimental reconstruction of genomes and acts as a focal point for experimental groups.[8] Numerous other databases store the sequences of protein molecules[9] and information about human genetic diseases.[10]

Included among the databases that have accelerated the development of bioinformatics is the Medline[11] database of the biomedical literature and its paper-based companion *Index Medicus* (see Chapter 15). Including articles as far back as 1966 and brought on-line free on the World Wide Web in 1997, Medline provides the glue that relates many high-level biomedical concepts to the low-level molecule, disease, and experimental methods. In fact, this "glue" role was the basis for creating the Entrez and Pub-MED systems for integrating access to literature references and the associated databases.

18.3.2 The Parallel Rise of Bioinformatics and Computers

Since 1994, the field of bioinformatics has emerged as an important component of the modern biomedical research enterprise. The computational technologies that have supported the growth of the discipline have revolutionized many other endeavors. In the context of the increasing availability of biological data, however, the field achieved a critical mass that has attracted significant attention (Marshall, 1996). Three key technological developments contributed to the rise of bioinformatics:

1. The availability of relatively inexpensive computer processing power (and graphical display technology) has enabled biologists and computer scientists to experiment with algorithms on real-world data sets within their own laboratories.
2. The spread of Internet technology, and the ability to share data either in point-to-point mode (through electronic mail and the File-Transfer Protocol [FTP])

---

[7]See http://db2.sdsc.edu/PDBObs/PDBObs.cgi.
[8]http://gdbwww.gdb.org/.
[9]The Protein Identification Resource: http://www.bis.med.jhmi.edu/Dan/proteins/pir.html; Swiss-Prot at http://expasy.hcuge.ch/sprot/sprot-top.html.
[10]Online Mendelian Inheritance in Man: http://www3.ncbi.nlm.nih.gov/omim/.
[11]See http://www.ncbi.nlm.nih.gov/PubMed/.

or in broadcast mode (through the World Wide Web and Hypertext Transfer Protocol, HTTP), have enabled data to be shared globally (also see Chapter 4).
3. The availability of virtually every important biological database on the Internet, in a publicly accessible form, and the development of efficient algorithms for searching the databases, have created a market for bioinformatics tools among scientists.

18.4 Current Application Successes from Bioinformatics

Biologists have embraced the World Wide Web in a remarkable way and have made Internet access to data a norm for doing business. Hundreds of databases curated by individual biologists create a haven for the developers of computational methods who can use these data to test and refine their analysis algorithms. With standard Internet search engines, most biological databases can be found and accessed within moments. The large number of databases has led to the development of meta-databases that combine information from individual databases to shield the user from the complex array that exists. There are various approaches to this task.

The Entrez system from the National Center for Biological Information (NCBI) gives integrated access to the biomedical literature, protein and nucleic-acid sequences, macromolecular and small-molecular structures, and genome project links (including both the Human Genome Project and sequencing projects that are attempting to determine the genome sequences for organisms that are either human pathogens or important experimental model organisms) in a manner that takes advantages of either explicit or computed links between these data resources.[12] The Sequence Retrieval System (SRS) from the European Molecular Biology Laboratory allows queries from one database to another to be linked and sequenced, thus allowing relatively complicated queries to be evaluated.[13] Newer technologies are being developed that will allow multiple heterogeneous databases to be accessed by search engines that can combine information automatically, thereby processing even more intricate queries requiring knowledge from numerous data sources.

18.4.1 Sequence Databases

The main types of sequence information that must be stored are DNA and protein. One of the largest **DNA sequence databases** is GENBANK, which is man-

[12]See http://www3.ncbi.nlm.nih.gov/Entrez/.
[13]See http://srs.ebi.ac.uk:5000/.

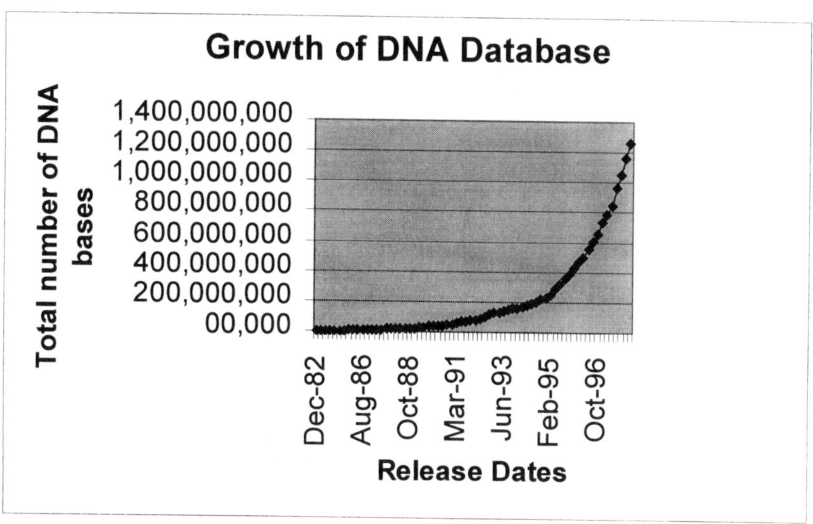

FIGURE 18.1. The great increase in biological sequence information, as evidenced by the number of DNA bases stored in the GENBANK database since inception in 1982.

aged by the NCBI.[14] GENBANK is growing rapidly as genome-sequencing projects feed their data (often in an automated procedure) directly into the database. Figure 18.1 shows the growth of data in GENBANK over the years. Table 18.1 shows a breakdown of organisms and number of bases sequenced within GENBANK. When you look at these impressive numbers, remember that a single human genome has 3 billion bases, and GENBANK contains DNA sequences from all organisms, so there is plenty of sequence information remaining to be determined and entered! GENBANK is still primarily distributed as a formatted flat file (often formatted for the World Wide Web) but can also be accessed in other formats. A GENBANK record contains information about the biological source of the sequence, reference information, and links to other biological databases (Fig. 18.2).

In addition to GENBANK, there are numerous special-purpose DNA databases for which the curators have taken special care to clean, validate, and annotate the data. The work required of such curators indicates the degree to which raw sequence data must be interpreted cautiously. GENBANK can be searched efficiently with a number of algorithms and is usually the first stop for a scientist with a new sequence who wonders "Has a sequence like this ever been observed before? If one has, what is known about it?" There are increasing numbers of stories about scientists using GENBANK to discover unanticipated relationships between DNA sequences, allowing their research programs to leap ahead while taking advantage of information collected on similar sequences.

---

[14]NCBI is part of the National Institutes of Health within the United States; GENBANK is at http://www.ncbi.nlm.nih.gov/Web/GENBANK/index.html.

Table 18.1. A listing of the species represented in GENBANK, release 110.0, December 1998.[a]

Number of entries	Total DNA bases	Species
1,676,931	1,084,135,266	*Homo sapiens*
416,959	200,554,172	*Mus musculus*
76,740	147,625,327	*Caenorhabditis elegans*
71,363	82,625,620	*Arabidopsis thaliana*
67,852	72,625,772	*Drosophila melanogaster*
46,235	28,943,917	*Rattus norvegicus*
10,595	28,693,027	*Saccharomyces cerevisiae*
56,789	28,385,949	*Oryza sativa*
52,126	22,002,992	*Rattus* sp.
4,972	18,095,876	*Escherichia coli*
32,195	16,636,036	*Fugu rubripes*
9,643	12,771,973	*Schizosaccharomyces pombe*
27,231	12,022,500	Human immunodeficiency virus type 1
1,094	9,985,595	*Bacillus subtilis*
4,832	7,969,885	*Plasmodium falciparum*
16,753	6,360,929	*Brugia malayi*
5,465	6,016,056	*Gallus gallus*
700	5,718,781	*Mycobacterium tuberculosis*
8,365	5,134,732	*Dictyostelium discoideum*
12,433	5,076,701	*Emericella nidulans*

[a]The number of gene sequences from each species and the total number of DNA bases in these sequences are as of early 1999. The Homo Sapiens genome has 3,000,000,000 bases of which approximately one-sixth are known. The finished genome sequence is expected around the year 2002 and a "rough draft" was released in mid-2000.

The **protein-sequence databases** contain the sequences of amino acids of proteins. In principle, it should be possible to analyze all the DNA sequences in GENBANK to infer the protein sequences of the genes within the DNA database. The problem, however, of identifying the protein-coding regions within a DNA sequence (in addition to determining the correct strand of DNA, which exists as a sequence and as a reverse-complement sequence, as proposed by Watson and Crick [1953]) is nontrivial, so sequences that have been determined reliably are placed into the special-purpose protein-sequence databases. Swiss-Prot, for example, is managed by Geneva University and the Geneva University Hospital and as of September 1997 contained over 60,000 protein sequences, for a total of over 22 million amino acids.[15] The ability to search the protein-sequence databases is critical, because these databases contain the sequence motifs that are often associated with particular functions.

In addition to looking for long stretches of similarity between two protein sequences (similar sequences usually indicate that the proteins have similar structures and functions), it is also increasingly possible to identify shared

[15]See http://expasy.hcuge.ch/sprot/sprot-top.html.

```
LOCUS       HSPCHYM         786 bp    RNA             PRI       12-JUN-1997
DEFINITION  Homo sapiens mRNA for pancreatic chymotrypsin.
ACCESSION   Y13697
NID         g2196867
KEYWORDS    chymotrypsin.
SOURCE      human.
  ORGANISM  Homo sapiens
            Eukaryotae; mitochondrial eukaryotes; Metazoa; Chordata;
            Vertebrata; Mammalia; Eutheria; Primates; Catarrhini; Hominidae;
            Homo.
REFERENCE   1  (bases 1 to 786)
  AUTHORS   Sziegoleit,A.
  TITLE     A human pancreatic chymotrypsin: biochemical and molecular
            characterization
  JOURNAL   Unpublished
REFERENCE   2  (bases 1 to 786)
  AUTHORS   Sziegoleit,A.
  TITLE     Direct Submission
  JOURNAL   Submitted (10-JUN-1997) A. Sziegoleit, Institute for Medical
            Microbiology, University of Giessen, Frankfurter Strasse 107,
            Giessen, D-35392, FRG
FEATURES             Location/Qualifiers
     source          1..786
                     /organism="Homo sapiens"
                     /db_xref="taxon:9606"
                     /tissue_type="pancreas"
                     /dev_stage="adult"
     exon            <1..759
                     /number=1
     CDS             <1..759
                     /EC_number="3.4.21.1"
                     /codon_start=1
                     /product="chymotrypsin"
                     /db_xref="PID:e321862"
                     /db_xref="PID:g2196868"
                     /translation="CGVPSFPPNLSARVVGGEDARPHSWPWQISLQYLKDDTWRHTCG
                     GTLIASNFVLTAAHCISNTWTYRVAVGKNNLEVEDEEGSLFVGVDTIHVHKRWNALLL
                     RNDIALIKLAEHVELSDTIQVACLPEKDSLLPKDYPCYVTGWGRLWTNGPIADKLQQG
                     LQPVVDHATCSRIDWWGFRVKKTMVCAGGDGVISACNGDSGGPLNCQLENGSWEVFGI
                     VSFGSRRGCNTRKKPVVYTRVSAYIDWINEKMQL"
BASE COUNT      157 a    229 c    249 g    151 t
ORIGIN
        1 tgtggggtgc ccagcttccc gcccaaccta tccgcccgag tggtgggagg agaggatgcc
       61 cggccccaca gctggccctg gcagatctcc ctccagtacc tcaaggacga cacgtggagg
      121 catacgtgtg gcgggacttt gattgctagc aacttcgtcc tcactgccgc ccactgcatc
      181 agcaacacct ggacctaccg tgtggccgtg ggaaagaaca acctggaggt ggaagacgaa
      241 gaaggatccc tgtttgtggg tgtggacacc atccacgtcc acaagagatg gaatgccctc
      301 ctgttgcgca atgatattgc cctcatcaag cttgcagagc atgtggagct gagtgacacc
      361 atccaggtgg cctgcctgcc agagaaggac tccctgctcc ccaaggacta cccctgctat
      421 gtcaccggct gggggcgcct ctggaccaac ggccccattg ctgataagct gcagcagggc
      481 ctgcagcccg tggtggatca cgccacgtgc tccaggattg actggtgggg cttcagggtg
      541 aagaaaacca tggtgtgcgc tgggggcgat ggcgttatct cagcctgcaa tggggactcc
      601 ggtggcccac tgaactgcca gttggagaac ggttcctggg aggtgtttgg catcgtcagc
      661 tttggctccc ggcggggctg caacacccgc aagaagccgg tagtctacac ccgggtgtcc
      721 gcctacatcg actggatcaa cgagaaaatg cagctgtgat ttgttgctgg gagcggcggc
      781 agcgag
//
```

FIGURE 18.2. The GENBANK entry for the digestive enzyme chymotrypsin. Basic information about the original report is provided, as well as some annotations of the key regions in the sequence and the complete sequence of DNA bases (a, g, t, and c). The translated protein sequence is also provided under "translation."

short motifs within sequences that are otherwise markedly different. These motifs often correspond to certain biological functions and can provide valuable information about the activity of a particular protein. The PROSITE database manages information about these sequence motifs,[16] and the BLOCKS database shows how these motifs can be aligned so that their key features can be found.[17]

---

[16]http://www.expasy.ch/sprot/PROSITE.html.

[17]http://blocks.fhcrc.org/.

18.4.2 Structure Databases

Although sequence information is obtained relatively easily, structural information remains expensive on a per-entry basis. The experimental protocols used to determine precise molecular structural coordinates are expensive in time, materials, and person-power. Therefore, we have only a small number of structures for all the molecules characterized in the sequence databases. The two main sources of structural information are the Cambridge Structural Database[18] for small molecules (usually less than 100 atoms) and the PDB[19] for macromolecules (see Section 18.3.1), including proteins and nucleic acids, and combinations of these macromolecules with small molecules (such as drugs, cofactors, and vitamins). The PDB has approximately 10,000 high-resolution structures, but this number is misleading because many of them are small variants on the same structural architecture (Fig. 18.3). If an algorithm is applied to the database to filter out redundant structures, less than 1,000 structures remain.

There are approximately 100,000 proteins in humans, so many structures remain unsolved. In the PDB, each structure is reported with its biological source, reference information, manual annotations of interesting features, and the Cartesian coordinates of each atom within the molecule. Given knowledge of the three-dimensional structure of molecules, the function sometimes becomes clear. For example, the ways in which the medication methotrexate interacts with its biological target have been studied in detail for two decades. Methotrexate is used to treat cancer and rheumatologic diseases, and it is an inhibitor of the protein dihydrofolate reductase, an important molecule for cellular reproduction. The three-dimensional structure of dihydrofolate reductase has been known for many years and has thus allowed detailed studies of the ways in which small molecules, such as methotrexate, interact at an atomic level of detail. As the PDB increases in size, it becomes important to have organizing principles for thinking about biological structure. SCOP[20] provides a classification based on the overall structural features of proteins (see Section 18.2.2). It is a useful method for accessing the entries of the PDB.

18.4.3 Molecular-Disease Databases

One excellent example of a database that may help to bridge the molecular biological databases with those of clinical importance is the Online Mendelian Inheritance in Man (OMIM) database,[21] which is a compilation of known human genes and genetic diseases, along with manual annotations describing the state

[18]http://www.ccdc.cam.ac.uk/.
[19]http://www.pdb.bnl.gov/.
[20]http://scop.mrc-lmb.cam.ac.uk/scop/.
[21]http://www3.ncbi.nlm.nih.gov/omim/.

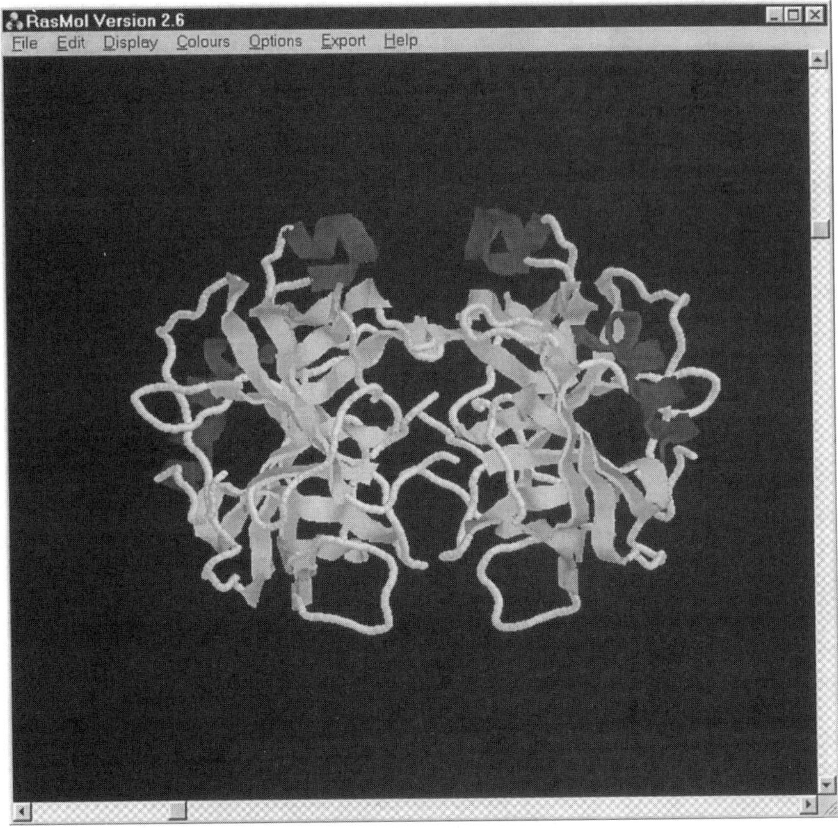

FIGURE 18.3. A stylized diagram of the structure of chymotrypsin, here shown with two identical subunits interacting. The red portion of the protein backbone shows α-helical regions, while the orange portion shows β-strands, and the white denotes connecting coils. The detailed rendering of all the atoms in chymotrypsin would make this view difficult to visualize because of the complexity of the spatial relationships between thousands of atoms.

of our understanding of individual genetic disorders. Each entry contains links to special-purpose databases and thus provides a bridge between clinical syndromes and basic molecular mechanisms (Fig. 18.4).

18.4.4 Key Bioinformatics Algorithms

There are a number of common computations that are performed in many contexts within bioinformatics. In general, these computations can be classified as sequence alignment, structure alignment, pattern analysis of sequence/structure, and pattern analysis of biochemical function.

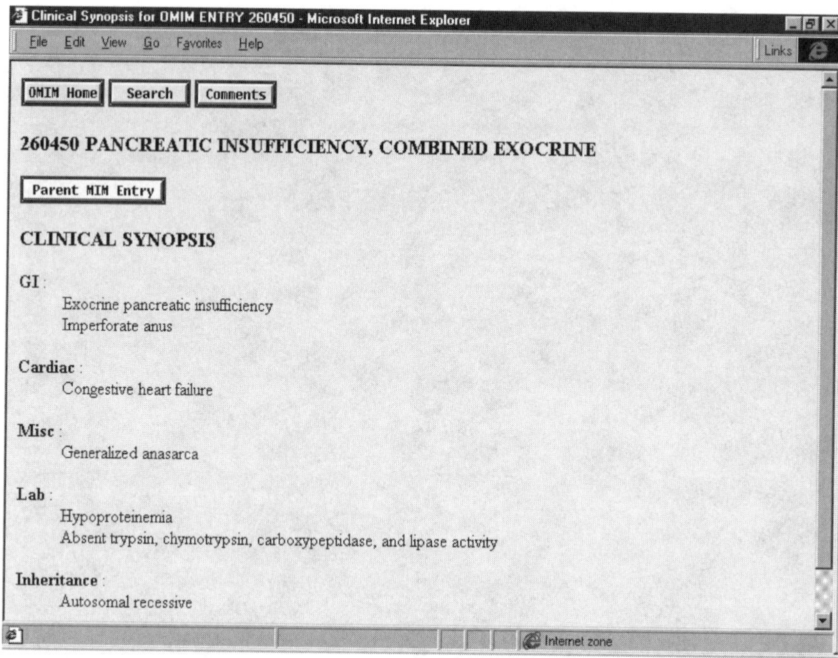

FIGURE 18.4. Screen from the Online Mendelian Inheritance in Man database showing an entry for pancreatic insufficiency, an autosomal recessive disease in which chymotrypsin (GENBANK entry shown in Fig. 18.2) is totally absent (as are some other key digestive enzymes).

Sequence Alignment

Perhaps the most basic activity in computational biology is comparing two biological sequences to determine (1) whether they are similar and (2) how to align them. The problem of alignment is not trivial but is based on a simple idea. Sequences that perform a similar function should, in general, be descendants of a common ancestral sequence, with mutations over time. These mutations can be replacements of one amino acid with another, deletions of amino acids, or insertions of amino acids. The goal of sequence alignment is to align two sequences so that the evolutionary relationship between the sequences becomes clear. If two sequences are descended from the same ancestor and have not mutated too much, then it is often possible to find corresponding locations in each sequence that play the same role in the evolved proteins. The problem of getting correct biological alignments is difficult (because it requires knowledge about the evolution of the molecules that we typically do not have). There are now, however, well-established algorithms for finding the mathematically-optimal alignment of two sequences. These algorithms require the two sequences and a scoring system based on (1) *exact matches* between amino acids that have not mutated in the two sequences and can be aligned perfectly; (2) *partial matches* between amino acids that have mutated in ways that have preserved their overall biophysical properties; and (3) *gaps in the alignment* signifying places where one sequence or the other has undergone a deletion or insertion of amino acids. The algorithms for determining optimal sequence alignments are based on a technique in computer science known as **dynamic programming** and are at the heart of many computational biology applications (Gusfield, 1997).

Unfortunately, the dynamic-programming algorithms are computationally expensive to apply, so a number of faster, more heuristic methods have been developed. The most popular algorithm is the Basic Linear Alignment and Search Technique (BLAST) (Altschul et al., 1990). BLAST is based on the observations that sections of proteins are often conserved without gaps (so the gaps can be ignored—a critical simplification for speed) and that there are statistical analyses of the occurrence of small subsequences within larger sequences that can be used to prune the search for matching sequences in a large database.

Structure Alignment and Docking of Drugs

When scientists investigate biological structure, they most commonly perform a task analogous to sequence alignment, called **structural alignment**. Given two sets of three-dimensional coordinates for a set of atoms, what is the best way to superimpose them so that the similarities and differences between the two structures are clear? Such computations are useful for determining whether two structures share a common ancestry and for understanding how the structures' functions have subsequently been refined during evolution. There are numerous published algorithms for finding good structural alignments. We can apply these algorithms in an automated fashion whenever a new structure is determined, thereby classifying the new structure into one of the protein families (such as those that SCOP maintains).

A related problem is that of using the structure of a large biomolecule and the structure of a small organic molecule (such as a drug or cofactor) to try to predict the ways in which the molecules will interact. An understanding of the structural interaction between a drug and its target molecule often provides critical insight into the drug's mechanism of action. The most reliable way to assess this interaction is to use experimental methods to solve the structure of a drug–target complex. Once again, these experimental approaches are expensive, so computational methods play an important role. Typically, we can assess the physical and chemical features of the drug molecule and can use them to find complementary regions of the target. For example, a highly electronegative drug molecule will be most likely to bind in a pocket of the target that has electropositive features.

Prediction of Structure and Function from Sequence

One of the primary challenges in bioinformatics is taking a newly determined DNA sequence (as well as its translation into a protein sequence) and predicting the structure of the associated molecules, as well as their function. Both problems are difficult, being fraught with all the dangers associated with making predictions without hard experimental data. Nonetheless, the available sequence data are starting to be sufficient to allow good prediction in a few cases. For example, there is a website devoted to the assessment of biological macromolecular structure-prediction methods.[22] Recent results suggest that, when two protein molecules have a high degree (more than 40 percent) of sequence similarity and one of the structures is known, then a reliable model of the other can be built by analogy. In the case that sequence similarity is less than 25 percent, however, performance of these methods is much less reliable.

Prediction of function often relies on use of sequential or structural similarity metrics and subsequent assignment of function based on similarities to molecules of known function. These methods can guess at general function for roughly 60 to 80 percent of all genes, but leave considerable uncertainty about the precise functional details even for those genes for which there are predictions, and have little to say about the remaining genes.

Analysis of Biological Pathways and Understanding of Disease Processes

The basic algorithms for analyzing sequence and structure are now leading to opportunities for more integrated analysis of the pathways in which these molecules participate and ways in which molecules can be manipulated for the purpose of combating disease. A detailed understanding of the role of a particular molecule in the cell requires knowledge of the context—of the other molecules with which it interacts—and of the sequence of chemical transformations that take place in the cell. Thus, major research areas in bioinformatics are elucidating the key pathways by which chemicals are transformed, defining the molecules that catalyze these transformations, identifying the input compounds and the output compounds, and linking these pathways into networks that we can then represent computationally and analyze to understand the significance of a particular molecule.

The ECOCYC project is an example of a computational resource that has comprehensive information about biochemical pathways.[23] ECOCYC is a knowledge base of the metabolic capabilities of *E. coli*; it has a representation of all the enzymes in the *E. coli* genome and of the compounds on which they work. It also links these enzymes to their position on the genome to provide a useful interface into this information. The network of pathways within ECOCYC provides an excellent substrate on which useful applications can be built. They could provide, for example, (1) the ability to guess the function of a new protein by assessing its similarity to *E. coli* genes with a similar sequence, (2) the ability to ask what the affect on an organism would be if a

[22]http://PredictionCenter.llnl.gov/.

[23]http://ECOCYC.pangeasystems.com/ECOCYC/.

critical component of a pathway were removed (would other pathways be used to create the desired function, or would the organism lose a vital function and die?), and (3) the ability to provide a rich user interface to the literature on *E. coli* metabolism.

18.4.5 Web-Based Storage, Search, and Retrieval

A critical technical challenge within bioinformatics is the interconnection of databases. As biological databases have proliferated, researchers have been increasingly interested in linking them to support more complicated requests for information. Some of these links are natural because of the close connection of DNA sequence to protein structure (a straightforward translation). Other links are much more difficult because the semantics of the data items within the databases are fuzzy or because good methods for linking certain types of data simply do not exist. For example, in an ideal world, a protein sequence would be linked to a database containing information about that sequence's function. Unfortunately, although there are databases about protein function, it is not always easy to assign a function to a protein based on sequence information alone, and so the databases are limited by gaps in our understanding of biology. Some excellent recent work in the integration of diverse biological databases has been done in connection with the NCBI Entrez/PubMed systems,[24] the SRS resource,[25] and the Biokleisli project.[26]

18.4.6 Molecular Visualization

Molecular visualization has attracted significant attention from computer scientists because it is one of the serious applications of technologies that are often developed for the purposes of entertainment. The three-dimensional coordinates stored in the PDB are difficult to understand as numbers, but certain features become crystal clear when rendered on a graphics screen. Most fundamentally, the ability to rotate molecules or biological structures gives users great assistance in understanding the structure. In addition, novel algorithms for highlighting regions of structural or functional significance are available to improve the visual analysis of molecular ensembles. They include algorithms for showing simple ball-and-stick models of molecular structure as well as space-filling models that approximate the real volume occupied by proteins. In addition, there are algorithms that define the spatial and electrical "surfaces" of molecules to see how these surfaces might be sensed by small molecules looking for a binding site.

---

[24]http://www.ncbi.nlm.nih.gov/Entrez/ and http://www.ncbi.nlm.nih.gov/PubMed/.

[25]http://www.embl-heidelberg.de/srs/srsc.

[26]http://sdmc.iss.nus.sg/kleisli/kleisli/kleisli.ht ml.

18.5 Future Challenges as Bioinformatics and Clinical Informatics Converge

The human genome sequencing projects will be complete within a decade, and if the only raison d'etre for bioinformatics is to support these projects, then the discipline is not well founded. If, on the other hand, we can identify a set of challenges for the next generations of investigators, then we can more comfortably claim disciplinary status for the field. Fortunately, there is a series of challenges for which the completion of the first human-genome sequence is only the beginning.

18.5.1 Completion of Multiple Human-Genome Sequences

With the first human genome in hand, the possibilities for studying the role of genetics in human disease multiply. A new challenge immediately emerges, however: collecting individual sequence data from patients who have disease. Researchers estimate that more than 99 percent of the DNA sequences within humans are identical, but the remaining sequences are different and account for our variability in susceptability to and development of disease states. It is not unreasonable to expect that, for particular disease syndromes, the detailed genetic information for individual patients will provide valuable information that will allow us to tailor treatment protocols and perhaps let us make more accurate prognoses. There are significant problems associated with obtaining, organizing, analyzing, and using this information.

18.5.2 Linkage of Molecular Information with Symptoms, Signs, and Patients

There is currently a gap in our understanding of disease processes. Although we have a good understanding of the principles by which small groups of molecules interact, we are not able to fully explain how thousands of molecules interact within a cell to create both normal and abnormal physiological states. As the databases continue to accumulate information ranging from patient-specific data to fundamental genetic information, a major challenge is creating the conceptual links between these databases to create an audit trail from molecular-level information to macroscopic phenomena, as manifested in disease. The availability of these links will facilitate the identification of important targets for future research and will provide a scaffold for biomedical knowledge, ensuring that important literature is not lost within the increasing volume of published data.

18.5.3 Computational Representations of the Biomedical Literature

An important opportunity within bioinformatics is the linkage of biological experimental data with the published papers that report them. Electronic publication of the biological literature provides exciting opportunities for making data easily available to scientists. Already, certain types of simple data that are produced in large volumes are expected to be provided with manuscripts, including new sequences that are required to be deposited in GENBANK and new structure coordinates that are deposited in the PDB. There are many other experimental data sources that are currently difficult to provide in a standardized way, however, because the data either are more intricate that those stored in GENBANK or PDB or they are not produced in a volume sufficient to fill a database devoted entirely to the relevant area. Knowledge-base technology can be used, however, to represent multiple types of highly interrelated data.

Knowledge bases can be defined in many ways (see, Chapter 16); for our purposes, we can think of them as databases in which (1) the ratio of the number of tables to the number of entries per table is high compared with usual databases, (2) the individual entries (or records) have unique names, and (3) the values of many fields for one record in the database are the names of other records, thus creating a highly interlinked network of concepts. The structure of knowledge bases often leads to unique strategies for storage and retrieval of their content. To build a knowledge base for storing information from biological experiments, there are some requirements. First, the set of experiments to be modeled must be defined. Second, the key attributes of each experiment that should be recorded in the knowledge base must be specified. Third, the set of legal values for each attribute must be specified, usually by creating a controlled terminology for basic data or by specifying the types of knowledge-based entries that can serve as values within the knowledge base.

The development of such schemes necessitates the creation of terminology standards, just as in clinical informatics. The RiboWeb project is undertaking this task in the domain of RNA biology (Chen et al., 1997). RiboWeb is a collaborative tool for ribosomal modeling, which has at its center a knowledge base of the ribosomal structural literature. RiboWeb links standard bibliographic references to knowledge-base entries that summarize the key experimental findings reported in each paper. For each type of experiment that can be performed, the key attributes must be specified. Thus, for example, a cross-linking experiment is one in which a small molecule with two highly reactive chemical groups is added to an ensemble of other molecules. The reactive groups attach themselves to two vulnerable parts of the ensemble. Because the molecule is small, the two vulnerable areas cannot be any further from each other than the maximum stretched-out length of the small molecule. Thus, an analysis of the resulting reaction gives information that one part of the ensemble is "close" to another part. This experiment can be summarized formally with a few features—for example, *target of experiment*, *cross-linked parts*, and *cross-linking agent*.

The task of creating connections between published literature and basic data is a difficult one because of the need to create formal structures and then to create the necessary content for each published article. The most likely scenario is that biologists will write and submit their papers along with the entries that they propose to add to the knowledge base. Thus, the knowledge base will become an ever-growing communal store of scientific knowledge. Reviewers of the work will examine the knowledge-base elements, perhaps will run a set of automated consistency checks, and will allow the knowledge base to be modified if they deem the paper to be of sufficient scientific merit. RiboWeb in prototype form can be accessed on the World Wide Web.[27]

18.5.4 A Complete Computational Model of Physiology

One of the most exciting goals for computational biology and bioinformatics is the creation of a unified computational model of physiology. Imagine a computer program that provides a comprehensive simulation of a human body. The simulation would be a complex mathematical model in which all the molecular details of each organ system would be represented in sufficient detail to allow complex "what if?" questions to be asked. For example, a new therapeutic agent could be introduced into the system, and its affects on each of the organ subsystems and on their cellular apparatus could be assessed. The side-effect profile, possible toxicities, and perhaps even the efficacy of the agent could be assessed computationally before trials are begun on laboratory animals or human subjects. The model could be linked to visualizations to allow the teaching of medicine at all grade levels to benefit from our detailed understanding of physiological processes—visualizations would be both anatomic (where things are) and functional (what things do). Finally, the model would provide an interface to human genetic and biological knowledge. What more natural user interface could there be for exploring physiology, anatomy, genetics, and biochemistry than the universally recognizable structure of a human that could be browsed at both macroscopic and microscopic levels of detail? As components of interest were found, they could be selected, and the available literature could be made available to the user.

The complete computational model of a human is not close to completion. First, all the participants in the system (the molecules and the ways in which they associate to form higher level aggregates) are not yet identified. Second, the quantitative equations and symbolic relationships that summarize how the systems interact have not been elucidated fully. Third, the computational representations and computer power to run such a simulation are not in place. Researchers are, however, working in each of these areas. The genome projects will soon define all the molecules that constitute each organism. Research in simulation and the new experimental technologies being developed will give us an understanding of how these molecules associate and perform their functions. Finally, research in both clinical informatics and bioinformatics will provide the computational infrastructure required to deliver such technologies.

[27]http://www.smi.stanford.edu/projects/helix/riboweb/.

18.5.5 Conclusion

Bioinformatics is closely allied to clinical informatics. It differs in its emphasis on a reductionist view of biological systems, starting with sequence information and moving to structural and functional information. The emergence of the genome sequencing projects and the new technologies for measuring metabolic processes within cells is beginning to allow bioinformaticians to construct a more synthetic view of biological processes, which will complement the whole-organism, top-down approach of clinical informatics. More importantly, there are technologies that can be shared between bioinformatics and clinical informatics because they both focus on representing, storing, and analyzing biological data. These technologies include the creation and management of standard terminologies and data representations, the integration of heterogeneous databases, the organization and searching of the biomedical literature, the use of machine learning techniques to extract new knowledge, the simulation of biological processes, and the creation of knowledge-based systems to support advanced practitioners in the two fields.

Suggested Readings

Altman R.B., Dunker A.K., Hunter L., Klein, T.E. (1998). *Pacific Symposium on Biocomputing '98*. Singapore: World Scientific Publishing.[28]
The proceedings of one of the principal meetings in bioinformatics, this is an excellent source for up-to-date research reports. Other important meetings include those sponsored by the International Society for Computational Biology (ISCB),[29] Intelligent Systems for Molecular Biology (ISMB),[30] and the RECOMB meetings on computational biology.[31] ISMB and PSB have their proceedings indexed in Medline.

Baldi P., Brunak S. (1998). *Bioinformatics: The Machine Learning Approach*. Cambridge, MA: MIT Press.
This introduction to the field of bioinformatics focuses on the use of statistical and artificial intelligence techniques in machine learning.

Bishop M., Rawlings C. (Eds.) (1997). *DNA and Protein Sequence Analysis—A Practical Approach*. New York: IRL Press at Oxford University Press.
This book provides an introduction to sequence analysis for the interested biologist with limited computing experience.

Durbin R., Eddy R., Krogh A., Mitchison G. (1998). *Biological Sequence Analysis: Probabilistic Models of Proteins and Nucleic Acids*. Cambridge, UK: Cambridge University Press.
This edited volume provides an excellent introduction to the use of probabilistic representations of sequences for the purposes of alignment, multiple alignment, and analysis.

---

[28]http://www.cgl.ucsf.edu/psb/.
[29]http://www.iscb.org/.
[30]http://www-lbit.iro.umontreal.ca/ISMB98/.
[31]http://www.mssm.edu/biomath/recomb98.html.

Gribskov M., Devereux J. (1991). *Sequence Analysis Primer.* New York: Stockton Press.
This primer provides a good introduction to the basic algorithms used in sequence analysis, including dynamic programming for sequence alignment.

Gusfield D. (1997). *Algorithms on Strings, Trees and Sequences: Computer Science and Computational Biology.* Cambridge: Cambridge University Press, 1997.
Gusfield's text provides an excellent introduction to the algorithmics of sequence and string analysis, with special attention paid to biological sequence analysis problems.

Hunter L. (1993). *Artificial Intelligence and Molecular Biology.* Menlo Park, CA: AAAI Press/MIT Press.
This volume shows a variety of ways in which artificial intelligence techniques have been used to solve problems in biology.

Salzberg S., Searls D., Kasif S. (Eds.) (1998). *Computational Methods in Molecular Biology.* New York: Elsevier Science.
This volume offers a useful collection of recent work in bioinformatics.

Setubal J., Medianis J. (1997). *Introduction to Computational Molecular Biology.* Boston: PWS Publishing Company.
Another introduction to bioinformatics, this text was written for computer scientists.

Stryer L. (1995). *Biochemistry.* New York: W.H. Freeman.
The textbook by Stryer is well written, is illustrated, and is updated on a regular basis. It provides an excellent introduction to basic molecular biology and biochemistry.

Questions for Discussion

1. In what ways will bioinformatics and medical informatics interact in the future? Will the research agendas of the two fields merge, or will they always remain separable?
2. Will the introduction of DNA and protein-sequence information change the way that medical records are managed in the future? Which types of systems will be most affected (laboratory, radiology, admission and discharge, financial, order entry)?
3. It has been postulated that clinical informatics and bioinformatics are working on the same problems, but in some areas one field has made more progress than the other. Identify three common themes. Describe how the issues are approached by each subdiscipline.
4. Why should an awareness of bioinformatics be expected of clinical informatics professionals? Should a chapter on bioinformatics appear in a clinical informatics textbook? Explain your answers.
5. One major problem with introducing computers into clinical medicine is the extreme time and resource pressure placed on physicians and other health-care workers. Will the same problems arise in basic biomedical research?
6. Why have biologists and bioinformaticians embraced the World Wide Web as a vehicle for disseminating data so quickly, whereas clinicians and clinical informaticians have been more hesitant to put their primary data on-line?

Unit III
Medical Informatics in the Years Ahead

19 Health Care and Information Technology: Growing Up Together

SARA J. SINGER, ALAIN C. ENTHOVEN, AND ALAN M. GARBER

After reading this chapter, you should know the answers to these questions:

- How did healthcare insurance contribute to rapid growth in healthcare spending during the 1970s through the 1980s? How has health insurance evolved in the past decade?
- How has healthcare financing influenced the development of healthcare information technology?
- What are health-maintenance organizations, prepaid group practices, preferred-provider organizations, point-of-service plans, and physician-hospital organizations? How do these groups provide incentives to reduce healthcare costs?
- How have employers and managed-care organizations acted to improve healthcare quality and to reduce healthcare spending?
- How have changes in fiscal designs and incentives affected the development and adoption of healthcare information technology?
- How can healthcare information systems help healthcare institutions to respond to the changing financial environment?

19.1 Introduction

Why is a chapter on healthcare financing and delivery included in a book about computer applications in medicine? In much the same way that financing is an important factor in determining the organization of healthcare delivery in general, financing may be the single most important driver of developments in the field of healthcare information.

Fiscal issues have become increasingly important to the study of medical informatics, with growing pressures on hospitals and other healthcare providers to deliver care more efficiently, to generate and use information more effectively, and to deal optimally with a complex array of reimbursement schemes. Information technology has become an essential part of these functions, and new approaches to collecting and using data and to providing information will have a profound effect on the ability of the healthcare community to respond to this increasingly challenging financial environment.

In this chapter, we provide an overview of the U.S. healthcare economy and describe how healthcare institutions are reimbursed for the services that they provide. We describe how the public and private healthcare financing and delivery systems have evolved from an era of open-ended spending through the decades of the 1980s and 1990s to an era of accountability and its current organizational forms. The remainder of the chapter explores the relationships among healthcare finance, healthcare delivery, and healthcare information technology. We address the implications of changes in healthcare financing on healthcare information technology and how these changes have affected both its introduction and its use. We also examine the implications of new information technology for healthcare delivery, management, and administrative functions and conclude by acknowledging the challenges healthcare organizations face in implementing and capturing value from technological innovation.

19.2 The Era of Open-Ended Spending

The period from 1960 to 1980 can be characterized as the era of open-ended financing in health care. During those two decades, national healthcare spending increased from about $27 billion to nearly $250 billion (Table 19.1A), from 5.1 percent of the gross domestic product (GDP) to 8.9 percent (Table 19.1A). Public-sector spending on health care increased from $6.6 billion to $104.8 billion. Aggregate private healthcare insurance premiums increased from $1.2 billion to $11.8 billion. In this section, we consider the ways in which patients managed to pay for their care as costs soared dramatically during the 20-year period.

19.2.1 Private (Employer-Paid) Healthcare Insurance

Although the antecedents to modern health insurance began in the nineteenth century, and several formative decisions were made in the 1930s, health insurance in the United States did not become a large-scale enterprise until World War II. About 12 million people had insurance for healthcare expenses in 1940; nearly 77 million had insurance by 1950 (Fig. 19.1) (Health Insurance Associa-

TABLE 19.1A. National health expenditures (in billions) by year.[a]

Spending category	1960	1970	1980	1990	1994	1995	1996	1997	1998
National health expenditures	26.9	73.2	247.2	699.4	937.1	988.5	1039.4	1088.2	1149.1
Public	6.6	27.7	104.8	283.2	419.9	456.4	480.4	502.2	522.7
Private	20.2	45.5	142.5	416.2	517.2	532.1	559.0	586.0	626.4
Cost of private health insurance	1.2	2.7	11.9	40.5	50.6	47.7	52.1	50.3	57.7

TABLE 19.1B. National health expenditures (NHE) as a percentage of the gross domestic product (GDP)

Spending category	1960	1970	1980	1990	1994	1995	1996	1997	1998
NHE as %GDP	5.1%	7.1%	8.9%	12.2%	13.5%	13.7%	13.6%	13.4%	13.5%
Average annual % change in NHE	—	10.6%	12.9%	11.0%	5.1%	7.3%	4.6%	4.7%	5.6%
GDP	$527	$1,036	$2,784	$5,744	$6,936	$7,270	$7,662	$8,111	$8,511
Average annual % change in GDP	—	7.0%	10.4%	7.5%	5.8%	4.8%	5.4%	5.9%	4.9%

[a]Table 19.1 tracks the dramatic growth of national health expenditures and its relationship to the growth in the gross domestic product.

Source: HCFA Office of the Actuary: National Health Statistics. Levit, K. (2000). Health spending. In 1998: Signals of Change, *Health Affairs*, January/February 2000.

tion of America, 1983). Most were insured through their employers. Several trends encouraged this development. Collective bargaining was an important factor, as union leaders considered employer-paid health insurance to be an attractive bargaining prize. Employers of nonunionized personnel also generally were willing to provide insurance because they wished to avoid grievances that would encourage unionization. Perhaps the most influential factor was that employer-paid health insurance was excluded from the taxable incomes of employees; thus, health insurance was a form of tax-free compensation. Health insurance as a fringe benefit continued to grow rapidly in the 1950s. In 1959, legislation was enacted to cover all federal employees. By 1960, about 123 million people were covered, at least for hospital expenses.

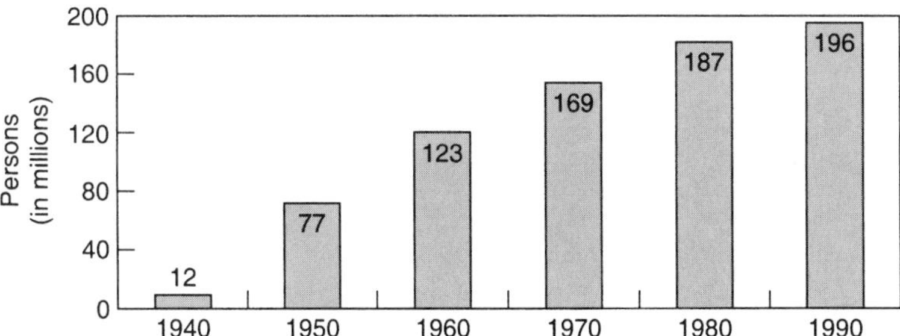

FIGURE 19.1. Persons with private health insurance coverage. Health insurance, through a variety of favorable incentives, became widespread after World War II. (*Source*: Health Insurance Association of America.)

During this period, health insurance generally was of two types. Commercial insurance companies offered **indemnity insurance**, modeled on casualty insurance. The typical form was payment of a specified amount for a hospital day or for each of a list of surgical procedures. Commercial insurance companies had no contractual link to providers. Their role was to indemnify patients for medical expenses as part of a package that included group life and disability insurance. As time went by, coverage became more comprehensive. Frequently, it was backed up by **major medical insurance** that paid 80 percent of all the patient's outlays after the patient had paid a specified amount or **deductible**.

The other type of health insurance was called **service benefit**, offered by Blue Cross and Blue Shield. Blue Cross plans were independent local nonprofit insurance companies sponsored by hospital associations. Blue Shield plans were sponsored by medical societies. These organizations were created to ensure that the providers would be paid in the manner most acceptable to those providers—that is, they could choose to be paid through cost reimbursement or through payment of billed charges to hospitals and fee-for-service payment to physicians. Most hospitals and physicians participated in Blue Cross and Blue Shield (the "Blues"). In the former case, participation usually meant that hospitals would give Blue Cross a discount from the fees charged for patients who were insured by other carriers. In the latter case, it usually meant agreement to accept Blue Shield fees as payment in full.

These insurance systems share certain features. First, they reimburse physicians for services based on **usual, customary, and reasonable fees**. They pay hospitals on the basis of billed charges or of retrospective cost reimbursement. Thus, they assign providers no responsibility for the total cost of care. They do not create incentives to analyze or control costs. On the contrary, they pay providers more for doing more whether or not more is necessary or beneficial to the patient. If outlays exceed premium revenues, future premiums are raised to make up the difference. Second, these insurance systems were based on the principle that at all times the patient must have free choice of provider. It was even against the law for the insurer to influence the patient's choice of provider. In such an arrangement, the insurer has no bargaining power with providers and thus no way to control prices or costs. Third, these financing systems generally covered entire employee groups. They were not conceived as competitors in situations in which individual employees would have a choice among healthcare-financing plans.

During the era of open-ended spending, the number of persons covered and the scope of private health-insurance coverage increased markedly. The number of people with private insurance protection increased from 123 million in 1960 to 187 million by 1980 (Health Insurance Association of America, 1983) (Fig. 19.1). This increase was encouraged by federal and state tax laws. The inflation that started in the late 1960s and intensified in the 1970s pushed people into higher and higher income-tax brackets. As this shift occurred, it became increasingly advantageous for employers and employees to agree that an employer would pay for comprehensive health insurance with before-tax dollars rather than paying the same amount in cash to employees and letting them pay for the insurance with net after tax dollars.

By 1980, the average taxpayer was in about the 40 percent marginal tax bracket, counting both income and payroll taxes. That is, of the final dollar earned by an average taxpayer, about 40 percent went to federal and state income and payroll taxes. In 1981, this tax subsidy for health insurance (in which employers used nontaxed dollars to purchase insurance for employees) cost the federal government about $20 billion in foregone tax revenues (Fig. 19.2) (Ginsburg, 1982). The same subsidy continues today and was calculated to reduce federal income and payroll tax revenues by $85 billion in 1997 (Congressional Budget Office, 1996).

In the 1970s, high interest rates made it more advantageous for large employers to self-insure. Instead of paying a premium to an insurance company that would keep the money for perhaps 3 or 4 months before paying the bills, a growing number of large employers decided to pay their employees' medical bills directly, to hire insurance companies to perform claims processing or **administrative services only** (ASO), and perhaps to buy insurance for only truly catastrophic cases. Under the Employee Retirement Income Security Act of 1974 (ERISA), these **self-insured plans** were also exempted from state regulation of insurance, which could be cumbersome and expensive. In effect, being self-insured means the employer takes on the health insurance function and risk directly. Although most practical for large employers, the availability of reinsurance or **stop-loss coverage**, which shifts the risk of a catastrophic case to an insurance company, has made it possible for small employers to self-insure as well. By 1998, about 68 percent of all employers, including 55 percent of firms with between 500 and 1,000 employees, self-insured their indemnity coverage (Mercer/Foster Higgins, 1998) (Fig. 19.3).

The most important exception to the private-sector, fee-for-service system of healthcare finance was **prepaid group practice**, in which members paid an annual fee set in advance and received comprehensive healthcare during the year.

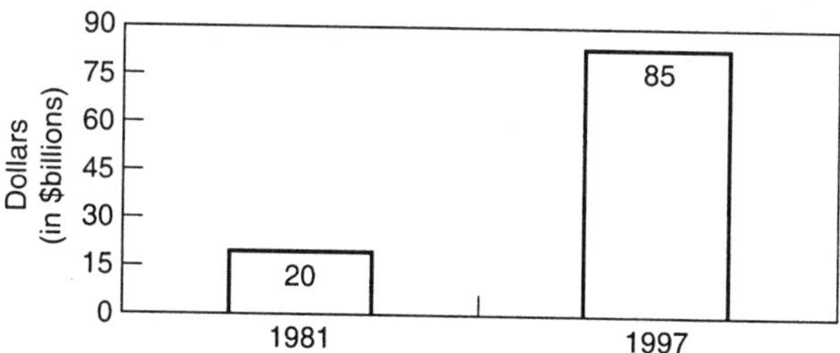

FIGURE 19.2. Foregone federal tax revenue. By allowing employers to purchase tax-free health insurance, the government foregoes billions of dollars in tax revenues. (*Source*: Ginsburg P. [1982]. *Containing Medical Care Costs through Market Forces* and Congressional Budget Office [1996] *Reducing the Deficit: Spending and Revenue Options*.)

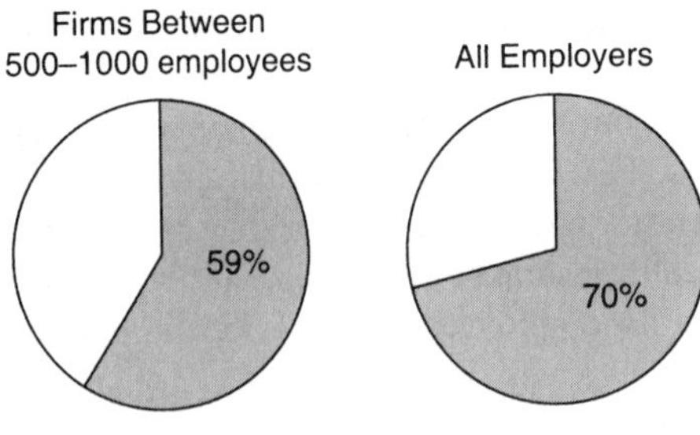

Figure 19.3. Percentage of firms that were self-insured in 1995. To realize the benefits from interest accrued on insurance premiums rather than handing it over to insurance companies and to avoid state regulation, many employers choose to self-insure. (*Source*: A. Foster Higgins & Co. [1997]. *Foster Higgins National Survey of Employer-Sponsored Health Plans*.)

In 1960, membership in prepaid group-practice plans was small (about 1 million nationwide). The plans' importance lay in the concepts on which they were based. Kaiser Permanente, the largest and most successful of these organizations, adopted the following principles (Somers, 1971):

- Multispecialty group practice
- Integrated inpatient and outpatient facilities
- Direct prepayment to the medical-care organization
- Reversal of economics: Providers are better off if the patients remain well or have their medical problems solved promptly
- Voluntary enrollment: Every enrollee should have a choice among competing alternatives
- Physician responsibility for quality and cost of care

The principle of voluntary enrollment was the beginning of the competition among healthcare financing and delivery plans that became widespread by the mid-1980s. Direct prepayment could reflect the overall efficiency of the provider organization, as well as the health risks and problems present in the enrolled population. Direct prepayment implies a reversal of the economic incentives in the fee-for-service system, such that doctors prosper by keeping patients healthy and by diagnosing and solving their patients' medical problems promptly and effectively. Tertiary care (e.g., open heart surgery and organ transplants, which are usually done in regional referral centers), seen as a major profit center in the traditional system, became a cost center. Under the traditional paradigm, filled beds were an indicator of success; under the new paradigm, it was better to minimize hospital utilization. In theory, direct prepayment holds providers accountable for costs and for the costs of poor quality. If a procedure is done poorly and leads to complications and the need for more treatment, providers, rather than insurers or patients, pay the extra costs.

19.2.2 Public-Sector Insurance

In 1965, Congress enacted the Medicare and Medicaid programs, Titles XVIII and XIX of the Social Security Act. **Medicare** is the federal program of hospital and medical insurance for Social Security retirees. In 1972, legislation added coverage for the long-term disabled and for patients suffering from chronic renal failure. By 1980, Medicare covered 25.5 million aged and 3 million disabled persons (Fig. 19.4).

Medicare was based on the same principles of payment as were Blue Cross and Blue Shield (reimbursement of reasonable cost to hospitals and fees to physicians). Patients were given unlimited free choice of provider, so a Medicare beneficiary received no financial advantage from going to a less costly hospital. The Medicare law did provide for certain deductibles and co-insurance to be paid by the patient who was receiving services. For example, under the 1997 Medicare system, the hospitalized patient is charged a deductible that approximates 1 day's cost at the average hospital's per diem rate. After an annual deductible, Medicare pays 80 percent of the doctor's usual and customary fee; the patient is responsible for the rest. The **co-insurance** is the remaining 20 percent that the Medicare beneficiary is responsible for paying. However, any cost consciousness that cost sharing might encourage is attenuated, because about 66 percent of Medicare beneficiaries purchase private supplemental insurance that helps to pay the co-insurance and deductibles. Another 9 percent have resources that place them below the federally defined poverty level and thus are jointly covered by Medicaid, which has no co-insurance and deductibles. Four percent receive supplemental coverage through the Defense and Veterans' Affairs Departments' programs (CHAMPUS and VA) and thus also have full coverage (Employee Benefit Research Institute, 1995). Thus, about 80 percent of elderly Americans have supplemental insurance that offsets or removes the cost sensitivity intended by the cost-sharing features of Medicare.

Medicaid is a program of federal grants to help states pay for the medical care of welfare recipients and of other people who resemble welfare recipients (people in welfare categories, above the welfare income line). Only about one-half of the population below the poverty line is covered by Medicaid. For example, care for *medically indigent adults* has remained the responsibility of local—usu-

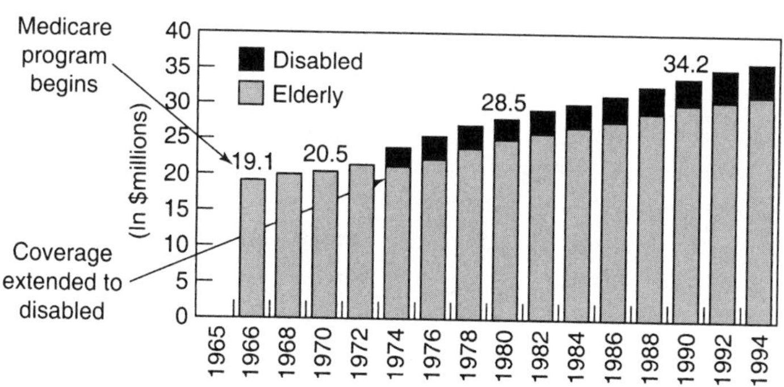

FIGURE 19.4. Growth of Medicare enrollment. With the enactment of the Medicare program, elderly Americans were ensured access to health care. (*Source*: Enthoven A.C. [1997]. *Market Based Reform of US Health Care Financing and Delivery.*)

ally county—governments. Under Medicaid, the federal government set elaborate standards that a state program must meet to be eligible for federal subsidies. The federal government pays a share of the cost (minimum 50 percent; average 55 percent), depending on the state's per capita income. Like Medicare, Medicaid was based on the principles of fee for service, cost reimbursement, and free choice of provider. Many physicians, however, choose not to participate in Medicaid because reimbursement is low.

In an effort to slow the growth of federal and state healthcare outlays for Medicare and Medicaid, the federal government imposed numerous regulatory restraints during the 1970s, with little success. Examples include institution of reimbursement limits on daily routine hospital care, creation of local nonprofit physicians' organizations called Professional Standards Review Organizations (PSROs) to review use of Medicare and Medicaid services and to deny payment for unnecessary services, and tying of the growth in reimbursable physician fees to an index of wages. These restraints were ineffective; Medicare and Medicaid outlays grew by about 17 percent per year through the 1970s.

19.3 Cost Growth and Strategies for Reform in the 1980s and 1990s

The cost-increasing incentives in the fee-for-service model, fueled by information and medical technology, continued to increase the costs of health care in the 1980s at rates faster than inflation. National health expenditures increased as a percentage of GDP from 8.9 percent to 12.2 percent, from $247.2 billion in 1980 to $699.4 billion in 1990—an average annual increase of 11 percent (see Table 19.1). Private-sector spending on health care increased from $142.5 to $416.2 billion, and public-sector spending increased from nearly $105 billion to $283.2 billion. From 1980 to 1990, Medicare outlays grew from $37.5 billion to $111.5 billion, or 11.5 percent per year (Table 19.2). Medicaid outlays grew from $26.1 billion to $75.4 billion, or 11.2 percent per year between 1980 and 1990. By comparison, the GDP grew about 7.5 percent per year between 1980 and 1990.

Despite the similarities in the problems they faced, the public and private sectors responded differently. Legislators attempted to control spending in the Medicare and Medicaid programs by making changes to the existing programs but leaving their fee-for-service incentives intact, whereas private-sector purchasers more willingly embraced the logic of the incentives inherent in the prepaid group-practice model.

19.3.1 Public-Sector Reform

Fiscal pressures in the early 1980s led to a great deal of legislative activity, the general thrust of which was to change the government's commitment from open-ended, cost-unconscious retrospective payment to limited, cost-conscious prospec-

TABLE 19.2. Medicare and Medicaid expenditures aggregate (in billions) by year.[a]

Spending category	1960	1970	1980	1990	1994	1995	1996	1997	1998
Medicare	—	7.7	37.5	111.5	166.9	185.3	199.4	211.3	216.6
Average annual % change in Medicare	—	—	17.2%	11.5%	11.2%	10.7%	7.6%	6.0%	2.5%
Medicaid	—	5.4	26.1	75.4	123.4	146.2	154.1	160.0	170.6
Average annual % change in Medicaid	—	—	17.1%	11.2%	7.7%	14.2%	3.8%	4.6%	6.6%
Average annual % change in GDP	—	7.0%	10.4%	7.5%	5.8%	4.8%	5.4%	5.9%	4.9%

[a]Medicare and Medicaid expenditures continue to grow faster than the gross domestic product (GDP). (*Source*: HCFA Office of the Actuary: National Health Statistics Group. Levit, K. (2000). Health Spending in 1998: Signals of Change. *Health Affairs*, January/February 2000.

tive payment. There was also a move from free choice of provider toward limited choice of provider, with limitations based on cost. These efforts, however, were not generally successful.

The Omnibus Budget Reconciliation Act of 1981 (OBRA 81) included many changes in Medicare and Medicaid. Two changes in Medicaid were particularly significant. First, federal matching payments to each state were reduced. States could avoid part of these reductions if they took certain actions to control costs. Second, Congress granted states more discretion in changing the features of their Medicaid programs to control costs. In particular, the law provided that the Secretary of Health and Human Services (HHS) could waive the provision for freedom of choice of provider in the Medicaid law and could thus allow states to engage in selective provider contracting. This flexibility led certain states, such as California, to enact legislation to require their Medicaid programs to contract selectively on the basis of price and to seek competitive bids from hospitals.

The Tax Equity and Fiscal Responsibility Act of 1982 (TEFRA) put two new constraints on the all-inclusive cost per case for Medicare. First, it placed a limit on total inpatient operating costs, applied on a cost-per-case basis, adjusted for each hospital's severity of case mix. Second, it placed a new limit on each hospital's rate of increase in cost per case, based on an index of the wages and prices that hospitals pay. The same law provided that Medicare could contract with health maintenance organizations or with other "competitive medical plans" to care for Medicare beneficiaries. Medicare paid these plans on the basis of a fixed prospective per capita payment equal to 95 percent of the adjusted average per capita cost to Medicare of similar patients who remained with fee-for-service providers.

In the Social Security Amendments of 1983, Congress enacted the **prospective payment system** (PPS) for Medicare inpatient cases. Under PPS, Medicare pays hospitals a uniform national fixed payment per case based on about 468 **diagnosis-related groups** (DRGs), adjusted for area hospital wage levels. The DRG classification system was derived empirically; diagnoses were assigned to a group based on major diagnostic category, secondary diagnosis, surgical procedure, age, and types of services required. The DRG classification system was intended to produce homogeneous groups from the point of view of resource use. Within each DRG, the average length of stay was expected to be similar. The PPS created hospital responsibility for effectively integrating the pieces of the inpatient-care process and powerful incentives to reduce the cost of inpatient cases. The PPS thus successfully slowed the growth of cost of inpatient services, but its introduction was followed by a rapid acceleration in the growth of outpatient services and, later on, home health agency services.

In the Omnibus Budget Reconciliation Act of 1989 (OBRA 89), Congress embarked on the **Resource-Based Relative Value Scale** (RBRVS) and **Volume Performance Standard** (VPS) systems for paying for Medicare physicians' services. RBRVS was intended to correct the large inequities and perverse incentives in Medicare's **"customary, prevailing, and reasonable"** (CPR) payment system. Medicare's CPR payment system reimbursed practitioners generously for doing procedures but poorly for providing cognitive services such as history taking and advice giving. RBRVS was intended to produce relative prices for physicians' services that approximated what would exist in an effective market system—that is, prices proportional to marginal costs. The intention of RBRVS was to diminish the incentives that providers had to perform expensive procedures. VPS was intended to control volume but may have instead motivated an increase in physician services as doctors sought to protect their real incomes in the face of controlled prices and a surplus of doctors.

The legislative changes in the 1980s did little to stem growth in the overall costs of Medicare and Medicaid. From 1990 to 1995, Medicare expenditures continued to grow at 10.7 percent—almost the same rate as the previous decade—to $185.3 billion. Medicaid outlays increased faster than they had in the 1980s, by 14.2 percent during 1990 and 1995, to $146.2 billion by 1995. In contrast, the GDP slowed during this period, growing by only 4.8 percent per year (see Table 19.2).

19.3.2 Private-Sector Reform

Pressure for changes in the private sector intensified as costs increased. Rather than trying to improve on the inherently flawed incentives intrinsic in the existing fee-for-service model, the private sector turned to managed care for cost relief.

Managed care is a complex bundle of innovative solutions to the problems that characterized the traditional fee-for-service system. The essential principles of managed care follow. There is great variation among individual managed-care organizations in the extent to and success with which these principles are applied in practice:

- *Selective provider contracting.* Insurers can select providers for quality and economy. Quality is important because people demand high quality of care; employers care about the health and satisfaction of their employees (if they do not, their trade unions are likely to care); because insurers care about their reputations; and because mistakes cost money. Historically, quality and economy have often gone hand in hand. Providers are also chosen for their willingness to cooperate with the managed-care organization's quality and utilization-management programs and reporting requirements.
- *Utilization management.* This principle varies from the crude to the sophisticated. For example, some managed-care organizations have retained actuarial consulting firms to develop guidelines for how long various types of patients should be hospitalized, and these guidelines are translated into limits on what the insurance will pay. Many employ **primary-care gatekeepers**—primary-care physicians who control referrals to specialists. Many managed-care organizations dealing with doctors from the fee-for-service sector who are thought to be overutilizers require prior authorization before a patient with a non-emergent problem can be hospitalized. An insurance contract may include, for example, a $200 deductible for hospitalizations, waived if the patient obtains authorization. Some managed-care organizations employ concurrent review, whereby utilization-management professionals check regularly on the hospital inpatient's condition and plan prompt discharges.

  The more advanced form of utilization management is based on the recognition that medical uncertainty is often great and practice variations are wide. Teams of physicians study particular medical conditions, review the medical literature, analyze and study their own data, and develop recommended practice guidelines based on professional consensus within the team. Typically, the guidelines reflect the least costly way of achieving the best obtainable outcomes.
- *Negotiated payment.* The basic idea of negotiated payment is to trade higher patient volume for lower prices. Compared with the usual and customary fees in the fee-for-service system, managed-care organizations typically obtain discounts in the range of 20 to 40 percent. These negotiated payments often include some bundling of services—for example, all-inclusive payments per inpatient day (for different types of patient) or per inpatient hospital case.
- *Quality management.* For example, a managed care organization is likely to survey patient satisfaction and to reward with bonuses those providers who score well. Providers who score poorly may not be offered a renewal of their contracts. Sophisticated organizations attempt to measure outcomes of care, or performance of processes of care, and report these measurements to consumers and purchasers.

In some communities, prepaid group practices, such as Kaiser Permanente, were successful and growing. The term **health maintenance organization** (HMO) was coined in 1970 by Paul Ellwood to describe prepaid group practices, which are the earliest form of managed care (Ellwood et al., 1971).

In general, an HMO is an health-insurance carrier that covers a comprehensive list of healthcare services: physician, hospital, laboratory, diagnostic imaging, and usually prescription drugs. The coverage provides for nominal co-payments at the point-of-service (e.g., $10 per doctor office visit), but there is no deductible and in general, no limit on the amount that the HMO will pay. Co-payments are not supposed to be so large as to constitute a barrier to care.

Health maintenance organizations contract with employers and individual subscribers on the basis of per capita prepayment. In this contract, the HMO bears the full risk for the cost of medical care. The amount and type of risk sharing that the HMO then arranges with providers varies widely, but usually the HMO shares some risk, explicitly or implicitly. An explicit risk-sharing arrangement might be a contract with a medical group to provide all necessary professional services for a fixed per capita payment. An implicit risk-sharing arrangement might pay individual doctors on a discounted fee-for-service basis, but the HMO would then keep track of the per patient costs of each doctor, adjusted for age, gender, and possibly diagnosis; doctors whose costs consistently exceed norms might receive extra counseling on practice patterns or might not have their contracts renewed (Table 19.3).

Originally, HMOs were of several types. **Group-model HMOs** are based on contracts between physicians organized in a medical group and the HMO. The medical group accepts risks of costs of care and usually rewards the partners if the group is successful in managing costs. **Staff-model HMOs**, in contrast, retain doctors on staff and pay them as salaried employees. Although the two are usually considered to be substantially similar organizational forms, there is an important difference. The doctors in group-model HMOs are more likely to see themselves as part owners of the enterprise and to feel more responsible for its success. Both types attempt to organize comprehensive care systems. Their doctors care exclusively for patients enrolled in their affiliated health-insurance plan. They generally care for patients in HMO-owned or HMO-leased facilities.

Doctors in fee-for-service solo practice, feeling competitive pressure from prepaid group practices, formed **individual practice associations** (IPAs), also known as **network-model HMOs**, through which they could offer patients the financial equivalent of the prepaid group practices. Independent medical group practices and individual doctors generally contract with several insurance carrier IPA HMOs to see the patients enrolled with those carriers while also continuing

Table 19.3. Comparisons between fee-for-service and managed care.[a]

Fee-for-service	Managed care
• Providers are paid a fee for each service provided	• Providers are paid a fixed payment per member per month
• Potential incentive for unnecessary services	• Potential incentive for underprovision of services
• Patients see any provider	• Patients see selected providers
• Little or no quality or utilization management	• Features quality and utilization management

[a] Managed care constitutes a reversal of the economic incentives in fee-for-service insurance.

to see patients enrolled in traditional insurance, Medicare, Medicaid, or other or no coverage. The doctors continue to practice in their own offices. The medical groups are paid on a per capita basis for professional services under contracts that include incentives for efficient hospital use. A typical contract might provide a fixed-dollar monthly amount per enrolled person for professional services plus a risk-sharing arrangement for hospital costs. Individual doctors are paid negotiated fees for services, with incentives for economical behavior, and are usually monitored for the economy of their practice patterns. A typical contract might pay primary-care doctors 80 percent of their fees soon after delivery of services, with the other 20 percent withheld to be sure that there is enough money in the pool. At the end of the year, the doctors are paid in proportion to their billings if there is money left over. In addition, the pool of primary-care doctors may share in the savings from efficient specialist referrals and hospital use.

In response to the early development and acceptance of HMOs, in 1973 Congress passed the Health Maintenance Organizations (HMO) Act. The HMO Act (1) defined HMOs as being of either the group practice or the individual practice variety; (2) provided grants and loans to help start nonprofit HMOs; and (3) required that all employers of 25 or more employees, subject to the Fair Labor Standards Act, who were offering traditional insurance also offer to their employees the choice of one group-practice and one individual-practice HMO as alternatives to traditional health insurance if such HMOs served the areas where their employees lived and asked to be offered; and (4) overruled state laws that inhibited HMO growth.

The HMO Act had an important effect in opening up the market to competition. These provisions also helped to expand access to HMOs and thus the number of HMOs. By 1978, there were 7.3 million members in 195 operating HMOs. At that time, the HMO industry was made up almost entirely of local nonprofit HMOs and of Kaiser Permanente, which was then a large national organization serving 3.5 million enrollees in six states—a multistate or national HMO. By 1995, 35 national HMO firms with 385 branches served 42.7 million of the industry's 53.8 million enrollees (Table 19.4). Since 1978, HMO annual enrollment growth has exceeded 12.5 percent. Analysts expect continued 12 to 13 percent annual growth in the near term (Abramowitz, 1996).

Some employers wanted to be able to offer employees health insurance based on selective provider contracting—that is, insurance that resembled the traditional model except that employees would be offered preferential terms of coverage if they would use contracting providers. Then, employers and insurers would be able to negotiate prices and utilization controls with providers. Until 1982, however, in compliance with the principle of free choice of independently practicing providers, this kind of insurance was illegal under the insurance codes in most states. In 1982, a major legislative battle erupted in California. Employers, insurers, and labor unions teamed up to defeat the California Medical Association and to secure the enactment of new legislation permitting insurers to contract selectively and to pass on the savings to the insured. Most other states

Table 19.4. Health maintenance organization growth: local and national firms by year.[a]

	1978	1985	1995
HMOs			
Local	183	298	192
Branches of national	12	187	385
Total	195	485	577
Members (millions)			
Local	3.7	10.1	11.0
Branches of national	3.6	10.9	42.7
Total	7.3	21.0	53.8
Members by model type			
Staff	—	3.0	8.0
IPA	0.6	6.4	22.1
Network	—	5.0	3.3
Group	6.7	6.6	9.1
Mixed	—	—	18.1
Members by tax status			
Nonprofit	—	13.6	22.1
For-profit	—	7.4	31.2

[a]Both the number of and enrollment in HMOs have grown rapidly since 1978.
Source: Enthoven A.C. (1997). *Market based reform of US health care financing and delivery: Managed care and managed competition.*

followed. Thus, the states authorized **preferred provider insurance** (PPI), another form of managed care.

Preferred provider insurance represents less change from the traditional fee-for-service model than do HMOs. Some people use the term **preferred provider organization** (PPO) to parallel the better-established term "HMO." These entities are not, however, medical-care organizations; they are insurance companies that contract with large numbers of providers that are not otherwise related to one another (Boland, 1985).

The typical preferred-provider insurer contracts with a large number of doctors, hospitals, laboratories, home-health agencies, and so on. It creates incentives for insured patients to choose contracting providers. For example, the insurance contract might pay in full the negotiated fee for the services of contracting providers but pay only 80 percent of what it would have paid contracting providers for the services of noncontracting providers, with the patient liable to pay the rest. The insurer negotiates discounted fees, and the provider agrees to accept those fees as payment in full from contracting patients; that is, providers agree to no *balance billing*. Finally, the insurer adopts utilization-management tools, such as prior authorization for hospital admissions, length-of-stay guidelines, and review of provider credentials.

Some preferred-provider insurers cover comprehensive healthcare services. Others specialize, carving out a subset of comprehensive services, such as mental health, pharmacy, cardiology, or radiology. They serve as subcontractors to insurers that cover comprehensive services. They can offer greater detailed knowledge of their particular specialty. They may also contract with several insurers that cover comprehensive care and subcontract the components.

Health maintenance organization providers differ from contracting PPI providers in that the former bear the financial risk associated with members' use of services, whereas the latter do not. The HMO agrees to provide all necessary services for a comprehensive per capita payment set in advance, independent of the number of services actually used. Contracting PPI providers do not suffer financially if the use of services increases, and they are not directly rewarded for reducing the use of services or for treating patients in less costly ways (Table 19.5).

In the 1980s, PPI was introduced at a rapid rate, and participation in PPI grew dramatically. Ninety-one million people were enrolled in PPOs in 1995 (American Association of Health Plans, 1995).

In the long run, PPI should be less effective at reducing costs than are HMOs because the providers retain fee-for-service incentives and are not financially constrained by a per capita budget. The PPI format does not reward providers for keeping patients out of the hospital, and keeping them out may be the single most important source of cost savings in health care. Preferred-provider insurance does not organize the healthcare system for efficiency; it merely tries to shop for the lowest price in an inefficient system.

Preferred-provider insurance was viewed as an important part of the transition from the traditional unmanaged fee-for-service system to HMOs that use per capita prepayment. A group of doctors may begin with a discounted fee-for-service contract, acquire experience on which they can base a per capita payment, and then eventually convert to per capita prepayment.

For consumers, managed care, especially HMOs, requires a change in patterns of access to doctors, from complete free choice to choice limited to the managed-care plan's contracting providers. People who are accustomed to the traditional

TABLE 19.5. Characteristics of managed-care organizations.[a]

Health maintenance organization (HMO)	Preferred provider organization (PPO)	Point-of-service plan (POS)	Physician-hospital organization (PHO)
• Insures via prepayment for comprehensive health services	• Arranges discounted fee-for-service rates with contracted providers	• Adds PPO option to HMO plan	• Hospitals work with their medical staffs to offer comprehensive health services and accept per capita prepayment
• Choice of provider limited to those within HMO • Providers bear risk for the cost of care	• Offers incentives for enrollees to use contracted providers • Providers do not bear risks for the cost of care	• Allows for free choice of provider with financial incentive to use HMO providers	

[a]Different organizational forms present trade-offs between cost and access.

system often do not understand this change and the reasons for it, although experience shows that people get used to the new pattern and are satisfied with HMOs (California Managed Health Care Improvement Task Force, 1998). When they are seriously ill, however, some patients want to be able to go to a famous regional or national referral center and to take their insurance with them. In the mid-1980s, HMOs introduced the **point-of-service** (POS) plan to address these concerns.

A POS HMO functions as an HMO for those who wish to stay with the medical group that they have chosen within their HMO but adds a PPI plan that the member can access by paying a deductible (typically, the first several hundred dollars of expense) and a fraction of each medical bill and also a traditional insurance plan with an even stronger financial disincentive. This plan gives the covered person the full range of choice of provider but offers more favorable financial terms for sticking to the HMO primary physician network. Most people in these arrangements stay with their primary-care group for more than 90 percent of the services that they use. Point-of-service options are popular. It appears that people simply want the comfort of knowing they have the option to choose. In March 1987, 11 HMOs reported POS enrollment of nearly 400,000. By July 1995, 318 HMOs served over 5 million enrollees in POS plans (American Association of Health Plans, 1995).

Some HMOs are working to improve customer service. For example, they may offer convenient access to **advice nurses** who can help patients to make good decisions about the care they seek. Some HMOs are developing call centers to shorten telephone waiting time and to expedite appointments. The emerging standard of access to doctors is same-day appointments (with a doctor, if not with your own doctor) for people who think they need immediate care. Some HMOs have designed open-access insurance plans that allow members to see a doctor of any specialty within an HMO network without a referral. Innovations in information systems that allow plans to keep the primary-care physicians informed of interactions throughout the delivery system make feasible such open-access plans. In addition, as has been the experience with POS plans, there seems to be less-than-expected use of the open-access option among customers.

In the 1990s, the **physician-hospital organization** (PHO) emerged. In PHOs, one or a group of hospitals team up with their medical staffs to offer subscribers comprehensive health services for a per capita prepayment. Physicians and hospitals are motivated to form PHOs by what appear to them to be large profit margins of for-profit carrier HMOs and by the opportunity to avoid the rules and requirements established by HMOs that some providers feel have usurped their autonomy and authority. Physician-hospital organizations reflect a desire by providers to control their own destinies and to eliminate the insurers' role and share of the premium dollar.

The PHOs, however, need to develop functions and capabilities that are associated with insurance companies, such as the abilities to enroll members, to collect premiums, to set prices on their services, to make actuarial estimates of the costs of caring for different groups of people, to make arrangements for covered services that are beyond their capabilities (e.g., to contract with national or regional centers for advanced care), to provide insurance coverage for enrolled members who are outside the PHO's direct service area when they fall ill, and to reinsure exceptional medical costs. They also need financial reserves to cover unplanned losses. Thus, PHOs must create or partner with an insurance company.

19.4 The Era of Accountability

The 1990s, especially the years after 1994, can be characterized as the era of accountability in healthcare delivery. Although accountability had been creeping into the healthcare system through managed care for several decades, the year 1994 seems an appropriate point of demarcation because it is the year that Congress and the nation debated President Clinton's Health Security Act. The **Health Security Act** was a bold—some would say brazen—attempt to overhaul the healthcare financing and delivery system and to provide universal coverage for all Americans.

For a variety of reasons, no legislation passed. The Administration's work, however, did have several important effects. First, the Clinton plan focused the nation's attention on health care, and people around the country learned about how the healthcare system works and how it might change. Second, the Clinton proposal served as a strong impetus for change on the part of the private sector. Many private-sector healthcare organizations feared being worse off, rather than better off, under the proposed reforms, so they responded by reforming themselves to preempt legislation or at least to be positioned to respond to it. The Clinton plan also paved the way for the passage of less comprehensive healthcare legislative initiatives.

Accountability in health care takes several forms. Employers, fearing potentially expensive and cumbersome government regulation of the healthcare system, became willing to accept greater accountability for their role in managing their healthcare benefits. They, in turn, started holding health plans more accountable for costs, service, and care outcomes. The health plans responded by lowering their prices and improving their care management (Table 19.6).

During the 1990s, national health expenditures increased from $699.4 to $1149.1 billion in 1998, from 12.2 percent to 13.5 percent of the GDP (Table

Table 19.6. Comparison of fee-for-service and HMO insurance.[a]

Fee-for-service insurers	Health maintenance organizations
• Traditionally not cost accountable • Providers are paid more for their services	• Accountable for cost and quality • Fixed reimbursement regardless of service quantity

[a]HMOs attempt to create accountability for cost and quality by decoupling the financing from the quantity of services provided.

19.1). The increase in overall private national health expenditures between 1990 and 1998 was greatly reduced compared with that in the previous decade. Private expenditures grew from $416.2 billion in 1990 to $626.4 billion in 1998—an annual average growth rate of 6.4 percent, approximately 1 percent faster than the GDP. Between 1993 and 1998, private health expenditures remained flat as a percentage of the GDP. Public-sector expenditures grew from $283.2 to $522.7 billion between 1990 and 1998. Medicare outlays grew from $111.5 to $216.6 billion, and Medicaid outlays grew from $75.4 to $170.6 billion, growth rates of 8.0 and 5.0 percent per year, respectively (Levit et al., 1996) (Table 19.2).

19.4.1 Medicare and Medicaid

The component of the healthcare system most resistant to the general trend toward accountability has been the Medicare program. Medicare builds in virtually no quality management or improvement and requires little accountability on the part of doctors, hospitals, or other providers. Although Medicare's risk-basis contracting program has made HMO alternatives available to some beneficiaries, the government's reimbursement policy of 95 percent of the average adjusted per capita fee-for-service costs (AAPCC) deprives the government of the full potential savings. If an HMO can provide Medicare's standard benefit package at lower cost than 95 percent of the AAPCC, the HMO must provide more benefits rather than offering a lower price. In addition, if the HMO enrolls a healthier than average population, government payments may greatly exceed 95 percent of the expenditures that the HMO enrollees would have generated if they had chosen the fee-for-service option. As of 1995, only 3.1 million, or 10 percent of, Medicare beneficiaries were enrolled in managed-care plans compared with 57 percent of the total U.S. population. (Levit et al., 1996) (Fig. 19.5). This pace, however, appears to have accelerated.

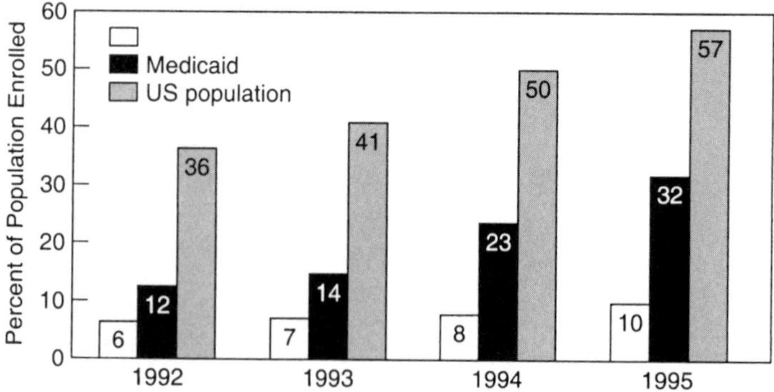

FIGURE 19.5. Proportion of population in managed care. Enrollment in managed care plans has grown sharply for Medicaid recipients, but slowly for the Medicare population. (*Source*: Health Care Financing Review [1996]. *Statistical Supplement*.)

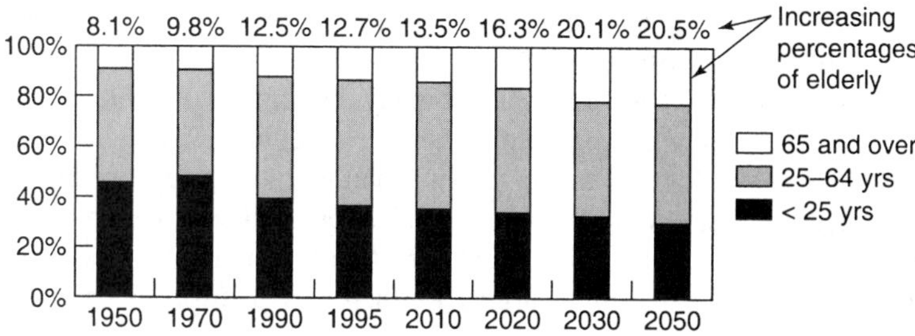

FIGURE 19.6. U.S. aging population. As the baby-boom generation approaches retirement age, problems with Medicare will grow dramatically. (*Source*: U.S. Bureau of Census, Committee on Ways and Means, 1997.)

In contrast to Medicare, Medicaid has seen a rapid expansion of managed care, particularly in the form of risk-based programs. In 1995, Medicaid managed care enrollment was 11.6 million, up 46 percent per year from 3.7 million in 1992 (Health Care Financing Review, 1996). As of 1997, only two states—Alaska and Wyoming—had no Medicaid managed care.

By 1996, the Medicare program was in dire need of reform. The trustees of the program predicted the impending expiration of the Medicare Trust Funds (Medicare Board of Trustees Reports, 1996). Federal outlays for Medicare were expected almost to double as a percentage of the nation's GDP, to 4.2 percent by 2010 (the year 78 million baby boomers start to become eligible for Medicare benefits), up from 2.3 in 1995 (Federal Hospital Insurance Trust Fund, 1996; Congressional Budget Office, 1996). Medicare would thus become the federal government's single largest expense. By 2015, the elderly population will have increased to 43.7 million. By 2030 there will be just over two workers to support the costs of each beneficiary; in 1997, there were four. The proportion of elderly in the population is expected to be nearly 20 percent—more than twice the proportion when the program was initiated (Committee on Ways and Means, 1997) (Fig. 19.6).

In response to these grave predictions, Congress enacted major reforms to the Medicare program through the Balanced Budget Act of 1997 (O'Sullivan et al., 1997). Among its main features, the Balanced Budget Act establishes the Medicare+Choice program, which expands private plan options to Medicare beneficiaries. Although this legislation should encourage beneficiaries' transition to managed care, it will not solve the long-run problems of the program.

19.4.2 Managed Competition and Purchaser Initiatives

Popular employer interventions to reduce costs in a cost-unconscious environment dominated by forms of fee-for-service insurance include requiring employees to pay a share of the cost for health insurance, consolidating the number of plans an employer offers so as to consolidate purchasing clout, and using self-insurance to eliminate administrative costs and to maximize the time value of money. Although these interventions may have reduced employer healthcare costs in the short term, they had no effect on health delivery and therefore could not reduce healthcare costs in the long run.

Dissatisfaction with these methods led many employers to embrace managed care. Initial efforts were only modestly effective at reducing costs, because most employers were unwilling or unable to make their employees responsible for premium price differences. Managed-care organizations that competed with fee-for-service plans recognized that they could attract customers by offering better service or benefits rather than by charging lower prices. Thus costs declined only modestly.

In contrast, some employers chose to hold health plans accountable for both the cost and the quality of the care delivered, thus intervening in ways that would affect care delivery and long-term costs. **Managed competition** (Enthoven, 1993) is a strategy used to varying degrees by some purchasers of healthcare services intended (1) to create health services delivery organizations capable of acquiring appropriate healthcare resources, obtaining value for money, deploying the resources to care for an enrolled population, designing and executing care processes that produce good outcomes and value for money, and measuring and monitoring performance (outcomes, satisfaction, and cost) and continuously improving it (i.e., managing care); (2) to create a framework of incentives for such organizations to improve quality and reduce cost; and (3) to use market forces to transform the healthcare delivery system from its former fragmented, nonaccountable mode to efficient integrated comprehensive-care organizations constantly striving to improve. In brief, *managed competition* refers to the rules of the game within which managed care organizations play (Table 19.7).

To manage competition, a "sponsor," either an employer or group of employers, continuously structures and adjusts the market to overcome attempts by health plans to avoid price competition. The sponsor offers its members a choice of standardized healthcare coverage options and provides them with information and incentives to choose a health plan that provides them the greatest value for money. The sponsor selects the managed-care organizations or insurance carriers that compete; sets equitable rules for pricing and enrollment within which all health plans must compete and monitors compliance; organizes a coordinated annual open enrollment during which members have an opportunity to consider alternative health plans; and provides comparative information about health-plan prices, performance, quality, and service.

Table 19.7. Principles of managed competition.

- Sponsor establishes equitable rules within which multiple plans compete and administers an open enrollment process
- Individual is responsible for premium difference among competing plans
- Standardizes coverage contracts between sponsored groups
- Provides for individual choice of plan rather than group choice
- Information on quality, plans, and providers is accessible and understandable
- Risk selection is managed by providing a single point of entry and standard coverage contracts, and by risk-adjusting premiums

Under managed competition, sponsors also require members to pay the full premium differences if they choose a plan whose premium is higher than the low-priced plan. This gives members an incentive to seek value for money and, more importantly, gives plans an incentive to offer the greatest value. In 1995, this principle was employed by only about 7 percent of employers, accounting for about 20 percent of employees (Singer et al., 1997). A complicating factor in creating subscriber premium responsibility is the fact that employer-based health insurance contributions are still tax free to the employee without limit. The effect is that, at the margin, choices of more costly health plans are subsidized by the government. This could be corrected by a limit on the tax-free amount, set at the premium of the low-priced plan.

The sponsor should also design solutions to offset the profitability of "risk selection" to ensure that healthcare organizations focus on giving better care at lower cost rather than selecting only healthy enrollees.

Managed competition has been introduced most extensively in California, mainly led by a few large employers and **purchasing coalitions**—groups of employers that together structure their healthcare-benefits program and negotiate with health plans. Most employers, even in California, have not applied all or even most of the principles outlined here. Examples of each component of the strategy, however, do exist. The Pacific Business Group on Health, a private large-employer purchasing coalition, negotiates health-plan premiums on behalf of member employers and requires participating health plans to meet performance standards on quality of care, customer service, and data provision. The HMOs each put a total of 2 percent of premiums at risk for all performance standards, weighted according to each health plan's relative weaknesses. Pacific Health Advantage, formerly the Health Insurance Plan of California, a state-sponsored small-employer purchasing coalition, adjusts payments to health plans based on average risk profiles of enrollees, using diagnostic information to ensure that health plans that attract higher risk populations will be compensated for their additional costs.

The California Public Employees Retirement System provides comparative price and quality information to state and other California agency employees. It has also done special analyses of the people who had been hospitalized or were frequent users of care to see if they were as satisfied as the healthy customers. Some California universities require their employees who choose a more expensive plan to pay the full premium difference. All these sponsors offer a choice of health plans and provide an annual open enrollment during which members choose plans. With these organizations leading the way, competition has become active in California, and healthcare costs have decreased in response. In inflation-adjusted terms, the 1997 premiums for competitive HMOs were about 13 percent below their 1992 levels. Premiums are, however, increasing again.

Employers in other states are also taking an active role. Some have formed coalitions to bargain collectively for health-insurance premiums. Others support the National Committee for Quality Assurance, the Foundation for Accountability, and other organizations that measure the outcomes of care provided by health plans to provide information about quality. Increasing numbers of employers are offering their employees a choice of health plans, and, although most do not require their employees to pay the full difference in price, many make their employees aware of price differences and require them to pay a portion of the difference. As a result, in the mid-1990s, national average HMO-premium growth flattened, although premium increases have recurred. According to one survey, HMO average premiums fell by 0.2 percent between 1995 and 1996, down consistently from a 12.1 percent increase between 1990 and 1991 (Kaiser Family Foundation, 1999). Premiums increased thereafter through 1999, suggesting that there is a great deal of room for improvement in the competitive environment for healthcare purchasing.

19.4.3 Managed Care and Provider Initiatives

Under pressure from greater competition, managed-care organizations and providers have become more accountable. So that important gains in quality and economy can be realized, the healthcare financing and delivery system is being integrated more closely together than ever before. There are at least seven levels of integration. More often than not, integration occurs through contractual relationship rather than ownership (Table 19.8).

The first integration is between financial responsibility and delivery of care. It occurs with per capita prepayment by the purchaser to the chosen medical-care organization. Health-maintenance organizations translate the broad incentive of **capitated** payment into payment to doctors in a great variety of ways. Some pay salaries. Others pay salaries with bonuses for productivity, patient satisfaction, and overall economic success. Others pay various forms of fee for service with management controls. Health-maintenance organizations are empirically tuning their methods to find what works in their marketplaces. Modern IPAs select doctors and drive hard bargains. The best IPAs evaluate their primary-care providers continuously and pay them in a manner that provides appropriate financial incentives. Good performers win cash bonuses; poor performers are dropped from the program. Individual-practice associations contract with selected specialists on a discounted fee-for-service basis and give the primary-care doctors as a group a financial incentive to control specialist referrals.

Table 19.8. Seven integrations of managed care.[a]

- *Financing and delivery*: responsibility for costs of healthcare delivery
- *Providers and populations*: population-based medicine
- *Full spectrum of healthcare services*: care provided in least costly appropriate setting
- *Doctors and other healthcare professionals*: right numbers and types
- *Doctors and hospitals*: vertical integration
- *Hospitals*: horizontal integration
- *Information*: information management

[a]Greater integration can lead to better quality and lower costs.

Embedded in these reimbursement schemes are often incentives to improve quality. They motivate providers to "do it right the first time" because mistakes cost money. Patients with unsolved or poorly managed problems continue to impose costs on the healthcare system. Per-capita prepayment facilitates the alignment of incentives of doctors with the interests of patients in high-quality economical care. It pays for and rewards cost-effective preventive services, such as more outreach of prenatal care to reduce the costs of neonatology, or more effective management of chronic diseases to minimize acute episodes. It provides a framework for cost-benefit analysis, which helps to determine where the most effective place is to spend limited resources. It also rewards cost-reducing innovation, such as the many incremental changes that have reduced the length of hospital stays for total hip replacement operations from an average of 17 days in 1983 to 8 days in 1993, with several facilities achieving 3-or 4-day average stays (Keston & Enthoven, 1996).

The second integration is between providers and populations. This integration facilitates and encourages population-based medicine that adds an epidemiological perspective to encounter-based medicine. Providers look behind the encounters with patients to the underlying causes of the patients' complaints to see whether there are effective methods of prevention. One of the enduring legends of Kaiser Permanente is that the founding doctor, Sidney Garfield, who was treating construction-site workers who had nail-puncture wounds in their feet, went to the site with a hammer and pounded down the offending nails. Some HMOs now give children bicycle helmets and videotapes explaining why the helmets should always be used. Thus, HMOs can allocate resources to maximize the wellness of their enrolled populations through preventive and patient-education services. Also, the defined population base enables HMOs to match the numbers and types of doctors in their groups, and also other resources, to the needs of the enrolled population.

The third integration is the full spectrum of healthcare services: inpatient, outpatient, doctor offices, home nursing, and so on, as well as drugs and other services. Health-maintenance organizations have been putting resources into improved preventive services and outpatient care and are being more than compensated by reduced inpatient cost. They seek to deliver care in the least costly appropriate setting. They are motivated to organize seamless comprehensive care so that patients are not left to their own devices when they leave the hospital. In the best-managed HMOs, committees of doctors and pharmacists choose drug regimens to produce the best outcomes and to minimize total costs of care rather than merely minimizing the cost of drugs.

The fourth integration is among doctors and other health professionals. The goal is the right numbers and types of professionals, the right specialty mix to ensure that patients have good access and to ensure that the specialists are proficient in caring for their patients. It includes rational referral patterns and efficient specialist–generalist division of labor. For example, specialists may serve as consultants to generalists who deliver the care. It includes efficient use of para-

TABLE 19.9. Health plan enrollments by year.[a]

Health plan type	1992	1994	1996	1998	1999
HMO	22%	25%	33%	27%	28%
PPO	26%	25%	26%	35%	38%
POS	8%	15%	16%	24%	25%
Conventional with precertification	45%	35%	23%	14%	9%

[a]Enrollments in conventional fee-for-service plans decreased and in managed care plans increased in the 1990s. *Source:* The Kaiser Family Foundation and Health Research and Education Trust, *Employer Health Benefits* (1999), pp. 57.

medicals, such as nurse practitioners and social workers, who may work in teams with primary-care physicians.

The fifth integration is between doctors and hospitals: giving doctors a serious interest in reducing hospital costs. In a well-integrated system, doctors develop practice patterns that facilitate efficient hospital operations. They work with hospitals to reduce unnecessary record keeping, they support "value for money" investment decisions.

The sixth integration is horizontal integration among hospitals. Groups of hospitals in a region combine to share administrative support functions, including management personnel, and tend to consolidate volume-sensitive clinical services, such as open-heart surgery and neonatology and laboratories.

The seventh integration is information. We describe this integration and its benefits in the remainder of this chapter. We argue that information and its management are fundamental to successful integration of the delivery system.

Employers have struggled with health-care costs and have recognized that managed-care organizations have the potential to offer increased value. As a result, managed care has penetrated the markets of many states, and penetration is continuing to increase. With the growth of managed-care organizations, traditional, unmanaged fee for service has disappeared almost entirely in many areas. Even fee-for-service insurers began managing their plans to avail themselves of the same purchasing preferences for buying large quantities and other economies of scale. By 1999, health-plan enrollments in the private sector comprised 28 percent HMOs, 38 percent in PPOs, 25 percent in POS plans, and 9 percent in conventional fee-for-service plans (Table 19.9) (Kaiser Family Foundation, 1999). These trends are expected to continue.

19.5 Relationships Among Healthcare Financing, Healthcare Delivery, and Healthcare Technology

Healthcare financing, healthcare delivery, and healthcare technology are directly linked. The way in which healthcare professionals and healthcare organizations are paid creates incentives that have consequences both in the way they act and in the information that they seek.

19.5.1 Technology During the Era of Open-Ended Spending

The open-ended, third-party reimbursement that was widespread in both the public and the private sectors from the 1960s through the 1980s resulted, as we have said, in payments to doctors and hospitals for each service rendered. Logically, this system created an incentive for doctors and hospitals to maximize their income by performing—or at least billing for—as many services as possible, especially highly paid services and including services of questionable value. Evidence of wide variations in physician practice patterns supports this conclusion (Wennberg, 1998; Wennberg & Gittelsohn, 1973). As a result of this incentive, healthcare providers purchased computer applications for tracking and maximizing charges and for billing payers. Hospital financial systems that could do so thrived.

Fee-for-service reimbursement also gave hospitals an incentive to attract as many physicians as possible to use their facilities. More physicians admitted more patients. Each day that a hospital bed was filled, it generated additional income for the hospital. Thus, hospitals invested money and effort in pursuit of physicians who would keep their beds filled. More highly specialized physicians were more highly prized, because charges for the hospitalizations that their services required were higher. Hospitals often enticed specialists to use their facilities by acquiring high-technology equipment.

With the emphasis on reimbursement and high technology, administrative systems received limited attention and financial resources. Unlike most industries, which spend significant proportions of their budgets on quality control and administration, medical care viewed administration as wasteful. Selling, general, and administrative expenses in other industries range up to 44 percent of total expenditures (CFO, 1996). To this day, those who accuse HMOs of having high administrative costs fail to acknowledge the legitimate need for "administrative" expenditure on quality improvement and on cost and utilization management (Woolhandler & Himmelstein, 1997).

Some people view the healthcare information technology of this era as unsophisticated. By the 1980s, however, information technology, in general, was sophisticated. Computer systems in the banking industry, for example, reported trades of shares of public companies on a stock exchange almost immediately all around the world and allowed bankers to track the performance of multiple stocks over time at a glance. At least one, and often many, computer terminals sat atop the desks of most investment bankers during the 1980s.

Certain healthcare information technology was also extremely advanced. Healthcare technology in general—such as medical devices and equipment—used some of the most advanced technology in existence. Computer systems designed to track charges were extremely sophisticated. These technologies were perceived at the time as offering the greatest financial returns, so the most money and resources flowed in their direction. As the financial incentives in the healthcare system changed, these technologies became less useful. Similarly, tech-

TABLE 19.10. Fee-for-service and managed care systems generate different information needs.

Fee-for-service	Managed care
• Bill charges for services without awareness of costs • Charge-based information systems	• Need to understand and be accountable for the costs of delivering services • Cost and encounter-based information systems

nologies that enable healthcare organizations to respond to today's incentives were unnecessary in an era of open-ended spending and thus were underfunded or not developed at all.

As interest has shifted toward cost and quality management, information systems that track charges have become much less useful because the relationship between charges and costs is inexact at best (Table 19.10). An emphasis on charges was acceptable in the 1980s because then cost reduction was not an issue. Charge-based systems also grew less useful because they did not track information about provider performance or patient outcomes, excluding death in the hospital. Hospital computer systems could not assist in answering questions like whether a particular course of treatment improved a patient's functioning or whether a particular physician had greater success performing a procedure than one of her colleagues. Physicians impeded the flow of information by staunchly refusing to allow disclosure of physician-specific information and fighting proposals that would do so. Even hospital-level information was (and often still is) difficult to obtain (Singer, 1991).

19.5.2 New Incentives and Requirements in the Era of Accountability

With fundamental shifts from fee-for-service reimbursement toward per capita prepayment, from price insensitivity among providers and consumers toward cost and quality consciousness, from loosely organized care toward managed care, and from unquestioning trust in providers to demands for accountability, the healthcare financing and delivery system now faces a new set of incentives. These new incentives—particularly the demand for accountability—create a need for new types of technology and performance.

The most important incentives created by the transition to accountability fall into four broad categories: (1) incentives for purchasers to seek value, (2) incentives for health plans and providers to improve quality and to reduce costs, (3) potential incentives for providers to underserve patients, and (4) an incentive for health plans to attract the healthiest possible populations. The first two incentives are desirable and require information to implement; the second two are largely undesirable and require information to counteract.

Incentives for Purchasers to Seek Value

When individuals have an incentive to seek value for their money because they must pay some or all of the difference in the price of a health plan, they need information with which to compare plans. Individuals taking a more active role in their health and medical treatment also seek comparative quality information about doctors and hospitals. Large employers, seeking to reduce their own health-care costs, also have an incentive to provide comparative information for their employees. They can exploit their far greater resources and leverage with health plans and providers to obtain it.

Information currently available includes measures of satisfaction of members enrolled in health plans; measures of access to providers, whether for scheduled appointments, on the telephone, or on an unscheduled basis; and measures of compliance with guidelines for preventive services, such as providing immunizations for children or mammograms for women. More desirable, yet more difficult to obtain, are risk-adjusted, condition-specific, and population-based measures of outcomes. Although strong purchasers may demand this information, most providers have not yet been able to put in place systems that can track outcomes (other than death) of the care that they provide or the health of the population that they serve.

Incentives for Health Plans and Providers to Improve Quality and Reduce Costs

When health plans and providers become accountable for the cost and quality of the care that they provide and for the health of the populations that they serve, they need the ability to measure cost and quality and the information with which to improve healthcare delivery. These incentives make it necessary to collect information that was not required in the past.

The first area for which information is required is for process improvement. For example, measuring variation in processes, outcomes, and costs among physicians and their practices enable these physicians to compare themselves with their colleagues, to seek help from colleagues who have better results in certain areas, and to improve their practice patterns. In addition, the measurement of inputs and outputs allows healthcare managers to track and improve productivity. Availability of this type of information opens up new areas for improved care management processes, such as closer monitoring of patients who have chronic conditions and case management of patients who have catastrophic illnesses.

Second, to improve continuity of care, it is no longer adequate to track patients within a single hospital stay; providers need to track patients in different care settings across the health system. If a patient visits a primary-care physician in a clinic, has a series of outpatient visits, and then is admitted to the hospital for a procedure weeks later, information about that patient—including results of previous laboratory tests, prescription drugs, and so on—should be available to ensure continuity of care.

Third, given responsibility for populations as well as individual patients, health plans require information about enrollees even before those people receive medical care. This information is important not only to make health-plan comparisons but also to identify enrollees at high risk of illness and disease. Quality is enhanced and costs reduced if problems can be identified early or avoided completely because preventive measures are taken. Thus, health plans should want to have good information on the presence of chronic conditions even before patients present with complaints.

Fourth, information will be required to enable the assessment of new technologies. Before the introduction of new technologies, payers will want to consider both the costs and the benefits. This process requires detailed information on operating costs and productivity in practice. Technologies that are not cost effective or that do not provide significant benefit relative to technology that is already available will not be introduced.

Fifth, healthcare managers will have to do make-versus-buy analyses to evaluate, for example, whether they can obtain a test at less cost by contracting with an outside laboratory rather than by purchasing the testing equipment and running the tests themselves. Information about the costs associated with providing services, equipment, and facilities in-house will be vital for negotiating appropriate contracts with external vendors. Again, detailed information on operating costs is needed.

Finally, the needs to reduce costs and to improve quality so as to stay competitive require that health plans and providers evaluate both physicians and healthcare facilities to determine where consolidation is appropriate. For example, the American College of Cardiology recommends that teams of physicians at any particular healthcare facility perform a minimum of 200 to 300 open heart surgeries per year (California Office of Statewide Health Planning and Development, 1992). At a lower quantity, surgeons may not be proficient, and the facility risks providing low-quality care. Thus, hospitals performing open heart surgeries should track the number and outcomes of their procedures and should seek ways to concentrate such procedures at high-volume, high-quality centers. As value-for-money competition becomes more intense, it will be important to make these cost comparisons with increasing accuracy.

Potential Incentive for Providers to Underserve Patients

Per capita prepayment is a double-edged sword. It gives providers an incentive to hold down costs. Ideally, providers respond to this incentive by finding ways to become more productive, to keep people healthy, to avoid mistakes, and so on. Because they are also at financial risk for all services that enrollees consume, however, providers may also have an incentive to underserve. Patients who need the most care are most vulnerable to underprovision of care not only because plans or providers may save money by holding back services but also because plans benefit if such patients "vote with their feet" by leaving for another health plan. This is a widespread and important fear among consumers.

This fear has given rise to much experimentation by health plans and providers around financial incentives. For example, it seems prudent to base capitation payments on populations of patients rather than on individual patients. By the same reasoning, groups of providers are better able to share the risk of a few expensive cases than is an individual physician. In addition, combinations of per capita prepayment with bonuses for high-quality care may prevent abuses.

Nevertheless, these reimbursement schemes are unproven and in flux, so consumers continue to worry that their providers may benefit by withholding needed care. This potential creates not only the need to track blatant abuses (a possible role for government), but also the need to provide access to information for consumers. Technologies such as video and CD-ROM can be applied to describe the costs and benefits of particular procedures in ways that consumers can understand and use to choose the most appropriate courses of action for themselves. In addition, directories and databases that provide information about individual practitioners, including experience with procedures and other quality indicators, would benefit consumers.

Incentive for Health Plans to Attract the Healthiest Populations Possible

Health insurers have an incentive to attract to their plans the healthiest population possible. If a health plan is unable to charge higher prices because that will cause it to lose business to a competitor, it can increase its profits by reducing its costs. Health plans have found that an effective way to reduce costs is simply to enroll a healthier population that has less total need for medical services. Those plans least successful at this strategy may end up with the sickest or highest risk population. In this situation, even the most efficient plan may not be able to survive. In health insurance, competition exacerbates this problem.

Assuming quality is constant, it would be best if the most efficient health plans were also the most successful. This outcome requires that health plans with a sicker and higher risk population than average be compensated for the additional expected cost of care. A variety of risk-adjustment mechanisms have been developed, and several have been applied in practice. The successful implementation of a risk-adjustment mechanism requires substantial diagnostic and demographic information and coordination of information, which in turn requires large databases, analytical capability, and the ability to read information in multiple technology platforms. The best risk-adjustment models are notable for their comprehensive data requirements; they use both inpatient and outpatient data and repeated observations on the same individual over time.

19.5.3 Implications of Developing Information Technology for Healthcare Financing and Delivery

Just as the needs of the healthcare financing and delivery system direct development of new healthcare information technologies, new technologies enable significant improvements in healthcare financing and delivery. In this section, we describe a few of the most important advances in information technology and predict the progress that they will permit.

Cost-Accounting Systems

Based on cost-accounting applications in other industries, healthcare cost-accounting systems have been developed and have been adopted widely. In health care, the matter of accounting for costs is extremely complicated not only because there are so many costs in even the simplest hospital stay and so many ways to account for them but also because healthcare organizations have not traditionally accounted for costs and so lack a time-tested, broadly accepted basis for defining those costs. Difficulties in defining costs may be compounded by the large fixed costs of hospitals, which use expensive capital heavily, and the presence of joint production. Some resources are used for multiple activities, so allocation of their costs to any single activity is difficult and often arbitrary. Without a defined cost for items, even the most sophisticated cost-accounting systems cannot provide satisfactory answers to even the most basic questions. For a typical hospital, the process of defining costs accurately may take years.

Cost-accounting systems enable the measurement of costs—the first step toward being able to manage costs. They enable the assessment of technologies on the basis of costs relative to benefits, so decisions can be made about which technologies are cost effective and which should be used sparingly or not at all. Cost-accounting systems enable organizations to profile and compare the utilization patterns of physicians, clinics, and hospitals on the basis of which they can target practice improvements, select a network, and determine bonuses. They empower organizations with information on the basis of which to negotiate contracts that cover at least variable costs. They enable organizations to determine that the costs of providing a service are higher than those of contracting it out. The better the ability to measure costs, the greater the capacity of the healthcare organization to survive in a competitive managed-care environment. Cost-accounting systems, still new to many organizations, are an essential and important tool.

Internet or Intranet

The advent of the information superhighway has expanded the possibilities for information and communication in the healthcare industry, as it has in other industries (National Research Council, 2000). The Internet, and its proprietary counterpart—intranets—enable new forms of interaction that may have a profound effect on healthcare delivery and administration. As of this writing, however, Internet access is still far from universal.

The Internet provides an open, widely accepted standard for transferring information. In general, healthcare information technologies, not unlike information technologies in other sectors, have used proprietary technology, much of which has been unable to communicate with other technologies. The result is great difficulty in sharing information across organizations—a function that is vitally important in health care as patients move among organizations. In contrast, healthcare information technologies based on the Internet standard can more easily communicate with one another.

Health care is a global concern; healthcare delivery is a local business. The Internet opens up local communication on a worldwide basis. It gives healthcare organizations the potential to communicate at low cost, because the Internet infrastructure is already built and is publicly available. Physicians and healthcare organizations can communicate with other physicians in different settings; they can also communicate with patients where the patients live and work. This ability enhances home health care, HMO–patient communication, physician–patient communication, and internal communications within increasingly large and decentralized healthcare organizations (see Chapter 10). In addition, telemedicine (see Chapter 20) becomes much more practical with Internet technologies. Healthcare sites make up a large proportion of Internet traffic, with hundreds of sites available and more added every week.

Comprehensive Longitudinal Databases

Theoretically, medical records include detailed information about every interaction an individual has with the healthcare delivery system. In practice, information is difficult to retrieve, and too often it is lost. Over time, and for individuals with complex problems, medical records can become thick documents of loose notes from multiple sources, test results, and images (see Chapter 2). For decades, most of the reports included in medical records were handwritten. Now, more sophisticated organizations have transcription departments or rely on outsourced services to type medical records.

Paper-based medical records do not support continuity of care across physicians and across healthcare institutions. Healthcare organizations do not share medical records. Thus, an individual may have multiple, but incomplete, medical records in different doctors' offices, clinics, and hospitals, representing different portions of the patient's medical history. Even if medical records are shared in a multispecialty-group practice setting, paper records may be missing when they are needed. Finding relevant information in even the best-organized medical records is a difficult and time-consuming task. Using medical-record information for learning about patterns of care across multiple patients can be a Herculean task.

Comprehensive longitudinal databases—in effect, a paperless, complete medical record—have been viewed by many people as the holy grail in healthcare information technology (see Chapters 1 and 9). Integrated delivery of care requires comprehensive longitudinal records for each patient so that each provider who contacts patients as well as the patients themselves can have a complete picture of the patients' medical history, access that helps to avoid duplicate tests and unfavorable drug interactions. In addition, the information can serve as a basis for research on the relationships among diagnoses, treatments, and outcomes. Comprehensive patient records would also enable outcomes measurement, technology assessment, physician profiling, measurement of practice variation, identification of best practices, continuous quality improvement, utilization management, continuity of care, measurement of compliance with guidelines, and risk adjustment.

Projects to develop comprehensive, computer-based medical records were common in the 1980s; they still persist. (Refer to Chapter 9 for a detailed discussion of computer-based patient records.) They have raised concern among consumer advocates about the confidentiality of information (Editorial, 1997). That concern has created yet another opportunity for healthcare information-technology development: systems have been and continue to be developed to address data security concerns (see Chapters 4 and 7).

Longitudinal databases are also being used to achieve slightly less ambitious aims. Some information technology companies focus on tracking courses of treatment for particular conditions or in single settings. Automated drug order-entry systems, when used in hospitals, call attention to potential errors. These technologies represent a great improvement in healthcare management and information.

The likely evolution of a comprehensive computer-based medical record will include several phases: first, through the development of universal identifiers for enrollees and providers, the capability to exchange electronically enrollment and eligibility information; next, through standardization and expanded coding, the capability to exchange pharmacy, laboratory, and encounter records. This intermediate stage will represent a tremendous step forward, facilitating quality improvement and performance measurement. The third phase of evolution will be the comprehensive computer-based medical-record systems originally envisioned.

19.5.4 The Challenge of Implementation

The era of open-ended spending left many healthcare organizations with a legacy of substantial but antiquated infrastructure. Data-management systems are also typically plagued by incomplete data and a lack of quality control. Both the management systems and information technologies associated with fee-for-service reimbursement were ingrained through years of development and use. In general, technology that predates the 1990s was proprietary to particular institutions and therefore incompatible with technology in other institutions. This situation makes difficult not only the transfer of information across institutions but also the modernization of existing technology. The transition to new integrated systems and new technologies therefore is extremely challenging and costly. Converting or replacing existing systems requires substantial investment (see Chapter 10).

Nevertheless, these systems must evolve to support future quality improvement and performance measurement. Healthcare institutions today must constantly balance the trade-off between the cost of upgrading information capabilities and collecting and disseminating information and the value that the additional information can provide. Nevertheless, with accountability for the health of patients and of populations, investment in new technology by health plans and providers makes more sense than ever before.

Acknowledgments. The authors thank Matt D. Solomon, Administrative Assistant for Health Care Management in the Graduate School of Business, Stanford University, for his skillful and enthusiastic assistance in the preparation of this chapter.

Suggested Readings

Ellwood P.M. (1988). Shattuck Lecture—outcomes management: A technology of patient experience. *The New England Journal of Medicine*, 318(23):1549–1556.

The author describes the destabilizing and democratizing effects in terms of choices and decisions of HMOs on patients, payers, and healthcare organizations. He coins the term "health maintenance organization" and makes the case for outcomes measurement.

Enthoven A.C. (1993). The history and principles of managed competition. *Health Affairs*, 12:24–48, Suppl.

The author articulates the principles of managed competition, a plan for comprehensive health reform that combines microeconomics with careful observation and analysis of what works. Managed competition relies on a sponsor to structure and adjust the market for competing health plans, to establish equitable rules, to create price-elastic demand, and to avoid uncompensated risk selection.

Fuchs V.R. (1983). *Who Shall Live?* (2nd ed.) New York: Basic Books.

The author presents an excellent introduction to the structure of the healthcare delivery system. The roles of the main players and the relationship between medical care and health are discussed.

Fuchs V.R. (1993). *The Future of Health Policy*. Cambridge, MA: Harvard University Press.

The author provides the reader with the necessary concepts, facts, and analyses to clarify complicated issues of health policy. The book addresses cost containment, managed competition, technology assessment, poverty and health, children's health, and national health insurance.

Glowniak J.W., Bushway, M.K. (1994). Computer networks as a medical resource: accessing and using the Internet. *Journal of the American Medical Association*, 271(24): 1934–1940.

This article provides an introduction to the Internet. It includes important principles for accessing and using this resource to obtain information relevant for medical practice, education, and research.

Weller C.D. (1984). "Free choice" as a restraint of trade in American health care delivery and insurance. *Iowa Law Review*, 69(5):1351–1378, 1382–1392.

This article explains in simple yet powerful terms many of the issues raised by the fundamental restructuring of the healthcare industry from the era of open spending to the era of accountability by providing a historical account of the transition from "guild free choice," which prevented doctors from organizing into groups and offering discounts, to "market free choice," which permits competition.

Questions for Discussion

1. Define the following terms, each of which is relevant to current healthcare financing:
   a. Usual, customary, and reasonable fees
   b. Health maintenance organization

   c. Diagnosis-related group
   d. Preferred provider insurance
2. Compare HMOs, PPOs, POS plans, and PHOs. What are the strengths and potential limitations of each with respect to cost and quality of care?
3. How will the differences in incentives for providers under each of the following payment systems affect providers' assessments of new medical technologies, such as patient-monitoring systems?
   a. An HMO
   b. An individual physician participating in a PPO arrangement
   c. A hospital with a large number of patients treated under Medicare's prospective-payment system
   d. A standard fee-for-service arrangement
4. Compare information-system needs in a hospital that treats mostly private-pay patients with those in one that is owned and operated by an HMO.
5. You are the new administrator of the Health Care Financing Administration, the agency responsible for Medicare and for the federal component of Medicaid. You are about to authorize a new program for healthcare financing for the elderly. The program offers elderly beneficiaries a choice of all health plans on the market.
   a. With what information do you think it is important to provide beneficiaries so that they can choose among plans?
   b. What data would you want to collect to evaluate the performance of plans?
   c. What mechanisms would you implement to collect these data?
6. Describe at least three ways in which healthcare organizations can use the Internet to improve patient care.

20 The Future of Computer Applications in Health Care

Lawrence M. Fagan and Edward H. Shortliffe

After reading this chapter, you should know the answers to these questions:

- What are possible future directions for medical informatics?
- What are the forces that are driving these changes?

In this book, we have summarized the current state of medical informatics in a variety of application areas and have reflected on the development of the field during the past 40 years. To provide a background for our discussions, we opened the book with a glimpse into the future—a vision of medical practice when individual physicians routinely and conveniently use network-based computers to help with information management, communication, and clinical decision-making. In this chapter, we again look forward, this time concentrating on likely trends in medical applications of computers, on current avenues of research, and on the issues that will determine along which paths medical informatics will develop.

20.1 Progress in Health Care Computing

We begin by looking back at the changes in medical computing since the first edition of this book was published in 1990. Then we look ahead to the not-too-distant future—presenting a few scenarios that we can extrapolate from the current trends in medical computing. These scenarios provide perspective on the ways that computers may pervade medical practice. A key aspect of the scenarios is the extent to which, unlike most specialized medical paraphernalia of today, medical-computing applications are integrated into routine medical practice rather than used on an occasional basis. The realization of a highly integrated environment depends on the solution of technological challenges, such as integrating information from multiple data sources and making the integrated information accessible to health professionals when, where, and in the form that it is needed. Integration of medical information also encompasses social issues, such as defining the appropriate role of computers in the workplace, resolving questions of legal liability and ethics related to medical computing, and assessing the effects of computer-based technology on healthcare costs. The chance that our hypothetical scenarios will become reality thus depends on the resolution of a number of technological and social issues that will be debated during the coming years.

20.1.1 Looking Back to 1990

In the first edition of our book, the closing chapter included two future scenarios of medical care and discussed emerging topics such as the Unified Medical Language System (UMLS), integrated academic information management systems (IAIMS), and the medical information bus (MIB). Today the UMLS is employed in information-retrieval systems as a tool for converting textual medical information into standardized terms taken from coding schemes and vocabularies such as MeSH and ICD and to help translate from one vocabulary to another (McCray & Miller, 1998). IAIMS sites are now scattered around the country with many different models being implemented. The MIB has been approved as the IEEE 1073 family of standards for medical device interconnection (Stead, 1997b) and has been incorporated into multiple instruments at the bedside (see Chapter 13).

The scenarios we discussed in the first edition included computer-based support during both cardiac-bypass surgery and long-term care of a patient with a chronic disease. Although the information-support capabilities have changed considerably in the decade since the first version of this chapter was written, it is possible that the practice of medicine has changed just as much. For example, less invasive alternatives to open-chest bypass surgery have become more common. Stricter criteria for admission to the hospital and shorter lengths of stay once hospitalized mean that sicker patients are routinely cared for in outpatient settings. In such situations, the need for computer-based tracking of a patient's medical status is increased. This need has led to experiments such as the use of wireless pen-based computers by home healthcare nurses for logging patient conditions and Internet-based disease management interactions between clinicians and patients in their homes.

Significant advances have been made in raw computing power (e.g., hardware and software for the manipulation of three-dimensional images); interconnectivity (e.g., high-speed network backbones and wireless connections to palm-sized hand-held computing devices); the ability to store very large amounts of data (e.g., the terabyte data storage device shown in Fig. 20.1); and the development of infrastructure—particularly in the area of communication standards (e.g., HL7 and object broker architectures). On the other hand, the anticipated level of seamless integration between applications, highly interconnected medical databases with embedded decision-support tools, and ubiquitous computing support have not come to pass.

20.1.2 Looking to the Future

During testimony before the U.S. House of Representatives Committee on Science in 1997 concerning the future role of the Internet, we laid out a set of long-

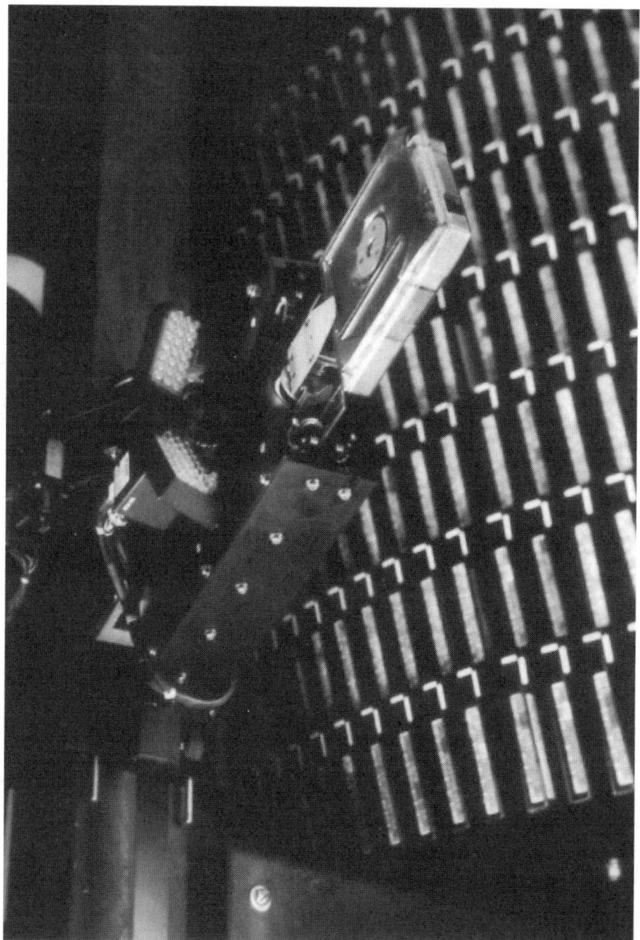

FIGURE 20.1. Multi-terabyte mass storage in a tape robot facility. (*Source*: Reprinted by permission from StorageTek, Louisville, CO. 1998.)

term goals for medical informatics. Like the scenarios we depicted nearly a decade ago, these goals depend on the occurrence of both technical and social changes for their fulfillment. If the assumptions identified in Section 20.1.3 prove valid, medical practice in the future will incorporate aspects of the following scenarios:

- **Telemedicine**: Today's early telemedicine experiments, dependent on specialized equipment and expensive communications lines, will have evolved such that the Internet is the standard vehicle for linking medical experts with other clinicians and patients at a distance (National Research Council, 2000). Clear video images will be transferred routinely, high-fidelity audio links will support listening to the heart and lungs, and common computing platforms at both ends of the links will make telemedicine a cost-effective form of medical practice. Patients will avoid unnecessary travel from rural settings to major medical centers, primary-care clinicians will have expert consultation delivered to them in their offices in a highly personalized fashion, and patients will accomplish in single office visits what now often requires multiple visits and major inconvenience.

- **Remote consultation**: Quick and easy electronic access between medical providers to discuss medical cases will improve access to expert patient care and enhance patient satisfaction. For example, an attending physician, residents, and medical students in a community clinic who treat a patient with an unusual skin lesion will obtain immediate teleconsultation with a dermatologist at a regional medical center. The remote medical team will learn from the dermatologist, the expert will receive clear, diagnostic-quality images of the lesion, and the patient will promptly receive a specialist's assessment. All too often today, patients, when referred to major centers, experience significant delays or fail to keep their appointments due to travel problems. Instead of sending patients to the experts, we will improve their care by using the Internet to bring the experts to them.
- **Integrated health records**: We envision the day when citizens no longer will have multiple records of their healthcare encounters scattered thoughout the offices of numerous physicians and the medical record rooms of multiple hospitals. Instead, their records will be linked electronically over the Internet so that each person has a single "virtual health record"—the distributed, but unified, summary of all the health care they have received in their lives. Furthermore, this record will be secure, treated with respect and confidentiality, and released to providers only with the patient's permission or during times of medical emergency according to strictly defined and enforced criteria (National Research Council, 1997).
- **Computer-based learning**: Soon, a medical student on her orthopedics rotation, preparing to observe her first arthroscopic knee surgery, will be able to go the school's electronic learning center and use the Internet to access and manipulate a three-dimensional "virtual reality" model of the knee on a computer at the National Institutes of Health. She will use new immersive technologies to "enter" the model knee, to look from side to side to view and learn the anatomic structures and their spatial relationships, and to manipulate the model with a simulated arthroscope, thus giving her a surgeon's-eye view of the procedure before she experiences the real thing.
- **Remote computing for bioinformatics**: Someday, a pharmaceutical researcher, working on problems related to drug discovery, will regularly use the Internet to work with three-dimensional molecular models on a supercomputer that is located hundreds of miles away. The researcher manipulates the model, visualizing it on a local display screen, and is able to examine the relationships among atoms or the shape of the active site of an agent or a receptor, all without moving the data from the supercomputer to a local machine.
- **Patient and provider education**: Eventually, clinicians will be able to prescribe specially selected video educational programs for patients that will be delivered to home television sets by a direct Internet connection. Our hospi-

tals and clinics will use video servers over the Internet not only to deliver such materials to patients but also to provide continuing medical and nursing education to their staffs. Health-science schools will similarly provide distance-learning experiences via the Internet for postgraduate education, refresher courses, and home study by health-science students.

- **Disease management**: We anticipate that high-speed Internet access soon will be available in most homes. Clinicians will move beyond the simple use of telephones for managing patient problems at a distance to using their visual senses as well via two-way video links. The infirm will receive "home visits" via video links, thus avoiding unnecessary office or emergency room visits, and care managers will have important new tools for monitoring patients that emphasize prevention rather than crisis management. Early experiments show remarkable enthusiasm by patients when familiar physicians and nurses provide such videoconferencing interactions in the home.

20.1.3 Assumptions Underlying the Scenarios

To help you evaluate these scenarios of the future, we must make explicit the assumptions on which these speculations are based. In particular, we assume that healthcare workers will work increasingly with computers in their daily lives and that improvements in computer technology will continue, independent of technological advances in medical science. Furthermore, we assume that concerns about healthcare cost containment and the threat of malpractice litigation will not be resolved in the near term.

The technological development of medical computing depends in large part on advances in general computing capabilities. Except in the area of medical imaging, little computer technology is first developed for medical applications and then applied to the rest of industry. This is especially true now that a few general-purpose microprocessors and operating systems have become standard for all personal computers. Specialized computer chips will continue to be created for computationally intensive medical applications, such as signal processing. In these image-processing applications, rotation, filtering, enhancement, and reconstruction algorithms must handle more data than can be processed with the standard microprocessors; thus, a market exists for specialized machines.

It is difficult to predict whether the development of new general-purpose computer products will continue to follow an evolutionary trend or will undergo a *paradigm shift*—defined by Kuhn in his book on the nature of scientific discovery as a complete change in perspective, such as occurred with the revelation that the earth is not flat (Kuhn, 1962). Computer processing has gone through some major shifts in direction over the last 30 years: from single-user batch processing, to timesharing on a central resource, and then back to single-user processing, this time on local machines with access to specialized machines through a network. As more and more people try to access key Internet sites, we have moved back to a version of the timesharing model of 30 years ago.

The human–machine interaction style has changed dramatically, with graphical interfaces for novices almost completely replacing command-line interfaces. Pen, speech, and three-dimensional interfaces have been built but have not been widely deployed, except in the case of pen-based datebook applications. For example, Figure 20.2 shows a prototype design of a three-dimensional literature retrieval application built at Xerox's Palo Alto Research Center. There also has been a significant change from electrical to optical methods of network transmission (fiberoptic cables) as well as a steady progression from analog to digital recording of information, best illustrated by the slow switch from film to digital images in radiology, the widespread introduction of high-speed fiber networks, and the development of satellite communication networks. For the purposes of this chapter, we shall assume the continued progression of current trends rather than a significant paradigm shift. An unanticipated discovery that is just around the corner could, of course, quickly invalidate the assumptions.

Another subtle, but pervasive, assumption underlies this book, much of which is written by researchers in medical informatics. We tend to believe that more technology, thoughtfully introduced, is usually better and that computers can enhance almost any aspect of medical practice—especially information access and

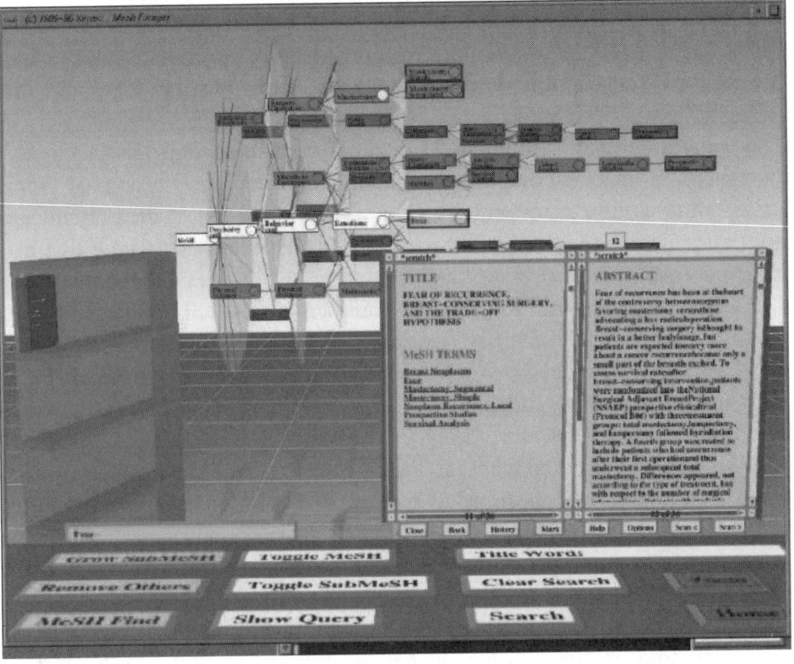

FIGURE 20.2. Three-dimensional representation of the MeSH tree using the Information Visualizer Toolkit created at Xerox PARC. A portion of a citation about breast cancer is shown in the foreground. (*Source*: Reprinted from Hearst/Karadi, SIGIR'97, Courtesy of *ACM*.)

the diagnostic and therapeutic components of the decision-making process. For example, paper documents are still the mainstay of medical records in many medical settings. Still, we strive to eliminate the paper-based components and assume that a well-designed interface (e.g., one that allows handwritten or continuous-speech input) applied to a sufficiently fast computer can significantly improve the overall process of recording and retrieving clinical data. This assumption, however, has yet to be verified.

People frequently criticize medical professionals for being technocrats—for encouraging an increase in mechanization and electronic gadgetry that tends to alienate both workers and patients. Such increases fuel the concern that modern medicine is becoming increasingly impersonal and sterile. How do we meld the automated environments proposed in this chapter's introductory scenarios with our wistful memories of kindly family doctors making house calls and attending their patients' weddings, christenings, bar mitzvahs, and the like? The reality, of course, is that the trend away from such traditional images predated the introduction of computers in medicine and has resulted more from modern pressures on healthcare financing and the need for subspecialization to deal with an increasingly complex subject area. The role for computers and other information technologies results as much from these pressures as it does from a blind faith that all technology is good, useful, and worth the associated costs.

Once medical-computing applications have been shown to be effective, the technologies will need to be evaluated carefully and consistently before their routine adoption. We need to know that the benefits exceed the costs, both financial and sociological. The debate about where and how computers should be used is even more complex in developing countries, where advanced technology might partially compensate for shortages in medical expertise but where scarce healthcare resources might be more effectively employed to provide sanitation, antibiotics, and basic medical supplies. Nonetheless, the scenarios above were painted with the assumptions that there will be an increased application of computers in all aspects of medicine and that the key difference between the future and today will be that computers will become ubiquitous and that they will have a high degree of interconnection and an increased ability to interoperate.

20.2 Integration of Computer-Based Technologies

Most of the individual capabilities described in the preceding scenarios exist today in prototype form. What does not exist is an environment that brings together a large variety of computer-based support tools. The removal of barriers to integration requires both technological advances, such as the development of common hardware-communication protocols, and a better understanding of sociological issues, such as when computer use may be inappropriate or how the need for coordinated planning can overcome logistical barriers to connecting heterogeneous resources in a seamless fashion.

We can begin to assess the degree of connectivity in a medical center by asking simple questions. Can the laboratory computer communicate results to the computer that provides decision support, without a person having to reenter the data? Do the programs that provide decision support use the same terms to describe symptoms as do those that professionals use to perform electronic searches of citation databases? Do physicians use computers to get information without thinking about the fact that they are using a computer system, just as they pick up a medical chart and use it without first thinking about the format of the paper documents?

Computer systems must be integrated into the medical setting in three ways. First, applications must fit the existing information flow in the settings where they are to be used. If the terminal sits in a corner of the clinic, out of the normal traffic flow, and if there is another way to accomplish the specific task, then the computer system is likely to be ignored. Likewise, programs that arbitrarily constrain physicians to unnatural procedures for entering and accessing information are less likely to be used. User interfaces should be flexible and intuitive; just as the fields of a paper medical form can be completed in an arbitrary order, data-entry programs should allow users to enter information in any order.

A surgeon attempting so-called telepresence surgery over the Internet, bringing specialized expertise to an operating room possibly hundreds of miles away, will be unable to assist in the procedure if the movements she makes with hand devices at her end are not instantly reflected in what she sees happening with the actual instruments at the other end of the link. How do we ensure interoperability across the many networks that now span our country (National Research Council, 2000)? Can we guarantee adequate response time for the telesurgery application not only on the major backbone networks but also on the last segments of wire, cable, or wireless network that come into offices and other remote settings?

Second, computer systems should provide common access to all computer-based resources, so a user cannot tell where one program ends and another starts. In this book, we have described such diverse applications as computed tomographic scanning and bibliographic searching. Many of these systems have been developed independently, and most are completely incompatible. In the future, the radiologists' PACS workstation should deliver more than just images—for example, a radiologist may wish also to search easily for references on unusual presentations of a specific disease process and to include these references in a paper that he is composing with a text editor. Ideally, users should not have to switch between computers, to stop one program and to start another, or even to use different sets of commands to obtain all the information they need. That the desired information resources may exist on multiple machines in different parts of the medical center or the country should be invisible to the user.

Third, the user interface must be both consistent across applications and easy to use, which may require multiple interface modalities, such as pointing, flexible spoken natural-language interfaces, and text input. Both at the user interface and internally, programs should use a common terminology to refer to frequently used concepts, such as a diagnosis, a symptom, or a laboratory-test value.

Figure 20.3 shows a futuristic version of a computer system that is worn attached to the body. Using spoken input or a keypad mounted on the arm along with a heads-up display, the computer is inherently as mobile as the person using the system. Although this device may seem far in the future for medical care, a less sophisticated version of this equipment is used everyday in the rental car business to check-in returning cars and print receipts. Although the rental car business is far more structured than medical practice, the example shows that this type of technological change can be successfully integrated into the workplace.

Figure 20.4 shows another possible futuristic communication device: A liquid crystal display (LCD) worn around the neck could be used to provide computer-generated images during surgery or to provide hands-free computer access to support clinical activities in an office-based setting or in the hospital. Input to the device would be speech driven, using the continuous-speech-input methods that are beginning to be adopted.

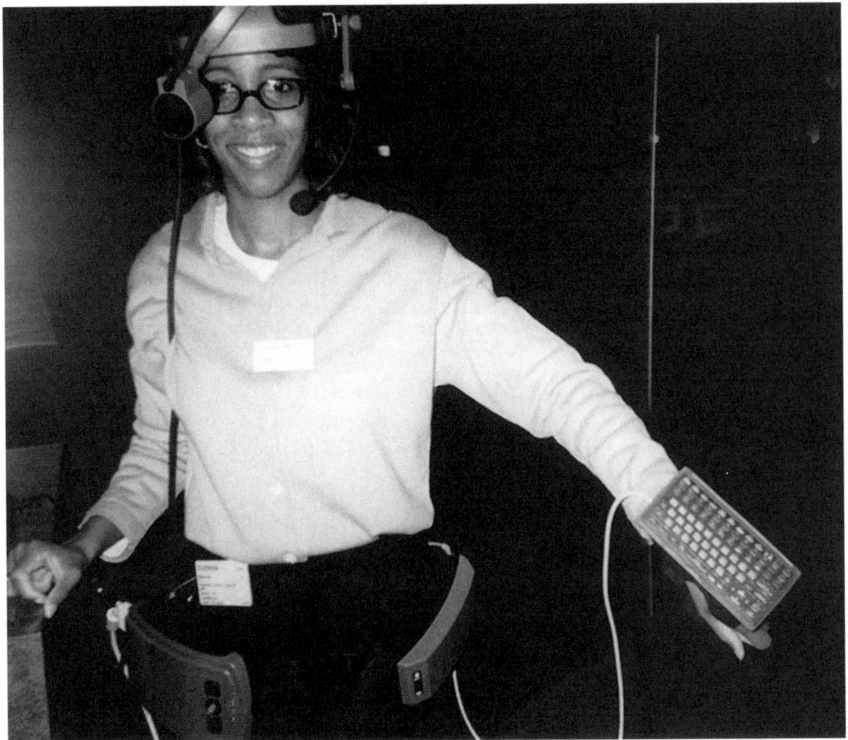

FIGURE 20.3. A wearable computer, including monacle display, voice input, belt-mounted central processing unit, and hand-mounted keypad. (*Source*: Photo by Lawrence M. Fagan. Xybernaut, Mobile Assistant, and MA IV are registered trademarks of Xybernaut Corporation.)

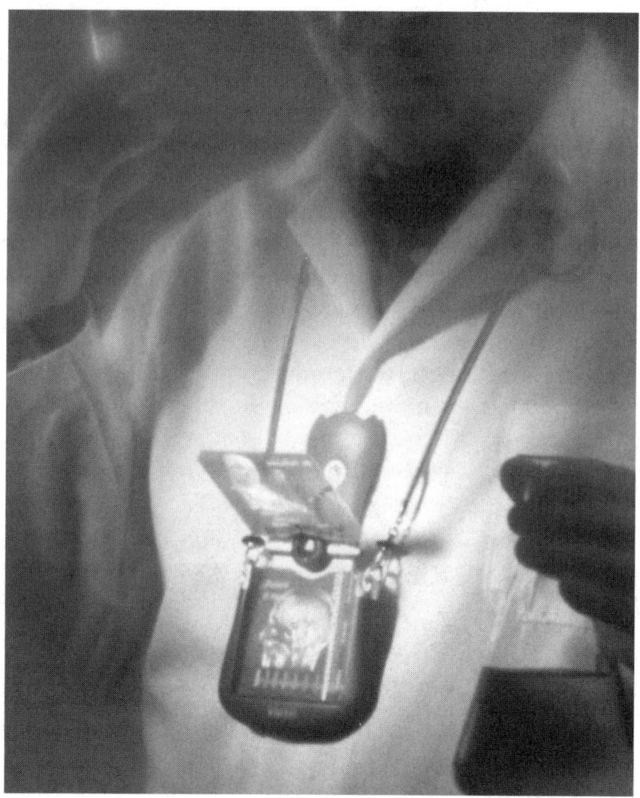

FIGURE 20.4. A possible futuristic personal computing device advances and combines the capabilities of laptop computers and cellular telephones. (*Source*: Reprinted with permission from the American College of Cardiology, *Journal of the American College of Cardiology*, 1998, 186(6):615–621.)

20.3 Future Role of Computers in Health Care

As we discussed in the previous section, fulfillment of the opening scenarios in this chapter will require significant technological changes. Equally important are the organizational and attitudinal changes that will be necessary to implement the new technologies as they emerge. Health professionals, health institutions, medical-system developers, and society as a whole must carefully consider the appropriate role of computers in medicine and assess the potential benefits of computers in terms of improved access to information, enhanced communication, increased efficiency of health-care delivery, and higher quality of medical care.

Although the potential benefits of using computers are many, there are also potential costs, only some of which are monetary. For example, computer-based medical-record systems will never exactly replicate the flexibility of current paper-based systems. This flexibility includes the ability to create progress notes about patients, using any words in any order and in any format, with or without diagrams, to record the information. Computer-based systems limit flexibility in return for increased legibility and access to the information and for the ability to use the information for other purposes, such as clinical research studies that use multiple patient databases. We see the same pattern in the use of automated bank-teller machines. There are only a few ways to complete a cash-withdrawal transaction through a sequence of button pushes, but there is a large number of ways in which we can make this request of a human teller. Automated tellers are available at 3:00 A.M. in the morning, however; human tellers are not.

The idea that computer approaches would require the additional structuring of medical records was perceived by Lawrence Weed more than 30 years ago (Weed, 1969). Weed noted that, for medical records to be useful, they had to be indexed such that important information could be extracted. In particular, he proposed that the medical record be organized according to the patient's current problems—the problem-oriented medical record (POMR). Variations on the POMR have become a standard feature of medical record keeping, regardless of whether computers are used. In the Problem-Oriented Medical Information System (PROMIS), a computer-based implementation of the POMR, such rigid and time-consuming indexing of patient problems was required that clinicians ultimately proved reluctant to use the system. Standardization provides benefits but exacts costs in terms of decreased flexibility; it makes information more accessible but restricts freedom to pursue alternate means to accomplish the same result. It is unlikely that new computer innovations will ever eliminate this trade-off.

Similarly, the use of computers requires trade-offs with respect to confidentiality of medical information. Legitimate users can more conveniently access computer-based records in well-designed systems. Without sufficient security measures, however, unauthorized users may threaten the confidentiality and integrity of databases. Fortunately, with adequate attention to security issues, modern methods backed by effective security policies can ensure that patient data are kept with greater confidentiality in computer systems than they are in paper charts on hospital wards. The growing volume of clinical data stored electronically, widespread remote access capabilities, and the trend toward secondary and tertiary uses of clinical information result in the need for ongoing attention to concerns of security and confidentiality.

Earlier fears that computers could replace physicians have not been borne out, and computers are likely to remain decision-support tools rather than substitute decision-makers (Shortliffe, 1989). It is more likely that computers will be used increasingly to monitor the quality of health care delivered and to help evaluate physician performance. Greater automation will therefore change the nature of medical practice in nontrivial ways. The challenge for system developers and users will be to identify the solution that provides the optimal balance between flexibility and standardization.

20.4 Forces Affecting the Future of Medical Computing

In this book, we have identified several important factors that affect the current and future role of computers in medicine. These factors include advances in biotechnology and computer hardware and software, changes in the background of health professionals, changes in the medicolegal climate, and changing strategies for healthcare reimbursement. The relative strengths of these forces will determine how likely it is that the scenarios we proposed will take place and how quickly we can expect such changes to occur.

20.4.1 Changes in Computers and Biomedical Technology

Modern computers are smaller, less expensive, and more powerful than were their predecessors. Although microchip designers are approaching the physical limits on how close together electronic elements can be placed, these trends will continue. By the time a new microprocessor chip or memory chip is adapted for use in new computer systems, manufacturers are creating samples of the next generation of chips. The most important ramification of current trends in microcomputer technology is that it is now possible to include a microprocessor and memory in most pieces of medical equipment.

The ability to connect multiple devices over high-speed networks has enabled a dramatic change in the way medical computer systems are designed. It is now practical to develop systems in which multiple data-storage devices are accessed by complex computers that sort and abstract the numerous patient data that are generated. This design contrasts with the traditional approach in which health professionals would need to gather information from many different devices or locations in the medical center to obtain a complete picture of a patient's status. Relatively low-cost computer workstations or network-based terminals now allow information to be manipulated at each patient's bedside, as well as at other work areas in medical centers and ambulatory clinics.

High-speed networks and private intranets allow physicians in private offices to connect to computers in the hospitals where they admit patients or to repositories of data from multiple care settings and systems.

We have many more data to transmit over the network, such as those from digitized radiology images, on-line reports, and computer-based charting of the patient's condition. In the future, even faster networks and larger storage devices will be necessary to manage the overwhelming volume of data that will be created by all-digital medical data systems.

20.4.2 Changes in the Background of Health Professionals

Computers will continue to be made faster and less expensive and will have more features; however, sufficient computing power now exists for most applications. Thus, the limitations on the pervasiveness of computers in medicine do not hinge as crucially on the development of new hardware as they did in the past. The availability of relatively inexpensive and powerful computers is changing healthcare workers' familiarity with machines by exposing these people to computers in all aspects of their daily lives. This increased familiarity in turn increases acceptance of computers in the workplace, another crucial determinant of how computers will fare in the next 15 years.

Since the early 1970s, people have increasingly interacted with computers in their daily lives to perform financial transactions, to make travel arrangements, and even to purchase groceries. In many situations, people do not use the computer themselves but rather talk to an intermediary, such as an airline-reservation agent or bank clerk. Large computer systems are so deeply integrated into many business practices that it is not uncommon to hear, "I can't help you—the computer is down." This switch to computer-based record keeping for most financial transactions is so pervasive that you would be surprised and concerned if you were to receive a monthly bank statement that was written out in longhand. Within the last 10 years, many mediated computer-based transactions have been replaced by direct contact between a consumer and a computer system. We can withdraw cash from automated bank tellers, request a trip routing from a computer at the rental-car stand, or obtain an account balance by a touch-tone telephone. As described in almost every chapter in this book, the acceptance of the Internet model of interaction is cutting out intermediary steps and allowing users to directly access large on-line databases from home or work.

Young healthcare workers today have been exposed to computers throughout their education. Many college courses assign projects that must be carried out using the computer. It is difficult to determine how the current hodgepodge of computers in the medical setting will bias these users. It may be that, when the integrated system becomes available, healthcare professionals will not use the system fully because of previous negative experiences in less sophisticated environments. On the other hand, familiarity with computers and with their operation may prepare users to accept well-designed, easy-to-use systems.

20.4.3 Legal Considerations

The number of malpractice lawsuits and the sizes of the settlements have increased in recent years. Today, the specter of potential legal action hangs over every medical interaction. Computers can either exacerbate or alleviate this situation. The computer-based diagnostic system may provide a reminder of a rare but life-threatening disease that might have been overlooked in the differential diagnosis. On the other hand, decision-support systems might generate warnings that, if ignored by healthcare workers, could be used as evidence against those workers in a court action.

20.4.4 Healthcare Financing

Some people assume that the continuing evolution of computer hardware and software is the most important force influencing the development of medical computing. Social issues such as healthcare financing and the legal aspects of medicine, however, probably outweigh the technological factors. Perhaps the strongest force at work today is the pressure to control healthcare costs. Healthcare financing influences all choices regarding the acquisition and maintenance of high-technology equipment and information systems.

Current schemes for healthcare financing have been designed to slow the rate of growth of healthcare costs. These policies translate into pressure to reduce costs in every aspect of medical diagnosis and treatment, such as to substitute ambulatory care for hospitalizations, to shorten hospital stays, to select less expensive surgical procedures, and to order fewer laboratory tests. As incentives for making optimal decisions in these areas increase, there is a greater need for computers that can collect, store, interpret, and present data during the decision-making process.

Order-entry systems routinely screen test orders against criteria for test ordering and question or cancel tests that do not meet the criteria. A more sophisticated clinical decision-support system might serve as an adjunct to an order-management system, assessing which tests are most appropriate to order for specific patients who require expensive workups (e.g., custom-tailored evaluation of thyroid function). Such a system might also evaluate drug orders and suggest less expensive substitutes that are equally effective while checking for drug–drug interactions, and so on.

It is now common that computers are used by health plans to enforce a particular style of care through concurrent or post hoc review of the medical decision-making process, including decisions about length of stay and tests performed. Thus, one force promoting the use of computers by clinicians is the knowledge that computers are often used by insurers to review these clinicians' decisions after the fact. The clinicians may prefer to know what the computer system will advise beforehand so that they can be prepared to justify intentional deviations from the norm. Increasingly, healthcare administrators and medical practice directors are requiring use of clinical systems by clinicians to understand and manage clinical interventions and outcomes in response to decreasing reimbursement for services and managed care contracting arrangements.

Although the use of computer technology can help health professionals to cope with the growing complexity of medical practice, it also contributes to the increasing cost of health care, and it is not always easy to demonstrate corresponding benefits. It is difficult to show that use of computers can lead to a decrease in patient morbidity or mortality, especially in complex environments such as operating rooms or intensive-care units. Large numbers of devices are already being used in these settings, and patients are often treated for multiple concurrent problems. Even if patient-monitoring equipment could help healthcare workers to recognize potentially dangerous situations earlier than they otherwise would, showing that the computer system affected the outcome would be difficult. At the other extreme are devices that can be shown to make a difference, but whose cost is very high, such as computed tomography and magnetic-resonance imaging systems. Because they replace invasive techniques (which have a significant potential for causing harm) or provide information that is available from no other source, there has been little debate about the utility of these new modalities. Instead, the high cost of this equipment has focused attention on how best to distribute these new resources. Demonstrating the return on investment in computer technology is a major challenge to widespread implementation of health-care computer systems in light of their often staggering capital cost and the expense of staff resources required to support the many clinical users and to implement, integrate, manage, and maintain increasingly complex distributed systems and networks. No matter how computer systems are used in the future, we will need to evaluate the influence of the computer application on healthcare financing and to assess the new technology in light of alternative uses of resources.

20.5 Looking Back: What Have We Learned?

An introductory book can only scratch the surface of a field as varied and complex as medical informatics. In each topic, we have examined technical questions about how a system works (or ought to work); we must also view each area in light of the healthcare trends and the social and fiscal issues that shape the ways in which medical care is delivered now and in the future. In this chapter, we have emphasized the rich social and technological context in which medical informatics moves ahead both as a scientific discipline and as a set of methodologies, devices, and complex systems that serve healthcare workers and, through them, their patients. Glimpses of the future can be at once both exciting and frightening—exciting when we see how emerging technologies can address the frequently cited problems that confound current healthcare practices but frightening when we realize that methodologies must be applied wisely and with sensitivity if patients are to receive the humane and cost-sensitive health care that they have every right to expect. The question is not whether computer technologies will play a pervasive role in the healthcare environment of the future, but how we can ensure that future systems are designed and implemented effectively to optimize technology's role as a stimulus and support for the healthcare system and for individual practitioners. The outcomes of the process will depend as much on healthcare planners, practitioners, and policy-makers as they will on the efforts of system developers and medical informatics professionals. It is accordingly to all such individuals that this book has been dedicated.

Suggested Reading

Stead W.W. et al. (Eds.) (1998). Focus on an agenda for biomedical informatics. *Journal of the American Medicial Informatics Association*, 5(5):395–420. Special Issue.

The 1998 Scientific Symposium of the American College of Medical Informatics (ACMI) was devoted to developing visions for the future of health care and biomedicine and a strategic agenda for health and biomedical informatics in support of those visions. The first five articles contained in this special issue illustrate these findings.

Questions for Discussion

1. Select an area of medicine with which you are familiar. Based on what you have learned in this book, propose a scenario for that area that takes place 20 years in the future. Be sure to think about how issues of system integration, networking, and changes in workflow will affect the evolution of computers in the setting you describe.
2. Imagine that you are a patient visiting a healthcare facility at which the physicians have made a major commitment to computer-based tools. How would you react to the following situations?
   a. Before you are ushered into the examining room, the nurse takes your blood pressure and pulse in a work area. He then enters the information into a computer terminal located in the nursing station adjacent to the waiting room.
   b. While the physician interviews you, she occasionally types information into a computer workstation that is facing her; you cannot see the screen.
   c. While the physician interviews you, she occasionally uses a mouse pointing device to enter information into a computer workstation located such that, when facing her, you cannot see the screen.
   d. While the physician interviews you, she occasionally uses a mouse pointing device to enter information into a computer workstation that you both can see. As she does so, she explains the data she is reviewing and entering.
   e. While the physician interviews you, she enters information into a clipboard-sized computer terminal that responds to finger touch and requires no keyboard typing.
   f. While the physician interviews you, she occasionally stops to dictate a phrase. A speech-understanding interface processes what she says and stores the information in a medical-record system.
   g. There is no computer in the examining room, but you notice that between visits, the physician uses a workstation in her office to review and enter patient data.

   Now imagine that you are the physician in each situation. How would you react in each case? What do your answers to these questions tell you about the potential effect of computers on patient–physician rapport? What insight have you gained regarding how interactive technologies could affect the patient–physician encounter? Did you have different reactions to scenarios c and d? Do you believe that most people would respond to these two situations as you did?
3. You are the medical director of a 30-physician multispecialty group practice. The practice is physician-owned and managed and maintains a tight affiliation with a nearby academic medical center. You are considering implementing an ambulatory medical record system to support your practice operations. Discuss at least eight significant challenges you will face, considering technology, user, legal, and financial factors. How will you address each issue?
4. Defend or refute the following proposition: "Knowledge-based clinical systems will be widely used and generally accepted by clinician users within the next 5 years."

Bibliography

3M Health Information Systems (updated annually). *AP-DRGs: All Patient Diagnosis Related Groups*. Wallingford, CT: 3M Health Care.

A. Foster Higgins & Co. Inc. (1997). *Foster Higgins National Survey of Employer-Sponsored Health Plans.*

Abbey L.M., Zimmerman J. (Eds.) (1991). *Dental Informatics, Integrating Technology into the Dental Environment*. New York: Springer-Verlag.

Abromowitz K. (1996). *HMO's: Cycle Bottoming; Secular Opportunity Undiminished.* Berstein Research.

Ackerman M.J. (1991). The Visible Human project. *Journal of Biocommunication*, 18(2): 14.

ADAM (1995). ADAM Software [CD-ROM]. ADAM Scholar Series.

Adams I.D., Chan M., Clifford P.C., Cooke W.M., Dallos V., de Dombal F.T., Edwards M.H., Hancock D.M., Hewett D.J., McIntyre N. (1986). Computer aided diagnosis of acute abdominal pain: a multicenter study. *British Medical Journal*, 293(6550):800–804.

Adderley D., Hyde C., Mauseth P. (1997). The computer age impacts nurses. *Computers in Nursing*, 15(1):43–46.

Aine C.J. (1995). A conceptual overview and critique of functional neuroimaging techniques in humans: I. MRI/fMRI and PET. *Critical Reviews in Neurobiology*, 9(2–3): 229–309.

Allaërt F.A., Dusserne L. (1992). Decision support systems and medical liability. In Frisse, M.E. (Ed.) *Proceedings of the 16th Annual Symposium on Computer Applications in Medical Care*, (pp. 750–753). Baltimore, MD.

Alpert S.A. (1998). Health care information: access, confidentiality, and good practice. In Goodman K.W. (Ed.), *Ethics, Computing, and Medicine: Informatics and the Transformation of Health Care* (pp. 75–101) Cambridge: Cambridge University Press.

Altman R.B. (1997). Informatics in the care of patients: ten notable challenges. *Western Journal of Medicine*, 166(6):118–122.

Altman R.B., Dunker A.K., Hunter L., Klein T.E. (Eds.) (1998). *Pacific Symposium on Biocomputing '98*. Singapore: World Scientific Publishing.

Altschul S.F., Gish W., Miller W., Myers E.W., Lipman D.J. (1990). Basic local alignment search tool. *Journal of Molecular Biology*, 215(3):403–410.

American Association of Health Plans (1995). AAHP HMO and PPO Trends Report. *AMCRA Census Database and AAHP Sample Survey of HMOs and PPOs*. Washington DC: American Association of Health Plans.

American College of Pathologists (1982). *SNOMED*. Skokie, IL: College of American Pathology.

American Medical Association (updated annually). *Current Procedural Terminology*. Chicago, IL: The American Medical Association.

American Nurses Association (1995). *Scope of Practice for Nursing Informatics*. Washington, DC: American Nurses Publishing.

American Nurses Association (1997). *NIDSEC Standards and Scoring Guidelines*. Washington, DC: American Nurses Publishing.

American Psychiatric Association Committee on Nomenclature and Statistics (1987). *Diagnostic and Statistical Manual of Mental Disorders* (rev. 3rd ed.). Washington, DC: The American Psychiatric Association.

American Psychiatric Association Committee on Nomenclature and Statistics (1994). *Diagnostic and Statistical Manual of Mental Disorders* (4th ed.). Washington, DC: The American Psychiatric Association.

American Society for Testing and Materials (1989). *Standard Guide for Nosologic Standards and Guides for Construction of New Biomedical Nomenclature* (Standard E1284–89). Philadephia: ASTM.

American Society for Testing and Materials (1994). *A Standard Specification for Representing Clinical Laboratory Test and Analyte Names* (Standard E3113.2 [draft]). Philadelphia: ASTM.

American Society for Testing and Materials (1999). *Standard Guide for Properties of a Universal Healthcare Identifier (UHID)* (E1714–95) West Conshohocken, PA: American Society for Testing and Materials.

Amir M., Shabot M.M., Karlan B.Y. (1997). Surgical intensive care unit care after ovarian cancer surgery: an analysis of indications. *American Journal of Obstetrics and Gynecology*, 176(6):1389–1393.

Anderson J.G., Aydin C.E. (1994). Overview: theoretical perspectives and methodologies for the evaluation of health care information systems. In Anderson J.G., Aydin C.E., Jay S.J. (Eds.), *Evaluating Health Care Information Systems: Methods and Applications.* Thousand Oaks, CA: Sage.

Anderson J.G., Aydin C.E. (1998). Evaluating medical information systems: social contexts and ethical challenges. In Goodman K.W. (Ed.), *Ethics, Computing, and Medicine: Informatics and the Transformation of Health Care* (pp. 57–74). Cambridge: Cambridge University Press.

Anderson J.G., Aydin C.E., Jay S.J. (Eds.) (1994). *Evaluating Health Care Information Systems: Methods and Applications*. Thousand Oaks, CA: Sage.

Anderson J.G., Aydin C.E., Jay S.J. (Eds.) (1995). *Computers in Health Care: Research and Evaluation* Newbury Park, CA: Sage.

Anderson J.G., Jay S.J. (Eds.) (1987). *Use and Impact of Computers in Clinical Medicine*. New York: Springer-Verlag.

Anonymous (1993a). *Draft Application Protocol for Electronic Exchange in Health Care Environments* (Version 2.2, HL7).

Anonymous (1993b). *Standard for Health Care Data Interchange—Information Model Methods.* Draft P1157.1, IEEE.

Anonymous (1994). *NCPDP Data Dictionary.* June 1.

Arenson R.L. (1984). Automation of the radiology management function. *Radiology*, 153:65–68.

Arenson R.L., Gitlin J.N., London J.W. (April 1982). The formation of a radiology computer consortium. In *Proceedings of the 7th Conference on Computer Applications in Radiology*, (pp. 153–164). Boston, MA: American College of Radiology.

Arenson R.L., Seshadri S., Kundel H.L., DeSimone D., Van der Voorde F., Gefter W.B., Epstein D.M., Miller W.T., Aronchick J.M., Simson M.B. (1988). Clinical evaluation of a medical image management system for chest images. *American Journal of Roentgenology*, 150(1):55–59.

Ash J. (1997). Organizational factors that influence information technology diffusion in academic health centers. *Journal of the American Medical Informatics Association*, 4(2):102–111.

Association of American Medical Colleges (1984). Physicians for the twenty-first century (Report of the Project Panel on the General Professional Education of the Physician and College Preparation for Medicine). *Journal of Medical Education*, 59(11):(Part 2)1–208.

Association of American Medical Colleges (1986). *Medical Education in the Information Age, Proceedings of the Symposium on Medical Informatics*. Washington D.C.: Association of American Medical Colleges.

Axford R., Carter B. (1996). Impact of clinical information systems on nursing practice: Nurses' perspectives. *Computers in Nursing*, 14(3):156–163.

Ayers S. (1983). NIH consensus conference. Critical care medicine. *Journal of the American Medical Association*, 250(6):798–804.

Babior B.M., Matzner Y. (1997). The familial Mediterranean fever gene—cloned at last. *New England Journal of Medicine*, 337(21):1548–1549.

Bachant J., McDermott J. (1984). R1 revisited: four years in the trenches. *AI Magazine*, 5:3.

Bachrach C., Charen T. (1978). Selection of MEDLINE contents, the development of its thesaurus, and the indexing process. *Medical Informatics*, 3(3):237–254.

Bader S. (1993). Recognition of computer-based materials in the promotion guidelines of U.S. medical schools. *Academic Medicine*, 68:S16–S17.

Bai C., Elledge S.J. (1997). Gene identification using the yeast two-hybrid system. *Methods of Enzymology*, 283:141–156.

Baker E.L., Friede A., Moulton A.D., Ross D.A. (1995). CDC's information network for public health officials (INPHO): A framework for integrated public health information and practice. *Journal of Public Health Management and Practice*, 1:43–47.

Balas E.A., Austin S.M., Mitchell J.A., Ewigman B.G., Bopp K.D., Brown G.D. (1996). The clinical value of computerized information services. A review of 98 randomized clinical trials. *Archives of Family Medicine*, 5(5):271–278.

Ball M. (Ed.) (1995). *Introduction to Nursing Informatics*. New York: Springer.

Bansler J.P., Bødker K. (1993). A reappraisal of structured analysis: design in an organizational context. *Proceedings of the ACM Transactions on Information Systems*, 11: 165–193.

Barfield W., Furness T. (Eds.) (1995). *Virtual Environments and Advanced Interface Design*. New York: Oxford University Press.

Barnett G.O. (1976). *Computer-Stored Ambulatory Record (COSTAR)* (DHEW (HRA) 76–3145). Washington, DC: Department of Health, Education, and Welfare.

Barnett G.O. (1984). The application of computer-based medical-record systems in ambulatory practice. *New England Journal of Medicine*, 310(25):1643–1650.

Barnett G.O., Cimino J.J., Hupp J.A., Hoffer E.P. (1987). DXplain. An evolving diagnostic decision-support system. *Journal of the American Medical Association*, 258(1): 67–74.

Barrows R.C. Jr., Clayton P.D. (1996). Privacy, confidentiality, and electronic medical records. *Journal of the American Medical Informatics Association*, 3(2):139–148.

Bass D.M., McClendon M.J., Brennan P.F., McCarthy C. (1998). The buffering effect of a computer support network on caregiver strain. *Journal of Aging and Health*, 10(1):20–43.

Bates D.W., Spell N., Cullen D.J., Burdick E., Laird N., Petersen L.A., Small S.D., Sweitzer B.J., Leape L.L. (1997). The costs of adverse drug events in hospitalized patients. *Journal of the American Medical Association*, 277(4):307–311.

Bauman R.A., Arenson R.L., Barnett G.O. (March 1975a). Computer-based master folder tracking and automated file room operations. In *Proceedings of the 4th Conference on Computer Applications in Radiology*, (pp. 469–480). Las Vegas, NV: American College of Radiology.

Bauman R.A., Arenson R.L., Barnett G.O. (March 1975b). Fully automated scheduling of radiology appointments. In *Proceedings of the 4th Conference on Computer Applications in Radiology*, (pp. 461–468). Las Vegas, NV: American College of Radiology.

Bauman R.A., Gell G., Dwyer S.J. 3rd. (1996). Large picture archiving and communication systems of the world-Part 2. *Journal of Digital Imaging*, 9(4):172–177.

Bauman R.A., Pendergrass H.P., Greenes R.A. (1972). Further development of an on-line computer system for radiology reporting. In *Proceedings of the Conference on Computer Applications in Radiology* (pp. 409–422). Las Vegas, NV: American College of Radiology.

Beck J.R., Pauker S.G. (1983). The Markov process in medical prognosis. *Medical Decision Making*, 3(4):419–58.

Bell D.S., Greenes R.A. (1994). Evaluation of UltraSTAR: Performance of a collaborative structured data entry system. In *Proceedings of the 18th Annual Symposium on Computer Applications in Medical Care (SCAMC), JAMIA, Symposium Supplement* (pp. 216–221). Washington, DC: Hanley & Belfus, November.

Bentt L.R., Santora T.A., Leyerle B.J., LoBue M., Shabot M.M. (1990). Accuracy and utility of pulse oximetry in a surgical ICU. *Current Surgery*, 47(4):267–268.

Berenson R. (1984). *Health Technology Case Study 28: Intensive Care Units (ICUs)—Clinical Outcomes, Costs and Decisionmaking*. Washington, DC: Office of Technology Assessment.

Berg M. (1997). *Rationalizing Medical Work: Decision Support Techniques and Medical Practices*. Cambridge, MA: MIT Press.

Bergeron B.P., Greenes R.A. (1989). Clinical skill-building simulations in cardiology: HeartLab and EKGLab. *Computer Methods and Programs in Biomedicine*, 30(2–3): 111–126.

Berners-Lee T., Cailliau R., Luotonen A., Nielsen H., Secret A. (1994). The World-Wide-Web. *Communications of the Association for Computing Machinery*, 37:76–82.

Bero L., Rennie D. (1996). The Cochrane Collaboration: preparing, maintaining, and disseminating systematic reviews of the effects of health care. *Journal of the American Medical Association*, 274:1935–1938.

Bickel R.G. (1979). The TRIMIS concept. In Dunn, R.A. *Proceedings of the 3rd Annual Symposium for Computer Applications in Medical Care* (pp. 839–842). Washington, DC: IEEE. October 14–17.

Bidgood W.D., Horii S.C., Prior F.W., Van Syckle D.E. (1997). Understanding and using DICOM, the data interchange standard for biomedical imaging. *Journal of the American Medical Informatics Association*, 4(3):199–212.

Bishop M., Rawlings C. (Eds.) (1997). *DNA and Protein Sequence Analysis—A Practical Approach*. New York: IRL Press at Oxford University Press.

Blaine G.J., Hill R.L., Cox J.R. (1983). PACS workbench at Mallinckrodt Institute of Radiology (MIR). In *Proceedings of the SPIE (Society of Photo-optical Instrumentation Engineers)* (pp. 80–86). Kansas City, MO, 418 (PACSII). IEEE Computer Society.

Bleich H. (1972). Computer-based consultation: electrolyte and acid-base disorders. *American Journal of Medicine*, 53:285–291.

Bleich H.L., Beckley R.F., Horowitz G.L., Jackson J.D., Moody E.S., Franklin C., Goodman S.R., McKay M.W., Pope R.A., Walden T. (1985). Clinical computing in a teaching hospital. *New England Journal of Medicine*, 312(12):756–764.

Bleich H.L., Safran C., Slack W.V. (1989). Departmental and laboratory computing in two hospitals. *MD Computing*, 6(3):149–155.

Bliss-Holtz J. (1995). Computerized support for case management: ISAACC. *Computers in Nursing*, 13(6):289–294.

Blois M.S. (1984). *Information and Medicine: The Nature of Medical Descriptions*. Berkeley: University of California Press.

Blum B.I. (1992). *Software Engineering, A Holistic Approach*. New York: Oxford University Press.

Blum B.I. (1986a). *Clinical Information Systems*. New York: Springer-Verlag.

Blum B.I. (1986b). Clinical information systems: a review. *Western Journal of Medicine*, 145(6):791–797.

Boehm B., Egyed A., Kwan J., Port D., Shah A., Madachy R. (1998). Using the Win Win Spiral Model: a case study. *IEEE Computer*, 31(7):33–44.

Boland P. (1985). *The New Healthcare Market: A Guide to PPOs for Purchasers, Payers and Providers*. Homewood, IL: Dow Jones Irwin.

Bone R.C. (1995). Standards of evidence for the safety and effectiveness of critical care monitoring devices and related interventions. *Critical Care in Medicine*, 23(10):1756–1763.

Booch G. (1994). *Object-Oriented Design with Applications*. (2nd ed.): Redwood City, CA: Benjamin-Cummins.

Bookstein F.L. (1989). Principal warps: thin-plate splines and the decomposition of deformations. *IEEE Transactions on Pattern Analysis and Machine Intelligence*, 11(6): 567–585.

Bowden D.M., Martin R.F. (1995). Neuronames brain hierarchy. *Neuroimage*, 2:63–83.

Bradshaw K.E., Gardner R.M., Clemmer T.P., Orme J.F., Thomas F., West B.J. (1984). Physician decision-making: evaluation of data used in a computerized ICU. *International Journal of Clinical Monitoring and Computing*, 1(2):81–91.

Bradshaw K.E., Sittig D.F., Gardner R.M., Pryor T.A., Budd M. (1988). Improving efficiency and quality in a computerized ICU. *Proceedings of the 12th Annual Symposium on Computer Applications in Medical Care*, Washington, DC, 763–767.

Brahams D., Wyatt J.C. (1989). Decision aids and the law. *Lancet*, 2(8663):632–634.

Brannigan V.M. (1991). Software quality regulation under the safe medical devices act of 1990: hospitals are now the canaries in the software mine. In Clayton, P.D. (Ed.) *Proceedings of the 15th Annual Symposium on Computer Applications in Medical Care* (pp. 238–242). Washington, DC. New York: McGraw-Hill

Brennan P.F. (1996). The future of clinical communication in an electronic environment. *Holistic Nursing Practice*, 11(1):97–104.

Brennan P.F., Moore S.M., Smyth K.A. (1995). The effects of a special computer network on caregivers of persons with Alzheimer's disease. *Nursing Research*, 44(3): 166–172.

Brennan P.F., Ripich S. (1994). Use of a home care computer network by persons with AIDS. *International Journal of Technology Assessment in Health Care*, 10(2):258–272.

Brigham C.R., Kamp M. (1974). The current status of computer-assisted instruction in the health sciences. *Journal of Medical Education*, 49(3):278–279.

Brimm J. (1987). Computers in critical care. *Critical Care Nursing Quarterly*, 9(4):53.

Brinkley J.F. (1991). Structural informatics and its applications in medicine and biology. *Academic Medicine*, 66:589–591.

Brinkley J.F. (1993). The potential for three-dimensional ultrasound. In: Chervenak F.A., Isaacson G.C., Campbell S. (Eds.), *Ultrasound in Obstetrics and Gynecology* (chap. 5, pp. 61–72). Boston: Little, Brown and Company.

Brinkley J.F., Moritz W.E., Baker D.W. (1978). Ultrasonic three-dimensional imaging and volume from a series of arbitrary sector scans. *Ultrasound in Medicine and Biology*, 4:317–327.

Brinkley J.F., Myers L.M., Prothero J.S., Heil G.H., Tsuruda J.S., Maravilla K.R., Ojemann G.A., Rosse C. (1997). A structural information framework for brain mapping. In Koslow S.H., Huerta M.F. (Eds.), *Neuroinformatics: An Overview of the Human Brain Project* (pp. 309–334). Mahwah, NJ: Lawrence Erlbaum.

Brinkley J.F., Rosse C. (1997). The Digital Anatomist distributed framework and its applications to knowledge based medical imaging. *Journal of the American Medical Informatics Association*, 4(3):165–183.

Brody B.A. (1989). The ethics of using ICU scoring systems in individual patient management. *Problems in Critical Care*, 3:662–670.

Bryant G.D., Norman G.R. (1980). Expressions of probability: words and numbers. *The New England Journal of Medicine*, 302:411.

Buchman T.G. (1995). Computers in the intensive care unit: promises yet to be fulfilled. *Journal of Intensive Care Medicine*, 10:234–240.

Bulecheck G.M., McCloskey J.C., Donahue W.J. (1995). Nursing Interventions Classification (NIC): a language to describe nursing treatments. In *Nursing Data Systems: The Emerging Framework* (pp. 115–131). Washington, DC: American Nurses Publishing.

California Managed Health Care Improvement Task Force (1998). Public Perceptions and Experiences with Managed Care, Background Paper and Literature Review. *Improving Managed Health Care in California.* Vols. 2:13–42 and Vol. 3:207–212. Sacramento, CA.

California Office of Statewide Health Planning and Development (1992). *Volume of Coronary Artery Bypass Grafts for 1989–1992 from the Patient Discharge Data Set.* California Office of Statewide Health Planning & Development.

Campbell J.R., Carpenter P., Sneiderman C., Cohn S., Chute C.G., Warren J. (1997). Phase II evaluation of clinical coding schemes: completeness, taxonomy, mapping, definitions, and clarity. CPRI Work Group on Codes and Structures. *Journal of the American Medical Informatics Association*, 4(3):238–251.

Campbell K.E., Tuttle M.S., Spackman K.A. (1998). A "lexically-suggested logical closure" metric for medical terminology maturity. In Chute, C.G. *Proceedings of the 1998 AMIA Annual Fall Symposium (Formerly SCAMC)* (pp. 785–789) Orlando, FL, November 7–11.

Capin T.K., Noser H., Thalmann D., Pandzic I.S., Thalmann N.M. (1997). Virtual human representation and communication in VLNet. *IEEE Computer Graphics and Applications*, 17(2):42–53.

CFO (1996). The Third Annual Survey: Holding the Line on SG&A. *CFO*, December 1996:28–36.

Chalmers I., Altman D. (Eds.) (1995). *Systematic Reviews.* London: BMJ Publishing Group.

Chandra M., Wagner W.H., Shabot M.M. (1995). ICU care after infra-inguinal arterial surgery: a critical analysis of outcomes. *The American Surgeon*, 61(10):904–907.

Chapman K.A., Moulton A.D. (1995). The Georgia Information Network for Public Health Officials: a demonstration of the CDC INPHO concept. *Journal of Public Health Management & Practice*, 1(2):39–43.

Chen R., Felciano R., Altman R.B. (1997). RIBOWEB: linking structural computations to a knowledge base of published experimental data. *Intelligent Systems for Molecular Biology*, 5:84–87.

Christensen G.E., Miller M.I., Vannier M.W. (1996). Individualizing neuroanatomical atlases using a massively parallel computer. *IEEE Computer*, 29(1):32–38.

Chute C.G. (1998). *Electronic Medical Record Infrastructures: An Overview of Critical Standards and Classifications*. New York: Springer-Verlag.

Chute C.G., Cohn S.P., Campbell K.E., Oliver D.E., Campbell J.R. (1996). The content coverage of clinical classifications. *Journal of the American Medical Informatics Association*, 3:224–233.

Cimino J.J., Johnson S.B., Aguirre A., Roderer N., Clayton P.D. (1992). The MEDLINE button. In Frisse, M.E. *Proceedings of the 16th Annual Symposium on Computer Applications in Medical Care*, (pp. 81–85). Baltimore, MD.

Clancey W. (1984). The epistemology of a rule-based expert system: a framework for explanation. In Frisse, M.E. *Artificial Intelligence*, McGraw Hill, Inc. 20:215–251.

Clancey W. (1989). Viewing knowledge bases as qualitative models. *IEEE Expert*, 4(2):9–23.

Clancey W.J. (1986). From GUIDON to NEOMYCIN and HERACLES in twenty short lessons: ONR final report 1979–1985. *AI Magazine*, 7(3):40–60.

Clark J., Lang N.M. (1992). Nursing's next advance: an international classification for nursing practice. *International Nursing Review*, 39(4):109–112.

Clarysse P., Riboulet D., Magnin I.E. (1997). Tracking geometrical descriptors on 3–D deformable surfaces: application to the left-ventricular surface of the heart. *IEEE Transactions on Medical Imaging*, 16(4):392–404.

Classen D.C., Pestotnik S.L., Evans R.S., Lloyd J.F., Burke J.P. (1997). Adverse drug events in hospitalized patients. Excess length of stay, extra costs, and attributable mortality. *Journal of the American Medical Association*, 277(4):301–306.

Cohen P.R. (1995). *Empirical Methods for Artificial Intelligence*. Cambridge, MA: MIT Press.

College of American Pathologists (1971). *Systematized Nomenclature of Pathology*. Chicago: The College of American Pathologists.

Collen M.F. (1983). The functions of an HIS: an overview. In: Fokkens O. *Proceedings of the MEDINFO 83 Seminars* (pp. 61–64). Amsterdam: North Holland.

Collen M.F. (1995). *A History of Medical Informatics in the United States: 1950 to 1990*. Bethesda, MD: American Medical Informatics Association, Hartman Publishing.

Collins D.L., Neelin P., Peters T.M., Evans A.C. (1994). Automatic 3–D intersubject registration of MR volumetric data in standardized Talairach space. *Journal of Computer Assisted Tomography*, 18(2):192–205.

Commission on Professional and Hospital Activities (1978). *International Classification of Diseases, Ninth Revision, with Clinical Modifications (ICD-9–CM)*. Ann Arbor: American Hospital Association.

Committee on Ways and Means (1997). *Medicare and Health Care Chartbook*. U.S. House of Representatives.

Congressional Budget Office (1996). *Reducing the Deficit: Spending and Revenue Options*. Washington, DC: U.S. Government Printing Office.

Connolly D. (Ed.) (1997). *XML: Principles, Tools, and Techniques*. Cambridge, MA: O'Reilly & Associates.

Cooke J.T., Barie P.S. (1998). Information management and decision support systems in the intensive care unit. *Surgical Technology International*, VI: 25–42.

Côté R.A., Robboy S. (1980). Progress in medical information management: systematized nomenclature of medicine (SNOMED). *Journal of the American Medical Association*, 243:756.

Côté R.A., Rothwell D.J., Palotay J.L., Beckett R.S., Brochu L. (Eds.) (1993). *The Systematized Nomenclature of Medicine: SNOMED International*. Northfield, IL: College of American Pathologists.

Covell D.G., Uman G.C., Manning P.R. (1985). Information needs in office practice: are they being met? *Annals of Internal Medicine*, 103(4):596–599.

Cox Jr. J. (1972). Digital analysis of the electroencephalogram, the blood pressure wave, and the electrocardiogram. *Proceedings of the IEEE*, 60:1137.

Cunneen S.A., Shabot M.M., Wagner W.H. (1998). Outcomes from abdominal aortic aneurysm resection: does SICU length of stay make a difference? *American Surgeon*, 64(2):196–199.

Curran W.J., Stearns B., Kaplan H. (1969). Privacy, confidentiality, and other legal considerations in the establishment of a centralized health-data system. *New England Journal of Medicine*, 281(5):241–248.

Cushing H. (1903). On routine determination of arterial tension in operating room and clinic. *Boston Medical Surgical Journal*, 148:250.

Dager S.R., Steen R.G. (1992). Applications of magnetic resonance spectroscopy to the investigation of neuropsychiatric disorders. *Neuropsychopharmacology*, 6(4):249–266.

Dalto J.D., Johnson K.V., Gardner R.M., Spuhler V.J., Egbert L. (1997). Medical Information Bus usage for automated IV pump data acquisition: evaluation of usage patterns. *International Journal of Clinical Monitoring and Computing*, 14(3):151–154.

David J.M., Krivine J.P., Simmons R. (Eds.) (1993). *Second Generation Expert Systems*. Berlin: Springer-Verlag.

Davis W.S. (1994). *Business Systems Design and Analysis*. Belmont, CA: Wadsworth Publishing.

Day H. (1963). An intensive coronary care area. *Diseases of the Chest*, 44:423.

Dayhoff M.O., Barker W.C., McLaughlin P.J. (1974). Inferences from protein and nucleic acid sequences: early molecular evolution, divergence of kingdoms and rates of change. *Origins of Life*, 5(3):311–330.

Dean A.G., Dean J.A., Burton A.H., Dicker R.C. (1991). EpiInfo: a general purpose microcomputer program for public health information systems. *American Journal of Preventitive Medicine*, 7(3):178–182.

DeBakey M.E. (1991). The National Library of Medicine: evolution of a premier information center. *Journal of the American Medical Association*, 266(9):1252–1258.

de Bliek R., Friedman C.P., Blaschke T.F., France C.L., Speedie S.M. (1988). Practitioner preferences and receptivity for patient-specific advice from a therapeutic monitoring system. In Greenes, R.A. *Proceedings of the 12th Annual Symposium on Computer Applications in Medical Care* (pp. 225–228). Washington, DC: IEEE.

de Dombal F.T. (1987). Ethical considerations concerning computers in medicine in the 1980s. *Journal of Medical Ethics*, 13(4):179–184.

de Dombal F.T., Leaper D.J., Staniland J.R., McCann A.P., Horrocks J.C. (1972). Computer-aided diagnosis of acute abdominal pain. *British Medical Journal*, 1:376–380.

Degoulet P., Phister B., Fieschi M. (1997). *Introduction to Clinical Informatics*. New York: Springer-Verlag.

Deibel S.R., Greenes R.A. (1995). An infrastructure for the development of health care information systems from distributed components. *Journal of the American Society for Information Science*, 26:765–771.

Deibel S.R., Greenes R.A. (1996). Radiology systems architectures. *Radiology Clinics of North America*, 34(3):681–696.

Detmer W.M., Barnett G.O., Hersh W.R. (1997). MedWeaver: integrating decision support, literature searching, and Web exploration using the UMLS Metathesaurus. In Masys D.R. *Proceedings of the 1997 AMIA Annual Fall Symposium (Formerly SCAMC)* (pp. 490–494). Nashville, TN: Hanky & Belfus, October 25–29.

Detmer W.M., Friedman C.P. (1994). Academic physicians' assessment of the effects of computers on health care. In *Proceedings of the 18th Annual Symposium on Computer Applications in Medical Care* (pp. 558–562). Washington, DC. Hanky & Belfus,

Detmer W.M., Shortliffe E.H. (1995). A model of clinical query management that supports integration of biomedical information over the World Wide Web. In Gardner RM *Proceedings of the 19th Annual Symposium on Computer Applications in Medical Care* (pp. 898–902). New Orleans, LA. Hankey & Belfus.

Detmer W.M., Shortliffe E.H. (1997). Using the Internet to improve knowledge diffusion in medicine. *Communications of the ACM*, 40:101–108.

Dev P., Pichumani R., Walker D., Heinrichs W.L., Karadi C., Lorie W. (1998). Formative design of a virtual learning environment. In *Medicine Meets Virtual Reality* (pp. 6). Amsterdam: IOS Press.

Dick R., Steen E. (Eds.) (1991 [Revised 1997]). *The Computer-Based Patient Record: An Essential Technology for Health Care*. Washington, DC: Institute of Medicine, National Academy Press.

Donabedian A. (1996). Evaluating the quality of medical care. *Millbank Memorial Quarterly*, 44:166–206.

D'Orsi C.J., Kopans D.B. (1997). Mammography interpretation: the BI-RADS method. *American Family Physician*, 55(5):1548–1550.

Drazen E., Metzger J. (1999). *Strategies for Integrated Health Care*. San Francisco: Jossey-Bass Publishers.

Duda R.O., Shortliffe E.H. (1983). Expert systems research. *Science*, 220(4594):261–268.

Durfy S.J. (1993). Ethics and the Human Genome Project. *Archives of Pathology and Laboratory Medicine*, 117(5):466–469.

Dwyer S.J. 3rd. (1996). Imaging system architectures for picture archiving and communication systems. *Radiology Clinics of North America*, 34(3):495–503.

East T.D., Bohm S.H., Wallace C.J., Clemmer T.P., Weaver L.K., Orme Jr. J.F., Morris A.H. (1992). A successful computerized protocol for clinical management of pressure control inverse ratio ventilation. *Chest*, 101(3):697–710.

Eddy D.M. (1992). *A Manual for Assessing Health Practices and Designing Practice Policies. The Explicit Approach.* Philadelphia: American College of Physicians.

Editorial (1997). Electronic threats to medical privacy. *New York Times,* March 11, A14.

Egan D., Remde J., Gomez L., Landauer T., Eberhardt J., Lochbaum C. (1989). Formative design-evaluation of Superbook. *ACM Transactions on Information Systems*, 7:30–57.

Eisner E.W. (1991). *The Enlightened Eye: Qualitative Inquiry and the Enhancement of Educational Practice*. New York: McMillan Publishing Co.

Eliot C.R., Williams K.A., Woolf B.P. (1996). An intelligent learning environment for advanced cardiac life support. In Cimino, J.J. *Proceedings of the AMIA Annual Fall Symposium (formerly SCAMC)* (pp. 7–11). Washington, DC: Hanley & Belfus, October 28–30.

Ellwood P.M. (1988). Shattuck lecture—outcomes management. A technology of Patient Experience. *New England Journal of Medicine*, 318(23):1549–1556.

Ellwood P.M. Jr., Anderson N.N., Billings J.E., Carlson R.J., Hoagberg E.J., McClure W. (1971). Health maintenance strategy. *Medical Care*, 9(3):291–298.

Elstein A.S., Shulman L.S., Sprafka S.A. (1978). *Medical Problem Solving: An Analysis of Clinical Reasoning*. Cambridge, MA: Harvard University Press.

Employee Benefit Research Institute (1995). *Sources of Health Insurance and Characteristics of the Uninsured: Analysis of the March 1994 Current Population Survey.*

Enthoven A.C. (1993). The history and principles of managed competition. *Health Affairs*, 12(Suppl):24–48.

Enthoven A.C. (1997). Market based reform of US health care financing and delivery: managed care and managed competition. In *Proceedings of the Innovations in Health Care Financing: Proceedings of a World Bank Conference* (pp. 195–214). March 10–11.

Enthoven A.C., Singer S.J. (1997). *Reforming Medicare before it's too late.* (Research Paper Series, No. 1411.) Stanford University Graduate School of Business.

Eriksson H., Musen M. (1993). Metatools for knowledge acquisition. *IEEE Software*, 10(3):23–29.

Eriksson H., Puerta A.R., Musen M.A. (1994). Generation of knowledge-acquisition tools from domain ontologies. *International Journal of Human-Computer Studies*, 41:425–453.

Eriksson H., Shahar Y., Tu S.W., Puerta A.R., Musen M.A. (1995). Task modeling with reusable problem-solving methods. *Artificial Intelligence*, 79(2):293–326.

EUCLIDES Foundation International (1994). *EUCLIDES Coding System Version 4.0*: The EUCLIDES Foundation.

Evans D., Patel V. (Eds.) (1989). *Cognitive Science in Medicine*. London: MIT Press.

Evans R.S., Larson R.A., Burke J.P., Gardner R.M., Meier F.A., Jacobson J.A., Conti M.T., Jacobson J.T., Hulse R.K. (1986). Computer surveillance of hospital-acquired infections and antibiotic use. *Journal of the American Medical Association*, 256(8): 1007–1011.

Evans R.S., Pestotnik S.L., Classes D.C., Clemmer T.P., Weaver L.K., Orme J.F. Jr., Lloyd J.F., Burke J.P. (1998). A computer-assisted management program for antibiotics and other antiinfective agents. *New England Journal of Medicine*, 338(4):232–238.

Fafchamps D., Young C.Y., Tang P.C. (1991). Modelling work practices: input to the design of a physician's workstation. In Clayton, P.D. *Proceedings of the 15th Annual Symposium on Computer Applications in Medical Care* New York: McGraw Hill (pp. 788–792).

Federal Hospital Insurance Trust Fund (1996). Annual Report of the Board of Trustees.

Feinstein A.R. (1995). Meta-analysis: statistical alchemy for the 21st century. *Journal of Clinical Epidemiology*, 48(1):71–79.

Field M.J. (Ed.) (1996). *Telemedicine: A Guide to Assessing Telecommunications in Health Care*. Washington, DC: National Academy Press.

Fielding N.G., Lee R.M. (1991). *Using Computers in Qualitative Research.* Newbury Park, CA: Sage.

Finkel A. (Ed.) (1977). *CPT4: Physician's Current Procedural Terminology* (4th ed.). Chicago: American Medical Association.

Flexner A. (1910). *Medical Education in the United States and Canada: A Report to the Carnegie Foundation for the Advancement of Teaching*. Boston, MA: Merrymount Press.

Flickner M., Sawhney H., Niblack W., Ashley J., Huang Q., Dom B., Gorkani M., Hafner

J., Lee D., Petkovic D., Steele D., Yanker P. (1995). Query by image and video content: the QBIC system. *IEEE Computer*, 28(9):23–32.

Foley D.D., Van Dam A., Feiner S.K., Hughes J.F. (1990). *Computer Graphics: Principles and Practice*. Reading, MA: Addison-Wesley.

Forrey A.W., McDonald C.J., DeMoor G., Huff S.M., Leavelle D., Leland D., Fiers T., Charles L., Griffin B., Stalling F., Tullis A., Hutchins K., Baenziger J. (1996). Logical observation identifier names and codes (LOINC) database: a public use set of codes and names for electronic reporting of clinical laboratory test results. *Clinical Chemistry*, 42(1):81–90.

Forsythe D.E. (1992). Using ethnography to build a working system: rethinking basic design assumptions. In Frisse, M.E. *Proceedings of the 16th Annual Symposium on Computer Applications in Medical Care* (pp. 505–509). McGraw Hill, Inc.

Forsythe D.E., Buchanan B.G. (1992). Broadening our approach to evaluating medical information systems. In Frisse, M.E. *Proceedings of the 16th Annual Symposium on Computer Applications in Medical Care* (pp. 8–12). McGraw Hill, Inc.

Fox E.A., Marchionini G. (1998). Toward a worldwide digital library. *Communications of the ACM*, 41(4):29–98.

Frakes W.B., Baeza-Yates R. (1992). *Information Retrieval: Data Structures and Algorithms*. Englewood Cliffs, NJ: Prentice-Hall.

Frank S.J. (1988). What AI practitioners should know about the law. *AI Magazine*, Part One, 9: 63–75; Part Two, 9:109–114.

Freiman J.A., Chalmers T.C., Smith H., Kuebler R.R. (1978). The importance of beta, the type II error and sample size in the design and interpretation of the randomized controlled trial. *New England Journal of Medicine*, 299:690–694.

Friede A., Freedman M.A., Paul J.E., Rizzo N.P., Pawate V.I., Turczyn K.M. (1994a). DATA2000: a computer system to link HP2000 objectives, data sources, and contacts. *American Journal of Preventive Medicine*, 10:230–234.

Friede A., McDonald M.C., Blum H. (1995). Public health informatics: how information-age technology can strengthen public health. *Annual Revised Public Health*, 16:239–252.

Friede A., O Carroll P.W. (1996). CDC and ATSDR Electronic Information Resources for Health Officers. *Journal of Public Health Practice Management*, 2:10–24 (the full text may be found at http://www.cdc.gov/elecinfo.htm).

Friede A., O'Carroll P.W. (1998). Public health informatics. In Last J.M. (Ed.), Maxcey-Rosenau-Last Public Health and Preventive Medicine (14th ed.). (pp. 59–65). Norwalk, CT: Appleton & Lange.

Friede A., O'Carroll P.W., Thralls R.B., Reid J.A. (1996). CDC WONDER on the Web. In Cimino, J.J. *Proceedings of the AMIA Annual Fall Symposium (formerly SCAMC)* (pp. 408–412). Washington, DC: Hanley and Belfus, October 28–30.

Friede A., Rosen D.H., Reid J.A. (1994b). CDC WONDER: cooperative processing for public health informatics. *Journal of the American Medical Informatics Association*, 1(4):303–312.

Friedman B., Dieterle M. (1987). The impact of the installation of a local area network on physicians and the laboratory information system in a large teaching hospital. In Stead, W.W. *Proceedings of the 11th Annual Symposium on Computer Applications in Medical Care* (pp. 783–788). Washington, DC: IEEE. November 1–4.

Friedman C.P. (1995). Where's the science in medical informatics? *Journal of the American Medical Informatics Association*, 2(1):65–67.

Friedman C.P., Dev P., Dafoe B., Murphy G., Felciano R. (1993). Initial validation of a test of spatial knowledge in anatomy. *Proceedings of the 17th Annual Symposium of*

Computer Applications in Medical Care (SCAMC) (pp. 791–795). Washington, DC, October 30 to November 3.

Friedman C.P., Wyatt J.C. (1997a). *Evaluation Methods in Medical Informatics.* New York: Springer-Verlag.

Friedman C.P., Wyatt J.C. (1997b). Studying clinical information systems. In Friedman C.P., Wyatt, J.C., (Ed.), *Evaluation Methods in Medical Informatics* (pp. 41–64). New York: Springer-Verlag.

Friedman R.B. (1973). A computer program for simulating the patient-physician encounter. *Journal of Medical Education*, 48(1):92–97.

Friedman R.B., Gustafson D.H. (1977). Computers in clinical medicine: a critical review. *Computers and Biomedical Research*, 10(3):199–204.

Friedman R.B., Korst D.R., Schultz J.V., Beatty E., Entine S. (1978). Experience with the simulated patient-physician encounter. *Journal of Medical Education*, 53(10):825–830.

Fries J.F. (1974). Alternatives in medical record formats. *Medical Care*, 12(10):871–881.

Frisse M.E., Braude R.M., Florance V., Fuller S. (1995). Informatics and medical libraries: changing needs and changing roles. *Academic Medicine*, 70(1):30–35.

Fuchs V.R. (1983). *Who Shall Live?* New York: Basic Books.

Fuchs V.R. (1993). *The Future of Health Policy.* Cambridge, MA: Harvard University Press.

Fuchs V.R., Garber A.M. (1990). The new technology assessment. *New England Journal of Medicine*, 323(20):673–677.

Fuller S. (1997). Regional health information systems: applying the IAIMS model. *Journal of the American Medical Informatics Association*, 4(2):S47–S51.

Funk M.E., Reid C.A., McGoogan L.S. (1983). Indexing consistency in MEDLINE. *Bulletin of the Medical Library Association*, 71(2):176–183.

Gabrieli E.R. (1989). A new electronic medical nomenclature. *Journal of Medical Systems*, 13(6):355–373.

Garber A.M., Owens D.K. (1994). Paying for evaluative research. In Gelijns A.C., Dawkins H.V. (Eds.), *Medical Innovations at the Crossroads, Volume IV: Adopting New Medical Technology* (pp. 172–192.) Washington, DC: National Academy Press.

Gardner R.M. (1997). Fidelity of recording: improving the signal-to-noise ratio. In Tobin M.J. (Ed.), *Principles and Practice of Intensive Care Monitoring* (pp. 123–132). New York: McGraw-Hill.

Gardner R.M., Hawley W.H., East T.D., Oniki T.A., Young H.F. (1992). Real time data acquisition: recommendations for the medical information bus (MIB). *International Journal of Clinical Monitoring and Computing*, 8(4):251–258.

Gardner R.M., Lundsgaarde H.P. (1994). Evaluation of user acceptance of a clinical expert system. *Journal of the American Medical Informatics Association*, 1(6):428–438.

Gardner R.M., Monis S., Oehler P. (1986). Monitoring direct blood pressure: algorithm enhancements. *IEEE Computers in Cardiology*, 13:607.

Gardner R.M., Sittig D.F., Clemmer T.P. (1995). Computers in the intensive are unit: a match meant to be! In Shoemaker W.C. (Ed.), *Textbook of Critical Care* (3rd ed., pp. 1757–1770). Philadelphia: W.B. Saunders.

Garibaldi R.A. (1998). Editorial: computers and the quality of care: a clinician's perspective. *New England Journal of Medicine*, 338(4):259–260.

Geissbuhler A.J., Miller R.A. (1997). Desiderata for product labeling of medical expert systems. *International Journal of Medical Informatics*, 47(3):153–163.

George J.S., Aine C.J., Mosher J.C., Schmidt D.M., Ranken D.M., Schlitz H.A., Wood C.C., Lewine J.D., Sanders J.A., Belliveau J.W. (1995). Mapping function in human brain with magnetoencephalography, anatomical magnetic resonance imaging, and functional magnetic resonance imaging. *Journal of Clinical Neurophysiology*, 12(5): 406–431.

Gibson K., Scheraga H. (1967). Minimization of polypeptide energy. I. Preliminary structures of bovine pancreatic ribonuclease S-peptide. *Proceedings of the National Academy of Sciences USA*, 58(2):420–427.

Giger M., MacMahon H. (1996). Image processing and computer-aided diagnosis. *Radiology Clinics of North America*, 34(3):565–596.

Ginsburg P. (1982). *Containing Medical Care Costs Through Market Forces*. Washington, DC: Congressional Budget Office.

Ginzton L.E., Laks M.M. (1984). Computer aided ECG interpretation. *M.D. Computing*, 1(3):36–44.

Glaeser D.H., Thomas, L.J. Jr. (1975). Computer monitoring in patient care. *Annual Review of Biophysics and Bioengineering*, 4:449–76.

Glowniak J.W., Bushway M.K. (1994). Computer networks as a medical resource: accessing and using the Internet. *Journal of the American Medical Association*, 271(24): 1934–1940.

Gold M.R., Siegel J.E., Russell L.B., Weinstein M.C. (Eds.) (1996). *Cost Effectiveness in Health and Medicine*. New York: Oxford University Press.

Goldberg M.A. (1996). Teleradiology and telemedicine. In Greenes R.A., Bauman R.A. (Eds.) Imaging and information management: computer systems for a changing health care environment. *Radiology Clinics of North America*, 34(3):647–665.

Goodman K.W. (1996). Ethics, genomics and information retrieval. *Computers in Biology and Medicine*, 26(3):223–229.

Goodman K.W. (Ed.) (1998a). *Ethics, Computing, and Medicine: Informatics and the Transformation of Health Care*. Cambridge: Cambridge University Press.

Goodman K.W. (1998b). Bioethics and health informatics: an introduction. In Goodman K.W. (Ed.), *Ethics, Computing, and Medicine: Informatics and the Transformation of Health Care* (pp. 1–31). Cambridge: Cambridge University Press.

Goodman K.W. (1998c). Outcomes, futility, and health policy research. In Goodman K.W. (Ed.), *Ethics, Computing, and Medicine: Informatics and the Transformation of Health Care* (pp. 116–138). Cambridge: Cambridge University Press.

Goodwin J.O., Edwards B.S. (1975). Developing a computer program to assist the nursing process: phase I-From systems analysis to an expandable program. *Nursing Research*, 24(4):299–305.

Gordon M. (1982). Nursing Diagnoses: Process and Application. New York: McGraw-Hill.

Gorman P.N. (1995). Information needs of physicians. *Journal of the American Society for Information Science*, 46:729–736.

Gorman P.N., Ash J., Wykoff L. (1994). Can primary care physicians' questions be answered using the medical literature? *Bulletin of the Medical Library Association*, 82(2):140–146.

Gorman P.N., Helfand M. (1995). Information seeking in primary care: how physicians choose which clinical question to pursue and which to leave unanswered. *Medical Decision Making*, 15(2):113–119.

Graves J.R., Corcoran S. (1989). The study of nursing informatics. *Image: Journal of Nursing Scholarship*, 21:227–231.

Greenes R.A. (1982). OBUS: a microcomputer system for measurement, calculation, reporting, and retrieval of obstetrical ultrasound examinations. *Radiology*, 144:879–883.

Greenes R.A. (1989). The radiologist as clinical activist: a time to focus outward. In Mun, S.K. *Proceedings of the First International Conference on Image Management and Communication in Patient Care: Implementation and Impact (IMAC 89)* (pp. 136–140). Washington, DC: IEEE Computer Society Press. June.

Greenes R.A., Barnett G.O., Klein S.W., Robbins A., Prior R.E. (1970). Recording, retrieval, and review of medical data by physician-computer interaction. *New England Journal of Medicine*, 282(6):307–315.

Greenes R.A., Bauman R.A., Robboy S.J., Wieder J.F., Mercier B.A., Altshuler B.S. (1978). Immediate pathologic confirmation of radiologic interpretation by computer feedback. *Radiology*, 127(2):381–383.

Greenes R.A., Bauman R.A. (Eds.) (1996). Imaging and information management: computer systems for a changing health care environment. *Radiology Clinics of North America*, 34(3):463–697.

Greenes R.A., Deibel S.R. (1996). Constructing workstation applications: component integration strategies for a changing health-care system. In Van Bemmel J.H., McCray A.T. (Eds.), *IMIA Yearbook of Medical Informatics '96* (pp. 76–86). Rotterdam, The Netherlands: IMIA.

Greenes R.A., Shortliffe E.H. (1990). Medical informatics: an emerging academic discipline and institutional priority. *Journal of the American Medical Association*, 263(8): 1114–1120.

Greenlick M.R. (1992). Educating physicians for population-based clinical practice. *Journal of the American Medical Association*, 267(12):1645–1648.

Gribskov M., Devereux J. (1991). *Sequence Analysis Primer*. New York: Stockton Press.

Griffith H.M., Robinson K.R. (1992). Survey of the degree to which critical care nurses are performing current procedural terminology-coded services. *American Journal of Critical Care*, 1(2):91–98.

Grigsby J., Sanders J.H. (1998). Telemedicine: where it is and where it's going. *Annals of Internal Medicine*, 129(2):123–127.

Grimm R.H., Shimoni K., Harlan W.R., Estes E.H.J. (1975). Evaluation of patient-care protocol use by various providers. *New England Journal of Medicine*, 282(10):507–511.

Grobe S.J. (1996). The nursing intervention lexicon and taxonomy: implications for representing nursing care data in automated records. *Holistic Nursing Practice*, 11(1):48–63.

Gross M.S., Lohman P. (1997). The technology and tactics of physician integration. *Journal of the Healthcare Information and Management Systems Society*, 11(2):23–41.

Gusfield D. (1997). *Algorithms on Strings, Trees, and Sequences: Computer Science and Computational Biology*. Cambridge, England: Cambridge University Press.

Gustafson D.H., Taylor J.O., Thompson S., Chesney P. (1993). Assessing the needs of breast cancer patients and their families. *Quality Management in Health Care*, 2(1): 6–17.

Hamilton D., Macdonald B., King C., Jenkins D., Parlett M. (Eds.) (1977). *Beyond the Numbers Game*. Berkeley, CA: McCutchan.

Hammond W.E., Stead W.W., Straube M.J., Jelovsek F.R. (1980). Functional characteristics of a computerized medical record. *Methods of Information in Medicine*, 19(3): 157–162.

Hanlon W.B., Fene E.F., Davi S.D., Downs J.W. (1996). Project BRAHMS: PACS Implementation at Brigham and Women's Hospital. In *Proceedings of the S/CAR96* Denver, CO: Symposia Foundation (pp. 489–490).

Haralick R.M., Shapiro L.G. (1992). *Computer and Robot Vision.* Reading, MA: Addison-Wesley.

Harless W.G., Drennon G.G., Marxer J.J., Root J.A., Miller G.E. (1971). CASE: A computer-aided simulation of the clinical encounter. *Journal of Medical Education*, 46(5): 443–448.

Harless W.G., Zier M.A., Duncan R.C. (1986). Interactive videodisc case studies for medical education. In Orthner, H. *Proceedings of the 10th Annual Symposium on Computer Applications in Medical Care* (pp. 183–187). Washington, DC, IEEE Computer Society Press. October 25–26.

Harris J.R., Caldwell B., Cahill C. (1998). HEDIS in perspective: measurement to improve the public's health in an era of accountability. *American Journal of Preventive Medicine* 14(3 Suppl): 9–13.

Hayes-Roth F., Waterman D., Lenat D. (Eds.) (1983). *Building Expert Systems*. Reading, MA: Addison-Wesley.

Haynes R.B., McKibbon K.A., Walker C.J., Ryan N., Fitzgerald D., Ramsden M.F. (1990). Online access to MEDLINE in clinical settings. *Annals of Internal Medicine*, 112(1):78–84.

Haynes R.B., Wilczynski N., McKibbon K.A., Walker C.J., Sinclair J.C. (1994). Developing optimal search strategies for detecting clinically sound studies in MEDLINE. *Journal of the American Medical Informatics Association*, 1(6):447–458.

Health Care Financial Management Association (1992). *Implementation Manual for the 835 Health Care Claim Payment/Advice*: The Health Care Financial Management Association.

Health Care Financial Management Association (1993). *Implementation Manual for the 834 Benefit Enrollment and Maintenance.* The Health Care Financial Management Association.

Health Care Financing Administration (1980). *The International Classification of Diseases 9th Revision, Clinical Modification, ICD-9–CM.* (PHS 80–1260). Washington, DC: U.S. Department of Health and Human Services.

Health Care Financing Review (1996). *Medicare and Medicaid Statistical Supplement.* Baltimore: U.S. Department of Health and Human Services.

Health Insurance Association of America (HIAA) (1983). *Source Book of Health Insurance Data 1982–1983.* Washington, DC: HIAA.

Heathfield H.A., Wyatt J.C. (1993). Philosophies for the design and development of clinical decision-support systems. *Methods of Information in Medicine*, 32(1):1–8.

Heathfield H.A., Wyatt J.C. (1995). The road to professionalism in medical informatics: a proposal for debate. *Methods of Information in Medicine*, 34(5):426–433.

Heckerman D., Horvitz E. (1986). The myth of modularity in rule-based systems for reasoning with uncertainty. In Lemmer J., Kanal L. (Eds.), *Uncertainty in Artificial Intelligence 2*, pp. 115–121. Amersterdam, the Netherlands: North Holland.

Heckerman D., Horvitz E., Nathwani B. (1989). Update on the Pathfinder project. In L.C. Kingsland III *Proceedings of the Thirteenth Annual Symposium on Computer Applications in Medical Care* (pp. 203–207). Washington, DC: IEEE Computer Society Press. November 5–8.

Heckerman D., Nathwani B. (1992). An evaluation of the diagnostic accuracy of Pathfinder. *Computers and Biomedical Research*, 25:56–74.

Henderson S., Crapo R.O., Wallace C.J., East T.D., Morris A.H., Gardner R.M. (1991). Performance of computerized protocols for the management of arterial oxygenation in an intensive care unit. *International Journal of Clinical Monitoring and Computing*, 8(4):271–280.

Hennessy J.L., Patterson D.A. (1994). *Computer Architecture, A Quantitative Approach* (2nd ed.). San Francisco: Morgan Kaufmann.

Henry S.B., Holzemer W.L., Randell C., Hsieh S.F., Miller T.J. (1997). Comparison of nursing interventions classification and current procedural terminology codes for categorizing nursing activities. *Image: Journal of Nursing Scholarship*, 29(2):133–138.

Henry S.B., Holzemer W.L., Reilly C.A., Campbell K.E. (1994). Terms used by nurses to describe patient problems: can SNOMED III represent nursing concepts in the patient record? *Journal of the American Medical Informatics Association*, 1(1):61–74.

Henry S.B., Holzemer W.L., Tallberg M., Grobe S. (Eds.). (1995). Informatics: infrastructure for quality assessment and improvement in nursing. In *Proceedings of the 5th International Nursing Informatics Symposium Post-Conference*. San Francisco, CA: U.C. Nursing Press.

Henry S.B., Mead C.N. (1997). Nursing classification systems: necessary but not sufficient for representing "what nurses do" for inclusion in computer-based patient record systems. *Journal of the American Medical Informatics Association*, 4(3):222–232.

Hersh W.R. (1991). Evaluation of Meta-1 for a concept-based approach to the automated indexing and retrieval of bibliographic and full-text databases. *Medical Decision Making*, 11(4 Suppl):S120–S124.

Hersh W.R. (1994). Relevance and retrieval evaluation: perspectives from medicine. *Journal of the American Society for Information Science*, 45:201–206.

Hersh W.R. (1996). *Information Retrieval: A Health Care Perspective*. New York: Springer-Verlag.

Hersh W.R., Brown K.E., Donohoe L.C., Campbell E.M., Horacek A.E. (1996a). CliniWeb: managing clinical information on the World Wide Web. *Journal of the American Medical Informatics Association*, 3:273–280.

Hersh W.R., Elliot D.L., Hickam D.H., Wolf S.L., Molnar A., Leichtenstein C. (1995). Towards new measures of information retrieval evaluation. In Fox, E.A., Ingwersen, P., and Fidel, R. (eds.). *Proceedings of the 18th Annual International ACMSIGIR Conference on Research and Development in Information Retrieval*. New York: ACM Press, 164–170.

Hersh W.R., Hickam D. (1994). Use of a multi-application computer workstation in a clinical setting. *Bulletin of the Medical Library Association*, 82(4):382–389.

Hersh W.R., Pentecost J., Hickam D. (1996b). A task-oriented approach to information retrieval evaluation. *Journal of the American Society for Information Science*, 47:50–56.

Hickam D.H., Shortliffe E.H., Bischoff M.B., Scott A.C., Jacobs C.D. (1985a). The treatment advice of a computer-based cancer chemotherapy protocol advisor. *Annals of Internal Medicine*, 103(6 Pt 1):928–936.

Hickam D.H., Sox H.C., Sox C.H. (1985b). Systematic bias in recording the history in patients with chest pain. *Journal of Chronic Diseases*, 38:91.

Hinshaw K.P., Brinkley J.F. (1997). Using 3-D shape models to guide segmentation of MR brain images. In Masys D.R. *Proceedings of the 1997 AMIA Annual Fall Symposium (Formerly SCAMC)* (pp. 469–478). Nashville, TN: Hanley & Belfus. October 25–29.

Hodge M.H. (1990). History of the TDS medical information system. In Blum B.I., Duncan K. (Eds.), *A History of Medical Informatics* (pp. 328–344). New York: ACM Press.

Hoffer E.P., Barnett G.O. (1986). Computer-aided instruction in medicine: 16 years of MGH experience. In Salamon R., Blum B., Jorgensen M. (Eds.), *MEDINFO 86*. Amsterdam: Elsevier North-Holland.

Hohne K.H., Pflesser B., Riemer M., Schiemann T., Schubert R., Tiede U. (1995). A new representation of knowledge concerning human anatomy and function. *Nature Medicine*, 1(6):506–510.

Horii S.C. (1996). Image acquisition: sites, technologies and approaches. *Radiology Clinics of North America*, 34(3):469–494.

House E.R. (1980). *Evaluating with Validity*. Beverly Hills, CA: Sage.

Hoy J.D., Hyslop A.Q. (1995). Care planning as a strategy to manage variation in practice: from care planning to integrated person-based record. *Journal of the American Medical Informatics Association*, 2(4):260–266.

Hripcsak G., Ludemann P., Pryor T.A., Wigertz O.B., Clayton P.D. (1994). Rationale for the Arden syntax. *Computers and Biomedical Research*, 27:291–324.

Hsu H.L. (1996). *Interactivity of Human-Computer Interaction and Personal Characteristics in a Hypermedia Learning Environment.* Unpublished doctoral dissertation, Stanford University.

Hubbs P.R., Tsai M., Dev P., Godin P., Olyarchuk, J.G., Nag D. (1997). The Stanford Health Information Network for Education: integrated information for decision making and learning. In Masys D.R. (Ed.) *Proceedings of the 1997 AMIA Annual Fall Symposium (formerly SCAMC)* (pp. 505–508). Nashville, TN, October 25–29: Hanley & Belfus, Inc.

Hudson L. (1985). Monitoring of critically ill patients. Conference summary. *Respiratory Care*, 30:628.

Huff S.M., Rocha R.A., McDonald C.J., De Moor G.J., Fiers T., Bidgood W.D. Jr., Forrey A.W., Francis W.G., Tracy W.R., Leavelle D., Stalling F., Griffin B., Maloney P., Leland D., Charles L., Hutchins K., Baenziger J. (1998). Development of the Logical Observation Identifier Names and Codes (LOINC) vocabulary. *Journal of the American Informatics Association*, 5(3):276–292.

Humphreys B.L. (Ed.) (1990). *UMLS Knowledge Sources—First Experimental Edition Documentation*. Bethesda, MD: National Library of Medicine.

Humphreys B.L., Lindberg D.A. (1993). The UMLS project: making the conceptual connection between users and the information they need. *Bulletin of the Medical Library Association*, 81(2):170–177.

Hunter L. (1993). *Artificial Intelligence and Molecular Biology*. Menlo Park: AAAI Press/MIT Press.

IAIMS (1996). *Proceedings of the 1996 IAIMS Symposium*. Nashville, TN: Vanderbilt University.

Institute of Medicine (1985). *Assessing Medical Technologies*. Washington, DC: National Academy Press.

Institute of Medicine Committee on Improving the Patient Record (1997). *The Computer-Based Patient Record: An Essential Technology for Health Care* (2nd ed.). Washington, DC: National Academy Press.

International Standards Organization (1987). *Information Processing Systems—Concepts and Terminology for the Conceptual Schema and the Information Base* (ISO TR 9007:1987). International Standards Organization.

Ivers M.T., Timson G.F. (1985). The applicability of the VA integrated clinical CORE information system to the needs of other health care providers. *MUG Quarterly*, 14:19–21.

Jain R. (1991). *The Art of Computer Systems Performance Analysis: Techniques for Experimental Design, Measurement, Simulation, and Modeling*. New York: John Wiley & Sons, Inc.

Jakobovits R.M., Modayur B., Brinkley J.F. (1996). A Web-based manager for brain mapping data. In Cimino J.J. *Proceedings of the 1996 AMIA Annual Fall Symposium (formerly SCAMC)* (pp. 309–313). Washington, DC: Hanley & Belfus. October 28–30.

Johnson P. (1983). What kind of expert should a system be? *Journal of Medicine and Philosophy*, 8:77–97.

Johnston M.C., Langton K.B., Haynes R.B., Mathieu A. (1994). Effects of computer-based clinical decision support systems on clinician performance and patient outcome. A critical appraisal of research. *Annals of Internal Medicine*, 120(2):135–142.

Jolesz F.A. (1997). 1996 RSNA Eugene P. Pendergrass New Horizons Lecture. Image-guided procedures and the operating room of the future. *Radiology*, 204(3):601–612.

Jollis J.G., Ancukiewicz M., DeLong E.R., Pryor D.B., Muhlbaier L.H., Mark D.B. (1993). Discordance of databases designed for claims payment versus clinical information systems. Implications for outcomes research. *Annals of Internal Medicine*, 119(8):844–850.

Jydstrup R.A., Gross M.J. (1966). Cost of information handling in hospitals. *Health Services Research*, 1(3):235–271.

Kahn M.G. (1994). Clinical databases and critical care research. *Critical Care Clinics*, 10(1):37–51.

Kaiser Family Foundation and Health Research and Educational Trust (1999). *Employer Health Benefits.*

Kalet I.J., Austin-Seymour M.M. (1997). The use of medical images in planning and delivery of radiation therapy. *Journal of the American Medical Informatics Association*, 4(5):327–339.

Kaplan B. (1997). Addressing organizational issues into the evaluation of medical systems. *Journal of the American Medical Informatics Association*, 4(2):94–101.

Kaplan B., Duchon D. (1988). Combining qualitative and quantitative methods in information systems research: a case study. *MIS Quarterly*, 4:571–586.

Karplus M., Weaver D.L. (1976). Protein-folding dynamics. *Nature*, 260(5550):404–406.

Kass M., Witkin A., Terzopoulos D. (1987). Snakes: active contour models. *International Journal of Computer Vision*, 1(4):321–331.

Kassirer J.P., Gorry G.A. (1978). Clinical problem solving: a behavioral analysis. *Annals of Internal Medicine*, 89(2):245–255.

Keen P.G.W. (1981). Information systems and organizational change. *Communications of the ACM*, 24:24.

Kennelly R.J., Gardner R.M. (1997). Perspectives on development of IEEE 1073: the Medical Information Bus (MIB) standard. *International Journal of Clinical Monitoring and Computing*, 14(3):143–149.

Keston V., Enthoven A.C. (1996). Total hip replacement: a history of innovations to improve quality while reducing costs. *Stanford University Working Paper Number 1411*, October 29, 1996.

Kevles B. (1997). *Naked to the Bone: Medical Imaging in the Twentieth Century*. New Brunswick, NJ: Rutgers University Press.

Khorasani R., Lester J.M., Davis S.D., Hanlon W.B., Fener E.F., Seltzer S.E., Adams D.F., Holman B.L. (1998). Web-based digital radiology teaching file: facilitating case input at time of interpretation. *AJR American Journal of Roentgenology*, 170(5):1165–1167.

Kim D., Constantinou P.S., Glasgow E. (1995). *Clinical Anatomy: Interactive Lab Practical.* St. Louis: Mosby-Year Book, CD-ROM.

Kingsland L.C., Harbourt A.M., Syed E.J., Schuyler P.L. (1993). Coach: applying UMLS knowledge sources in an expert searcher environment. *Bulletin of the Medical Library Association*, 81(2):178–183.

Kirby M., Miller N. (1986). MEDLINE searching on Colleague: reasons for failure or success of untrained users. *Medical Reference Services Quarterly*, 5:17–34.

Kirkpatrick D.L. (1994). *Evaluating Training Programs*. San Francisco, CA: Berrett-Koehler Publishers.

Knaus W.A., Wagner D.P., Lynn J. (1991). Short-term mortality predictions for critically ill hospitalized adults: science and ethics. *Science*, 254(5030):389–394.

Komaroff A., Black W., Flatley M. (1974). Protocols for physician assistants: management of diabetes and hypertension. *New England Journal of Medicine*, 290:370–312.

Koslow S.H., Huerta M.F. (1997). *Neuroinformatics: An Overview of the Human Brain Project*. Mahwah, NJ: Lawrence Erlbaum.

KPMG Peat Marwick (1996). Health benefits in 1996. *KPMG Survey of Employer Sponsored Health Benefits*.

Kuhn I.M., Wiederhold G., Rodnick J.E., Ramsey-Klee D.M., Benett S., Beck D.D. (1984). Automated ambulatory medical record systems in the U.S. In B. Blum (Ed.), *Information Systems for Patient Care*. (pp. 199–217). New York: Springer-Verlag.

Kuhn T. (1962). *The Structure of Scientific Revolutions*. Chicago: University of Chicago Press.

Kulikowski C.A. (1997). Medical imaging informatics: challenges of definition and integration. *Journal of the American Medical Informatics Association*, 4(3):252–253.

Kulikowski C.A., Jaffe C.C. (1997). Focus on imaging informatics. *Journal of the American Medical Informatics Association*, 4(3).

Kuperman G., Gardner R., Pryor T.A. (1991). *HELP: A Dynamic Hospital Information System*. New York: Springer-Verlag.

Kupiers B., Kassirer J. (1984). Causal reasoning in medicine: analysis of a protocol. *Cognitive Science*, 8:363–385.

Kurtzke J.F. (1979). ICD-9: a regression. *American Journal of Epidemiology*, 108(4):383–393.

Lange L.L. (1996). Representation of everyday clinical nursing language in UMLS and SNOMED. In Cimino, J.J. *Proceedings of the 1996 AMIA Annual Fall Symposium (formerly SCAMC)* (pp 140–144). Washington, DC: Hanley & Belfus, October 28–30.

Langridge R. (1974). Interactive three-dimensional computer graphics in molecular biology. *Federal Proceedings*, 33(12):2332–2335.

Lanzola G., Quaglini S., Stefanelli M. (1995). Knowledge-acquisition tools for medical knowledge-based systems. *Methods of Information in Medicine*, 34(1–2):25–39.

Laskkari D.A., DeRisi J.L., McCusker J.H., Namath A.F., Gentile C., Hwang S.Y., Brown P.O., Davis R.W. (1997). Yeast microarrays for genome wide parallel genetic and gene expression analysis. In *Proceedings of the National Academy of Science USA*, 94(24): 13057–13062.

Lederberg J. (1978). Digital communications and the conduct of science: the new literacy. *Proceedings of the IEEE*, 66(11):1314–1319.

Ledley R., Lusted L. (1959). Reasoning foundations of medical diagnosis. *Science*, 130:9–21.

Ledley, R. (1965). *Use of Computers in Biology and Medicine*. New York: McGraw-Hill.

Lee C.C., Jack C.R.J., Riederer S.J. (1996). Use of functional magnetic resonance imaging. *Neurosurgery Clinics of North America*, 7(4):665–683.

Leeming B.W.A., Simon M. (1982). CLIP: a 1982 update. In *Proceedings of the 7th Conference on Computer Applications in Radiology* (pp. 273–289). Boston, MA: American College of Radiology April.

Lehr J.L., Lodwick G.S., Nicholson B.F., Birznieks F.B. (1973). Experience with MARS (Missouri Automated Radiology System). *Radiology*, 106(2):289–294.

Leiner F., Haux R. (1996). Systematic planning of clinical documentation. *Methods of Information in Medicine*, 35:25–34.

Leitch D. (1989). Who should have their cholesterol measured? What experts in the UK suggest. *British Medical Journal*, 298:1615–1616.

Lenert L.A., Michelson D., Flowers C., Bergen M.R. (1995). IMPACT: an object-oriented graphical environment for construction of multimedia patient interviewing software. In: Gardner RM *Proceedings of the Annual Symposium of Computer Applications in Medical Care* (pp. 319–323). New Orleans: Hanley & Belfus.

Levit K.R., Lazenby H.C., Braden B.R., Cowan C.A., McDonnell P.A., Sivarajan L., Stiller J.M., Won D.K., Donham C.S., Long A.M., Stewart M.W. (1996). Data View: National Health Expenditures, 1995. *Health Care Financing Review*, 18:175–214.

Levitt M. (1983). Molecular dynamics of native protein. I. Computer simulation of trajectories. *Journal of Molecular Biology*, 168(3):595–617.

Libicki M.C. (1995). *Information Technology Standards: Quest for the Common Byte*: Digital Press.

Lincoln Y.S., Guba E.G. (1985). *Naturalistic Inquiry*. Beverly Hills, CA: Sage.

Lindberg D.A. (1965). Operation of a hospital computer system. *Journal of the American Veterinary Medical Association*, 147(12):1541–1544.

Lindberg D.A., Humphreys B.L., McCray A.T. (1993). The Unified Medical Language System. *Methods of Information in Medicine*, 32(4):281–291.

Lorenzi N.M., Riley R.T., Blyth A.J., Southon G., Dixon B.J. (1997). Antecedents of the people and organizational aspects of medical informatics. *Journal of the American Medical Informatics Association*, 4(2):79–93.

Lou S.L., Huang H.K., Arenson R.L. (1996). Workstation design: image manipulation, image set handling, and display issues. *Radiology Clinics of North America*, 34(3):525–544.

Lowe H.J., Barnett G.O. (1994). Understanding and using the medical subject headings (MeSH) vocabulary to perform literature searches. *Journal of the American Medical Association*, 271(14):1103–1108.

Lyon H.C. Jr., Healy J.C., Bell J.R., O'Donnell J.F., Shultz E.K., Moore-West M., Wigton R.S., Hirai F., Beck J.R. (1992). PlanAlyzer, an interactive computer-assisted program to teach clinical problem solving in diagnosing anemia and coronary artery disease. *Academic Medicine*, 67(12):821–828.

Maas M.L., Johnson M., Moorhead S. (1996). Classifying nursing-sensitive patient outcomes. *Image: Journal of Nursing Scholarship*, 28(4):295–301.

Macklin R. (1992). Privacy and control of genetic information. In Annas G.J., Elias S. (Eds.), *Gene Mapping: Using Law and Ethics as Guides*. New York: Oxford University Press.

Maloney J. Jr. (1968). The trouble with patient monitoring. *Annals of Surgery*, 168(4): 605–619.

Mant J., Hicks N. (1995). Detecting differences in quality of care: the sensitivity of measures of process and outcome in treating acute myocardial infarction. *British Medical Journal*, 311(7008):793–796.

Margulies S.I., Wheeler P.S. (1972). Development of an automated reporting system. In *Proceedings of the Conference on Computer Applications in Radiology* (pp. 423–440). Columbia, MO, September. Dept of HEW.

Marrone T.J., Briggs J.M., McCammon J.A. (1997). Structure-based drug design: computational advances. *Annual Review of Pharmacology and Toxicology*, 37(71–90).

Marshall E. (1996). Hot property: biologists who compute [news]. *Science*, 272(5269): 1730–1732.

Martin K.S., Scheet N.J. (1992). *The Omaha System: Applications for Community Health Nursing*. Philadelphia: W.B. Saunders.

Martin K.S., Scheet N.J. (Eds.) (1995). *The Omaha System: Nursing Diagnoses, Interventions, and Client Outcomes*. Washington, DC: American Nurses Publishing.

Masys D.R. (1992). An evaluation of the source selection elements of the prototype UMLS information sources map. In Frisse M.E. *Proceedings of the 16th Annual Symposium on Computer Applications in Medical Care* (pp. 295–298). Baltimore, MD. McGraw-Hill, Inc.

McCloskey J.C., Bulecheck G.M. (1996). *Nursing Interventions Classification* (2nd ed.). St. Louis: C.V. Mosby.

McCormick K.A., Lang N., Zielstorff R., Milholland D.K., Saba V., Jacox A. (1994). Toward standard classification schemes for nursing language: recommendations of the American Nurses Association Steering Committee on Databases to Support Clinical Nursing Practice. *Journal of the American Medical Informatics Association*, 1(6):421–427.

McCray A.T., Miller R.A. (1998). Focus on the Unified Medical Language System. *Journal of the American Medical Informatics Association*, 5(1):1–138.

McDaniel A.M. (1997). Developing and testing a prototype patient care database. *Computers in Nursing*, 15(3):129–136.

McDonald C.J. (1976). Protocol-based computer reminders, the quality of care and the non-perfectibility of man. *New England Journal of Medicine*, 295(24):1351–1355.

McDonald C.J. (Ed.) (1987). *Tutorials (M.D. Computing: Benchmark Papers)*. New York: Springer-Verlag.

McDonald C.J. (1997). The barriers to electronic medical record systems and how to overcome them. *Journal of the American Medical Informatics Association*, 4(3):213–221.

McDonald C.J., Hui S.L., Smith D.M., Tierney W.M., Cohen S.J., Weinberger M., McCabe G.P. (1984a). Reminders to physicians from an introspective computer medical record. A two year randomized trial. *Annals of Internal Medicine*, 100(1):130–138.

McDonald C.J., Overhage J.M., Dexter P., Takesue B.Y., Dwyer D.M. (1997). A framework for capturing clinical data sets from computerized sources. *Annals of Internal Medicine*, 127(8 Pt.2):675–682.

McDonald C.J., Tierney W.M. (1986a). Research uses of computer-stored practice records in general medicine. *Journal of General Internal Medicine*, 1(4 Suppl):S19–S24.

McDonald C.J., Tierney W.M. (1986b). The medical gopher: a microcomputer system to help find, organize and decide about patient data. *The Western Journal of Medicine*, 145(6):823–829.

McDonald C.J., Tierney W.M., Overhage J.M., Martin D.K., Wilson G.A. (1992). The Regenstrief Medical Record System: 20 years of experience in hospitals, clinics, and neighborhood health centers. *MD Computing*, 9(4):206–217.

McDonald C.J., Wiederhold G., Simborg D., Hammond E., Jelovsek F., Schneider K. (1984b). A discussion of the draft proposal for data exchange standards for clinical laboratory results. In *Proceedings of the 8th Annual Symposium on Computer Applications in Medical Care* (pp. 406–413). November 4–7.

McDonald C.J. (Ed.) (1988). Computer-stored medical record systems. *M.D. Computing*, 5(5):1–62.

McFarland G.K., McFarlane E.A. (1993). *Nursing Diagnosis & Intervention: Planning for Patient Care*. (2nd ed.). St. Louis: Mosby.

McGrath J.C., Wagner W.H., Shabot M.M. (1996). When is ICU care warranted after carotid endarterectomy? *American Surgeon*, 62(10):811–814.

McKinin E.J., Sievert M.E., Johnson E.D., Mitchell J.A. (1991). The Medline/full-text research project. *Journal of the American Society for Information Science*, 42:297–307.

McNeer J.F., Wallace A.G., Wagner G.S., Starmer C.F., Rosati R.A. (1975). The course of acute myocardial infarction: feasibility of early discharge of the uncomplicated patient. *Circulation*, 51:410–413.

McPhee S.J., Bird J.A., Fordham D., Rodnick J.E., Osborn E.H. (1991). Promoting cancer prevention activities by primary care physicians: results of a randomized, controlled trial. *Journal of the American Medical Association*, 266(4):538–544.

Medicare Board of Trustees (1996). *1996 Annual Report of the Board of Trustees of the Federal Hospital Insurance Trust Fund and of the Federal Supplementary Medical Insurance Trust Fund.* Washington, DC.

Meigs J., Barry M., Oesterling J., Jacobsen S. (1996). Interpreting results of prostate-specific antigen testing for early detection of prostate cancer. *Journal of General Internal Medicine*, 11(9):505–512.

Mercer/Foster-Higgins, Inc. (1998). *National Survey of Employer-Sponsored Health Plans.*

Michaelis J., Wellek S., Willems J.L. (1990). Reference standards for software evaluation. *Methods of Information in Medicine*, 29(4):289–297.

Michel A., Zorb L., Dudeck J. (1996). Designing a low-cost bedside workstation for intensive care units. In Cimino J.J. *Proceedings of the AMIA Annual Fall Symposium (formerly SCAMC)* (pp. 777–781). Washington, DC: Hanley & Belfus October 28–30.

Miles W. (1982). *A History of the National Library of Medicine: The Nation's Treasury of Medical Knowledge*. Bethesda, MD: U.S. Department of Health and Human Services.

Miller P. (1986). *Expert Critiquing Systems: Practice-Based Medical Consultation by Computer*. New York: Springer-Verlag.

Miller P. (1988). *Selected Topics in Medical Artificial Intelligence*. New York: Springer-Verlag.

Miller R., Masarie F. (1990). The demise of the Greek oracle model for medical diagnosis systems. *Methods of Information in Medicine*, 29:1–2.

Miller R., Pople H. Jr., Meyers J. (1982). INTERNIST-1: an experimental computer-based diagnostic consultant for general internal medicine. *New England Journal of Medicine*, 307:468–476.

Miller R., Schaffner K., Meisel A. (1985). Ethical and legal issues related to the use of computer programs in clinical medicine. *Annals of Internal Medicine*, 102(4):529–537.

Miller R.A. (1989). Legal issues related to medical decision support systems. *International Journal of Clinical Monitoring and Computing*, 6:75–80.

Miller R.A. (1990). Why the standard view is standard: people, not machines, understand patients' problems. *Journal of Medicine and Philosophy*, 15(6):581–591.

Miller R.A., Gardner R.M. (1997a). Summary recommendations for responsible monitoring and regulation of clinical software systems. *Annals of Internal Medicine*, 127(9): 842–845.

Miller R.A., Gardner R.M. (1997b). Recommendations for responsible monitoring and regulation of clinical software systems. *Journal of the American Medical Informatics Association*, 4(6):442–457.

Miller R.A., Gieszczykiewicz F.M., Vries J.K., Cooper G.F. (1992). CHARTLINE: providing bibliographic references relevant to patient charts using the UMLS Metathesaurus knowledge sources. In Frisse M.E. *Proceedings of the 16th Annual Symposium on Computer Applications in Medical Care* (pp. 86–90). Baltimore, MD: McGraw-Hill.

Miller R.A., Goodman K.W. (1998). Ethical challenges in the use of decision-support software in clinical practice. In Goodman K.W. (Ed.), *Ethics, Computing, and Medi-*

cine: Informatics and the Transformation of Health Care. Cambridge: Cambridge University Press.

Miller R.A., McNeil M.A., Challinor S.M., Masarie F.E. Jr., Myers J.D. (1986). The INTERNIST-1/Quick Medical Reference project: status report. *Western Journal of Medicine*, 145(6):816–822.

Modayur B., Prothero J., Ojemann G., Maravilla K., Brinkley J. (1997). Visualization-based mapping of language function in the brain. *Neuroimage*, 6(4):245–258.

Mohr D.N., Offord K.P., Owen R.A., Melton L.J. (1986). Asymptomatic microhematuria and urologic disease. A population-based study. *Journal of the American Medical Association*, 256(2):224–229.

Monson-Haefel R. (1999). *Enterprise JavaBeans.* Cambridge, MA: O'Reilly & Associates.

Mortensen R.A., Nielsen G.H. (1996). *International Classification of Nursing Practice (version 0.2).* Geneva, Switzerland: International Council of Nursing.

Moses L.E., Littenberg B., Shapiro D. (1993). Combining independent studies of a diagnostic test into a summary ROC curve: data-analytic approaches and some additional considerations. *Statistics in Medicine*, 12(4):1293–1316.

Mulrow C.D. (1987). The medical review article: state of the science. *Annals of Internal Medicine*, 106:485–488.

Munnecke T., Kuhn I. (1989). Large-scale portability of hospital information system software with the Veteran Administration. In Orthner H., Blum B. (Ed.), *Implementing Health Care Information Systems.* New York: Springer-Verlag.

Musen M. (1997). Modeling for decision support. In van Bemmel J., Musen M. (Eds.), *Handbook of Medical Informatics* (pp. 431–448). Heidelberg: Springer-Verlag.

Musen M. (1998). Domain ontologies in software engineering: Use of PROTÉGÉ with the EON architecture. *Methods of Information in Medicine*, 37(4–5):540–550.

Musen M.A. (1993). An overview of knowledge acquisition. In David J.M., Krivine J.P., Simmons R. (Eds.), *Second Generation Expert Systems* (pp. 415–438). Berlin: Springer-Verlag.

Musen M.A., Carlson R.W., Fagan L.M., Deresinski S.C. (1992). T-HELPER: automated support for community-based clinical research. In Frisse M.E. *Proceedings of the 16th Annual Symposium on Computer Applications in Medical Care* (pp. 719–723). Baltimore, MD: McGraw-Hill.

Musen M.A., Fagan L.M., Combs D.M., Shortliffe E.H. (1987). Use of a domain model to drive an interactive knowledge-editing tool. *International Journal of Man-Machine Studies*, 26(1):105–121.

Musen M.A., Gennari J.H., Eriksson H., Tu S.W., Puerta A.R. (1995). PROTÉGÉ-II: computer support for development of intelligent systems from libraries of components. In *Proceedings of the MEDINFO '95: The Eighth World Congress on Medical Informatics* (pp. 766–770). Vancouver, British Columbia.

Musen M.A., Tu S.W., Das A.K., Shahar Y. (1996). EON: a component-based approach to automation of protocol-directed therapy. *Journal of the American Medical Informatics Association*, 3(6):367–388.

National Committee for Quality Assurance (1997). *HEDIS 3.0.* Washington, DC: National Committee for Quality Assurance; see also www.ncqa.org.

National League for Nursing (1987). *Guidelines for basic computer education in nursing.* New York: National League for Nursing.

National Library of Medicine (updated annually). *Medical Subject Headings.* Bethesda, MD: The National Library of Medicine.

National Priority Expert Panel on Nursing Informatics (1993). *Nursing Informatics: En-*

hancing Patient Care. Bethesda, MD: U.S. Department of Health and Human Services, U.S. Public Health Service, National Institutes of Health.

National Research Council (1997). *Assessment of Performance Measures for Public Health, Substance Abuse, and Mental Health*. Washington, DC: National Academy Press.

National Research Council (1997). *For the Record: Protecting Electronic Health Information*. Washington, DC: National Academy Press.

National Research Council (2000). *Networking Health: Prescriptions for the Internet*. Washington, D.C.: Natioal Academies Press.

NCPDP Telecommunication (1992). *NCPDP Telecommunicatio Standard Format* (Version 3.20.

Nease R.F. Jr., Kneeland T., O'Connor G.T., Sumner W., Lumpkins C., Shaw L., Pryor D., Sox H.C. (1995). Variation in patient utilities for the outcomes of the management of chronic stable angina. Implications for clinical practice guidelines. *Journal of the American Medical Association*, 273(15):1185–1190.

Nease R.F. Jr., Owens D.K. (1994). A method for estimating the cost-effectiveness of incorporating patient preferences into practice guidelines. *Medical Decision Making*, 14(4):382–392.

Nease R. F. Jr., Owens D.K. (1997). Use of influence diagrams to structure medical decisions. *Medical Decision Making*, 17(13):263–275.

Needleman S.B., Wunsch C.D. (1970). A general method applicable to the search for similarities in the amino acid sequence of two proteins. *Journal of Molecular Biology*, 48(3):443–453.

New York Academy of Medicine (1961). *Standard Nomenclature of Diseases and Operations* (5th ed.). New York: McGraw-Hill.

Nguyen J.H., Shahar Y., Tu S.W., Das A.K., Musen M.A. (1997). A temporal database mediator for protocol-based decision support. In Masys D.R. *Proceedings of the 1997 AMIA Annual Fall Symposium (formerly SCAMC)* (pp. 298–302). Nashville, TN: Hanley & Belfus, October 25–29.

NHS Centre for Coding and Classification (1994a). *Read Codes, Version 3*. London: NHS Management Executive, Department of Health.

NHS Centre for Coding and Classification (1994b). *Read Codes and the Terms Projects: A Brief Guide*. Leicestershire, Great Britain: NHS Management Executive, Department of Health.

Nielsen G.H., Mortensen R.A. (1996). The architecture for an International Classification of Nursing Practice (ICNP). *International Nursing Review*, 43(6):175–182.

O'Connell E.M., Teich J.M., Pedraza L.A., Thomas D. (1996). A comprehensive inpatient discharge system. In Cimino, JJ. *Proceedings of the AMIA Annual Fall Symposium (formerly SCAMC)* (pp. 699–703). Washington, DC, Hanley & Belfus, October 28–30.

O'Donnell-Maloney M.J., Little D.P. (1996). Microfabrication and array technologies for DNA sequencing and diagnostics. *Genetic Analysis*, 13(6):151–157.

Office of Technology Assessment (1980). *The Implications of Cost-Effectiveness Analysis of Medical Technology*. Washington DC: Congress of the United States, U.S. Government Printing Office.

Oldendorf W.H., Oldendorf W.H. Jr. (1991). *MRI Primer*. New York: Raven Press.

Orthner H.F., Blum B.I. (Eds.) (1989). *Implementing Health Care Information Systems*. New York: Springer-Verlag.

Osheroff J. (Ed.) (1995). *Computers in Clinical Practices. Managing Patients, Information, and Communication*. Philadelphia: American College of Physicians.

O'Sullivan J., Franco C., Fuchs B., Lyke B., Price R., Swendiman K. (1997). *Medicare Provisions in the Balanced Budget Act of 1997.* Congressional Research Service Report for Congress BBA 97, P.L. 105–33.

Overhage J.M. (Ed.) (1998). *Proceedings of the Fourth Annual Nicholas E. Davies CPR Recognition Symposium.* Schaumburg, IL: Computer-based Patient Record Institute.

Owens D., Harris R., Scott P., Nease R.F. Jr. (1995). Screening surgeons for HIV infection: a cost-effectiveness analysis. *Annals of Internal Medicine*, 122(9):641–652.

Owens D.K. (1998a). Spine update. Patient preferences and the development of practice guidelines. *Spine*, 23(9):1073–1079.

Owens D.K. (1998b). Interpretation of cost-effectiveness analyses. *Journal of General Internal Medicine*, 13(10):716–717.

Owens D.K., Holodniy M., Garber A.M., Scott J., Sonnad S., Moses L., Kinosian B., Schwartz J.S. (1996a). The polymerase chain reaction for the diagnosis of HIV infection in adults: a meta-analysis with recommendations for clinical practice and study design. *Annals of Internal Medicine*, 124(9):803–815.

Owens D.K., Holodniy M., McDonald T.W., Scott J., Sonnad S. (1996b). A meta-analytic evaluation of the polymerase chain reaction (PCR) for diagnosis of human immunodeficiency virus (HIV) infection in infants. *Journal of the American Medical Association*, 275(17):1342–1348.

Owens D.K., Nease R.F. Jr. (1993). Development of outcome-based practice guidelines: a method for structuring problems and synthesizing evidence. *Joint Commission Journal on Quality Improvement*, 19(7):248–263.

Owens D.K., Nease R.F. Jr. (1997). A normative analytic framework for development of practice guidelines for specific clinical populations. *Medical Decision Making*, 17(4): 409–426.

Owens D.K., Sanders G.D., Harris R.A., McDonald K.M., Heidenreich P.A., Dembitzer A.D., Hlatky M.A. (1997a). Cost-effectiveness of implantable cardioverter defibrillators relative to amiodarone for prevention of sudden cardiac death. *Annals of Internal Medicine*, 126(1):1–12.

Owens D.K., Shachter R.D., Nease R.F. Jr. (1997b). Representation and analysis of medical decision problems with influence diagrams. *Medical Decision Making*, 17(3):241–262.

Ozbolt J.F., Schultz II S., Swain M.A., Abraham I.I. (1985). A proposed expert system for nursing practice: a springboard to nursing science. *Journal of Medical Systems*, 9(1–2):57–68.

Ozbolt J.G. (1996). From minimum data to maximum impact: using clinical data to strengthen patient care. *Advanced Practice Nursing Quarterly*, 1(4):62–69.

Ozbolt J.G., Fruchnicht J.N., Hayden J.R. (1994). Toward data standards for clinical nursing information. *Journal of the American Medical Informatics Association*, 1(2): 175–185.

Ozbolt J.G., Russo M., Stultz M.P. (1995). Validity and reliability of standard terms and codes for patient care data. In Gardner R.M. *Proceedings of the 19th Symposium on Computer Applications in Medical Care* (pp. 37–41). New Orleans: American Medical Informatics Association, October 28 to November 1.

Pabst M.K., Scherubel J.C., Minnick A.F. (1996). The impact of computerized documentation on nurses' use of time. *Computers in Nursing*, 14(1):25–30.

Paddock S.W. (1994). To boldly glow . . . applications of laser scanning confocal microscopy in developmental biology. *Bioessays*, 16(5):357–365.

Palda V.A., Detsky A.S. (1997). Perioperative assessment and management of risk from coronary artery disease. *Annals of Internal Medicine*, 127(4):313–328.

Patel V.L., Groen C.G. (1986). Knowledge-based solution strategies in medical reasoning. *Cognitive Science*, 10:91–116.

Patten S.F., Lee J.S., Nelson A.C. (1996). NeoPath, Inc. NeoPath AutoPap 300 Automatic Pap Screener System. *Acta Cytologica*, 40(1):45–52.

Pauker S.G., Gorry G.A., Kassirer J.P., Schwartz W.B. (1976). Towards the simulation of clinical cognition. Taking a present illness by computer. *American Journal of Medicine*, 60(7):981–996.

Pauker S.G., Kassirer J.P. (1980). The threshold approach to clinical decision making. *New England Journal of Medicine*, 302(20):1109–1117.

Pauker S.G., Kassirer J.P. (1981). Clinical decision analysis by computer. *Archives of Internal Medicine*, 141(13):1831–1837.

Peabody G. (1922). The physician and the laboratory. *Boston Medical Surgery Journal*, 187:324.

Perreault L.E., Metzger J.B. (1999). A pragmatic framework for understanding clinical decision support. *Heathcare Information Management* 13(2):5–21.

Peterson W., Birdsall T. (1953). *The Theory of Signal Detectability.* (Technical Report No. 13). Electronic Defense Group, University of Michigan, Ann Arbor.

Piemme T.E. (1988). Computer-assisted learning and evaluation in medicine. *Journal of the American Medical Association*, 260(3):367–372.

Pinciroli F. (1995). Virtual Reality for Medicine. *Computers in Biology and Medicine*, 25(2):81–83.

Pople H. (1982). Heuristic methods for imposing structure on ill-structured problems: the structuring of medical diagnosis. In Szolovits P. (Ed.), *Artificial Intelligence in Medicine.* Boulder, CO: Westview Press.

Prothero J.S., Prothero J.W. (1986). Three-dimensional reconstruction from serial sections IV. The reassembly problem. *Computers and Biomedical Research*, 19(4):361–373.

Pryor T.A. (1988). The HELP medical record system. *M.D. Computing*, 5(5):22–33.

Pryor T.A., Gardner R.M., Clayton P.D., Warner H.R. (1983). The HELP system. *Journal of Medical Systems*, 7(2):87–102.

Public Health Service (1991). *Healthy People 2000: National Health Promotion and Disease Prevention Objectives—Full Report, with Commentary.* (DHHS publication No. [PHS]91–50212.). Washington, DC: U.S. Department of Health and Human Services, Public Health Service.

Quarterman J.S. (1990). *The Matrix: Computer Networks and Conferencing Systems Worldwide.* Digital Press.

Raiffa H. (1970). *Decision Analysis: Introductory Lectures on Choices Under Uncertainty.* Reading, MA: Addison-Wesley.

Ransohoff D.F., Feinstein A.R. (1978). Problems of spectrum and bias in evaluating the efficacy of diagnostic tests. *New England Journal of Medicine*, 299(17):926–930.

Read J.D. (1990). Computerising medical language. *British Journal of Health Care Computing*, 203–208.

Read J.D., Benson T.J. (1986). Comprehensive coding. *British Journal of Health Care Computing*, May:22–25.

Rector A.L., Glowinski A.J., Nowlan W.A., Rossi-Mori A. (1995). Medical-concept models and medical records: an approach based on GALEN and PEN & PAD. *Journal of the American Medical Informatics Association*, 2(1):19–35.

Reggia J., Turhim S. (Eds.) (1985). *Computer-Assisted Medical Decision Making*. New York: Springer-Verlag.

Reiser S. (1991). The clinical record in medicine. Part 1: Learning from cases. *Annals of Internal Medicine*, 114(10):902–907.

Reiser S.J., Anbar M. (Eds.) (1984). *The Machine at the Bedside: Strategies for Using Technology in Patient Care*. Cambridge: Cambridge University Press.

Richardson J.S. (1981). The anatomy and taxonomy of protein structure. *Advances in Protein Chemistry*, 34:167–339.

Ritchie C.J., Edwards W.S., Cyr D.R., Kim Y. (1996). Three-dimensional ultrasonic angiography using power-mode Doppler. *Ultrasound in Medicine and Biology*, 22(3):277–286.

Robbins A.H., Vincent M.E., Shaffer K., Maietta R., Srinivasan M.K. (1988). Radiology reports: assessment of a 5,000–word speech recognizer. *Radiology*, 167(3):853–855.

Roethligsburger F.J., Dickson W.J. (1939). *Management and the Worker*. Cambridge, MA: Harvard University Press.

Rose M.T. (1989). *The Open Book, A Practical Perspective on OSI*. Englewood Cliffs, NJ: Prentice Hall.

Rosse C., Mejino J.L., Jakobovits R.M., Modayur B.R., Brinkley J.F. (1997). Motivation and organizational principles for anatomical knowledge representation: the digital anatomist symbolic knowledge base. *Journal of the American Medical Informatics Association*, 5(1):17–40.

Rossi P.H., Freeman H.E. (1989). *Evaluation: A Systematic Approach* (4th ed.). Newbury Park, CA: Sage.

Rothschild M.A., Wett H.A., Fisher P.R., Weltin G.G., Miller P.L. (1990). Exploring subjective vs. objective issues in the validation of computer-based critiquing advice. *Computer Methods and Programs in Biomedicine*, 31(1):11–18.

Rothwell D.J., Côté R.A., Cordeau J.P., Boisvert M.A. (1993). Developing a standard data structure for medical language: the SNOMED proposal. In Safran C. *Proceedings of the 17th Annual Symposium for Computer Applications in Medical Care (SCAMC)* (pp. 695–699). Washington, DC: McGraw-Hill, October 30 to November 3.

Rothwell D.J., Côté R.A. (1996). Managing information with SNOMED: understanding the model. In Cimino J.J. *Proceedings of the AMIA Annual Fall Symposium (formerly SCAMC)* (pp 80–83) Washington, DC: Hanley & Belfus, Inc., October 28–30.

Rotman B.L., Sullivan A.N., McDonald T.W., Brown B.W., DeSmedt P., Goodnature D., Higgins M.C., Suermondt H.J., Young C., Owens D.K. (1996). A randomized controlled trial of a computer-based physician workstation in an outpatient setting: implementation barriers to outcome evaluation. *Journal of the American Medical Association*, 3(5):340–348.

Saba V.K. (1992). The classification of home health care nursing: diagnoses and interventions. *Caring Magazine*, 11(3):50–56.

Saba V.K. (1994). *Home Health Care Classification of Nursing Diagnoses and Interventions*. Washington, DC: Georgetown University.

Saba V.K. (1995). Home Health Care Classifications (HHCCs): Nursing diagnoses and nursing interventions In *Nursing Data Systems: The Emerging Framework* (pp. 61–103). Washington, DC: American Nurses Publishing.

Saba V.K., McCormick K. (1996). *Essentials of Computers for Nurses*. New York: McGraw-Hill.

Sackett D.L., Richardson W.S., Rosenberg W.M., Haynes R.B. (Eds.) (1997). *Evidence-Based Medicine: How to Practice and Teach EBM*. New York: Churchill Livingstone.

Safran C., Porter D., Lightfoot J., Rury C.D., Underhill L.H., Bleich H.L., Slack W.V. (1989). ClinQuery: a system for online searching of data in a teaching hospital. *Annals of Internal Medicine*, 111(9):751–756.

Safran C., Rind D.M., Davis R.B., Ives D., Sands D.Z., Currier J., Slack W.V., Makadon H.J., Cotton D.J. (1995). Guidelines for management of HIV infection with computer-based patient's record. *Lancet*, 346(8971):341–346.

Safran C., Rury C., Rind D.M., Taylor W.C. (1991). A computer-based outpatient medical record for a teaching hospital. *M.D. Computing*, 8(5):291–299.

Safran C., Slack W.V., Bleich H.L. (1989). Role of computing in patient care in two hospitals. *M.D. Computing*, 6(3):141–148.

Sailors R.M., East T.D. (1997). Role of computers in monitoring. In Tobin M.J. (Ed.), *Principles and Practice of Intensive Care Monitoring* (pp. 1329–1354). New York: McGraw-Hill.

Salpeter S.R., Sanders G.D., Salpeter E.E., Owens D.K. (1997). Monitored isoniazid prophylaxis for low-risk tuberculin reactors older than 35 years of age: a risk-benefit and cost-effectiveness analysis. *Annals of Internal Medicine*, 127(12):1051–1061.

Salton G. (1983). *Introduction to Modern Information Retrieval.* New York: McGraw-Hill.

Salton G. (1991). Developments in automatic text retrieval. *Science*, 253:974–980.

Salton G., Buckley C. (1990). Improving retrieval performance by relevance feedback. *Journal of the American Society for Information Science*, 41:288–297.

Salzberg S., Searls D., Kasif S. (Eds.) (1998). *Computational Methods in Molecular Biology*. New York: Elsevier Science.

Sanders G.D., Hagerty C.G., Sonnenberg F.A., Hlatky M.A., Owens D.K. (1999). Distributed dynamic decision support using a Web-based interface for prevention of sudden cardiac death. *Medical Decision Making*, 19(2):157–166.

Sanford M.K., Hazelwood S.E., Bridges A.J., Cutts J.H. 3rd, Mitchell J.A., Reid J.C., Sharp G. (1996). Effectiveness of computer-assisted interactive videodisc instruction in teaching rheumatology to physical and occupational therapy students. *Journal of Allied Health*, 25(2):141–148.

Saracevic T. (1991). Individual differences in organizing, searching, and retrieving information. In *Proceedings of the 54th Annual Meeting of the American Society for Information Science*, Washington, DC.

Scherrer J.R., Baud R.H., Hochstrasser D., Ratib O. (1990). DIOGENE: an integrated hospital information system in Geneva. *M.D. Computing*, 7(2):81–89.

Scherrer J.R., Lovis C., Borst F. (1995). DIOGENE 2: a distributed hospital information system with an emphasis on its medical information content. In van Bemmel J.H., McCray A.T. (Eds.), *Yearbook of Medical Informatics* (pp. 86–97). Stuttgart: Schattauer.

Schreiber G., Wielinga B., Breuker J. (Eds.) (1993). *KADS: A principled Approach to Knowledge-Based System Development.* London: Academic Press.

Schulz K.F., Chalmers I., Hayes R.J., Altman D.G. (1995). Empirical evidence of bias. Dimensions of methodological quality associated with estimates of treatment effects in controlled trials. *Journal of the American Medical Association*, 273(5):408–412.

Schwartz R.J., Weiss K.M., Buchanan A.V. (1985). Error control in medical data. *M.D. Computing*, 2(2):19–25.

Schwartz W. (1970). Medicine and the computer: the promise and problems of change. *New England Journal of Medicine*, 283(23):1257–1264.

Science (1997). Special issue on bioinformatics. *Science*, 278(Oct. 24):541–768.

Scriven M. (1973). Goal free evaluation. In House E.R. (Ed.), *School Evaluation.* Berkeley, CA: McCutchan Publishers.

Selden C., Humphreys B.L., Friede A., Geisslerova Z. (1996). *Public Health Informatics, January 1980 Through December 1995: 471 Selected Citations* (pp. 1–21). Bethesda, MD: National Institutes of Health, National Library of Medicine.

Senior Medical Review (1987). Urinary tract infection. *Senior Medical Review*.

Severinghaus J.W., Astrup P.B. (1986). History of blood gas analysis IV. Oximetry. *Journal of Clinical Monitoring*, 2(4):270–288.

Sewell W., Teitelbaum S. (1986). Observations of end-user online searching behavior over eleven years. *Journal of the American Society for Information Science*, 37(4):234–245.

Shabot M.M. (1982). Documented bedside computation of cardiorespiratory variables with an inexpensive programmable calculator. In DeAngelis J. (Ed.), *Debates and Controversies in the Management of High Risk Patients* (pp. 153–163). San Diego, CA: Beach International.

Shabot M.M. (1989). Standardized acquisition of bedside data: The IEEE P1073 medical information bus. *International Journal of Clinical Monitoring and Computing*, 6(4): 197–204.

Shabot M.M. (1995). Computers in the intensive care unit: Was Pogo correct? *Journal of Intensive Care Medicine*, 10:211–212.

Shabot M.M. (1997a). Automated clinical pathways for surgical services. *Surgical Services Management*, (June):19–23.

Shabot M.M. (1997b). The HP CareVue clinical information system. *International Journal of Clinical Monitoring and Computing*, 14(3):177–184.

Shabot M.M., Shoemaker W.C., State D. (1977). Rapid bedside computation of cardiorespiratory variables with a programmable calculator. *Critical Care Medicine*, 5(2): 105–111.

Shahar Y. (1997). A framework for knowledge-based temporal abstractions. *Artificial Intelligence*, 90:79–133.

Shahar Y., Miksch S., Johnson P.D. (1988). The Asgaard Project: a task-specific framework for the application and critiquing of time-oriented clinical guidelines. *Artificial Intelligence in Medicine*, 14:29–51.

Shahar Y., Musen M.A. (1996). Knowledge-based temporal abstractions in clinical domains. *Artificial Intelligence in Medicine*, 8(3):267–298.

Shea S., DuMouchel W., Bahamonde L. (1996). A meta-analysis of 16 randomized controlled trials to evaluate computer-based clinical reminder systems for preventive care in the ambulatory setting. *Journal of the American Medical Informatics Association*, 3(6):399–409.

Shlaer S., Mellor S.J. (1992). *Object Life Cycles, Modeling the World in States*. Englewood Cliffs, NJ: Prentice-Hall.

Shortliffe E.H. (1976). *Computer-Based Medical Consultations: MYCIN*. New York: Elsevier/North Holland.

Shortliffe E.H. (1984). Coming to terms with the computer. In Reiser S., Anbar M. (Eds.), *The Machine at the Bedside: Strategies for Using Technology in Patient Care* (pp. 235–239). Cambridge, MA: Cambridge University Press.

Shortliffe E.H. (1986). Medical expert systems: knowledge tools for physicians. *Western Journal of Medicine*, 145:830–839.

Shortliffe E.H. (1989). Testing reality: the introduction of decision-support technologies for physicians. *Methods of Information in Medicine*, 28:1–5.

Shortliffe E.H. (1993). Doctors, patients, and computers: will information technology dehumanize healthcare delivery? *Proceedings of the American Philosophical Society*, 137(3):390–398.

Shortliffe E.H. (1994). Dehumanization of patient care: are computers the problem or the solution. *Journal of the American Medical Informatics Association*, 1(1):76–78.

Shortliffe E.H. (1995a). Medical informatics meets medical education. *Journal of the American Medical Association*, 273(13):1061–1065.

Shortliffe E.H. (1995b). Medical informatics training at Stanford University School of Medicine. In van Bemmel J.H., McCray A.T. (Eds.), *IMIA Yearbook of Medical In-*

formatics (vol. 1995, pp. 105–110). Stuttgart, Germany: Schattauer Publishing Company.

Shortliffe E.H. (1998a). Health care and the Next Generation Internet [editorial]. *Annals of Internal Medicine*, 129(2):138–140.

Shortliffe E.H. (1998b). The Next Generation Internet and health care: a civics lesson for the informatics community. In Chute C.G. *Proceedings of the 1998 AMIA Annual Fall Symposium (formerly SCAMC)* (pp. 8–14). Orlando, FL: Henley & Belfus, November 7–11, 1998.

Shortliffe E.H. (1998c). The evolution of health-care records in the era of the Internet [semi-plenary talk]. In *Proceedings of Medinfo 98.* Amsterdam: IOS Press.

Shortliffe E.H., Buchanan B.G., Feigenbaum E. (1979). Knowledge engineering for medical decision making: a review of computer-based clinical decision aids. *Proceedings of the IEEE*, 67:1207–1224.

Shubin H., Weil M.H. (1966). Efficient monitoring with a digital computer of cardiovascular function in seriously ill patients. *Annals of Internal Medicine*, 65(3):453–460.

Siegel E., Cummings M., Woodsmall R. (1990). Bibliographic retrieval systems. In Shortliffe E., Perreault L. (Eds.), *Medical Informatics: Computer Applications in Health Care* (pp. 434–465). Reading, MA: Addison-Wesley.

Siegel E.L., Protopapas Z., Reiner B.I., Pomerantz S.M. (1997). Patterns of utilization of computer workstations in a filmless environment and implications for current and future picture archiving and communication systems. *Journal of Digital Imaging*, 10(3 Suppl 1):41–43.

Silberg W.M., Lundberg G.D., Musacchio R.A. (1997). Assessing, controlling, and assuring the quality of medical information on the Internet: caveat lector et viewor—let the reader and viewer beware. *Journal of the American Medical Association*, 277(15): 1244–1245.

Simborg D.W., Chadwick M., Whiting-O'Keefe Q.E., Tolchin S.G., Kahn S.A., Bergan E.S. (1983). Local area networks and the hospital. *Computers and Biomedical Research*, 16(3):247–259.

Simmons D.A. (1980). *A Classification Scheme for Client Problems in Community Health Nursing: Nurse Planning Information Series.* (vol. 14, Pub No.[HRP] 501501). Springfield, VA: National Technical Information Service.

Singer S.J. (1991). Problems in gaining access to hospital information. *Health Affairs*, 10(2):148–151.

Singer S.J., Hunt K., Gabel J., Liston D., Enthoven A.C. (1997). New research shows how to save money on employee health benefits. *Managing Employee Health Benefits*, 5(4):1–9.

Sittig D. (1987). Computerized management of patient care in a complex, controlled clinical trial in the intensive care unit. In Stead W.W. *Proceedings of the 11th Annual Symposium on Computer Applications in Medical Care* (pp. 225–232). Washington, DC: November 1–4.

Smith L. (1985). Medicine as an art. In Wyngaarden J., Smith L. (Eds.), *Cecil Textbook of Medicine.* Philadelphia: W.B. Saunders, p. 3.

Smith R. (1992). Using a mock trial to make a difficult clinical decision. *British Medical Journal*, 305(6864):1284–1287.

Smith T., Waterman M. (1981). Identification of common molecular subsequences. *Journal of Molecular Biology*, 147(1):195–197.

Somers A.R. (1971). The Kaiser Permanente Medical Care program. *Commonwealth Fund.* New York.

Sonnenberg F.A., Beck J.R. (1993). Markov models in medical decision making: a practical guide. *Medical Decision Making*, 13(4):322–338.

Southon F.C., Sauer C., Dampney C.N. (1997). Information technology in complex health services: organizational impediments to successful technology transfer and diffusion. *Journal of the American Medical Informatics Association*, 4(2):112–124.

Sox H.C. (1986). Probability theory in the use of diagnostic tests. An introduction to critical study of the literature. *Annals of Internal Medicine*, 104(1):60–66.

Sox H.C. (1987). Probability theory in the use of diagnostic tests: application to critical study of the literature. In Sox H.C. (Ed.), *Common Diagnostic Tests: Use and Interpretation* (pp. 1–17). Philadelphia: American College of Physicians.

Sox H.C., Blatt M.A., Higgins M.C., Marton K.I. (1988). *Medical Decision Making*. Boston, MA: Butterworth Publisher.

Spee J.H., de Vos W.M., Kuipers O.P. (1993). Efficient random mutagenesis method with adjustable mutation frequency by use of PCR and dITP. *Nucleic Acids Research*, 21(3):777–778.

Stallings W. (1987a). *The Open Systems Interconnection (OSI) Model and OSI-Related Standards* (vol. 1). New York: Macmillian.

Stallings W. (1987b). *Handbook of Computer-Communications Standards*. New York: Macmillan Publishing Company.

Stallings W. (1997). *Data and Computer Communications*. Englewood Cliffs, NJ: Prentice Hall.

Starr P. (1982). *The Social Transformation of American Medicine*. New York: Basic Books.

Stead W. (1997a). 1996 IAIMS Symposium. Building infrastructure for integrated health systems. Proceedings. Nashville, TN, September 27, 1996. Dedicated to Richard T. West. *Journal of the American Medical Informatics Association*, 4(2 Suppl):S1–76.

Stead W.W. (1997b). The evolution of the IAIMS: lessons for the next decade. *Journal of the American Medical Informatics Association*, 4(2 Suppl):S4–9.

Stead W.W., Borden R., Bourne J., Giuse D., Giuse N., Harris T.R., Miller R.A., Olsen A.J. (1996). The Vanderbilt University fast track to IAIMS: Transition from planning to implementation. *Journal of the American Medical Informatics Association*, 3(5): 308–317.

Stead W.W., Hammond W.E. (1988). Computer-based medical records: the centerpiece of TMR. *M.D. Computing*, 5(5):48–62.

Steedman D. (1990). *Abstract Syntax Notation One: The Tutorial and Reference*. Great Britain: Technology Appraisals, Ltd.

Steen E.B. (Ed.) (1996). *Proceedings of the Second Annual Nicholas E. Davies CPR Recognition Symposium*. Schaumburg, IL: Computer-Based Patient Record Institute.

Stewart B.K., Langer S.G., Hoath J.I., Tarczy-Hornuch P. (1997). DICOM image integration into a Web-browsable electronic medical record. In *RSNA 1997 Scientific Program supplement to Radiology* (p. 205).

Strasberg H.R., Hubbs P.R., Rindfleisch T.C., Melmon, K.L. (1999). Analysis of information needs of users of the Stanford Health Information Network for Education. In Lorenzi N.M. (Ed.) *Proceedings of the AMIA Annual Fall Symposium*, (pp. 965–969). Washington, DC: Hanley and Belfus, Inc. November 6–10.

Stringer W.A. (1997). MRA image production and display. *Clinical Neuroscience*, 4(3):110–116.

Strong D.M., Lee Y.W., Wang R.T. (1997). 10 potholes in the road to information quality. *IEEE Computer*, 31:38–46.

Stryer L. (1995). *Biochemistry.* New York: WH Freeman.

Sumner W., Nease Jr. R.F., Littenberg B. (1991). U-titer: a utility assessment tool. In Clayton P.D. *Proceedings of the 15th Annual Symposium on Computer Applications in Medical Care* (pp. 701–705). Washington, DC. New York: McGraw-Hill.

Sweeney L. (1996). Replacing personally-indentifying information in medical records, the SCRUB system. In Cimino J.J. *Proceedings of the AMIA Annual Fall Symposium (formerly SCAMC)* (pp. 333–337). Washington, DC, October 28–30. Hanley & Belfus, Inc.

Swets J.A. (1973). The relative operating characteristic in psychology. *Science*, 182:990.

Szolovits P. (Ed.) (1982). *Artificial Intelligence in Medicine.* Boulder, CO: Westview Press.

Szolovits P., Pauker S.G. (1979). Computers and clinical decision making: whether, how much, and for whom? *Proceedings of the IEEE*, 67:1224–1226.

Tagare H.D., Jaffe C.C., Duncan J. (1997). Medical image databases: a content-based retrieval approach. *Journal of the American Medical Informatics Association*, 4(3):184–198.

Tagare H.D., Vos F.M., Jaffe C.C., Duncan J.S. (1995). Arrangement: a spatial relation between parts for evaluating similarity of tomographic section. *IEEE Transactions on Pattern Analysis and Machine Intelligence*, 17(9):880–893.

Tanenbaum A.S. (1987). *Computer Networks* (2nd ed.). Englewood Cliffs, NJ: Prentice Hall.

Tanenbaum A.S. (1996). *Computer Networks* (3rd. ed.). Englewood Cliffs, NJ: Prentice Hall.

Tang P.C., Annevelink J., Suermondt H.J., Young C.Y. (1994a). Semantic integration in a physician's workstation. *International Journal of Bio-Medical Computing*, 35(1):47–60.

Tang P.C., Fafchamps D., Shortliffe E.H. (1994b). Traditional medical records as a source of clinical data in the outpatient setting. In *Proceedings of the 18th Annual Symposium on Computer Applications in Medical Care* (pp. 575–579). Washington, DC: Hanley & Belfus.

Tang P.C., Marquardt W.C., Boggs B., Fellencer C.A., Gorden S., Jaworski M.A., et al. (1999). NetReach: Building a clinical infrastructure for the enterprise. In Overage J.M. (Ed.) *Fourth Annual Davies Award Proceedings of the CPR Recognition Symposium*, (pp. 25–68). Chicago: McGraw-Hill.

Tang P.C., Patel V.L. (1993). Major issues in user interface design for health professional workstations: summary and recommendations. *International Journal of Bio-Medical Computing*, 34(1–4):139–148.

Tarczy-Hornuch P., Kwan-Gett T.S., Fouche L., Hoath J., Fuller S., Ibrahim K.N., Ketchell D.S., LoGerfo J.P., Goldberg H. (1997). Meeting clinician information needs by integrating access to the medical record and knowledge sources via the Web. In Masys D.R. *Proceedings of the 1997 AMIA Annual Fall Symposium (formerly SCAMC)* (pp. 809–813). Nashville, TN: Hanley & Belfus, Inc., October 25–29.

Tatro D., Briggs R., Chavez-Pardo R., L. F., Hannigan J., Moore T., Cohen S. (1975). Online drug interaction surveillance. *American Journal of Hospital Pharmacy*, 32:417.

Teach R.L., Shortliffe E.H. (1981). An analysis of physician attitudes regarding computer-based clinical consultation systems. *Computers and Biomedical Research*, 14(6):542–558.

Teich J.M. (Ed.) (1997). *Proceedings of the Third Annual Nicholas E. Davies CPR Recognition Symposium.* Schaumburg, IL: Computer-based Patient Record Institute.

Teich J.M., Glaser J.P., Beckley R.F. (1996). Toward cost-effective, quality care: the Brigham Integrated Computing System. In E.B. Steen (Ed.), *Proceedings of the Second Annual Nicholas E. Davies CPR Recognition Symposium.* (vol. 2, pp. 3–34). Schaumburg, IL: Computer-Based Patient Record Institute.

Teich J.M., Kuperman G.J., Bates D.W. (1997). Clinical decision support: making the transition from the hospital to the community network. *Healthcare Information Management*, 11(4):27–37.

NCPDP Telecommunication. (1992). *NCPDP Telecommunication Standard Format.* (Version 3.2).

Templeton A.W., Dwyer S.J., Johnson J.A., Anderson W.H., Hensley K.S., Rosenthal S.J., Lee K.R., Preston D.F., Batnitzky S., Price H.I. (1984). An on-line digital image management system. *Radiology*, 152(2):321–325.

Thompson P., Toga A.W. (1996). A surface-based technique for warping three-dimensional images of the brain. *IEEE Transactions on Medical Imaging*, 15(4):402–417.

Tierney W.M., Miller M.E., Overhage J.M., McDonald C.J. (1993). Physician inpatient order writing on microcomputer workstations. Effects on resource utilization. *Journal of the American Medical Association*, 269(3):379–383.

Torrance G.W., Feeny D. (1989). Utilities and quality-adjusted life years. *International Journal of Technology Assessment in Health Care*, 5(4):559–575.

Tsien C.L., Fackler J.C. (1997). Poor prognosis for existing monitors in the intensive care unit. *Critical Care Medicine*, 25(4):614–619.

Tu S., Musen M.A. (1996). The EON model of intervention protocols and guidelines. In Cimino J.J. *Proceedings of the AMIA Annual Fall Symposium (formerly SCAMC)* (pp. 587–591). Washington, DC, Hanley & Belfus, Inc., October 28–30.

Tu S.W., Eriksson H., Gennari J.H., Shahar Y., Musen M.A. (1995). Ontology-based configuration of problem-solving methods and generation of knowledge-acquisition tools: application of PROTÉGÉ-II to protocol-based decision support. *Artificial Intelligence in Medicine*, 7(3):257–289.

Tu S.W., Kemper C.A., Lane N.M., Carlson R.W., Musen M.A. (1993). A methodology for determining patients' eligibility for clinical trials. *Methods of Information in Medicine*, 32(4):317–325.

Turing A.M. (1950). Computing machinery and intelligence. *Mind*, 59:433–460.

Tversky A., Kahneman D. (1974). Judgment under uncertainty: heuristics and biases. *Science*, 185:1124–1131.

Tysyer D.A. (1997). Copyright law: databases. *Bitlaw*, http://www.bitlaw.com/copyright/database.htm.

Ullman J.D., Widom J. (1997). *A First Course in Database Systems*. Englewood Cliffs, NJ: Prentice Hall Engineering, Science & Math.

United States General Accounting Office (1993). *Automated Medical Records: Leadership Needed to Expedite Standards Development: Report to the Chairman/Committee on Governmental Affairs*. Washington, DC: U.S. Senate, USGAO/IMTEC-93-17.

U.S. Preventive Services Task Force (1996). *Guide to Clinical Preventive Services* (2nd. ed.). Baltimore: Williams & Wilkins.

van Bemmel J.H., Musen M.A. (1997). *Handbook of Medical Informatics*. New York: Bohn Stafleu Van Loghum, Houten, and Springer-Verlag.

van der Lei J., Musen M.A. (1991). A model for critiquing based on automated medical records. *Computers and Biomedical Research*, 24(4):344–378.

van der Lei J., Musen M.A., van der Does E., Man in 't Veld A.J., van Bemmel J.H. (1991). Comparison of computer-aided and human review of general practitioners' management of hypertension. *Lancet*, 338(8781):1504–1508.

van Heijst G., Falasconi S., Abu-Hanna A., Schreiber G., Stefanelli M. (1995). A case study in ontology library construction. *Artificial Intelligence in Medicine*, 7(3):227–255.

Vannier M.W., Marsh J.W. (1996). Three-dimensional imaging, surgical planning, and image-guided therapy. *Radiology Clinics of North America*, 34(3):545–563.

Vetterli M., Kovarevic J. (1995). *Wavelets and Subband Coding*. Englewood Cliffs, NJ: Prentice Hall.

Vosniadou S., DeCorte E., Glaser R., Mandl H. (Eds.) (1996). *International Perspectives on the Design of Technology-Supported Learning Environments.* Mahwah, NJ: L. Erlbaum Associates.

Wake M.M., Murphy M., Affara F.A., Lang N.M., Clark J., Mortensen R. (1993). Toward an International Classification for Nursing Practice: a literature review and survey. *International Nursing Review*, 40(3):77–80.

Warner H.R. (1979). *Computer-Assisted Medical Decision-Making*. New York: Academic Press.

Warner H.R., Gardner R.M., Toronto A.F. (1968). Computer-based monitoring of cardiovascular function in postoperative patients. *Circulation*, 37(4 Suppl):II68–II74.

Warner H.R., Toronto A.F., Veasy L. (1964). Experience with Bayes' theorem for computer diagnosis of congenital heart disease. *Annals of the New York Academy of Science*, 115:2–16.

Warren J.J., Hoskins L.M. (1995). NANDA's Nursing diagnosis taxonomy: a nursing database. In *Nursing Data Systems: The Emerging Framework* (pp. 49–59). Washington, DC: American Nurses Publishing.

Watson J., Crick F. (1953). A structure for deoxyribose nucleic acid. *Nature*, 171:737.

Watson R.J. (1977). A large-scale professionally oriented medical information system: five years later. *Journal of Medical Systems*, 1:3–16.

Weed L.L. (1969). *Medical Records, Medical Education and Patient Care: The Problem-Oriented Record as a Basic Tool.* Chicago, IL: Year Book Medical Publishers.

Weed L.L. (1975). Problem-Oriented Medical Information System (PROMIS) Laboratory. In Giebin G.A., Hurst L.L. (Eds.), *Computer Projects in Health Care.* Ann Arbor, MI: Health Administration Press.

Weinberg A.D. (1973). CAI at the Ohio State University College of Medicine. *Computers in Biology and Medicine*, 3(3):299–305.

Weinfurt P.T. (1990). Electrocardiographic monitoring: an overview. *Journal of Clinical Monitoring*, 6(2):132–138.

Weinstein M.C., Fineberg H. (1980). *Clinical Decision Analysis.* Philadelphia: W. B. Saunders.

Weller C.D. (1984). "Free choice" as a restraint of trade in American health care delivery and insurance. *Iowa Law Review*, 69(5):1351–1378, 1382–1392.

Wennberg J. (1998). *The Dartmouth Altas of Health Care in the United States.* Dartmouth Medical School, American Hospital Publishing Inc.

Wennberg J., Gittelsohn A. (1973). Small area variations in health care delivery. *Science*, 182(117):1102–1108.

Werley H.H., Lang N.M. (Eds.) (1988). *Identification of the Nursing Minimum Data Set.* New York: Springer.

Westwood J.D., Hoffman H.M., Stredney D., Weghorst S.J. (1998). *Medicine Meets Virtual Reality.* Amsterdam: IOS Press.

Whitely W.P., Rennie D., Hafner A.W. (1994). The scientific community's response to evidence of fraudulent publication: the Robert Slutsky case. *Journal of the American Medical Association*, 272(2):170–173.

Whiting-O'Keefe Q.E., Simborg D.W., Epstein W.V. (1980). A controlled experiment to evaluate the use of a time-oriented summary medical record. *Medical Care*, 18(8):842–852.

Whiting-O'Keefe Q.E., Simborg D.W., Epstein W.V., Warger A. (1985). A computerized summary medical record system can provide more information than the standard medical record. *Journal of the American Medical Association*, 254(9):1185–1192.

Widman L.E., Tong D.A. (1997). Requests for medical advice from patients and families to health care providers who publish on the World Wide Web. *Archives of Internal Medicine*, 15(2):209–212.

Wiederhold G. (1981). *Databases for Health Care*. New York: Springer-Verlag.

Wiederhold G., Bilello M., Sarathy V., Qian X. (1996). A security mediator for health care information. In Cimino J.J. *Proceedings of the AMIA Annual Fall Symposium (formerly SCAMC)* (pp. 120–124). Washington, DC: Hanley & Belfus, October 28–30.

Wiederhold G., Clayton P.D. (1985). Processing biological data in real time. *M.D. Computing*, 2(6):16–25.

Williams R.M., Baker L.M., Marshall J.G. (1992). *Information Searching*. Thorofare, NJ: Slack.

Winograd T., Flores F. (1987). *Understanding Computers and Cognition: A New Foundation for Design*. Reading, MA: Addison-Wesley.

Winston P.H., Narasimhan S. (1996). *On to Java*. Reading, MA: Addison Wesley.

Wittenber J., Shabot M.M. (1990). Progress report: the medical device data language for the IEEE 1073 medical information bus. *International Journal of Clinical Monitoring and Computing*, 7(2):91–98.

Wood E.H. (1994). MEDLINE: the options for health professionals. *Journal of the American Medical Informatics Association*, 1(5):372–380.

Woods J.W. (Ed.) (1991). *Subband Image Coding*. Boston, MA: Kluwer Academic Computer Publishers.

Woolhandler S., Himmelstein D.U. (1997). Costs of care and administration at for-profit and other hospitals in the United States. *New England Journal of Medicine*, 336(11): 769–774.

World Health Organization (1977). *Ninth Edition. International Classification of Diseases Index. Manual for the International Statistical Classification of Diseases*. Geneva: The World Health Organization.

World Health Organization (1992). *International Classification of Diseases Index. Tenth Revision. Volume 1: Tabular List*. Geneva: The World Health Organization.

Wyatt J.C. (1989). Lessons learned from the field trial of ACORN, an expert system to advise on chest pain. In Barber B., Cao D., Quin D. *Proceedings of the Sixth World Conference on Medical Informatics* (pp. 111–115). North Holland Press, Amsterdam.

Wyatt J.C. (1991a). *A Method for Developing Medical Decision-Aids Applied to ACORN, a Chest Pain Advisor*. Unpublished DM thesis, Oxford University.

Wyatt J.C. (1991b). Use and sources of medical knowledge. *Lancet*, 338(8779):1368–1373.

Wyatt J.C., Altman D.G. (1995). Prognostic models: clinically useful, or quickly forgotten? *British Medical Journal*, 311:1539–1541.

Wyatt J.C., Spiegelhalter D. (1990). Evaluating medical expert systems: what to test and how? *Medical Informatics*, 15(3):205–217.

Young D.W. (1980). An aid to reducing unnecessary investigations. *British Medical Journal*, 281(6225):1610–1611.

Young F. (1987). Validation of medical software: present policy of the Food and Drug Administration. *Annals of Internal Medicine*, 106:628.

Young W.H., Gardner R.M., East T.D., Turner K. (1997). Computerized ventilator charting: artifact rejection and data reduction. *International Journal of Clinical Monitoring and Computing*, 14(3):165–176.

Youngner S.J. (1988). Who defines futility? *Journal of the American Medical Association*, 260(14):2094–2095.

Yu V.L., Buchanan B.G., Shortliffe E.H., Wraith S.M., Davis R., Scott A.C., Cohen S.N. (1979a). Evaluating the performance of a computer-based consultant. *Computer Programs in Biomedicine*, 9(1):95–102.

Yu V.L., Fagan L.M., Wraith S.M., Clancey W.J., Scott A.C., Hannigan J., Blum R.L., Buchanan B.G., Cohen S.N. (1979b). Antimicrobial selection by a computer. A blinded evaluation by infectious disease experts. *Journal of the American Medical Association*, 242(12):1279–1282.

Zachary W.W., Strong G.W., Zaklad A. (1984). Information systems ethnography: integrating anthropological methods into system design to insure organizational acceptance. In Hendrick H.W., Brown O. (Eds.), *Human Factors in Organizational Design and Management* (pp. 223–227). Amsterdam: North Holland Press.

Zielstorff R.D., Barnett G.O., Fitzmaurice J.B., Estey G., Hamilton G., Vickery A., Welebob E., Shahzad C. (1996). A decision support system for prevention and treatment of pressure ulcers based on AHCPR guidelines. In Cimino J.J. *Proceedings of the AMIA Annual Fall Symposium (formerly SCAMC)* (pp. 562–566). Washington, DC: Hanley & Belfus, Inc., October 26–30.

Zielstorff R.D., Hudgings C.I., Grobe S.J. (1993). *Next-Feneration Nursing Information Systems: Essential Characteristics for Nursing Practice*. Washington, DC: American Nurses Publishing.

Glossary

Key chapters in which a term is used are indicated in square brackets.

Abstraction: A level of medical data encoding that entails examining the recorded data and selecting an item from a terminology with which to label the data. [6]

Accountability: Security function that ensures users are responsible for their access to and use of information based on a documented need and right to know. [4]

Acquired immunodeficiency syndrome (AIDS): A disease of the immune system caused by a retrovirus and transmitted chiefly through blood or blood products, characterized by increased susceptibility to opportunistic infections, certain cancers, and neurological disorders. [3,11,17]

Active storage: In a hierarchical data-storage scheme, the devices used to store data that have long-term validity and that must be accessed rapidly. [4]

Address: In a computer system, a number or symbol that identifies a particular cell of memory. [4]

Administrative services only (ASO): The practice by employers of paying their employees' medical bills directly (self-insurance) and hiring insurance companies only to process claims. [19]

Admission-discharge-transfer (ADT): The core component of a hospital information system that maintains and updates the hospital census. [10]

Advanced Research Projects Agency Network (ARPANET): A large wide-area network created in the 1960s by the U.S. Department of Defense Advanced Research Projects Agency for the free exchange of information among universities and research organizations; the precursor to today's Internet. [1,4]

Advice nurse: A health professional, typically trained in nursing, who is available by telephone to answer patients' questions and to help them to make appropriate use of health services. [19]

Aggregate content: Information from multiple sources, which can be viewed within an information-retrieval system using a single interface. [15]

Alert message: A computer-generated output that is created when a record meets prespecified criteria; for example, receipt of a new laboratory test result with an abnormal value. [9]

Algorithm: A well-defined procedure or sequence of steps for solving a problem. [1]

Allocation bias: Overestimation of the effects of an intervention caused by systematic assignment of favorable subjects to the study group by investigators. [8]

Alphabetic ranking: A common ranking criterion used by information-retrieval systems; for a particular field in the database, results are output based on the order of the field's first word in the alphabet. [15]

Ambulatory medical record system (AMRS): A computer information system designed to support all information requirements of an outpatient clinic, including registration, appointment scheduling, billing, order entry, results reporting, and clinical documentation. [10]

American Standard Code for Information Interchange (ASCII): A 7-bit code for representing alphanumeric characters and other symbols. [4]

Analog signal: A signal that takes on a continuous range of values. [4]

Analog-to-digital conversion (ADC): Conversion of sampled values from a continuous-valued signal to a discrete-valued digital representation. [4,13]

Anchoring and adjustment: A heuristic used when estimating probability, in which a person first makes a rough approximation (the anchor) and then adjusts this estimate to account for additional information. [3]

Angiography: A technique used to increase the contrast resolution of X-ray images of the blood vessels by injection of radiopaque contrast material into the vessels. [14]

Antibiotic-assistant program: Computer program developed at LDS Hospital to assist physicians in ordering antibiotics for patients who have or who are suspected of having an infection. [13]

Applets: Small computer programs that can be embedded in an HTML document that will execute on the user's computer when referenced. [4]

Application program: A computer program designed to accomplish a user-level task. [4]

Applications research: Systematic investigation or experimentation with the goal of applying knowledge to achieve practical ends. [1]

Arc: A diagrammatic element of an influence diagram, which appears between two chance nodes and indicates that a probabilistic relationship may exist between the chance nodes. [3]

Archival storage: In a hierarchical data-storage scheme, the devices used to store data for backup, documentary, or legal purposes. [4]

Arden Syntax: A programming language that provides a canonical means for writing rules (Medical Logic Modules) that relate specific patient situations to appropriate actions for practitioners to follow. The Arden Syntax standard is maintained by HL7. [6,16]

Art-criticism approach: An evaluation approach that relies on the review and opinions of an experienced and respected critic to highlight an information resource's strengths and weaknesses. [8]

Artificial intelligence (AI): The branch of computer science concerned with endowing computers with the ability to simulate intelligent human behavior. [1,16,17]

Artificial neural network (ANN): A computer program that performs classification by taking as input a set of findings that describe a given case, propagating calculated weights through a network of several layers of interconnected nodes, and generating as output a set of numbers in which each output corresponds to the likelihood of a particular classification that could explain the findings. [16]

Assembler: A computer program that translates assembly-language programs into machine-language instructions. [4]

Assembly language: A low-level language for writing computer programs using symbolic names and addresses. [4]

Assessment bias: Overestimation (or underestimation) of the effects of an intervention caused by systematic favorable (or unfavorable) evaluations of results by the investigators. [8]

Asynchronous transfer mode (ATM): A network protocol designed for sending streams of small, fixed length cells of information over very high-speed, dedicated connections, often digital optical circuits. [4]

ATTENDING: A standalone decision-support program that critiqued a patient-specific plan for anesthetic selection, induction, and administration after that plan had been proposed by the anesthesiologist who would be managing the case. [16]

Audit trail: A chronological record of all accesses and changes to data records, often used to promote accountability for use of medical data. [4]

Augmented reality: A user-interface method in which a computer-generated scene is superimposed on the real world, usually by painting the scene on semi-transparent goggles that track the motion of the head. [14]

Authentication: A process for positive and unique identification of users, implemented to control system access. [4]

Authoring system: In computer-aided instruction, a specialized, high-level language used by educators to create computer-based teaching programs. [17]

Authorization: A process for controlling user activities within a system to only actions defined as appropriate based on the user's role. [4]

Automated indexing: The most common method of full-text indexing; words in a document are stripped of common suffixes, entered as items in the index, then assigned weights based on their ability to discriminate among documents (*see* Vector-space model). [15]

Availability: In decision making, a heuristic method by which a person estimates the probability of an event based on the ease with which similar events can be recalled. [3] In security systems, a function that ensures delivery of accurate and up-to-date information to authorized users when needed. [4]

Averaging out at chance nodes: The process by which each chance node of a decision tree is replaced by the expected value of the event that it represents. [3]

Backbone links: Sections of high-capacity trunk (backbone) network that interconnect regional and local networks. [4]

Backbone network: A high-speed communication network that carries major traffic between smaller networks. [1]

Back-projection: A method for reconstructing images, in which the measured attenuation along a path is distributed uniformly across all pixels along the path. [14]

Bandwidth: The capacity for information transmission; the number of bits that can be transmitted per unit of time. [1,4]

Baseband transmission: A data-transmission technique in which bits are sent without modulation (*see* Modem). [4]

Baseline measurement: An observation collected prior to an intervention and used for comparison with an associated study observation. [8]

Baseline rate, individual: The frequency, rate, or degree of a condition before an intervention or other perturbation; **population:** The prevalence of the condition under consideration in the population from which the subject was selected. [2]

Basic research: Systematic investigation or experimentation with the goal of discovering new knowledge, often by proposing new generalizations from the results of several experiments. [1]

Basic science: The enterprise of performing basic research. [1]

Batch mode: A noninteractive mode of using a computer, in which users submit jobs for processing and receive results on completion (*see* Time-sharing mode). [4]

Baud rate: The rate of information transfer; at lower speeds, baud rate is equal to the number of bits per second being sent. [4]

Bayesian diagnosis program: A computer-based system that uses Bayes' theorem to assist a user in developing and refining a differential diagnosis. [16]

Bayes' theorem: An algebraic expression for calculating posttest probability of a condition (for example, a disease) if the pretest probability (prevalence) of the condition, as well as the sensitivity and specificity of the test, are known (also called Bayes' rule). [3]

Before-after study: An experiment that compares study measurements to the same (baseline) measurements collected prior to introduction of the resource of interest (*see* Historically controlled experiment). [8]

Belief network: A diagrammatic representation used to perform probabilistic inference; an influence diagram that has only chance nodes. [3,16]

Bias: A systematic difference in outcome between groups that is caused by a factor other than the intervention under study. [3]

Bibliographic content: In information retrieval, information abstracted from the original source. [15]

Binary: The condition of having only two values or alternatives. [4]

Bioinformatics: The study of how information is represented and transmitted in biological systems starting at the molecular level. [7,18]

Biomedical computing: The use of computers in biology or medicine. [1]

Biomedical engineering: An area of engineering concerned primarily with the research and development of medical instrumentation and medical devices. [1]

Business-logic layer: A conceptual level of system architecture that insulates the applications and processing components from the underlying data and the user interfaces that access the data. [10]

Bit: A digit that can assume the values of either 0 or 1. [4]

Bit map: A digital representation of an image in memory, in which there is a one-to-one correspondence between bits and pixels of a displayed image. [14]

Bit-mapped display: A display screen that is divided into a grid of tiny areas (pixels), each associated with a bit that indicates whether the area is on (black) or off (white). [14]

Bit rate: The rate of information transfer; a function of the rate at which signals can be transmitted and the efficacy with which digital information is encoded in the signal. [4]

Body (of E-mail)**:** The portion of a simple electronic mail message that contains the free-text content of the message. [4]

Boolean operators: The mathematical operators AND, OR, and NOT, which are used to combine index terms in information retrieval searching. [15]

Bootstrap: A small set of initial instructions that is stored in read-only memory and executed each time the computer is turned on. Execution of the bootstrap is called *booting* the computer. By analogy, the process of starting larger computer systems. [4]

Broadband transmission: A data-transmission technique in which multiple signals may be transmitted simultaneously, each modulated within an assigned frequency range. [4]

Browser: A user interface to the World Wide Web that allows users to search for and display remote information resources in a suitable format. [5]

Browsing: Scanning a database, a list of files, or the Internet, either for a particular item or for anything that seems to be of interest. [4]

Business services: Remote network services that are designed for controlled or contractual user access (also see informational services). [5]

Buttons: Graphic elements within a dialog box or user-selectable areas within an HTML document that, when activated, perform a specified function, such as invoking other HTML documents and services. [4]

Byte: A sequence of 8 bits often used to store an ASCII character. [4]

Capitated system: System of health-care reimbursement in which providers are paid a fixed amount per patient to take care of all the health-needs of a population of patients. [9,19]

Capitation: In health-care financing, the payment of premiums or dues directly to the provider organization in the form of a fixed periodic payment for comprehensive care, set in advance (also called per capita payment). [19]

Case manager: A health professional assigned to monitor and coordinate a patient's care across care providers and health settings throughout an episode of treatment. [12]

Cathode-ray tube (CRT): A data-output device that displays information by projecting streams of electrons onto a fluorescent screen to create programmed patterns of light and dark or color. [4,13]

Centers for Disease Control (and Prevention) **(CDC):** The United States government health agency responsible for monitoring and reporting incidences and trends in infectious disease, bacterial-resistance patterns, and other public health information. [2,11]

Central computer system: A single system that handles all computer applications in an institution using a common set of databases and interfaces. [10]

Central monitor: Computer-based monitoring system with waveform analysis capabilities and high-capacity data storage. [13]

Central processing unit (CPU): The "brain" of the computer. The CPU executes a program stored in main memory by fetching and executing instructions in the program. [4]

Certificate: Coded authorization information that can be verified by a certification authority to grant system access. [4]

Chance node: A symbol that represents a chance event. By convention, a chance node is indicated in a decision tree by a circle. [3]

Charge coupled device (CCD) camera: A device used to convert existing film-based images to digital form. [14]

Charges: In a health-care institution, the established prices for services. Often, charges do not reflect the cost of providing the service. [19]

Checklist effect: The improvement observed in decision making because of more complete and better structured data collection when paper- or computer-based forms are used to collect patient data. [8]

Chronology: The primary ranking criterion in many information-retrieval systems, in which the most recent entries are output first. [15]

Classification (of features)**:** In image processing, the categorization of segmented regions of an image based on the values of measured parameters, such as area and intensity. [14]

Client-server: Information processing interaction that distributes application processing between a local computer (the client) and a remote computer resource (the server). [4]

Clinically relevant population: The population of patients that is seen in actual practice. In the context of estimating the sensitivity and specificity of a diagnostic test, that group of patients in whom the test actually will be used. [3]

Clinical data repository (CDR): Clinical database optimized for storage and retrieval for information on individual patients and used to support patient care and daily operations. [10]

Clinical decision-support system: A computer-based system that assists physicians in making decisions about patient care. [16]

Clinical expert system: A computer program designed to provide decision support for diagnosis or therapy planning at a level of sophistication that an expert physician might provide. [7,16]

Clinical informatics: The application of medical informatics methods in the patient care domain; a combination of computer science, information science, and clinical science designed to assist in the management and processing of data, information, and knowledge to support the practice and delivery of clinical care. [12]

Clinical information system (CIS): The components of a health-care information system designed to support the delivery of patient care, including order communications, results reporting, care planning, and clinical documentation. [10]

Clinical judgment: Decision making by clinicians that incorporates professional experience and social, ethical, psychological, financial, and other factors in addition to the objective medical data. [7]

Clinical modifications: A published set of changes to the International Classification of Diseases that provides additional levels of detail necessary for statistical reporting in the United States. [6]

Clinical pathway: Disease-specific plan that identifies clinical goals, interventions, and expected outcomes by time period. [10,12]

Clinical prediction rule: A rule, derived from statistical analysis of clinical observations that is used to assign a patient to a clinical subgroup with a known probability of disease. [3]

Clinical research: The collection and analysis of medical data acquired during patient care to improve medical science and the knowledge physicians use in caring for patients. [7]

Clinical subgroup: A subset of a population in which the members have similar characteristics and symptoms, and therefore similar likelihood of disease. [3]

Clinical trials: Experiments in which data from specific patient interactions are pooled and analyzed in order to learn about the safety and efficacy of new treatments or tests and to gain insight into disease processes that are not otherwise well understood. [1]

Closed-loop control: Regulation of a physiological variable, such as blood pressure, by monitoring the value of the variable and altering therapy without human intervention. [13]

Coaching system: A computer-based education system that monitors the session and intervenes only when the student requests help or makes serious mistakes (*see* Tutoring system). [17]

Coded: Form of data that has been standardized and classified for processing by computer. [9]

Coding scheme: A system for classifying objects and entities (such as, diseases, procedures, or symptoms) using a finite set of numeric or alphanumeric identifiers. [2]

Coercion: A function of a computer language that provides for automatic conversion of data types when a mismatch is identified. [4]

Cognitive heuristics: Mental processes by which we learn, recall, or process information; rules of thumb. [3]

Cognitive science: Area of research concerned with studying the processes by which people think and behave. [1]

Coinsurance: The percentage of charges that is paid by the insuree rather than by the insurance company once the deductible has been satisfied. [19]

Color resolution: A measure of the ability to distinguish among different colors (indicated in a digital image by the number of bits per pixel). Three sets of multiple bits are required to specify the intensity of red, green, and blue components of each pixel color. [4]

Communication (computer)**:** Data transmission and information exchange between computers using accepted protocols via an exchange medium such as a telephone line or fiberoptic cable. [4]

Community Health Information Network (CHIN): A computer network developed for exchange of sharable health information among independent participant organizations in a geographic area (or community). [7,11]

Compact disk (CD): A round, flat piece of material used to encode data through the use of a laser that alters the material's reflectivity. [4]

Compact-disk read-only memory (CD-ROM): An optical-disk technology for storing and retrieving large numbers of prerecorded data. Data are permanently encoded through the use of a laser that marks the surface of the disk, then can be read an unlimited number of times using a finely focused semiconductor laser that detects reflections from the disk. [4]

Comparison-based approach: Evaluation approach that studies an experimental resource in contrast to a control resource or placebo. [8]

Compiler: A program that translates a program written in a high-level programming language to a machine-language program, which can then be executed. [4]

Comprehensibility and control: Security function that ensures that data owners and data stewards have effective control over information confidentiality and access. [4]

Computability theory: The foundation for assessing the feasibility and cost of computation to provide the complete and correct results to a formally stated problem. Many interesting problems cannot be computed in a finite time and require heuristics. [1]

Computed check: Procedure applied to entered data that verifies values based on calculation of a correct mathematical relationship; for example, white-blood-cell differential counts (reported as percentages) must sum to 100. [9]

Computed radiography: An imaging technique in which a latent image is recorded on a specially coated cassette that is then scanned by a computer to capture the image in digital form. [14]

Computed tomography (CT): An imaging modality in which X-rays are projected through the body from multiple angles and the resultant absorption values are analyzed by a computer to produce cross-sectional slices. [4,9,14]

Computer-aided instruction (CAI): The application of computer technology to education (also called computer-assisted learning and computer-based education). [17]

Computer architecture: The basic structure of a computer, including memory organization, a scheme for encoding data and instructions, and control mechanisms for performing computing operations. [4]

Computer-assisted learning: The application of computer technology to education (also called computer-based education and computer-aided instruction). [17]

Computer-based education (CBE): The application of computer technology to education (also called computer-assisted learning and computer-aided instruction). [17]

Computer-based monitoring: Use of computers to acquire, process, and evaluate analog physiological signals captured from patients. [13]

Computer-based patient monitor: A patient monitoring device that supports other data functions, such as database maintenance, report generation, and decision-making. [13]

Computer-based patient record (CPR): A repository of electronically maintained information about an individual's lifetime health status and health care, stored such that it can serve the multiple legitimate users of the record. [9]

Computer-based patient record system: The addition to a computer-based patient record of information-management tools that provide clinical alerts and reminders, linkages with external health knowledge sources, and tools for data analysis. [9]

Computer interpretation: Translation by computer of voice input into appropriate text, codes, or commands. [9]

Computer program: A set of instructions that tells a computer which mathematical and logical operations to perform. [4]

Computer system: An integrated arrangement of computer hardware and software operated by users to perform prescribed tasks. [5]

Concordant (test results): Test results that reflect the true patient state (true-positive and true-negative results). [3]

Conditional independence: Two events, *A* and *B*, are conditionally independent if the occurrence of one does not influence the probability of the occurrence of the other, when both events are conditioned on a third event *C*. Thus, $p[A \mid B,C] = p[A \mid C]$ and $p[B \mid A,C] = p[B \mid C]$. The conditional probability of two conditionally independent events both occurring is the product of the individual conditional probabilities: $p[A,B \mid C] = p[A \mid C] \times p[B \mid C]$. For example, two tests for a disease are conditionally independent when the probability of the result of the second test does not depend on the result of the first test, given the disease state. For the case in which disease is present, p[second test positive | first test positive and disease present] = p[second test positive | first test negative and disease present] = p[second test positive | disease present]. More succinctly, the tests are conditionally independent if the sensitivity and specificity of one test do not depend on the result of the other test (*see* Independence). [3]

Conditional probability: The probability of an event, contingent on the occurrence of another event. [3]

Conditioned event: A chance event the probability of which is affected by another chance event (the conditioning event). [3]

Conditioning event: A chance event that affects the probability of occurrence of another chance event (the conditioned event). [3]

Confidentiality: The ability of data owners and data stewards to control access to or release of private information. [4,7]

Consensus: With respect to medical care, general agreement regarding proper action. [8]

Consistency check: Procedure applied to entered data that detects errors based on internal inconsistencies; for example, recording of cancer of the prostate as the diagnosis for a female patient. [9]

Constructive (approach to learning)**:** An approach to teaching in which students learn through reassembly of separated parts; for example, learning anatomy by putting together body parts or by placing cross-sections at the correct location in the body. [17]

Consulting model: A style of interaction in a decision-support system, in which the program serves as an adviser, accepting patient-specific data, asking questions, and generating advice for the user about diagnosis or management. [16]

Consulting system: A computer-based system that develops and suggests problem-specific recommendations based on user input (*see* Critiquing system). [16]

Consumer health informatics (CHI): Applications of medical informatics technologies that focus on the patient as the primary user. [7,11]

Content: In information retrieval, media developed to communicate information or knowledge. [15]

Content structuring: The process by which distinct semantic regions of content, such as title, author names, and abstract, are identified. [15]

Contingency table: A 2×2 table that shows the relative frequencies of true-positive, true-negative, false-positive, and false-negative results. [3]

Continuity of care: The coordination of care received by a patient over time and across multiple health-care providers. [2]

Continuous-speech recognition: Translation by computer of voice input, spoken using a natural vocabulary and cadence, into appropriate text, codes, and commands. [9]

Continuum of care: The full spectrum of health services provided to patients, including health maintenance, primary care, acute care, critical care, rehabilitation, home care, skilled nursing care, and hospice care. [12]

Contract-management system: A computer system used to support managed-care contracting by estimating the costs and payments associated with potential contract terms and by comparing actual with expected payments based on contract terms. [10]

Contrast radiography: A technique used to increase the contrast resolution of X-ray images by injection of radiopaque contrast material into a body cavity or blood vessels. [14]

Contrast resolution: A measure of the ability to distinguish among different levels of intensity (indicated in a digital image by the number of bits per pixel). [4,14]

Controls: In an experiment, subjects who are not affected by the intervention of interest. [8]

Convolution: In image processing, a mathematical edge-enhancement technique used to sharpen blurred computed-tomographic images. [14]

Copyright law: Protection of written materials and intellectual property from being copied verbatim. [7]

Cost–benefit analysis (CBA): An analysis of the costs and benefits associated with alternative courses of action that is designed to identify the alternative that yields the maximum net benefit. CBA is generally used when it is possible to assign dollar values to all relevant costs and benefits. [8]

Cost center: An organizational department that does not have revenue associated with the services it provides (for example, administration, data processing, billing, and housekeeping). [19]

Cost–effectiveness analysis (CEA): An analysis of alternative courses of action, the objective of which is to identify either the alternative that yields the maximum effectiveness achievable for a given amount of spending, or the alternative that minimizes the cost of achieving a stipulated level of effectiveness. CEA is generally used when it is not possible to measure benefits in dollar units. [8]

Cost–effectiveness threshold: Threshold level in a cost–effectiveness analysis that reflects a decision maker's value judgment regarding a maximum (or minimum) value; for example, the maximum value of a quality-adjusted life year to be used in an analysis. [8]

Credentialing: Certification of a resource's quality by a recognized body such as a clinical professional association. [11]

Critical care: Monitoring and treatment of patients with unstable physiologic systems, life-threatening conditions, or at high-risk of developing life-threatening conditions, typically in an intensive-care unit. [7]

Critiquing model: A style of interaction in a decision-support system, in which the program acts as a sounding board for the user's ideas, expressing agreement or suggesting reasoned alternatives. [16]

Critiquing system: A computer-based system that evaluates and suggests modifications for plans or data analyses already formed by a user (*see* Consulting system). [16]

Cross-validation: Verification of the accuracy of data by comparison of two sets of data collected by alternate means. [13]

Cryptographic encoding: Scheme for protecting data through authentication and authorization controls based on use of keys for encrypting and decrypting information. [4]

Cursor: A blinking region of a display monitor, or a symbol such as an arrow, that indicates the currently active position on the screen. [4]

Customary, prevailing, and reasonable: The payment system used by Medicare (prior to implementation of the Resource-Based Relative Value Scale and Volume Performance Standard), which reimbursed practitioners generously for performing procedures and relatively poorly for providing cognitive services such as history taking and advice giving. [19]

Custom-designed system: A computer system designed and developed within an institution to meet the special needs of that institution. [5]

Customer: The user who interacts with the software and hardware of a computer system and uses the results.[5]

Data acquisition: The input of data into a computer system through direct data entry, acquisition from a medical device, or other means. [12]

Database: A collection of stored data—typically organized into fields, records, and files—and an associated description (schema). [2,4]

Database-management system (DBMS): An integrated set of programs that manages access to databases. [4]

Database mediator: A software component of the EON knowledge-based system that is used to insulate EON's problem solvers from the logistical issues associated with accessing the database of a clinical information system. [16]

Data bus: An electronic pathway for transferring data—for instance, between a CPU and memory. [4]

Data capture: The acquisition or recording of information. [9]

Data compression: A mathematical technique for reducing the number of bits needed to store data, with or without loss of information. [14]

Data flow: The input, processing, storage, and output of information in a computer system. [5]

Data flow diagram (DFD): A graphical representation for the sources, transformation processes, storage, and presentation of data in a computer system. [5]

Data independence: The insulation of applications programs from changes in data-storage structures and data-access strategies. [4]

Data-interchange standards: Adopted formats and protocols for exchange of data between independent computer systems. [6]

Data layer: A conceptual level of system architecture that insulates the data collected and stored in the enterprise from the applications and user interfaces used to access those data. [10]

Data overload: The inability to access crucial information due to the overwhelming number of irrelevant data or due to the poor organization of data. [13]

Data processing: The manipulation of data to convert it to some desired result (also called data transformation). [12]

Data recording: The documentation of information for archival or future use through mechanisms such as handwritten text, drawings, machine-generated traces, or photographic images. [2]

Data standard: A set of syntactic and semantic rules for defining elements of information to be recorded or exchanged. [6,12]

Data storage: The methods, programs, and structures used to organize data for subsequent use. [12]

Data transcription: The transfer of information from one data-recording system to another, such as the entry into a computer by clerical personnel of the handwritten or dictated notes or datasheets created by a health professional. [9]

Data transformation: The manipulation of data to convert it to some desired result (also called data processing). [12]

Data warehouse: Database optimized for long-term storage, retrieval, and analysis of records aggregated across patient populations, often serving the longer-term business and clinical analysis needs of an organization. [10]

Datum: Any single observation of fact. A medical datum generally can be regarded as the value of a specific parameter (for example, red-blood-cell count) for a particular object (for example, a patient) at a given point in time. [2]

Debugger: A system program that provides traces, memory dumps, and other tools to assist programmers in locating and eliminating errors in their programs. [4]

Decision analysis: A methodology for making decisions by identifying alternatives and assessing them with regard to both the likelihood of possible outcomes and the costs and benefits of the outcomes. [16]

Decision-facilitation approach: A formative evaluation approach designed to resolve issues important to system developers and administrators by asking and answering successive questions during the course of resource development. [8]

Decision node: A symbol that represents a choice among actions. By convention, a decision node is represented in a decision tree by a square. [3]

Decision tree: A diagrammatic representation of the outcomes associated with chance events and voluntary actions. [3]

Deductible: A set dollar amount of covered charges that must be paid by the insuree before the insurance company begins to reimburse for outlays. [19]

Deformable model: In image processing, a generic shape that is close in shape to a structure of interest, and which can be reshaped (deformed) until it matches the imaged structure. The deformation is controlled by an optimization procedure that minimizes a cost function. [14]

Delta check: Procedure applied to entered data that compares the values of new and previous results to detect large and unlikely differences in value; for example, a recorded weight change of 100 pounds in 2 weeks. [9]

Demonstration study: An experiment designed to draw inferences about performance, perceptions, or effects of an information resource. [8]

Denominator: The part of a fraction that is below the line; in public health, data on the population as a whole, which is used for comparison to the data of specific subpopulations. [11]

Deoxyribonucleic acid (DNA): The genetic material that is the basis for heredity. DNA is a long polymer chemical made of four basic subunits. The sequence in which these subunits occur in the polymer distinguishes one DNA molecule from another and in turn directs a cell's production of proteins and all other basic cellular processes. [18]

Dependent variable: In a statistical analysis, the variable that measures experimental outcome. Its value is assumed to be a function of the experimental conditions (independent variables). [8]

Derived parameter: A parameter that is calculated indirectly from multiple parameters that are measured directly. [13]

Descriptive (or uncontrolled) **study:** Experiment in which there is no control group for comparison. [8]

Diagnosis: The process of analyzing available data to determine the pathophysiologic explanation for a patient's symptoms. [1,7,16]

Diagnosis-related group (DRG): One of 468 categories based on major diagnosis, length of stay, secondary diagnosis, surgical procedure, age, and types of services required. Used to determine the fixed payment per case that the Health Care Financing Administration will reimburse hospitals for providing care to Medicare patients. [17,19]

Diagnostic process: The activity of deciding which questions to ask, which tests to order, or which procedures to perform, and determining the value of the results relative to associated risks or financial costs. [16]

Differential diagnosis: The set of active hypotheses (possible diagnoses) that a physician develops when determining the source of a patient's problem. [2]

Digital computer: A computer that processes discrete values based on the binary digit or bit. [4]

Digital image: An image that is stored as a grid of numbers, where each picture element (pixel) in the grid represents the intensity of a small area. [14]

Digital radiography: The process of producing X-ray images that are stored in digital form in computer memory rather than on film. [14]

Digital radiology: The use of digital radiographic methods for medical imaging. [14]

Digital signal: A signal that takes on discrete values from a specified set of values. [4]

Digital signal processing (DSP) chip: An integrated circuit designed for high-speed data manipulation and used in audio communications, image manipulation, and other data acquisition and control applications. [4]

Digital subscriber line (DSL): A digital telephone service that allows high-speed network communication using conventional (twisted pair) telephone wiring. [4]

Digital subtraction angiography (DSA): A radiologic technique for imaging blood vessels in which a digital image acquired before injection of contrast material is subtracted pixel by pixel from an image acquired after injection. The resulting image shows only the differences in the two images, highlighting those areas where the contrast material has accumulated. [14]

Digital video disk (DVD): Next generation optical disk storage technology that allows encoding and high-volume storage of video, audio, and computer data on a compact disk. [4,17]

Direct cost: A cost that can be directly assigned to the production of goods or services. For example, direct costs in the laboratory include the cost of the technician's salary, equipment, and supplies. [8]

Direct entry: The entry of data into a computer system by the individual who personally made the observations. [9]

Discounting: Calculation that accounts for time preference by reducing the value of expenditures and payments that accrue in the future relative to those that occur immediately. [8]

Discrimination learning: An approach to teaching in which students are presented with a series of examples of increasing complexity, thereby learning to detect subtle differences. [17]

Display: In information retrieval, the last step of the information-retrieval process, in which the final result set is shown to the user. [15]

Display monitor: A device for presenting output to users through use of a screen. (*see* cathode-ray tube.)[4]

Distributed computer system: A collection of independent computers that share data, programs, and other resources. [10]

DNA arrays: Small glass plates onto which specific DNA fragments can be affixed and then used to detect other DNA fragments present in a cell extract. [18]

DNA sequence database: A searchable, stored collection of known DNA sequences (GENBANK is one of the largest). Individual databases may also contain information about the biological source of the sequence, reference information, and annotations regarding the data. [18]

Domain: A unique corporate or institutional address that designates one or multiple hosts on the Internet. [1]

Domain Name System (DNS): A hierarchical name-management system used to translate computer names to Internet protocol addresses. [4]

Dot-matrix printer: Output device that prints patterns of small dots on paper to form characters or other marks. [4]

Double-blind: A clinical study methodology in which neither the researchers nor the subjects know to which study group a subject has been assigned. [2]

Drill and practice: An approach to teaching in which students are presented with a small amount of information, then are asked questions about the material, and thus receive immediate feedback to support the learning process. [17]

Dynamic (simulation program attribute)**:** A simulation program that models changes in patient state over time and in response to students' therapeutic decisions. [17]

Dynamic programming: A computationally intensive computer-science technique used to determine optimal sequence alignments in many computational biology applications. [18]

Edge-detection technique: A method, such as application of an edge-following algorithm, used to identify a region of interest from an overall image by delineating the borders of the region. [14]

Efficacy: The capacity for producing a desired result. [8]

Electrocardiogram (ECG): The graphic recording of minute differences in electric potential caused by heart action. [4,6,13]

Electronic Data Interchange (EDI): Electronic exchange of standard data transactions, such as claims submission and electronic funds transfer. [6,10]

Electronic textbook: An online reference containing non-patient-specific information. [16]

Emergent: Experimental design whereby the results of earlier stages of investigation are used to identify future issues for evaluation. [8]

Enterprise master patient index (EMPI): An architectural component that serves as the name authority in a health-care information system composed of multiple independent systems; the EMPI provides an index of patient names and identification numbers used by the connected information systems. [10]

Entry term: A synonym form for a subject heading in the Medical Subject Headings (MeSH) controlled, hierarchical vocabulary. [15]

Epidemiology: The study of the incidence, distribution, and causes of disease in a population. [1,11]

Escrow: Use of a trusted third party to hold cryptographic keys, computer source code, or other valuable information to protect against loss. [4]

Ethernet: A network standard that uses a bus or star topology and regulates communication traffic using the Carrier Sense Multiple Access with Collision Detection (CSMA/CD) approach. [4]

Ethics: A system of moral principles; the rules of conduct recognized in respect to a particular class of human actions or a particular group or culture. [7]

Ethnography: A branch of anthropology dealing with the scientific description of individual cultures. [8]

Evaluation: Data collection and analysis designed to appraise a situation, answer a question, or judge the success of an intervention. [8,15,17]

Evidence-based guidelines: Consensus approaches for handing recurring health-management problems aimed at reducing practice variability and improving health outcomes. Clinical guideline development emphasizes using clear evidence from the existing literature, rather than expert opinion alone, as the basis for the advisory materials. [1]

Evidence-based medicine (EBM): An approach to medical practice whereby the best possible evidence from the medical literature is incorporated in decision making. [7,15]

Evoking strength (ES): One of two numbers used by the Internist-1 decision-support system to reflect the strength of the relationship between a disease and a finding; the evoking strength is a number between 0 and 5 that reflects the likelihood that a patient with the finding has the disease in question (*see* Frequency weight). [16]

Expected value: The value that is expected on average for a specified chance event or decision. [3]

Expected-value decision making: A method for decision making in which the decision maker selects the option that will produce the best result on average (that is, the option that has the highest expected value). [3]

Experimental science: Systematic study characterized by posing hypotheses, designing experiments, performing analyses, and interpreting results to validate or disprove hypotheses and to suggest new hypotheses for study. [1]

Expert system: A computer program that symbolically encodes concepts derived from experts in a field and uses that knowledge to provide the kind of problem analysis and advice that the expert might provide. [7,16]

Expert witness: A person, such as a physician, who provides testimony at a legal proceeding in the form of professional opinions. [7]

Explosion: In information-retrieval systems, the process in which a general vocabulary term and the more specific terms beneath it in the hierarchy are combined using the or boolean operator. [15]

Extended Binary Coded Decimal Interchange Code (EBCDIC): An 8-bit code for representing alphanumeric characters and other symbols. [6]

External router: A computer that resides on multiple networks and that can forward and translate message packets sent from a local or enterprise network to a regional network beyond the bounds of the organization. [4]

External validity: Characteristic of a well-founded study methodology, such that the study conclusions can be generalized from the specific setting, subjects, and intervention studied to the broader range of settings that other people will encounter. [8]

False-negative rate (FNR): The probability of a negative result, given that the condition under consideration is true—for example, the probability of a negative test result in a patient who has the disease under consideration. [3]

False-negative result (FN): A negative result when the condition under consideration is true—for example, a negative test result in a patient who has the disease under consideration. [3]

False-positive rate (FPR): The probability of a positive result, given that the condition under consideration is false—for example, the probability of a positive test result in a patient who does not have the disease under consideration. [3]

False-positive result (FP): A positive result when the condition under consideration is false—for example, a positive test result in a patient who does not have the disease under consideration. [3]

Feature detection: In image processing, determination of parameters, such as volume or length, from segmented regions of an image. In signal processing, identification of specific waveforms or other patterns of interest in a signal. [13,14]

Feature extraction: Computer processing to identify patterns of interest and characteristics within imaged, waveforms, and other signals (*see* Feature detection). [13]

Feedback: In a computer-based education program, system-generated responses, such as explanations, summaries, and references, provided to further a student's progress in learning. [17]

Fee-for-service model: Unrestricted system of health-care reimbursement in which payers pay providers for all services the provider deemed necessary. [9]

Fiberoptic cable: A communication medium that uses light waves to transmit information signals. [4]

Field: The smallest named unit of data in a database. Fields are grouped together to form records. [4] In the context of an evaluation study, the setting or settings in which the activity under study is carried out. [8]

Field qualification: In information-retrieval systems, the designation of which index or field should be searched. [15]

File: In a database, a collection of similar records. [4]

File server: A computer that is dedicated to storing shared or private data files. [4]

File Transfer Protocol (FTP): The protocol used for copying files to and from remote computer systems on a network using TCP/IP. [4]

Filtering algorithm: A defined procedure applied to input data to reduce the effect of noise. [4]

Firewall: A security system intended to protect an organization's network against external threats by preventing computers in the organization's network from communicating directly with computers external to the network, and vice versa. [4]

Fixed cost: A cost that does not vary with the volume of production during a given period. Examples are expenses for plant, equipment, and administrative salaries. [19]

Fixed fee: Restricted system of health-care reimbursement in which payers pay providers a set amount for health services approved by the payer. [9]

Floppy disk: An inexpensive magnetic disk that can be removed from the disk-drive unit. [4]

Flowsheet: A tabular summary of information that is arranged to display the values of variables as they change over time. [9]

Fluoroscopy: An imaging method in which a screen coated with a fluorescent substance is used for viewing objects by means of X-ray or other radiation. [14]

Food and Drug Administration (FDA): Division of the Department of Health and Human Services that regulates medical devices, as well as food, drugs, and cosmetics. [7,13,16]

Formal systems analysis: A methodology for evaluating requirements and generating specifications for developing computer systems and other information resources. [8]

Formative decision: A decision made as a result of a study undertaken while a resource is being developed and that can affect future development of the resource. [8]

Formative evaluation: An assessment of a system's behavior and capabilities conducted during the development process and used to guide future development of the system. [17]

Frame relay: A high-speed network protocol designed for sending digital information over shared wide-area networks using variable length packets of information. [4]

Free text: Unstructured, uncoded representation of information in text format; for example, sentences describing the results of a patient's physical examination. [9]

Frequency-modulated (FM): A signal representation in which signal values are represented as changes in frequency rather than amplitude. [4]

Frequency weight (FW): One of two numbers used by the Internist-1 decision-support system to reflect the strength of the relationship between a disease and a finding; the frequency weight is a number between 1 and 5, where 1 means that the finding is seldom seen in the disease and 5 means it is essentially always seen (*see* Evoking strength). [16]

Front-end application: A computer program that interacts with a database-management system to retrieve and save data and accomplish user-level tasks. [4]

Full disclosure: In ECG monitoring, a process whereby all data regarding the full set of leads are stored and available for reconstruction of the complete cardiogram as it would have appeared during a period of abnormal rhythms. [13]

Full-text content: The complete textual information contained in a bibliographic source. [15]

Full-text database: A bibliographic database that contains the entire text of journal articles, books, and other literature, rather than only citations. [15]

Functional image: An image, such as a computed-tomographic image or a digital subtraction angiogram image, which is computed from derived quantities, rather than being measured directly. [14]

Functional mapping: An imaging method that relates specific sites on images to particular physiologic functions. [14]

Gateway: A computer that resides on multiple networks and that can forward and translate message packets sent between nodes in networks running different protocols. [4]

Genetic data: Information regarding a person or organism's genome and heredity. [7]

Genome: The total collection of DNA for a person or organism. [18]

Gigabits per second (Gbps): A common unit of measure for data transmission over high-speed networks. [4]

Gigabyte: 2^{30} or 1,073,741,824 bytes. [4]

Global processing: Any image-enhancement technique in which the same computation is applied to every pixel in an image. [14]

Goal-free approach: An evaluation approach in which evaluators are purposely unaware of the intended effects of an information resource and collect evidence to enable identification of all effects, intended or not. [8]

Gold-standard test: The test or procedure whose result is used to determine the true state of the subject—for example, a pathology test used to determine a patient's true disease state. [3]

Graphic editor: A program used to create and manipulate files of drawings or images.[4]

Graphic user interface (GUI): A type of environment that represents programs, files, and options by means of icons, menus, and dialog boxes on the screen.[4]

Gray scale: A scheme for representing intensity in a black-and-white image. Multiple bits per pixel are used to represent intermediate levels of gray. [4]

Group-model HMO: A type of HMO that is based on contracts between physicians organized in a medical group and the HMO; the medical group accepts risks of costs of care and usually rewards the partners if the group is successful in managing costs (*see* Staff-model HMO). [19]

Guidance: In a computer-based education program, proactive feedback, help facilities, and other tools designed to assist a student in learning the covered material. [17]

Hard disk: A magnetic disk used for data storage and typically fixed in the disk-drive unit. [4]

Hardware: The physical equipment of a computer system, including the central processing unit, data-storage devices, workstations, terminals, and printers. [4,5]

Hawthorne effect: The tendency for humans to improve their performance if they know it is being studied. [8]

Header (of E-mail)**:** The portion of a simple electronic mail message that contains information about the date and time of the message, the address of the sender, the addresses of the recipients, the subject, and other optional information. [4]

Health Care information system (HCIS): An information system used within a health-care organization to facilitate communication, integrate information, document health-care interventions, perform record keeping, or otherwise support the functions of the organization. [10]

Health Care team: A coordinated group of health professionals including physicians, nurses, case managers, dieticians, pharmacists, therapists, and other practitioners who collaborate in caring for a patient. [2]

Health Level 7 (HL7): An ad hoc standards group formed to develop standards for exchange of health-care data between independent computer applications; the health-care data messaging standard developed and adopted by the Health Level 7 standards group. [6,9]

Health-maintenance organization (HMO): A group practice or affiliation of independent practitioners that contracts with patients to provide comprehensive health care for a fixed periodic payment specified in advance. [6,19]

Health Security Act: The 1994 proposal (by then President Clinton) drafted to overhaul the health-care financing and delivery system and to provide universal coverage for all Americans. [19]

Hearsay evidence: Testimony based on what a witness has heard from another source rather than on direct personal knowledge or experience. [7]

Helpers (plug ins)**:** Applications that are launched by a Web browser when the browser downloads a file that it is not able to process itself. [4]

HELP sector: A decision rule encoded in the HELP system, a clinical information system that was developed by researchers at LDS Hospital in Salt Lake City. [16]

Heuristic: A rule of thumb; a cognitive process used in learning or problem solving. [2]

High-level process: A complex process comprising multiple lower-level processes. [1]

Histogram equalization: An image enhancement technique that spreads the image's gray levels throughout the visible range to maximize the visibility of those gray levels that are used frequently. [14]

Historically controlled experiment: A study that makes and compares the same measurements before and after the introduction of the resource of interest (*See* Before-after study). [8]

Hospital information system (HIS): Computer system designed to support the comprehensive information requirements of hospitals and medical centers, including patient, clinical, ancillary, and financial management. [1,4,5,6,9,10,12,14]

Human Genome Project: An international undertaking the goal of which is to determine the complete sequence of human deoxyribonucleic acid (DNA), as it is encoded in each of the 23 chromosomes. [18]

Human immunodeficiency virus (HIV): A retrovirus that invades and inactivates helper T-cells of the immune system and is a cause of AIDS and AIDS-related complex. [3,6,11,17]

Hypertext: Text linked together in a nonsequential web of associations. Users can traverse highlighted portions of text to retrieve additional related information. [4,15]

HyperText Markup Language (HTML): The document specification language used for documents on the World Wide Web. [4,5,15,16,17]

HyperText Transfer Protocol (HTTP): The client-server protocol used to access information on the World Wide Web. [4,15]

Hypothetico-deductive approach: In clinical medicine, an iterative approach to diagnosis in which physicians perform sequential, staged data collection, data interpretation, and hypothesis generation to determine and refine a differential diagnosis. [2]

ICD-9-CM: See Ninth International Classification of Diseases–Clinical Modification (ICD-9-CM). [6]

Icon: In a graphical interface, a pictorial representation of an object or function. [4]

IDF*TF weighting: A simple weighting measure used for document retrieval based on term frequency (TF) and inverse document frequency (IDF); terms that occur often in a small number of documents are given the highest weighting (*see* Inverse document frequency). [15]

Image enhancement: The use of global processing methods to improve the appearance of an image, either for human use or for subsequent processing by computer. [14]

Image generation: The process of producing images and converting them to digital form if they are not intrinsically digital. [14]

Image integration: The combination of images with other information needed for interpretation, management, and other tasks. [14]

Image management: The application of methods for storing, transmitting, displaying, retrieving, and organizing images. [14]

Image manipulation: The use of pre- and postprocessing methods to enhance, visualize, or analyze images. [14]

Image processing: The transformation of one or more input images, either into one or more output images, or into an abstract representation of the contents of the input images. [14]

Imaging informatics: A subdiscipline of medical informatics concerned with the common issues that arise in all image modalities and applications once the images are converted to digital form. [14]

Imaging modality: A method for producing images. Examples of medical applications are X-ray imaging, computed tomography, echosonography, and magnetic resonance imaging. [14]

Immersive simulated environment: A teaching environment in which a student manipulates tools to control simulated instruments, producing visual, pressure, and other feedback to the tool controls and instruments. [17]

Impact printer: Output device that uses typewriter, print chain, or drum technologies to contact paper, thus producing a character or mark. [4]

Implementation phase: A major step in the system life cycle in which the system is constructed based on the design specifications. [5]

Import number: A number used by the Internist-1 decision-support system; the import number captures the notion that some abnormalities have serious implications and must be explained, whereas others may be safely ignored. [16]

Inaccessibility: Unavailability; a limitation of traditional medical records, which can be used by only one person at a time. [9]

Incrementalist: Person who is able to make changes gradually, by degrees. [8]

Indemnity insurance: A type of insurance modeled on casualty insurance. Typically, an insuree is reimbursed a specified amount for a hospital day, or for each of a list of surgical procedures. [19]

Independence: Two events, A and B, are considered independent if the occurrence of one does not influence the probability of the occurrence of the other. Thus, $p[A \mid B] = p[A]$. The probability of two independent events A and B both occurring is given by the product of the individual probabilities: $p[A,B] = p[A] \times p[B]$. (*see* Conditional independence). [3]

Independent variable: A variable believed to affect the outcome (dependent variable) of an experiment. [8]

Index: In information retrieval, a shorthand guide to the content that allows users to find relevant content quickly. [15,17]

Index attribute: A term that describes some aspect of an index item, such as the document numbers where the item appears or the frequency of the item within a document. [15]

Indexing: In information retrieval, the assignment to each document of specific terms that indicate the subject matter of the document and that are used in searching. [15]

Index item: A unit of information used for matching with a query during searching. [15]

Index Medicus: The printed index used to catalog the medical literature. Journal articles are indexed by author name and subject heading, then aggregated in bound volumes. [15]

Index test: The diagnostic test whose performance is being measured. [3]

Indirect care: Activities of health professionals that are not directly related to patient care, such as teaching and supervising students, continuing education, and attending staff meetings. [12]

Individual (or independent) practice association (IPA): A group of individual physicians that has joined together to contract with one or more insurance carrier IPA-HMOs to see patients enrolled with those carriers. The physicians continue to practice in their own offices and continue to see patients with other forms of insurance coverage. The group is paid on a per capita basis for services delivered by member physicians under the IPA contracts. Individual physicians members agree to fee schedules, management controls, and risk-sharing arrangements (also known as network-model HMOs). [19]

Influence diagram: A belief network in which explicit decision and utility nodes are added. [3,16]

Information: Organized data or knowledge that provide a basis for decision making. [2]

Information need: In information retrieval, the searcher's expression, in her own language, of the information that she desires. [15]

Informational services: Remote network services that are designed to be broadly accessible (*see also* Business services). [5]

Information resources: In medical informatics, computer systems developed to collect, process, and disseminate health information. [8]

Information retrieval (IR): The science and practice of identification and efficient use of recorded media. [15]

Information retrieval (IR) database: An organized collection of stored bibliographic data, which contains both an index and the full original content. [15]

Information science: The field of study concerned with issues related to the management of both paper-based and electronically stored information. [1]

Information Sources Map (ISM): One component of the Unified Medical Language System, the Information Sources Map (ISM) is a database of available databases, indexed by terms in the Metathesaurus. [15]

Information theory: The theory and mathematics underlying the processes of communication. [1]

Ink-jet printer: Output device that uses a moveable head to spray liquid ink on paper; the head moves back and forth for each line of pixels. [4]

Input: The data that represent state information, to be stored and processed to produce results (output). [5]

Institute of Electrical and Electronics Engineers (IEEE): An international organization through which many of the world's standards in telecommunications, electronics, electrical applications, and computers have been developed. [6,13]

Integrated circuit (IC): A circuit of transistors, resistors, and capacitors constructed on a single chip and interconnected to perform a specific function. [4]

Integrated delivery network (IDN): A large conglomerate health-care organization developed to provide and manage comprehensive health-care services. [7,10,14]

Integrated Service Digital Network (ISDN): A digital telephone service that allows high-speed network communications using conventional (twisted pair) telephone wiring. [4]

Intellectual property: Software programs, knowledge bases, Internet pages, and other creative assets that require protection against copying and other unauthorized use. [7]

Intensive-care unit (ICU): A hospital unit in which critically ill patients are monitored closely. [1,6,13]

Interface engine: A computer system that translates and formats data for exchange between independent (sending and receiving) computer systems. [9]

Intermittent monitoring: The periodic measurement of a physiological parameter. [13]

Internal validity: Characteristic of a well-founded experiment; the ability to have confidence in an experiment's conclusions due to the quality of its methodology. [8]

Internet: A worldwide collection of gateways and networks that communicate with each other using the TCP/IP protocol, collectively providing a range of services including electronic mail and World Wide Web access. [4]

Internet 2: The initial project of the University Consortium for Advanced Internet Development (UCAID), Internet 2 is a testbed for high-bandwidth communications to support research and education that builds on existing federally funded or experimental networks. [1]

Internet Control Message Protocol (ICMP): A network-level Internet protocol that provides error correction and other information relevant to processing data packets. [4]

Internet Mail Access Protocol (IMAP): A protocol used by electronic mail programs to access messages stored on a mail server. [4]

Internet Protocol (IP): The protocol within TCP/IP that governs the creation and routing of data packets and their reassembly into data messages. [4]

Internet service provider (ISP): A commercial communications company that supplies Internet connectivity to individuals and organizations. [4]

Internet standards: The set of conventions and protocols all Internet participants use to enable data communications. [4]

Interpreter: A program that converts each statement in a high-level program to a machine-language representation and then executes the binary instruction(s). [4]

Interventional radiology: The use of needles, catheters, biopsy instruments, or other invasive methodologies with the aim of producing a diagnostic or therapeutic, or possibly palliative, effect. Examples are balloon angioplasty for coronary stenosis and cyst aspiration and drainage. [14]

Intranet: An enterprise-wide network that is managed and controlled by an organization for communication and information access within the organization by authorized users. [1]

Intuitionist–pluralist: A philosophical orientation whereby an observation depends on both the resource under study and the perspective of the observer. [8]

Invasive monitoring technique: A method for measuring a physiological parameter that requires breaking the skin or otherwise entering the body. [13]

Inverse document frequency (IDF): A measure of how infrequently a term occurs in a document collection. $IDF_i = 1 + \log(\text{number of documents}/\text{number of documents with term } i)$. [15]

Inverted index: In information retrieval, a simple guide to the content that includes items (such as words) and item attributes (such as documents that contain the words). [15]

Ionizing radiation: X-rays and other forms of radiation that penetrate cells, and, when sufficiently intense, inhibit cell division, thereby causing cell death. [14]

IP address: A 32-bit number that uniquely identifies a computer connected to the Internet. [4]

Job: A set of tasks submitted by a user for processing by a computer system. [4]

Joystick: A leverlike device (like the steering stick of an airplane) that a user moves to control the position of a cursor on a screen. [4]

Kernel: The core of the operating system that resides in memory and runs in the background to supervise and control the execution of all other programs and direct operation of the hardware. [4]

Keyboard: A data-input device used to enter alphanumeric characters through typing. [4]

Key field: A field in the record of a file that uniquely identifies the record within the file. [4]

Kilobyte: 2^{10} or 1024 bytes. [4]

Knowledge: Relationships, facts, assumptions, heuristics, and models derived through the formal or informal analysis (or interpretation) of data. [2]

Knowledge base: A collection of stored facts, heuristics, and models that can be used for problem solving. [2,16]

Knowledge-based system: A program that symbolically encodes facts, heuristics, and models derived from experts in a field—in a knowledge base—and uses that knowledge base to provide problem analysis or advice that the expert might provide. [16]

Laser printer: Output device that uses an electromechanically controlled laser beam to generate an image on a xerographic surface, which then is used to produce paper copies. [4]

Latency: The time required for a signal to travel between two points in a network. [1]

Legacy system: A computer system that remains in use after an organization installs new systems. [10]

Legal issues: The aspects of using software applications in clinical practice and in biomedical research that are defined by law, including liability under tort law, legislation governing privacy and confidentiality, and intellectual property issues. [7]

Level: One of a set of discrete values that can be assumed by a categorical variable. [8]

Light: Electromagnetic radiation that can be detected by the organs of sight. [14]

Light pen: A penlike photosensitive device with which a user can select and enter data by pointing at the screen of a video display terminal. [4]

Likelihood ratio (LR): A measure of the discriminatory power of a test. The LR is the ratio of the probability of a result when the condition under consideration is true to the probability of a result when the condition under consideration is false (for example, the probability of a result in a diseased patient to the probability of a result in a nondiseased patient). The LR for a positive test is the ratio of true-positive rate (TPR) to false-positive rate (FPR). [3]

Liquid-crystal-display (LCD): A display technology that uses rod-shaped molecules to bend light and alter contrast and viewing angle to produce images. [4,13]

Listserv: A distribution list for electronic mail messages. [4]

Local-area network (LAN): A network for data communication that connects multiple nodes—all typically owned by a single institution and located within a small geographic area. [4,14]

Logical link control (LLC): A sublayer of the data-link layer of the ISO Open Systems Interconnection model. [6]

Logical-positivist: A philosophical orientation that holds factual only that which has verifiable consequences in experience. [8]

Lossless compression: A mathematical technique for reducing the number of bits needed to store data that allows recreation of the original data. [14]

Lossy compression: A mathematical technique for reducing the number of bits needed to store data that results in loss of information. [14]

Low-level process: An elementary process that has its basis in the physical world of chemistry or physics. [1]

Machine code: The set of primitive instructions to a computer represented in binary code (machine language). [4]

Machine language: The set of primitive instructions represented in binary code. [4]

Macro: A reusable set of computer instructions. [4]

Magnetic disk: A round, flat plate of material that can accept and store magnetic charge. Data are encoded on magnetic disk as sequences of charges on concentric tracks. [4]

Magnetic resonance imaging (MRI): A modality that produces images by evaluating the differential response of atomic nuclei in the body when the patient is placed in an intense magnetic field. [4,14]

Magnetic tape: A long ribbon of material that can accept and store magnetic charge. Data are encoded on magnetic tape as sequences of charges along longitudinal tracks. [4]

Magnetism: The properties of attraction possessed by magnets. Many atomic nuclei within the body act like tiny magnets, a characteristic that is used in the creation of images through methods such as nuclear magnetic resonance spectroscopy. [14]

Mailing list: A set of mailing addresses used for bulk distribution of electronic or physical mail. [4]

Mainframe computer: A large, multiuser computer, operated and maintained by professional computing personnel. [4]

Maintenance phase: The final step in the system life cycle during which the system is in routine use and is periodically modified based on changing requirements. [5]

Major medical insurance: Comprehensive insurance for medical expenses. The insurer pays a certain percentage of covered charges once the insuree has satisfied the deductible. [19]

Malpractice: Class of litigation in health care based on negligence theory; failure of a health professional to render proper services in keeping with the standards of the community. [7]

Managed competition: A strategy used by health services purchasers intended to use market forces to transform the health-care delivery system, create integrated, efficient provider organizations capable of delivering high-value health services and good health outcomes, and create incentives for continuous quality improvement and cost reduction. [19]

Management: The process of treating a patient (or allowing the condition to resolve on its own) once the medical diagnosis has been determined. [16]

Marginal cost: The increase in total cost associated with the production of one more unit of a good or service. [19]

Marginal cost-effectiveness ratio: The relative value of two interventions, calculated as the difference in the measured costs of the two interventions divided by the difference in the measured benefits of the interventions. [8]

Markov cycle: The period of time specified for a transition probability within a Markov model. [3]

Markov model: A simulation model used to calculate the probabilities of future outcomes by specifying a set of alternative future states and the probabilities of transitioning between each pair of states in a specified time period, then running the model for a specified number of cycles. [3]

Markup: Labeling of distinct semantic regions of content in a document. [15]

Markup language: A document specification language that identifies and labels the components of the document's contents. [5]

Master patient index (MPI): The module of a health-care information system used to uniquely identify a patient within the system. The MPI stores patient-identification information, basic demographic data, and basic encounter-level data such as dates and locations of service. [10]

Matching: The first step of the information-retrieval process, in which a query is compared against an index to create a result set. [15]

Measurement: The process of assigning a value corresponding to presence, absence, or degree of a specific attribute in a specific object. [8]

Measurement study: An experiment that seeks to determine how accurately an attribute of interest can be measured in a population of objects. [8]

Measures of concordance: Measures of agreement in test performance: the true-positive and true-negative rates. [3]

Measures of discordance: Measures of disagreement in test performance: the false-positive and false-negative rates. [3]

Medicaid: A program of federal grants to help states pay for the medical care of welfare recipients and of other people who resemble welfare recipients (people in welfare categories, above the welfare income line). [19]

Medical computer science: The subdivision of computer science that applies the methods of computing to medical topics. [1]

Medical computing: The application of methods of computing to medical topics (*see* Medical computer science). [1]

Medical datum: Any single observation of medical fact; the value of a specific parameter (for example, red-blood-cell count) for a particular object (for example, a patient) at a given point in time. [2]

Medical informatics: A field of study concerned with the broad range of issues in the management and use of biomedical information, including medical computing and the study of the nature of medical information. [1]

Medical information bus (MIB): A data-communication system that supports data acquisition from a variety of independent devices. [6,13]

Medical information science: The field of study concerned with issues related to the management and use of biomedical information (see also medical informatics). [1]

Medical Literature Analysis and Retrieval System (MEDLARS): The initial electronic version of Index Medicus developed by the National Library of Medicine. [15]

Medical logic module (MLM): A single chunk of medical reasoning or decision rule encoded using the Arden Syntax. [16]

Medical management: Process employed by a health plan or integrated delivery network to manage patient care proactively and to ensure delivery of (only) appropriate health services. [10]

Medical record: A paper-based or computer-stored document in which are recorded the data gathered during a patient's encounters with the health-care system. [9]

Medical-record committee: An institutional panel charged with ensuring appropriate use of medical records within the organization. [7]

Medical spreadsheet: A tool within the Quick Medical Reference decision-support system used to determine how coexisting diseases might give rise to a user-specified combination of diseases or findings. [16]

Medical subject heading (MeSH): One of some 18,000 medical terms used to identify the subject content of the medical literature. The National Library of Medicine's MeSH vocabulary has emerged as the de facto standard for biomedical indexing. [6,11,15]

Medical technology: Techniques, drugs, equipment, and procedures used by health-care professionals in delivering medical care to individuals, and the system within which such care is delivered. [8]

Medicare: The federal program of hospital and medical insurance for Social Security retirees, the long-term disabled, and patients suffering from chronic renal failure. [19]

MEDLARS Online (MEDLINE): The National Library of Medicine's electronic catalog of the medical literature, which includes information abstracted from journal articles, including author names, article title, journal source, publication date, and medical subject heading. [15]

MedWeaver: A Web application designed to integrate functions from the DXplain decision-support system, the WebMedline literature-search system, and the CliniWeb clinical Web-search system using the UMLS Metathesaurus for vocabulary translation. [15]

Megabits per second (Mbps): A common unit of measure for specifying a rate of data transmission. [4]

Megabyte: 2^{20} or 1,048,576 bytes. [4]

Member checking: Step in a subjectivist study during which the investigator shares emerging thoughts and beliefs with the participants themselves in order to validate and reorganize the structure of the study. [8]

Memorandum of understanding: Document that represents the general goals, scope, methods, conditions, and expected outcomes of a research study. [8]

Memory: Areas that are used to store programs and data. The computer's working memory comprises read-only memory (ROM) and random-access memory (RAM). [4]

Menu: In a user interface, a displayed list of valid commands or options from which a user may choose. [4]

MeSH subheading: One of 76 qualifier terms that can be added to a MeSH entry term to specify the meaning further. [15]

Meta-analysis: A summary study that combines quantitatively the estimates from individual studies. [3]

Metacontent: Information that describes the content of an information resource and thus adds structure to the content. [17]

Metathesaurus: One component of the Unified Medical Language System, the Metathesaurus contains linkages in terms between Medical Subject Headings (MeSH) and dozens of controlled vocabularies. [15]

Meta-tool: A computer program used to generate automatically a domain-specific knowledge-elicitation tool based on a model of the intended application area for a decision-support system. [16]

Middleware: Software that resides between and translates information between two or more types of software. For example, middleware components may support access, processing, analysis, and composition of lower-level resources available through basic services, such as access to image data or clinical data. [14]

Mixed-initiative system: An educational program in which user and program share control of the interaction. Usually, the program guides the interaction, but the student can assume control and digress when new questions arise during a study session. [17]

Modeling: Task in the creation of a computer-based decision-support system that entails deciding what distinctions and data are relevant, identifying the concepts and relationships among concepts that bear on the decision-making task, and ascertaining a problem-solving strategy that can use the relevant knowledge to reach appropriate conclusions. [16]

Modem: A device used to modulate and demodulate digital signals for transmission to a remote computer over telephone lines; converts digital data to audible analog signals, and vice versa. [4]

Modular computer system: A system composed of separate units, each of which performs a specific set of functions. [10]

Morphometrics: The quantitative study of growth and development, a research area that depends on the use of imaging methods. [14]

Mouse (input device): A small boxlike device that is moved on a flat surface to position a cursor on the screen of a display monitor. A user can select and mark data for entry by depressing buttons on the mouse. [4]

Multidisciplinary care: A system of patient care characterized by the collaboration of health professionals, including physicians, nurses, therapists, technicians, dieticians, pharmacists, and other care providers. [12]

Multimedia content: Information sources that encompass all common computer-based forms of information, including texts, graphics, images, video, and sound. [15]

Multimodality image fusion: Image processing that uses multiple techniques of image manipulation to generate a composite visualization that combines images from more than one source. [14]

Multiprocessing: The use of multiple processors in a single computer system to increase the power of the system (*see* Parallel processing). [4]

Multiprogramming: A scheme by which multiple programs simultaneously reside in the main memory of a single central processing unit. [4]

Multipurpose Internet Mail Extensions (MIME): An extended standard for exchange of electronic mail that allows the direct transmission of video, sound, and binary data files by Internet electronic mail. [4]

Multiuser system: A computer system that shares its resources among multiple simultaneous users. [4]

Mutually exclusive: State in which one, and only one, of the possible conditions is true; for example, either A or not A is true, and one of the statements is false. When using Bayes' theorem to perform medical diagnosis, it is generally assumed that diseases are mutually exclusive, meaning that the patient has exactly one of the diseases under consideration. [3]

MYCIN: A computer-assisted decision support system developed in the 1970s, which used artificial intelligence techniques (production rules) to recommend appropriate therapy for patients with infections. [16]

Name authority: The component of a health-care information system that uniquely identifies a patient within the system. [10]

Name-server: In networked environments such as the Internet, computers that convert a host name into an IP address before the message is placed on the network. [4]

Naturalistic: In evaluation studies, an environment which is drawn from the real world and not constrained or externally controlled as a part of the study design. [8]

Natural-language query: A question expressed in unconstrained text, from which meaning must somehow be extracted or inferred so that a suitable response can be generated. [15]

Negative predictive value (PV−): The probability that the condition of interest is absent if the result is negative—for example, the probability that the disease is absent given a negative test result. [3]

Negligence law: Laws, such as those governing medical malpractice, that are based on negligence theory. [16]

Negligence theory: A concept from tort law that states that providers of goods and services are expected to uphold the standards of the community, thereby facing claims of negligence if individuals are harmed by substandard goods or services. [7]

Net present value (NPV): The difference between the present value of benefits and the present value of costs (*see* present value). [8]

Network-based hypermedia: The mechanism by which media of all types (text, graphics, images, audio, and video) are integrated, interlinked, and delivered via networks. [15]

Network-model HMO: A model whereby groups of physicians in private practice band together to offer contracted services, generally simulating a prepaid group practice approach (*see also* Individual practice associations). [19]

Network node: One of the interconnected computers or devices linked in a communications network. [4]

Network protocol: The set of rules or conventions that specifies how data are prepared and transmitted over a network and that governs data communication among the nodes of a network. [4]

Network stack: The method within a single machine by which the responsibilities for network communications are divided into different levels, with clear interfaces between the levels, thereby making network software more modular. [4]

Network topology: The configuration of the physical connections among the nodes of a communications network. [4]

Neuroinformatics: An emerging subarea of medical informatics in which the discipline's methods are applied to the management of neurological data sets and the modeling of neural structures and function. [14]

Next Generation Internet (NGI): A federally funded research program that seeks to provide technical enhancements to the Internet to support future applications that currently are infeasible or are incapable of scaling for routine use. [1]

Ninth International Classification of Diseases—Clinical Modification (ICD-9-CM): A coding system for medical diagnoses, symptoms, and nonspecific complaints. It is frequently used on insurance claim forms to identify the reasons for providing medical services. [6]

Node: In networking topologies, a machine on the network that sits at the intersection of incoming and outgoing communications channels. [4]

Noise: The component of acquired data that is attributable to factors other than the underlying phenomenon being measured (for example, electromagnetic interference, inaccuracy in sensors, or poor contact between sensor and source). [4]

Nomenclature: A system of terms used in a scientific discipline to denote classifications and relationships among objects and processes. [2,6]

Noninvasive monitoring technique: A method for measuring a physiological parameter that does not require breaking the skin or otherwise entering the body. [13]

Nonionizing radiation: Radiation that does not cause damage to cells; for example, the sound waves used in ultrasonography (*see* Ionizing radiation). [14]

Nonquantifiable benefits and costs: In a cost-benefit analysis, those elements that are important to consider but may defy formal numeric measurements. [19]

Notifiable disease: In communicable disease management, a disease that must be reported to a public health agency when a new case occurs. [11]

NP hard: A complexity class of problems that are intrinsically harder than those that can be solved in polynomial time. When a decision version of a combinatorial optimization problem is proven to belong to a class of well-known complex problems such as satisfiability, traveling salesman, and bin packing, an optimization version is said to be NP-hard. [8]

Nuclear magnetic resonance (NMR) spectroscopy: A spectral technique used in chemistry to characterize chemical compounds by measuring magnetic characteristics of their atomic nuclei. [14]

Nuclear-medicine imaging: A modality for producing images by measuring the radiation emitted by a radioactive isotope that has been attached to a biologically active compound and injected into the body. [14]

Null hypothesis: In evaluation studies, the negatively-stated hypothesis that is the subject of study, generally because of a suspicion that the hypothesis is incorrect. [8]

Nursing care plan: A proposed series of nursing interventions based on nursing assessments and nursing diagnoses. It identifies nursing care problems, states specific actions to address the problems, specifies the actions taken, and includes an evaluation of a client's response to care. [12]

Nursing informatics: The application of medical informatics methods and techniques to problems derived from the field of nursing. [12]

Nursing information system (NIS): A computer-based information system that supports nurses' professional duties in clinical practice, nursing administration, nursing research, and education. [12]

Nursing intervention: Any of a variety of interactions between nurse and client, including physical care, emotional support, and client education. [12]

Nyquist frequency: The minimum sampling rate necessary to achieve reasonable signal quality. In general, it is twice the frequency of the highest-frequency component of interest in a signal. [4]

Objectives-based approach: An evaluation methodology in which a study seeks to determine whether a resource meets its designers' objectives. [8]

Objectivist: A philosophy of evaluation which suggests that the merit and worth of an information resource—the attributes of most interest in evaluation—can in principle be measured with all observations yielding the same result. [8]

Object-oriented programming: An approach to computer programming in which individual concepts are modeled as objects that are acted upon by incoming messages and that act upon other objects by outgoing messages. [5]

Occam's razor: A philosophical and scientific rule that the simpler explanation is preferred to a more complicated one, all else being equal. [2]

Odds: An expression of the probability of the occurrence of an event relative to the probability that it will not occur. [3]

Odds-likelihood form: *See* odds-ratio form. [3]

Odds-ratio form: An algebraic expression for calculating the posttest odds of a disease, or other condition of interest, if the pretest odds and likelihood ratio are known (an alternative formulation of Bayes' theorem, also called the odds-likelihood form). [3]

Offline device: A device that operates independently of the processor; for example, a card to tape converter. [4]

ONCOCIN: An expert system built in the 1980s to assist physicians with the management of patients enrolled in cancer chemotherapy clinical trials. [16]

Online bibliographic searching: The use of computers to search electronically stored databases of indexed literature references. [15]

Online device: A device that is under the direct control of the processor; for example, a magnetic-disk drive. [4]

Ontology: A description (like a formal specification of a program) of the concepts and relationships that can exist for an agent or a community of agents. In biomedicine, such ontologies typically specify the meanings and hierarchical relationships among terms and concepts in a domain. [16]

OPAL: A knowledge-acquisition program, related to ONCOCIN, designed to allow clinicians to specify the logic of cancer clinical trials using visual-programming techniques. [16]

Open-loop control: A computer system that assists in regulation of a physiological variable, such as blood pressure, by monitoring the value of the variable and reporting measured values or therapy recommendations. Healthcare personnel retain responsibility for therapeutic interventions (*see* Closed-loop control). [13]

Open policy: In standards group, a policy that allows anyone to become involved in discussing and defining the standard. [6]

Operating system (OS): A program that allocates computer hardware resources to user programs and that supervises and controls the execution of all other programs. [4]

Opportunity cost: The value of the alternatives foregone that might have been produced with those resources (also called the economic cost). [19]

Optical disc: A round, flat plate of plastic or metal that is used to store information. Data are encoded through the use of a laser that marks the surface of the disc. [4]

Order entry: In a hospital or health-care information system, online entry of orders for drugs, laboratory tests, and procedures, usually by nurses or physicians. [10]

Orienting issues: Initial investigations that help to define the issues of interest in a subjectivist study design. [8]

Orienting questions: The aims of a study, defined at the outset and sometimes contractually mandated. [8]

Original content: Online information created and provided by the same organization. [15]

Outcome measure: A parameter for evaluating the success of a system; the parameter reflects the top-level goals of the system. [8]

Outcomes: In a study, the events or measurements that reflect the possible influences of the interventions being studied. [8]

Outcomes data: Formal information regarding the results of interventions. [7]

Outcome variable: *See* outcome measure. [8]

Output: The results produced when a process is applied to input. Some forms of output are hardcopy documents, images displayed on video display terminals, and calculated values of variables. [4,5]

Overhead: *See* indirect cost. [19]

Packet: In networking, a variable-length message containing data plus the network addresses of the sending and receiving nodes, and other control information. [4]

Page: A partitioned component of a computer users' programs and data that can be kept in temporary storage and are brought into main memory by the operating system as needed. [4]

Parallel processing: The use of multiple processing units running in parallel to solve a single problem (*see* Multiprocessing). [4]

Patent: A specific legal approach for protecting methods used in implementing or instantiating ideas (*see* Intellectual property). [7]

Pathfinder: A computer program that uses Bayesian methods in the diagnosis of lymph-node pathology. [16]

Pathognomonic: Distinctively characteristic, and thus, uniquely identifying of a condition or object (100 percent specific). [2,16]

Patient-care system: Comprehensive computer systems used by health workers in the management of individual patients, usually in hospital settings. [12]

Patient chart: Another name for the medical record of a patient. [9]

Patient monitor: An instrument that collects and displays physiological data, often for the purpose of watching for and warning against life-threatening changes in physiological state. [13]

Patient monitoring: Repeated or continuous measurement of physiological parameters for the purpose of guiding therapeutic management. [13]

Patient record: Another name for the medical record, but one often preferred by those who wish to emphasize that such records need to contain information about patients that extends beyond the details of their diseases and medical or surgical management. [9]

Patient-tracking application: A computer system used to monitor and manage the movement of patients through multistep processes, such as in the emergency department or imaging department. [10]

Patient triage: A computer system that helps health professionals to classify new patients and to direct them to appropriate health resources. [10]

Pattern check: A method for verifying the accuracy of an identifier by assuring that it follows a predefined pattern (e.g., that a Social Security Number must be 3 numbers followed by a hyphen, followed by 2 numbers followed by a hyphen, and then ending with 4 numbers). [9]

Pattern recognition: The process of organizing visual, auditory, or other data and identifying meaningful motifs. [13]

Peer review: In scientific publication, the process of requiring that articles be reviewed by other scientists who are peers of the author and that, before publication, the author subsequently revise the paper in response to comments and criticisms from such reviewers. [15]

Per capita payment: *See* Capitation. [19]

Perimeter definition: Specification of the boundaries of trusted access to an information system, both physically and logically. [4]

Personal computer (PC): A small, relatively inexpensive, single-user computer. [4,17]

Personal digital assistant (PDA): A small, relatively inexpensive, handheld device with electronic schedule, contact list, (modified) handwriting recognition capabilities, and other productivity tools. [10]

Phantom: In image processing, an object of known shape, used to calibrate imaging machines. The reconstructed image is compared to the object's known shape. [14]

Pharmacokinetic parameters: The drug-specific and patient-specific parameters that determine the shape of the mathematical models used to forecast drug concentrations as a function of drug regimen. [16]

Pharmacokinetics: The study of the routes and mechanisms of drug disposition over time, from initial introduction into the body, through distribution in body tissues, biotransformation, and ultimate elimination. [16]

Pharmacy information system: A computer-based information system that supports pharmacy personnel. [10]

Phased installation: The incremental introduction of a system into an institution. [5]

Physician-hospital organization (PHO): An approach wherein one or a group of hospitals team up with their medical staffs to offer subscribers comprehensive health services for a per-capita prepayment. [19]

Picture-archiving and communication system (PACS): An integrated computer system that acquires, stores, retrieves, and displays digital images. [14]

Picture-archiving and communication system (PACS) workbench: A set of tools to study PACS design and to conduct experiments related to image acquisition, transmission, archiving, and viewing. [6,14]

Pixel: One of the small picture elements that make up a digital image. The number of pixels per square inch determines the spatial resolution. Pixels can be associated with a single bit to indicate black and white or with multiple bits to indicate color or gray scale. [4,14]

Placebo effect: In some drug trials, simply giving patients an inactive tablet or other placebo can cause a measurable improvement in some clinical variables because patients feel good about receiving attention and potentially useful medication. This placebo effect may be more powerful than the drug effect itself, and may obscure a complete absence of pharmaceutical benefit. [8]

Plug ins: Software components that are added to web browsers or other programs to allow them a special functionality, such as an ability to deal with certain kinds of media (e.g., video or audio). [4]

Point-of-care system: A hospital information system that includes bedside terminals or other devices for capturing and entering data at the location where patients receive care. [10]

Point of service (POS): A type of health plan introduced by HMOs in the mid-1980s to allow patients, at some expense, to seek care outside of the network that includes their contracted providers. [19]

Positive predictive value (PV+): The probability that the condition of interest is true if the result is positive—for example, the probability that the disease is present given a positive test result. [3]

Posterior probability: The updated probability that the condition of interest is present after additional information has been acquired. [3]

Post Office Protocol (POP): A protocol used in the delivery of E-mail services to any of a number of client software packages used to read E-mail from a central server. [4]

Posttest probability: The updated probability that the disease or other condition under consideration is present after the test result is known (more generally, the posterior probability). [3]

Practice management system (PMS): A computer information system designed to support all information requirements of a physician's office, including registration, appointment scheduling, billing, and clinical documentation. [10]

Precision: The degree of accuracy with which the value of a sampled observation matches the value of the underlying condition, or the exactness with which an operation is performed. In bibliographic searching, a measure of a system's performance in retrieving relevant information (expressed as the ratio of relevant records to irrelevant records retrieved in a search). [4,15]

Predictive model: In evaluation studies, the unusual situation in which investigators have a mechanism to tell them what would have happened to patients if they had not intervened. Such models allow comparisons of what actually happens with what is predicted. [8]

Predictive value: The posttest probability that a condition is present based on the results of a test (see positive predictive value and negative predictive value). [2]

Preferred-provider insurance (PPI): In managed care, an insurance plan in which companies contract with large numbers of providers that are not otherwise related to one another. [19]

Preferred-provider organization (PPO): A method of health-care financing based on selective contracting in advance for the services of health-care providers. A PPO typically is composed of a panel of providers, a negotiated fee schedule that providers agree to accept as payment in full for their services, a mechanism for utilization control, and incentives for consumers to select providers from the panel, usually in the form of reduced coinsurance. [6,19]

Prepaid group practice: An affiliation of health-care providers that agree to provide comprehensive health care to members for a fixed annual fee set in advance. [19]

Presentation: The forms in which information is delivered to the end user after processing. [12]

Presentation layer: In software systems, the components that interact with the user. The term generally connotes an architecture in which the system components are modular and *layered* between the underlying data structures and the user interface. [14]

Present value (PV): The current value of a payment or stream of payments to be received in the future. The concept of present value generally reflects the fact that $1 received 1 year from now is not worth as much as $1 received today because it is not available to earn interest over the course of 1 year. [19]

Pressure transducer: A device that produces electrical signals proportional in magnitude to the level of a pressure reading. [13]

Pretest probability: The probability that the disease or other condition under consideration is present before the test result is known (more generally, the prior probability). [3]

Prevalence: The frequency of the condition under consideration in the population. For example, we calculate the prevalence of disease by dividing the number of diseased individuals by the number of individuals in the population. Prevalence is the prior probability of a specific condition (or diagnosis), before any other information is available. [2,3]

Primary care: The level of care normally provided by a personal physician or walk-in clinic. The point of entry to the health-care system. [9]

Primary-care gatekeepers: In managed care settings, those primary care physicians who provide all initial care and then make determinations about when referral of a patient to a specialist is necessary or appropriate. [19]

Primary literature: Scientific articles that present the initial research results, as opposed to review articles or textbooks that synthesize such studies into general coverage of a topic. [15]

Prior probability: The probability that the condition of interest is present before additional information has been acquired. In a population, the prior probability also is called the prevalence. [3]

Privacy: A concept that applies to people, rather than documents, in which there is a presumed right to protect that individual from unauthorized divulging of personal data of any kind. [4,7]

Privacy Enhanced Mail protocol (PEM): A protocol whereby electronic mail is encrypted to assure that only the sender and intended receiver can read it. [4]

Private branch exchange (PBX): A telephone switching center. PBXs can be extended to provide a local-area network in which digital data are converted to analog signals and are transmitted over an existing telephone system. [4]

Probabilistic relationship: Exists when the occurrence of one chance event affects the probability of the occurrence of another chance event. [3]

Probability: Informally, a means of expressing belief in the likelihood of an event. Probability is more precisely defined mathematically in terms of its essential properties. [3]

Problem-oriented medical record (POMR): A clinical record in which the data collected, the physician's assessment, and the proposed therapeutic plans are grouped by association with the patient's specific medical problems. [9]

Problem solver: A program designed to address a certain class of problems using a defined methodology. [16]

Process measure: A parameter for evaluating the success of a system; the parameter measures a byproduct of the system's function. [8]

Product: An object that goes through the processes of design, manufacture, distribution, and sale. [7]

Production: The process of executing a product's design in an ongoing, maintained manner. [17]

Production rule: A conditional statement that relates premise conditions to associated actions or inferences. [16]

Productivity cost: Costs that accrue because of changes in productivity due to illness or death. [8]

Professional-developed: A reference to educational and other resources created by health professionals and their organizations for direct use by patients. [11]

Professional-patient relationship: Refers to a set of assumptions regarding the primacy of patient's well-being rather than other external factors in the determination of actions by health professionals. [7]

Professional-review approach: An approach to evaluation in which panels of experienced peers spend several days in the environment where the resource or activity to be assessed is operational. [8]

Professional Standards Review Organization (PSRO): A physicians' organization created to review use of Medicare and Medicaid services and to deny payment for unnecessary services. [19]

Prognostic scoring system: An approach to prediction of patient outcomes based on formal analysis of current variables, generally through methods that compare the patient in some way with large numbers of similar patients from the past. [7]

Projection: In imaging systems, a measured attenuation or superposition. [14]

Prospective payment: A method of health-care reimbursement in which providers receive a set payment specified in advance for providing a global unit of care, such as a hospitalization for a specified illness or a hospital day. [19]

Prospective-payment system (PPS): A scheme for health-care financing enacted by Congress in 1983, in which hospitals receive from Medicare a fixed payment per hospital admission, adjusted for diagnosis-related group. [19]

Prospective study: An experiment in which researchers, before collecting data for analysis, define study questions and hypotheses, the study population, and data to be collected. [2,9]

Prosthesis: A device that replaces a body part—for example, an artificial hip or heart. [11]

Protégé: A software meta-tool used by developers to create automatically domain-specific knowledge-elicitation tools by taking as input analysts' models of the relevant applications areas. [16]

Protein-sequence database: A database that contains the known sequences of amino acids of proteins. [18]

Protocol: A standardized method or approach. [4,16]

Prototype system: A working model of a planned system that demonstrates essential features of the operation and interface. [5, 17]

Provider-profiling system: Computer system used to manage utilization of health resources by tracking and comparing physicians' resource utilization (for example, cost of drugs prescribed, laboratory tests ordered) compared to severity-adjusted outcomes of the providers' patients. [10]

Proximity searching: A technique used with full-text databases that retrieves documents containing the specified words when they are adjacent in the text or when they occur within a certain number of words of each other. [15]

Publication type: One of several classes of articles or books into which a new publication will fall (e.g., review articles, case reports, original research, textbook, and so on). [15]

Public health: The field that deals with monitoring and influencing trends in habits and disease in an effort to protect or enhance the health of the population. [7,11]

Public-key cryptography: In data encryption, a method whereby two keys are used, one to encrypt the information and a second to decrypt it. Because two keys are involved, only one need be kept secret. [4]

Purchasing coalitions: Groups of employers that together structure their health-care-benefits program and negotiate with health plans. [19]

Qualitative arrangement: An approach to image retrieval that looks at the relative relationships of regions in the image, without trying to identify them, and retrieves images that have similar relationships. [14]

Qualitative model: A method for capturing the characteristics of a process or phenomenon in descriptive terms without attempting to define or simulate it quantitatively. [16]

Quality-adjusted life-year (QALY): A measure of the value of a health outcome that reflects both longevity and morbidity; it is the expected length of life in years, adjusted to account for diminished quality of life due to physical or mental disability, pain, and so on. [3]

Quality assurance: A means for monitoring and maintaining the goodness of a service, product, or process. [19]

Quality management: A specific effort to let qualify of care be the goal that determines changes in processes, staffing, or investments. [12]

Quantitation: In imaging, global processing and segmentation to characterize meaningful regions of interest. [14]

Quasilegal approach: An evaluation method that establishes a *mock trial*, or other formal adversary proceeding, to judge a resource. [8]

Query: In a database system, a request for specific information that is stored in the computer. By extension, updates to the database. [9,15]

Query and retrieval: An approach to information retrieval in which the terms are selected by the user. Terms can be matched against a predetermined index or against a thesaurus that searches for synonyms, more global concepts, and more specific concepts. [17]

Query formulation: The process of stating information needs in terms of queries. Also, the process by which information needs are translated into queries suitable for searching. [15]

Queue: In a computer system, an ordered set of jobs waiting to be executed. [4]

Quick Medical Reference (QMR): A decision-support system that grew out of the Internist-1 program. QMR is now marketed commercially for use by both students and practitioners. [16,17]

Radioactive isotope: Chemical compounds used in nuclear medicine imaging techniques. Specific compounds are selected because they tend to concentrate in specific types of tissues. [14]

Radiography: The process of making images by projecting X rays through the patient onto X-ray-sensitive film. [14]

Radiology: The medical field that deals with the definition of health conditions through the use of visual images that reflect information from within the human body. [14]

Radiology information system (RIS): Computer-based information system that supports radiology department operations; includes management of the film library, scheduling of patient examinations, reporting of results, and billing. [6,14]

Random-access memory (RAM): The portion of a computer's working memory that can be both read and written into. It is used to store the results of intermediate computation, and the programs and data that are currently in use (also called variable memory or core memory). [4,14]

Randomization: A research technique for assigning subjects to study groups without a specific pattern. Designed to minimize experimental bias. [8]

Randomized clinical trial (RCT): A prospective experiment in which subjects are randomly assigned to study subgroups to compare the effects of alternate treatments. [2]

Randomly: Without bias. [2]

Range check: Verification that a clinical parameter falls in an expected (normal) range. [9]

Ranking: In information retrieval, the specification of a retrieved item's match to the query, based on some kind of sorting criteria. [15]

Raster-scan display: A pattern of closely spaced rows of dots that forms an image on the cathode-ray tube of a video display monitor. [14]

Read-only memory (ROM): The portion of a computer's working memory that can be read, but not written into. [4,13]

Real-time acquisition: The continuous measurement and recording of electronic signals through a direct connection with the signal source. [4]

Recall: In information retrieval, the ability of a system to retrieve relevant information (expressed as the ratio of relevant records retrieved to all relevant records in the database). [15]

Receiver: In data interchange, the program or system that receives a transmitted message. [6]

Receiver operating characteristic (ROC) curve: A curve that depicts the tradeoff between the sensitivity and specificity of a test as the criteria of their definition for that test are varied. [3]

Record: In a data file, a group of data fields that collectively represent information about a single entity. [4]

Referral bias: In evaluation studies, a bias that is introduced when the patients entering a study are in some way atypical of the total population, generally because they have been referred to the study based on criteria that reflect some kind of bias by the referring physicians. [3]

Refinement: In information retrieval, the adjustment of a search query in order to obtain more appropriate information than was initially retrieved. [15]

Regional Health Information Network (RHIN): A public–private alliance among health-care providers, pharmacies, public-health departments and payors, designed to share health information among all health participants, thereby improving community health and heath care (*see also* CHIN). [10,11]

Regional network: A network that provides regional access from local organizations and individuals to the major backbone networks that interconnect regions. [4]

Region-detection techniques: A technique in which structures are delineated by their composition on the image. [14]

Register: In a computer, a group of electronic switches used to store and manipulate numbers or text. [4]

Registration: One of the problems to solve in multi-modality image fusion, specifically the alignment of separately acquired image volumes. [14]

Relevance feedback: The process that allows a searcher to obtain more relevant documents by designating retrieved documents as relevant and adding terms from them into a new query. [15]

Relevance ranking: The degree to which the results are relevant to the information need specified in a query. [15]

Reliability: In networking, the ability of a networked resource to be available and to meet expectations for performance, as related to network bandwidth and quality of service. [1]

Reminder systems: A decision-support system that monitors a patient's care over time and uses encoded logic to generate warnings and reminders to clinicians when situations arise that require clinical attention. [16]

Remote access: Access to a system or to information therein, typically by telephone or communications network, by a user who is physically removed from the system. [4]

Remote-presence health care: The use of video teleconferencing, image transmission, and other technologies that allow clinicians to evaluate and treat patients in other than face-to-face situations. [7]

Report generation: A mechanism by which users specify their data requests on the input screen of a program that then produces the actual query, using information stored in a database schema, often at predetermined intervals [4]

Representation: A level of medical data encoding; the process by which as much detail as possible is coded. [6]

Representativeness: An heuristic by which a person judges the chance that a condition is true based on the degree of similarity between the current situation and the stereotypical situation in which the condition is true. For example, a physician might estimate the probability that a patient has a particular disease based on the degree to which the patient's symptoms matches the classic disease profile. [3]

Requirements analysis: An initial analysis performed to define a problem clearly and to specify the nature of the proposed solution (for example, the functions of a proposed system). [5]

Research protocol: In clinical research, a prescribed plan for managing subjects that describes what actions to take under specific conditions. [2]

Resource-based relative value scale (RBRVS): A system authorized by Congress for paying for Medicare physician's services, intended to correct the large inequities and perverse incentives in Medicare's "customary, prevailing, and reasonable" payment system. (*see also* Volume performance standard). [19]

Responsive-illuminative approach: An approach to evaluation that seeks to represent the viewpoints of both users of the resource and people who are an otherwise significant part of the clinical environment where the resource operates. [8]

Results reporting: In a hospital or health-care information system, online access to the results of laboratory tests and other procedures. [10]

Retrieval: A process by which queries are compared against an index to create results for the user who specified the query. [15]

Retrospective chart review: Extraction and analysis of data from medical records to investigate a question that was not a subject of study at the time the data were collected. [2]

Retrospective payment: A method of health-care financing in which providers are reimbursed based on charges for the services actually delivered. [19]

Retrospective study: An analysis of pre-existing sets of data to answer experimental questions. [9]

Revenue center: In a health-care institution, a department that charges patients directly for the services provided (*see also* Cost center). [10]

Review of systems: The component of a typical history and physical examination in which the physician asks general questions about each of the body's major organ systems to discover problems that may not have been suggested by the patient's chief complaint. [2]

Risk attitude: A person's willingness to take risks. [3]

Risk-neutral: Having the characteristic of being indifferent between the expected value of a gamble and the gamble itself. [3]

Role-limited access: The mechanism by which an individual's access to information in a database, such as a medical record, is limited depending upon that user's job characteristics and their need to have access to the information. [4]

Router: In networking, a device that sits on the network, receives messages, and forwards them accordingly to their intended destination. [4]

RS-232-C: A commonly used standard for serial data communication that defines the number and type of the wire connections, the voltage, and the characteristics of the signal, and thus allows data communication among electronic devices produced by different manufacturers. [4]

Rule interpreter: The software component of a rule-based system that assesses individual rules and determines their applicability in a specific case or situation. [16]

Sample attrition rate: The proportion of the sample population that drops out before the study is complete. [8]

Sampling rate: The rate at which the continuously varying values of an analog signal are measured and recorded. [4]

Schema: In a database-management system, a machine-readable definition of the contents and organization of a database. [4]

Screening: The use of global processing, segmentation, feature detection, and classification to determine whether an image should be flagged for careful review by a human being who is an expert in an image-processing domain. [14]

Script: In software systems, a keystroke-by-keystroke record of the actions performed for later reuse. [4]

Search intermediary: In information retrieval, a specially trained information specialist who interprets users' requests for information, formulates search requests in terms of the commands and vocabulary of the search systems, and carries out the search. [15]

Secondary care: The level of care normally provided by a typical hospital. [10]

Secret-key cryptography: In data encryption, a method whereby the same key is used to encrypt and to decrypt information. Thus, the key must be kept secret, known to only the sender and intended receiver of information. [4]

Security: The process of protecting information from destruction or misuse, including both physical and computer-based mechanisms. [4]

Segmentation: In image processing, the extraction of selected regions of interest from an image using automated or manual techniques. [14]

Selection bias: An error in the estimates of disease prevalence and other population parameters that results when the criteria for admission to a study produce systematic differences between the study population and the clinically relevant population. [8]

Selectivity: In data collection and recording, the process that accounts for individual styles, reflecting an ongoing decision-making process, and often reflecting marked distinctions among clinicians. [2]

Self-insured plans: The system whereby (large) employers pay their employee's medical bills directly, hire insurance companies to perform claims processing, and perhaps buy outside insurance for only truly catastrophic cases. [19]

Semantics: The meanings assigned to symbols and sets of symbols in a language. [4,15,16]

Semistructured interview: The process whereby an investigator specifies in advance a set of topics that he would like to address, but is flexible as to the order in which these topics are addressed and is open to discussion of topics not on the prespecified list. [8]

Sender: In data interchange, the program or system that sends a transmitted message. [6]

Sensitivity (of a test): The probability of a positive result, given that the condition under consideration is present—for example, the probability of a positive test result in a person who has the disease under consideration (also called the true-positive rate). [2,3]

Sensitivity analysis: A technique for testing the robustness of a decision analysis by repeating the analysis with a range of probability and utility estimates. [3]

Sensitivity calculation: An analysis to determine which parameters, scenarios, and uncertainties affect a decision, and by how much. [3]

Sequence information: Information from a database that captures the sequence of component elements in a biological structure (e.g., the sequence of amino acids in a protein or of nucleotides in a DNA segment). [18]

Server: A computer that shares its resources with other computers and supports the activities of many users simultaneously within an enterprise. [4]

Service: An intangible activity provided to consumers, generally at a price, by a (presumably) qualified individual or system. [7]

Service benefit: A type of health insurance benefit, created to ensure that the providers are paid in the manner most acceptable to them—that is, they can choose to be paid through cost reimbursement or through payment of billed charges to hospitals and fee-for-service payment to physicians. [19]

Service bureau: A data-processing business that produces bills, third-party invoices, and financial reports for medical practices from information recorded on encounter forms. [10]

Shadowgraph: In radiology, a superposition of all the structures traversed by each X-ray beam. The beams are differentially absorbed by the various body tissues, and the X-rays produce shadows on the radiographic film. [14]

Short-run cost: The cost of producing a good or service when the levels of some inputs (for example, plant and equipment) remain fixed. (*see* Long-run cost.) [19]

Signal artifact: A false feature of the measured signal caused by noise or other interference. [13]

Simple Mail Transport Protocol (SMTP): The standard protocol used by networked systems, including the Internet, for packaging and distributing E-mail so that it can be processed by a wide variety of software systems. [4]

Simulation: A system that behaves according to a model of a process or another system; for example, simulation of a patient's response to therapeutic interventions allows a student to learn which techniques are effective without risking human life. [17]

Simultaneous access: Access to shared computer-stored information by multiple concurrent users. [4]

Simultaneous controls: In an evaluation study, subjects who are not exposed to the intervention under consideration but who are subject to the other influences of the clinical environment in question. [8]

Single-user system: Computers designed for use by single individuals, such as personal computers, as opposed to servers or other resources that are designed to be shared by multiple people at the same time. [4]

Site visit: An evaluation method whereby experts visit the site of a study or experiment in order to assess the detailed local components of the study as well as the relevant expertise of the investigators. [8]

Situation-action rules: Rules in software environments that propose a specific action that should be taken when a situation arises. (*see* production rules). [16]

Software: Computer programs that direct the hardware how to carry out specific automated processes. [4,5]

Software engineering: The discipline concerned with organizing and managing the software-development process (the process of creating computer programs and documentation) to facilitate production of high-quality systems in a timely and cost-effective manner. [5]

Software-oversight committees: Groups within organizations that are constituted to oversee computer programs and to assess their safety and efficacy in the local setting. [7]

Spamming: The process of sending unsolicited E-mail to large numbers of unwilling recipients, to sell a product or make a political statement. [4]

Spatial resolution: A measure of the ability to distinguish among points that are close to each other (indicated in a digital image by the number of pixels per square inch). [4,14]

Specification phase: In system design, the stage during which general system requirements are analyzed and formalized. [5]

Specificity (of a test): The probability of a negative result, given that the condition under consideration is absent—for example, the probability of a negative test result in a person who does not have the disease under consideration (also called the true-negative rate). [2,3]

Spectrum bias: Systematic error in the estimate of a study parameter that results when the study population includes only selected subgroups of the clinically relevant population—for example, the systematic error in the estimates of sensitivity and specificity that results when test performance is measured in a study population consisting of only healthy volunteers and patients with advanced disease. [3]

Speech understanding: The field of computer science related to the development of computer programs that appropriately interpret and act upon information that is entered using human speech through a microphone. [4]

Spelling check: The software process whereby a specified selection of text is assessed for accuracy of the spelling of its words. [9]

Spiral model: A software-engineering model in which an initial prototype is presented to the customers, who assess it, and expand and modify requirements in an ongoing iterative process. [5]

Spirometry: Evaluation of the air capacity and physiologic function of the lungs. [13]

Staff-model HMOs: A health-maintenance organization in which doctors are retained as salaries employees on the organization's staff. (*see* group model HMOs). [19]

Staged evaluation: Incremental evaluation of a system, in which different criteria for success are applied at successive stages of development. [8]

Standard-gamble: A technique for utility assessment that enables an analyst to determine the utility of an outcome by comparing an individual's preference for a chance event when compared with a situation of certain outcome. [3]

Standardized coding and classification (SCC): A generic term describing any system that is used to define a standard for data coding. [12]

Standard of care: The community-accepted norm for management of a specified clinical problem. [7]

Standards development organizations (SDOs): An organization charged with developing a standard that is accepted by the community of affected individuals. [6]

Static: In patient simulations, a program that presents a predefined case in detail but which does not vary in its response depending on the actions taken by the learner. [17]

Statistical error: In a model relating x to y, the portion of the variance in the dependent variable that cannot be explained by variance in the independent variables. [8]

Statistical life: An anonymous individual, such as a person affected by a policy that saves "one life in a thousand." (*see* Identified life.) [8]

Statistical package: A collection of programs that implement statistical procedures. Used to analyze data and report results. [8]

Stemmed: The process of converting a word to its root form by removing common suffixes from the end. [15]

Stop-loss coverage: Reinsurance, which shifts the risk of a catastrophic case to an insurance company, thereby making it possible for small employers to self-insure (as large employers do). [19]

Stop-word list: In full text indexing, a list of words that are low in semantic content (e.g., "the", "a," "an") and are generally not useful as mechanisms for retrieving documents. [15]

Strict product liability: The principle which states that a product must not be harmful. [7,16]

Structural alignment: In biological sequences, the task of aligning a new structure against a database of known structures, to determine regions of identity or similarity. [18]

Structural informatics: The study of methods for organizing and managing diverse sources of information about the physical organization of the body and other physical structures. [14]

Structured content: The organization and labeling of text (or other information) according to subsections that represent coherent concepts. [17]

Structured encounter form: A form for collecting and recording specific information during a patient visit. [9]

Structured interview: An evaluation method that uses a schedule of questions that are always presented in the same words and in the same order. [8]

Structured programming: The composition of computer programs using only sequences of statements and formal constructs for iteration (*do while*) and selection (*if . . . then . . . else*); implies modularity, absence of *go to* statements, and the use of stylistic conventions, such as indentation and the use of meaningful variable and subroutine names. [5]

Structured Query Language (SQL): A commonly used syntax for retrieving information from relational databases. [4]

Study population: The population of subjects—usually a subset of the clinically relevant population—in whom experimental outcomes (for example, the performance of a diagnostic test) are measured. [3]

Study protocol: A prescribed plan for managing experimental subjects that describes what actions to take under what conditions. [8]

Subject: An individual about whom data are collected during the conduct of a study. [8]

Subject heading: In information retrieval, the standardized terms used to categorize documents in order to faciliate their retrieval when appropriate. [15]

Subjectivist: A philosophy of evaluation that suggests that what is observed about a resource depends in fundamental ways on the observer. [8]

Summary ROC curve: A composite ROC curve developed by using estimates from many studies. [3]

Summative decision: A decision made after a resource is installed in its envisioned environment; deals explicitly with how effectively the resource performs in that environment. [8]

Superbill: An itemized bill that summarizes the financial transactions occurring during a patient-physician encounter, including specification of the type of visit and a listing of the procedures performed and drugs administered; also, a checklist form for generating such a bill. [16]

Supervised learning: In automated neural networks, a process by which the values for weights are determined in an incremental fashion as the network is trained on a large collection of previously classified examples. [16]

Surface rendering: A visualization technique that provides an alternative to volume rendering. This is the primary technique used in computer graphics, and has been applied widely in the entertainment industry for movies such as *Toy Story*. Surface rendering requires that the surface of interest be segmented from the image volume, after which rendering speeds on standard workstations are much faster than those possible with volume rendering. [14]

Surveillance: In a computer-based medical-record system, systematic review of patients' clinical data to detect and flag conditions that merit attention. [9]

Symbolic-programming language: A language designed to support the representation of knowledge and semantic relationships, while deemphasizing numerical computations. [4]

Synoptic content: Information in computer systems and databases that is created by extracting important observations and principles from sources of original content, as well as from personal experience. [15]

Syntactic: That which relates to the *structure* of words, phrases, or sentences (as opposed to their meanings). [15]

Syntax: The rules that specify the legal symbols and constructs of a language. [4]

System: A set of integrated entities that operate as a whole to accomplish a prescribed task. [5]

Systematic classification of proteins (SCOP): A currently available online resource that classifies proteins based on shape and function. [18]

Systematic review: A type of journal article that reviews the literature related to a specific clinical question, analyzing the data in accordance with formal methods to assure that data are suitably compared and pooled. [15]

Systematized Nomenclature Of MEDicine (SNOMED): The expanded form of the diagnostic coding scheme, formerly known as SNOP (Systematized Nomenclature of Pathology). A multi-axial nomenclature system for the coding of several aspects of a diagnosis or other clinical entity. [2,6]

Systematized Nomenclature Of Pathology (SNOP): A widely-used diagnostic coding scheme, developed by pathologists. A nomenclature system of the College of American Pathologists based on four coding axes: topography, morphology, etiology, and function. A predecessor to SNOMED. [2,6]

System integration: The process by which software systems and components are brought together to work as a coherent whole. [5]

System programs: The operating system, compilers, and other software that are included with a computer system and that allow users to operate the hardware. [4]

System-review form: A paper form used during a physical examination to record findings related to each of the body's major systems. [2,9]

Systems aggregation: A situation in which functions from disparate and widely distributed information systems are brought together in one application. [15]

Task: An activity of study, when computers or people solve problems or work through clinical cases. [8]

Technical characteristics: The first stage in a technology assessment, in which the formal capabilities of a studied technology are defined and assessed. [8]

Technology assessment: Any process of examining and reporting properties of a medical technology used in health care, such as safety, efficacy, feasibility, and indication for use, cost, and cost-effectiveness, as well as social, economic, and ethical consequences, whether intended or unintended. [8]

Telemedicine: A broad term used to describe the delivery of health care at a distance, increasingly but not exclusively by means of the Internet. [1,7,14]

Telepresence: A technique of telemedicine in which a viewer can be physically removed from an actual surgery, viewing the abnormality through a video monitor that displays the operative field and allows the observer to participate in the procedure. [14]

Teleradiology: The provision of remote interpretations, increasing as a mode of delivery of radiology services. [14]

Telerobotics: A technique of telemedicine in which the manipulation of a biomedical device (e.g., a robot arm, a microscope, or an endoscope) is controlled at a distance by the hand movements of a remote operator. [14]

Temporal resolution: The time between acquisition of each of a series of images. Limited by the time needed to produce each image. [14]

Temporal subtraction: A technique of image enhancement that subtracts a reference image from later images that are registered to the first. A common use of temporal subtraction is digital-subtraction angiography (DSA), in which a background image is subtracted from an image taken following the injection of contrast material. [14]

Term frequency (TF): In information retrieval, a measurement of how frequently a term occurs in a document. [15]

Terminal: A simple device that has no processing capability of its own but allows a user to access a server. [4]

Terminal interface processor (TIP): A utility communications computer that is used to attach video display terminals and other communications devices to a LAN. [4]

Terminology: A set of terms representing the system of concepts of a particular subject field. [6]

Terminology authority: The component of a health-care information system that defines the vocabulary standard and valid terms within the system; the medical entities dictionary. [10]

Terminology services: A set of functions provided by a health-care information systems and used to link, translate, and cross reference diverse vocabulary terms for consistent use within the system. [10]

Tertiary care: The level of care normally provided only by a specialized medical center. [10]

Testing: The process of formally running a newly developed computer system or set of programs to exercise them fully and to determine their reliability, accuracy, and freedom from programming errors. [5]

Test-interpretation bias: Systematic error in the estimates of sensitivity and specificity that results when the index and gold-standard test are not interpreted independently. [3]

Test-referral bias: Systematic error in the estimates of sensitivity and specificity that results when subjects with a positive index test are more likely to receive the gold-standard test. [3]

Text editor: A program used to create files of character strings, such as other computer programs and documents. [4]

Text-scanning devices: A mechanical device that scans a paper document and converts text into computer-interpretable elements. [4]

Text-word searching: In a bibliographic database, retrieval of relevant articles based on the words that appear in titles and abstracts, rather than the index terms that have been assigned to each entry. [15]

Three-dimensional reconstruction and visualization: The process of producing three-dimensional models from uniform data (typically from slices through a structure) and rendering them for computer visualization and manipulation. [14]

Three-dimensional-structure information: In a biological database, information regarding the three-dimensional relationships among elements in a molecular structure. [18]

Tiled: A technique used in three-dimensional surface segmentation wherein a surface is applied over manually or automatically segmented two-dimensional contours which have been stacked together, creating a continuous surface. [14]

Time-sharing mode: An interactive mode for communicating with a computer in which the operating system switches rapidly among all the jobs that require CPU services (*see* batch mode). [4]

Time-tradeoff: A common approach to utility assessment, comparing a better state of health lasting a shorter time, with a lesser state of health lasting a longer time. The time-tradeoff technique provides a convenient method for valuing outcomes that accounts for gains (or losses) in both length and quality of life. [3]

Token Ring: A type of local area network, typically used by IBM systems. (*see also* Ethernet) [4]

Topology: In networking, the overall connectivity of the nodes in an network. [4]

Touch screen: A display screen that allows users to select items by touching them on the screen. [4]

Track ball: An interactive device that uses a mounted ball which, when rolled in its housing, manipulates a pointer on the computer screen. [4]

Transaction set: In data transfer, the full set of information exchanged between a sender and a receiver. [6]

Transcription: The conversion of dictated notes into ASCII text by a typist. [9]

Transducer: A device that produces electrical signals proportional in magnitude to the level of a measured parameter, such as blood pressure. [13]

Transition probabilities: The probabilities that a person will transit from one health state to another during a specified time period. [3]

Transmission Control Protocol/Internet Protocol (TCP/IP): The standard protocols used for data transmission on the Internet and other common local and wide-area networks. [4]

Treatment-threshold probability: The probability of disease at which the expected values of withholding or giving treatment are equal. Above the threshold treatment is recommended; below the threshold, treatment is not recommended and further testing may be warranted. [3]

Tree: In information retrieval, the hierarchically organized sets of index terms. [15]

Trigger event: In monitoring, events that cause a set of transactions to be generated. [6]

True-negative rate (TNR): The probability of a negative result, given that the condition under consideration is false—for example, the probability of a negative test result in a patient who does not have the disease under consideration (also called specificity). [3]

True-negative result (TN): A negative result when the condition under consideration is false—for example, a negative test result in a patient who does not have the disease under consideration. [3]

True-positive rate (TPR): The probability of a positive result, given that the condition under consideration is true—for example, the probability of a positive test result in a patient who has the disease under consideration (also called sensitivity). [3]

True-positive result (TP): A positive result when the condition under consideration is true—for example, a positive test result in a patient who has the disease under consideration. [3]

Turnaround document: A form that serves first as a summary form for presenting results and subsequently as a data-collection form. [9]

Turnkey system: A computer system that is purchased from a vendor and that can be installed and operated with minimal modification. [5]

Tutoring system: A computer program designed to provide self-directed education to a student or trainee. [17]

Twisted-pair wires: The typical copper wiring used for routine telephone service but adaptable for newer communication technologies. [4]

Type I error: A false positive error in an evaluation study such that the resource being studied is ineffective, but for some reason the study mistakenly shows that it is. [8]

Type II error: A false negative error in an evaluation study such that the resource being studied is effective, but for some reason the study mistakenly fails to show that it is. [8]

Type checking: In computer programming, the act of checking that the types of values, such as integers, decimal numbers, and strings of characters, match throughout their use. [4]

Typology: A classification scheme (e.g., of evaluation methods). [8]

Ultrasonography: The use of pulses of high-frequency sound waves, rather than ionizing radiation, to produce images of body structures. [14]

Ultrasound (US): A common energy source derived from high-frequency soundwaves. [14]

Ultrasound imaging: The transmission of sound waves through the body with analysis of the returning echos to produce images. [14]

Unified Medical Language System (UMLS): A terminology system, developed under the direction of the National Library of Medicine, to produce a common structure that ties together the various vocabularies that have been created for biomedical domains. [2,6,14,15,20]

Uniform Resource Locator (URL): The address of an information resource on the World Wide Web. [4]

Unit-dose dispensing: An approach to the distribution of drugs, whereby patients' drugs are packaged on a unit-of-dose basis to reduce wastage and to control drug use. [10]

Universal workstation: A computer of moderate size and cost that is used to access all computer resources connected to a network. [10]

Unobtrusive measures: Records or data for an evaluation that are accrued as part of a routine activity under study and therefore require no special intervention. [8]

Unsharp masking: A technique of image enhancement, in which a blurred image is subtracted from the original image to increase local contrast and to enhance the visibility of fine-detail (high-frequency) structures. [14]

Unstructured interview: An interview in an evaluation study in which there are no predefined questions to be asked. [8]

User-interface layer: A conceptual level of a system architecture that insulates the programs designed to interact with users from the underlying data and the applications that process those data. [10]

Usual, customary, and reasonable fee: The typical fee used as the basis for billed charges and retrospective cost reimbursement. [19]

Utility: In decision making, a number that represents the value of a specific outcome to a decision maker (*see*, for example, quality-adjusted life-years). [3,16]

Utilization review: In a hospital, inspection of patients' medical records to identify cases of inappropriate care, including excessive or insufficient use of resources. [10]

Validation: Verification of correctness. [5]

Validity check: In a database system or computer-based medical-record system, a test (such as a range check or a pattern check) that is used to detect invalid data values. [9]

Variable: In evaluations, specific characteristics of subjects that either are measured purposefully by the investigator or are self-evident properties of the subjects that do not require measurement. [8]

Variable cost: A cost that changes with the volume of goods or services produced during a given period. [19]

Variable memory: *See* random-access memory. [4]

Vector-space model: A method of full-text indexing in which documents can be conceptualized as vectors of terms, with retrieval based on the cosine similarity of the angle between the query and document vectors. [15]

Vendor system: A host computer system owned by a third party that provides users with access to multiple databases or other services. [5]

Video display terminal (VDT): An input–output device that is used for communication with a remote computer and that has a cathode-ray-tube display for viewing output and a keyboard for entering data. [4]

View: In a database-management system, a logical submodel of the contents and structure of a database used to support one or a subset of applications. [4,9]

View schemas: An application-specific description of a view that supports that program's activities with respect to some general database for which there are multiple views. [4]

Virtual addressing: A technique in memory management such that each address referenced by the CPU goes through an address mapping from the **virtual address** of the program to a physical address in main memory. [4]

Virtual memory: A scheme by which users can access information stored in auxiliary memory as though it were in main memory. Virtual memory addresses are automatically translated into actual addresses by the hardware. [4]

Virtual reality (VR): A collection of interface methods that simulate reality more closely than does the standard display monitor, generally with a response to user maneuvers that heighten the sense of being connected to the simulation. (*see also* augmented reality) [14]

Virus: A software program that is written for malicious purposes to spread from one machine to another and to do some kind of damage. Such programs are generally self replicating, which has led to the comparison with biological viruses. [4]

Visual-analog scale: A method for valuing health outcomes, wherein a person simply rates the quality of life with a health outcome on a scale from 0 to 100. [3]

Vital signs: A person's core temperature, pulse rate, respiratory rate, and arterial blood pressure. [13]

Vocabulary: A dictionary containing the terminology of a subject field. [6]

Volatile: A characteristic of a computer's memory, in that contents are changed when the next program runs and are not retained when power is turned off. [4]

Volume performance standard (VPS): A system authorized by Congress for paying for Medicare physicians' services, intended to control volume. This approach may have instead motivated an increase in physician services as doctors sought to protect their real incomes in the face of controlled prices and a surplus of doctors. (*see* resource-based relative value scale). [19]

Volume rendering: A method whereby a computer program projects a two-dimensional image directly from a three-dimensional voxel array by casting rays from the eye of the observer through the volume array to the image plane. [14]

von Neuman machine: A computer architecture that comprises a single processing unit, computer memory, and a memory bus. [4]

Voxel: A volume element or small cubic area of a three-dimensional digital image (see pixel). [14]

Waveform template: A wave pattern that is stored in a computer and compared to collected waveforms, such as those acquired from patients. Used to identify and classify abnormal wave patterns. [13]

Web browser: A computer program used to access and display information resources on the World Wide Web. [4]

WebMedline: The first World Wide Web interface developed for searching the MEDLINE database. [15]

Weights: Values associated with the nodes of an artificial neural network; the weights propagate through the layers of the network to perform classification based on a set of inputs. [16]

Wide-area network (WAN): A network that connects computers owned by independent institutions and distributed over long distances. [4,14]

Wildcard character: In search and retrieval applications, a method which allows unspecified single- or multiple-character expansion somewhere in a string that is being used as the basis for the search. [15]

Willingness to pay: An approach to valuing human life based on the values implied by the choices people make every day to change their probabilities of living or dying. For example, a person's implicit valuation for life could be calculated based on how much he is willing to pay for a car airbag that will reduce his chance of by death by a certain incremental amount. [3]

Word: In computer memory, a sequence of bits that can be accessed as a unit. [4]

Word size: The number of bits that define a word in a given computer. [4]

Workstation: A powerful desktop computer system designed to support a single user. Workstations provide specialized hardware and software to facilitate the problem-solving and information-processing tasks of professionals in their domains of expertise. [4]

World Wide Web (WWW): An application implemented on the Internet in which multimedia information resources are made accessible by any of a number of protocols, the most common of which is the HyperText Transfer Protocol (HTTP). [4]

Write-it-once system: A type of paper-based billing system that uses carbon paper or photocopying to generate bills from patient-encounter information that has been transcribed onto ledger cards. [9]

Write once, read many (WORM): A storage medium that is suitable for reuse but cannot be erased or rewritten. [4]

X-ray: A type of ionizing radiation which has been harnessed to provide a technique of medical imaging, allowing the capture of views of structures within the body. [14]

Name Index

E

F

G

N

O

P

Q

R

S

T

U

V

W

Y

Z

Subject Index

A

B

C

E

F

G

H

N

O

P

S

U

V

Health Informatics Series

(formerly Computers in Health Care)

Organizational Aspects of Health Informatics
Managing Technological Change
N.M. Lorenzi and R.T. Riley

Transforming Health Care Through Information
Case Studies
N.M. Lorenzi, R.T. Riley, M.J. Ball, and J.V. Douglas

Trauma Informatics
K.I. Maull and J.S. Augenstein

Advancing Federal Sector Health Care
A Model for Technology Transfer
P. Ramsaroop, M.J. Ball, D. Beaulieu and J.V. Douglas

Medical Informatics
Computer Applications in Health Care and Biomedicine, Second Edition
E.H. Shortliffe and L.E. Perreault

Filmless Radiology
E.L. Siegel and R.M. Kolodner

Knowledge Coupling
New Premises and New Tools for Medical Care and Education
L.L. Weed